D1257716

STEROIDS IN
NONMAMMALIAN VERTEBRATES

CONTRIBUTORS

D. Bellamy

Howard A. Bern

D. K. O. Chan

B. K. Follett

I. W. Henderson

D. R. Idler

I. Chester Jones

Brian Lofts

R. Ozon

J. G. Phillips

Thomas Sandor

R. S. Snart

B. Truscott

STEROIDS IN
NONMAMMALIAN VERTEBRATES

Edited by David R. Idler

Fisheries Research Board of Canada
Halifax, Nova Scotia, Canada

ACADEMIC PRESS   New York and London   1972

ACADEMIC PRESS, INC.
111 Fifth Avenue, New York, New York 10003

United Kingdom Edition published by
ACADEMIC PRESS, INC. (LONDON) LTD.
24/28 Oval Road, London NW1

LIBRARY OF CONGRESS CATALOG CARD NUMBER: 74-182615

PRINTED IN THE UNITED STATES OF AMERICA

CONTENTS

LIST OF CONTRIBUTORS

Numbers in parentheses indicate the pages on which the authors' contributions begin.

D. BELLAMY, Department of Zoology, University College, Cardiff, Wales (414)

HOWARD A. BERN, Department of Zoology and Its Cancer Research Genetics Laboratory, University of California, Berkeley, California (37)

D. K. O. CHAN, Department of Zoology, University of Hong Kong, Hong Kong, The Nationalist Republic of China (37)

B. K. FOLLETT, Department of Zoology, University College of North Wales, Bangor, Caernarvonshire, North Wales (44)

I. W. HENDERSON, Department of Zoology, University of Sheffield, Sheffield, England (414)

D. R. IDLER,* Fisheries Research Board of Canada, Halifax, Nova Scotia, Canada (1, 6, 126)

I. CHESTER JONES, Department of Zoology, University of Sheffield, Sheffield, England (414)

BRIAN LOFTS, Department of Zoology, University of Hong Kong, Hong Kong, The Nationalist Republic of China (37)

R. OZON, Laboratoire de Physiologie de la Reproduction, Université de Paris, Paris, France (328, 390)

*Present address: Marine Sciences Research Laboratory, Memorial University of Newfoundland, St. Johns, Newfoundland, Canada

J. G. PHILLIPS, Department of Zoology, University of Hull, Hull, England (414)

THOMAS SANDOR, Laboratoire d'Endocrinologie, Hôpital Notre-Dame, et Departement de Medicine, Université de Montréal, Montreal, Canada (6, 253)

R. S. SNART, Department of Zoology, University of Sheffield, Sheffield, England (414)

B. TRUSCOTT*, Fisheries Research Board of Canada, Halifax, Nova Scotia, Canada (126)

*Present address: Marine Sciences Research Laboratory, Memorial University of Newfoundland, St. Johns, Newfoundland, Canada

PREFACE

There have been several review articles written on the steroids of non-mammalian vertebrates, but this may be the first book on the subject. Valuable though the reviews have been, they have tended to establish as fact observations which should be reconsidered in light of the rapid advances in methodology during the past decade. A primary purpose of this volume is to provide the reader with a critical assessment of each identification and/or quantification of a steroid in nonmammalian vertebrates. It is hoped that this exercise will encourage a reexamination where reasonable doubt exists, point out where little or no information is available, and show where significant progress has been made.

A second goal is to encourage the use of nonmammalian vertebrates as experimental animals. There is such a diversity of life forms among "lower" vertebrates that there may well be one or more animals uniquely suited to an investigation of almost any problem concerned with steroidal hormones. Chapter 1 is intended to whet the reader's appetite for further exploration into these fascinating possibilities. Chapter 2 will provide a reference source for the scientist who may lack the necessary background in nonmammalian physiology to select and locate appropriate steroidogenic tissues. The function of hormones in "lower" vertebrates is examined in Chapter 8, and it is hoped that the reader will be stimulated to fill in some of the many voids on this subject.

I must accept some responsibility if any portion of Chapters 6 and 7 fails to adequately convey the thoughts of the author; this material was translated verbatim from the French, and I exercised considerable latitude in interpretation.

My appreciation is due Dr. R. Ozon for writing Chapter 7 in a very short time when the designated author failed to undertake the task. My

associates, Miss B. Truscott and Mrs. M. J. O'Halloran, worked very con-
scientiously to assist me with all chapters, and Mr. H. C. Freeman assisted
with the sections of Chapter 4 dealing with protein binding and corpuscles
of Stannius. Finally, my appreciation is due Mrs. S. B. Coombes and her
associates for performing stenographic and proofreading chores effectively
and cheerfully.

DAVID R. IDLER

Chapter 1

WHY COMPARATIVE ENDOCRINOLOGY?

D. R. IDLER

During a comparative endocrinology session at the Third International Congress of Endocrinology in Mexico City, the chairman, O. M. Hechter, asked this provocative question: Why comparative endocrinology? The writer was among the participants who sought meaningful answers. It might be useful to set forth a few thoughts, most of which occurred to me in retrospect.

In recent years comparative endocrinology has received increasing attention at international meetings of endocrinologists. From a casual examination of the programs for such meetings one might erroneously conclude that comparative endocrinology is practiced by scientists not concerned with the applicability of their research to mammals in general and man in particular. On the contrary, there have been instances in which a discovery was first made with nonmammalian species and subsequent comparative investigations were carried out on mammals. Studies on the mode of hormonal action in mammals were influenced and stimulated by results obtained on the action of molting hormones in insects. Another example was the discovery of 18-hydroxycorticosterone in amphibians and the subsequent elucidation of the key role played by this steroid in aldosterone biosynthesis in mammals. In 1920, P. Smith employed tadpoles to demonstrate atrophy of adrenocortical tissue following hypophysectomy and 10 years elapsed before this finding was confirmed in rats.

1

Special characteristics of nonmammalian vertebrates often facilitate the study of endocrine phenomena. Nonmammalian vertebrates have been extensively employed for the bioassay of hormones, e.g., chick oviduct (estrogens), chick blood pressure depression (oxytocin), pigeon crop sac (prolactin), weaver finch feather color (luteinizing hormone), cock's comb growth and fish sex characters (androgens), and amphibian ovulation or sperm release (human chorionic gonadotropin). Determination of the effect of steroids on ion transport has been expedited by the use of toad bladder, frog skin, the rectal gland of elasmobranchs, and the salt gland of birds. Some of these investigations have been extensive and have contributed to our understanding of the mammalian kidney. The anatomical separation of interrenal and medullary tissue in elasmobranchs offers interesting possibilities for study of the function of each tissue independent of the other *in vivo* as well as *in vitro*. Thus, in 1913, A. Biedl was able to demonstrate that the cortex of interrenal tissue is the segment essential to life. In a similar manner studies on the hormonal regulation of calcium have been facilitated by the availability of species in which parathyroid issue is separate from thyroid tissue. D. H. Copp and his co-workers have demonstrated calcitonin in a wide range of nonmammalian vertebrates. The biological potency of salmon calcitonin is much greater than that of the porcine hormone. The availability of calcitonin from abundant Pacific salmonids suggests its application in human therapy.

Sometimes the mode of action of a hormone can be so different in different life forms that it is hardly recognizable as belonging to the same substance or group of substances. Thus, prolactin is variously concerned with the regulation of ion balance, the stimulation of milk production, and the molting process, to name a few activities. Through comparative investigations additional functions may be found for this hormone, and perhaps a common mechanism may emerge to explain the seemingly unrelated phenomena.

There is evidence to suggest that target glands increase in specificity during evolutionary development. Thus, the thyroid of fishes responds to mammalian gonadotropin and thyrotropin as well as to fish thyroid-stimulating hormone, but the mammalian thyroid does not respond to mammalian gonadotropin and it responds only weakly to the thyroid-stimulating hormone of teleosts.

The chemist, searching at the molecular level for explanations of natural phenomena, is well advised to spend some time looking for a rich source of the active substance. Extremely high levels of cortisol and several of the intermediates in its biogenesis occur in the blood of some fish, and aldosterone is plentiful in birds and amphibians. It is interesting to speculate that progress relating to these steroids in mammals might have proceeded more rapidly had comparative studies received emphasis at an earlier date.

Nandi has observed that historically the comparative endocrinologist has asked in what way "lower" vertebrates are similar to higher vertebrates. This is certainly evident in much of the work on steroids; the presence or absence of mammalian hormones in nonmammalian vertebrates has too often been considered to be a sufficient goal. The search for differences has hardly begun. The bias toward searching for similarities has prompted several authors to emphasize the pathways of steroidogenesis in lower vertebrates that parallel the established pathways in mammals. Such conclusions do not adequately take certain facts into account; for example, although only a very small number of fish has been investigated to date, two unique steroids, 11-ketotestosterone and 1α-hydroxycorticosterone, have already been found. The first is an important androgen for some teleosts and the second is a principal corticoid of sharks, rays, and other elasmobranchs.

Perhaps of great significance is the observation that *in vitro* corticosterone undergoes substantial 17-hydroxylation in certain fish in contrast to many mammals; this could have a profound effect on the significance of a given pathway *in situ*, even if the various hydroxylases which occur in mammalian systems also occur in a given species of fish. For example, it has been demonstrated *in vitro* that 11-deoxycorticosterone can be converted to 18-hydroxy-11-deoxycorticosterone and corticosterone can be converted to 18-hydroxy-corticosterone and aldosterone by certain teleost fishes. But it would seem that the existence of these enzyme systems is of significance to the living animal only if substrates are available on which the enzyme can work competitively. If, as may be the case, a strong 17-hydroxylase system is competing for the available 17-deoxycorticosteroid precursors of aldosterone in certain teleosts, then aldosterone may not be produced in physiological concentrations even though the enzyme systems appropriate for its synthesis are present. Thus, a single alteration in enzyme substrate relations could result in major variations in the circulating steroids of the animal. Similarly, the sockeye salmon seems to maintain a relatively constant plasma level of testosterone plus 11-ketotestosterone throughout the period of sexual maturation, but the ratio of these two steroids has been shown to vary appreciably. The relative amounts of cortisol and cortisone in the blood also fluctuate and, although cortisol is normally the principal hormone, there are other occasions when cortisone predominates.

Those who are impressed with the similarities of enzyme systems throughout the vertebrates might consider the remarks of A. S. Parks in opening a Ciba colloquium entitled "Hormones in Blood"—"A hormone is not something that occurs in the urine or something knocked up by a chemist in his laboratory; a hormone is something that goes around in the blood to act in another part of the body." Thus, while nothing can happen without an enzyme, nothing will happen unless the enzyme and substrate get together under appropriate conditions. I strongly urge scientists to heed Parks' advice and place more emphasis on steroids in blood.

Finally, and certainly not least important, there is the need to understand the endocrinology of lower vertebrates for its own sake. Fish, chickens, and ducks come to mind. Let us again take fish as an example. In several countries salmon represent an important fishery and a renewable resource if they can be managed successfully. Some species (e.g., the sockeye salmon *Oncorhynchus nerka*) have not only an uncanny homing ability but an amazing timing with regard to sexual development and spawning migration. What triggers this migration? Hormones are almost certainly involved, but which ones and when? In one race of sockeye there are changes in certain androgens in the blood at this time. However, there are many different races of salmon and many different types of behavior. The salmon of one race (Great Central Lake, British Columbia) enter the river with small gonads, migrate 550 km to a lake, develop sexually in the lake, and spawn on the beaches. At the other extreme is the Stuart Lake (British Columbia) run where the fish enter the river with small gonads, migrate 1000 km, and arrive on the spawning grounds with only a few days to spare before spawning. Those of yet another race (Adams River, British Columbia) delay in brackish water until the gonads are in an advanced state of development and then make a frantic dash to the spawning grounds, 550 km distant, arriving with little or no time to spare. It is difficult to visualize a common endocrine mechanism operating in all these circumstances but it is a great challenge to search for one. It would be of economic value if the arrival of these fish could be predicted while the fish were still at sea. It seems likely that the initial trigger for the migration occurs well in advance of their arrival in estuarial waters. In 1957, the Stuart Lake fish were 10 calender days late in beginning the freshwater phase of the spawning migration but their sexual development as determined by the gonadosomatic index was exactly as in other years. For many of the important salmon runs the freshwater phase of the spawning migration is a race against energy reserves as well as sexual development. The ability of salmon to perform is legendary but construction of dams on major rivers has taxed even this animal to the limit. Its movement from salt to fresh water, capacity to maintain sustained activity, sexual maturation, requirements for periods of rest, and sublethal effects of pollutants are all phenomena which can be studied at the endocrine level. Finally, there is evidence that death after spawning is preceded by an impaired metabolism of steroids.

Endocrinology can also play an important role in the rearing and manipulation of fish. Hormones have already been used to improve methods of propagation of sturgeon, salmon, and other species. Any successful rearing of fish in captivity must take into account the influence of hormones on sexual maturation, color of the flesh, tolerance of salinity and temperature changes, growth, feeding habits, and related phenomena.

In summary, comparative endocrinology has contributed to progress in human medicine, the elucidation of evolutionary processes, and the utilization and manipulation of nonmammalian vertebrates for commericial purposes. There is good evidence to suggest that knowledge of vital endocrine processes would have advanced more rapidly if more investigators had directed some of their attention to nonmammalian vertebrates. I would particularly urge chemists and biochemists to enter this challenging field of research.

For those who wish to explore further the contributions of comparative endocrinology, various aspects are discussed in books, essays, and symposium lectures (e.g., Chester Jones, 1957; Gorbman, 1959; Deane, 1962; Takewaki, 1962; Barrington, 1963; Fontaine, 1967; Barrington and Jørgensen, 1968; Prasad, 1969).

REFERENCES

Barrington, E. J. W. (1963). "An Introduction to General and Comparative Endocrinology." Oxford Univ. Press (Clarendon). London and New York.
Barrington, E. J. W., and Jørgensen, C. B., eds. (1968). "Perspectives in Endocrinology: Hormones in the Lives of Lower Vertebrates." Academic Press, New York.
Chester Jones, I. (1957). "The Adrenal Cortex." Cambridge Univ. Press, London and New York.
Deane, H. W., ed. (1962). "The Adrenocortical Hormones: Their Origin, Chemistry, Physiology and Pharmacology," Vol. 14, Part 1. Springer-Verlag, Berlin and New York.
Fontaine, M. (1967). *Gen. Comp. Endocrinol.* **9**, 529.
Gorbman, A., ed. (1959). "Comparative Endocrinology." Wiley, New York.
Prasad, M. R. N., ed. (1969). *Gen. Comp. Endocrinol. Suppl.* **2**.
Takewaki, K., ed. (1962). *Gen. Comp. Endocrinol. Suppl.* **1**.

Chapter 2

STEROID METHODOLOGY

T. SANDOR and D. R. IDLER

I. Introduction

In a presidential address to the Endocrine Society, Greep (1966) observed that scientists in the field of endocrinology are a mixed breed with backgrounds in zoology, biochemistry, physiology, and other disciplines. A significant part of endocrinology is concerned with the isolation, identification, and quantification of steroids. This falls into the realm of chemistry and all the methods employed and criteria applied should conform to those utilized in other branches of chemistry. Scanning the literature, one is aware that in steroid biochemical work there is a lack of uniform criteria as to the chemical validity of published studies. Acceptable standards vary from one journal to another and, in addition, some laboratories establish arbitrary criteria of their own which sometimes find their way into world literature. On the occasion of a roundtable discussion held at Naples, Italy, May 30–31 1966, on steroid hormones in fishes (Chieffi and Bern, 1966), these problems were discussed with reference to the conflicting evidence concerning the occurrence of certain steroids in fish. Bern, who cochaired the roundtable with Chieffi, suggested that it would be a step forward if papers dealing with chemical aspects of steroids (identification, quantification, etc.) were examined in all instances by a referee with a background in chemistry. This recommendation was made to the editors of *General and Comparative Endocrinology*.

Discussions at Naples and elsewhere suggested the need for a critical review of the status of steroid hormones in nonmammalian vertebrates. Thus, one of the purposes of the present volume is to give a review of the literature dealing with occurrence and biosynthesis of androgens, estrogens, and corticoids in lower vertebrates. In view of the difficulties connected with the identification of small amounts of natural steroids, it was decided that this review should be not only a compilation and interpretation of published data, but also, to a certain extent, a critical analysis. This task proved to be a rather difficult and delicate one. However, there are many instances in the literature in which identifications are incomplete. This in itself is acceptable as long as the claims are qualified. However, such a qualification is not always apparent and it is sometimes very difficult to decide whether in a given species a particular steroid should be considered as positively identified. It must be emphasized that this critical assessment of published data does not represent a value judgment on the part of the reviewers. The assessment scheme, described in the next section, is simply meant to clarify, from the steroid chemist's point of view, the degree of confidence one can place in the reported identity and quantity of steroids isolated from nonmammalian sources and, in this way, to serve as a guide to newcomers in this field.

II. Criteria for the Identification of Steroids Isolated from Natural Sources

Steroid biochemistry is a relative latecomer among the different branches of biochemistry. Its development was hampered by methodological problems related directly to the minute amounts in which natural steroids are produced by endocrine tissue.

The recent important advances in our knowledge of the occurrence, biosynthesis, and metabolism of steroid hormones in vertebrates can be attributed, in large measure, to the development of new analytical techniques and to the adaptation of known techniques to the particular problems of steroid chemistry. Thus, for all practical purposes a new branch of ultramicrochemistry has emerged which relies heavily on tools such as chromatography in its different forms, spectrometry, and the use of isotopically labeled, high specific activity substrates and derivatizing agents. Highly efficient counters of radioactivity capable of the simultaneous and differential counting of radioactivity originating from more than one isotope are now available, as are spectrometers and fluorimeters which handle material in the 10^{-6} g range. However, in spite of the growing sophistication of the methodology, the proper identification or quantification of steroids present in microgram or nanogram quantities is by no means a simple feat. Thus, proper identification remains a crucial part of any work concerned with the isolation or quantification of natural steroid substances. In addition, workers in the nonmammalian vertebrate field often face additional handicaps. Biological material has to be obtained from animals which are sometimes very small or which have diffuse steroid-producing organs. Other difficulties occur when experiments involve rare animals or animals which cannot be easily maintained under laboratory conditions, thus excluding the possibility of multiple experiments.

The criteria by which the validity of an identification procedure can be evaluated, irrespective of the chemical nature of the substance, are the following. (1) The material to be identified has to be isolated in a form sufficiently pure to render subsequent work meaningful. (2) Once a homogeneous substance has been obtained, there are two possible ways open for identification: (a) by a detailed analysis of the chemical and physical properties of the compound and its derivatives or (b) by a comparison of the chemical and physical properties of the unknown compound with a reference compound of known structure. Identification by method 2a may be achieved by classical techniques, such as elemental analyses, melting point, solubility and partition coefficients, refractive indexes, and by instrumental analyses including X-ray crystallography and nuclear magnetic resonance spectrometry. Such methods usually require milligram amounts of material and are most useful in the characterization of a compound but rarely applicable to the identification of steroids isolated from biological sources. Identification by 2b can be achieved with samples in microgram or even nanogram quantities. This has become possible by the extensive application of chromatographic techniques and by the use of isotopically labeled substances. Mass spectrometry, particularly in combination with gas chromatography, is a more recent but excellent method for the identification of microquantities of steroid.

Chromatography in its original conception is a method of separation involving the multistage partition of material between liquid–liquid, liquid–solid, or gas–liquid. All three forms of chromatography are widely used in steroid biochemistry not only as methods of separation, but also because the migration rate of a steroid in a given system can be considered as a physical index of its structural identity. In addition, isopolarity (i.e., identical migration rate) of an unknown steroid with an authentic carrier can be interpreted under certain conditions as indicative of chemical identity of the two compounds. Chromatography, especially paper partition, thin-layer, and gas–liquid forms, is very well suited for handling submilligram amounts of material and it has found extensive use in the separation and identification of natural steroids.

Chromatography became an even more indispensable tool with the advent of commercially available high specific activity ^{14}C- and ^{3}H-labeled steroids. Thus, with efficient detecting and counting procedures, extensive chemical workup became possible on samples in the $10^{-8} - 10^{-9}$ g range.

These advances in methodology gave a big impetus to steroid research but on the other hand increased the number of pitfalls the individual researcher had to avoid. For example, there is sometimes a tendency to consider the results obtained by certain techniques, usually involving complicated instrumentation, as positive proof of structural identity, e.g., spectra obtained by microinfrared. It has to be realized that at the present time no single technique, instrumental or otherwise, is capable in itself of furnishing such evidence. Similarly, chromatographic isopolarity of an unknown steroid with an authentic carrier cannot be construed as evidence for the identity of the two compounds, unless this isopolarity continues to exist following derivative formation and/or molecular modification.

Work with radioactive steroids poses its own difficulties. One is the original homogeneity of the commercial product. This can become a real problem, especially with high specific activity tritiated substances, due to the intense self-destruction of the substance. Another problem involves establishing the criteria for the radiochemical purity of a radioactive substance diluted with its presumed nonradioactive analog. Usually, radiochemical purity is admitted after the obtention of three consecutive specific activities which have a coefficient of variation of less than $\pm 5\%$. However, crystallization to constant specific activity or isotope ratio (isomorphism) must be obtained with a radioactive substance that has been rigorously established to be isopolar with the authentic carrier in order to constitute convincing proof of identity between the radioactive and nonradioactive molecules. It should be remembered that isopolarity is a relative term and the onus is on the investigator to select solvent systems which will separate the most closely related steroids.

The above considerations, encompassing only a small fraction of the possible pitfalls and problems, explain the need for the critical survey of the literature dealing with the isolation and identification of steroids from lower vertebrates. This survey was approached in the following way. An assessment scheme was devised and every publication included in this volume and reporting isolation, identification, and/or quantification of steroid substances was evaluated. The publications were assessed from various viewpoints. These included the soundness of the experimental setup, the adequacy of the isolation and purification procedure, and finally the chemical validity of the structural identification. In practice, the assessment was performed by devising a detailed evaluation chart and each specific criterion described in this chart was evaluated by a point system. The overall rating of the work was determined by the total number of points awarded. The basic aim of this rating was by no means to make any judgment on the value of the paper but simply to determine the completeness of the reported isolation and identification of the given steroid.

A similar assessment has been made of publications reporting quantification of natural steroids from lower vertebrate sources. Problems related to the quantification of steroids are discussed in Section III. Tables I, II, and III give the description of the evaluation charts. Although these tables are self-explanatory, a few points may need clarification. Identification of a native steroid and its derivatives, as described in Table I, parts II,A and B, was based on the principle of comparing these substances, by the aid of mixed chromatograms, with authentic substances. The question of the chromatographic isopolarity of two substances has already been discussed. It might be added, however, that comparison of the migration rates of two substances can be adequately determined only if these two substances have been *intimately mixed* prior to chromatography. Similarly, whenever chemical derivatives of two substances are to be compared, the chemical reaction and subsequent chromatography should be performed on a mixture of the two substances. Such a procedure becomes extremely valuable if a radioactive steroid is compared to a nonlabeled one or if a radioactive substance is mixed with an authentic carrier which is labeled with a different isotope.

In this evaluation, identical importance has been given to procedures using either nonradioactive or radioactive steroids. In the last few years a certain unjustified bias has developed against so-called "cold experiments." While the use of radioactive steroids increased the scope and ease of experimentation, the "cold" experiments have not become by any means obsolete and, when used within their limitations, can give valid results.

Identification in part III of Table I refers to situations in which steroids could be characterized by the determination of their physical properties. Identification of this kind is still regarded by many as the only valid one. Undoubtedly, the description of the physical properties of a compound

TABLE I

Assessment of Steroid Identification

Criteria	Maximum points
I. Isolation of the steroid	16
A. Adequacy of starting material	6
General care in preparation of the biological material, reagents, purity, and quantity of eventual substrates; adequacy of the quantity of biological material, precursors, etc.	
B. Adequacy of experimental procedures	10
This section applies to both the isolated steroid and any product to which it was transformed	
Proper description of experimental procedures; suitability of techniques used for the purification of extracts and isolation steroids; proper selection of chromatographic systems, solvent pairs for partition, countercurrent distribution, etc.	
Detection of steroids on chromatograms or in liquid fractions	
II. Identification of the steroid	25
A. Steroid nonradioactive	
1. Identity of nonmodified compound	6
Isopolarity of native steroid in different chromatographic systems with authentic marker; partition coefficient in partition systems, etc.	
Application of group reactions (blue tetrazolium, Porter–Silber, *m*-dinitrobenzene, Kober, soda fluorescence for 4-ene–3-one etc.)	
or 2. Identity of nonmodified compound *and one* derivative or transformation product	15
Proper identification of transformation product or derivative; suitability of derivative (ether, ester, etc.) or molecule-modifying-reaction (chemical oxidation or reduction; enzymic reactions)	
Radioactive or nonradioactive derivative	
Assessment of degree of molecule modification	
or 3. Identity of nonmodified compound *and more than one* derivative and/or transformation product	25
Criteria identical to those listed under 2	
B. Steroid radioactive	
1. Isopolarity of nonmodified radioactive compound with authentic carrier in different systems (chromatography, partition, etc.)	6
or 2. Isopolarity of nonmodified compound and at least *one derivative* in different systems	10
or 3. Constant specific activities or isotope ratios (about $\pm 5\%$) obtained on one derivative or transformation product	
Specific activities were obtained by a method other than crystallization	15
or 4. Constancy of specific activities and/or isotope ratios through sequential derivations but not involving crystallizations	20
or 5. Isopolarity of original compounds and derivatives with authentic compounds; crystallization to constant specific activity and/or isotope ratio following dilution with authentic carriers	25

TABLE I (cont.)

Criteria	Maximum points
6. Double-isotope derivative assay; assessment can be made under 3 or 4	
III. Special techniques for identification	30
Criteria in this section can be used to confirm identifications performed under II, A or B; when complete chemical and physicochemical description of the steroid has been reported criteria can be used without reference to Section II	
A. Physical identification of functional groups	2
IR, NMR, ORD polarography, UV absorption, etc.	
B. Absorption spectra in strong mineral acids or alkali	4
C. Fingerprint identification	20
IR, NMR, mass spectra, etc. (max. 10 points for single technique)	
D. Special techniques for specific steroid	10
Aromatase, glucosaccharo-1,4-lactone, fluorescence at various acid concentrations, etc.	
E. Crystallization of the natural steroid	10
Quantitative data on chemical and/or physical properties (e_{max}, mp; mixed up, molecular rotation, carbon–hydrogen, etc.)	
F. Bioassay	4
Generally no points awarded, but could be if homogeneity of steroid established first; in very special cases, points could be increased to 10 if isopolarity established first	
IV. Modifying factors in the assessment of steroid identity	
A. Isolation of a known steroid from an unfamiliar source	-10%[a]
B. Isolation of a known steroid from an unfamiliar source, but well identified in closely related species	None[a]
C. Isolation of known steroid from a familiar source	$+20\%$[a]
D. Isolation of an unfamiliar steroid	-10%[a]

[a]Change in earned points

yields direct proof of structures, while the results obtained by comparing a substance with a carrier on the basis of their chromatographic behavior yield evidence which is in some cases circumstantial or negative. The use of physical identification procedures remains limited in steroid biochemistry, as some of these procedures, with a few exceptions (microinfrared, acid chromogens), require milligram amounts of purified material. The present concept of valid criteria for the identity of a steroid is essentially a compromise between the desirable and the possible. This has been taken into consideration in the point system in Table I. By identifying steroids under criteria described in parts II,A or II,B, one can arrive at a total of 41 points, i.e., "presumptive identification" (Table II). To obtain a rating of absolute identification, some criteria described in part III of Table I have to

TABLE II

Final Rating of Steroid Identification on the Basis of Points Earned in Table I

Rating	Code	Definition of rating	Points
Positive identification	Po	Rigorously identified (absolute identification)	45 and above
Presumptive identification	Pr	Can be considered adequate beyond reasonable doubt	31–45
Tentative identification	Te	Identification not complete but reported identity of compound probable	18–30
Suggestive identification	Su	Preliminary identification and can serve as working hypothesis	10–17
Exploratory identification	Ex	Suggested identity of steroid doubtful on the basis of evidence presented	to 10
Insufficient data	ID	Insufficient data to permit an assessment	

TABLE III

Assessment of Quantification Procedures of Steroids

Criteria	Rating	Code
Identity of measured steroid not established	Steroid not identified	SNI
Identity of measured steroid established	Rating in "identity" category	
Evaluation of analytical procedure as to its specificity, accuracy, precision, sensitivity	Positive *or* presumptive *or* tentative	Po Pr Te
Value of the method and the steroid levels reported to other investigators (this is mainly an evaluation of reproducibility of the method by its published description, especially in regard to the condition of the biological material or experimental animals)	Thorough *or* partial *or* sparse	T P S

be also fulfilled. Thus, a special category has been reserved for instances in which structures have been established by direct evidence. It is realized that these instances are very rarely encountered in nonmammalian steroid biochemistry and a rating of "presumptive identification" must generally be accepted as positve proof for structural identity of the isolated steroid.

Rating of the quantification procedures of steroids (Table III) became necessary since the quantification of these substances is intimately connected with their isolation and identification. Any quantitative value obtained for a natural steroid is meaningless unless the steroid has been properly isolated and purified and convincing evidence exists that the procedure quantifies nothing else but the substance in question.

In this connection, a word should be said about a technique which, although developed for the quantification of small amounts of material from biological sources, can furnish, if properly performed, proof of identity of the quantified compound. This procedure is the double-isotope derivative assay (Table I, part II,B,6). The natural steroid is quantified by derivatizing it with a radioactive reagent of known specific activity and is subjected to extensive purification. To correct for the losses incurred during this purification, a ring-labeled radioactive model compound of the steroid to be quantified is added to the biological material at the outset of the test. This model compound is labeled with a radioactive isotope different from that contained in the derivatizing agent. Thus, the radioactivity of one isotope serves as quantitative measure of the natural substance while the activity of the second isotope is used to correct for losses. In addition, the isotope ratio can be utilized to establish the radiochemical purity of the substance.

The evaluation of published data on the identification and/or quantification of natural steroids from nonmammalian vertebrate sources has been incorporated into tables in Chapters 4–7. The following information is given in these tables: species investigated; steroid isolated, identified, and/or quantified; the precise source of the natural steroid; the quantity obtained or, in experiments utilizing precursors, the yield of the steroid in question from the substrate; major criteria of identification; and the rating given for (a) the identification, (b) the quantification, and (c) the value of the quantification to other investigators (reproducibility, etc.). Under the heading "major criteria" are listed, in abbreviated form, the physical and chemical procedures used by the respective author(s) which led to the claim of identity of the steroid in question. In this way, the reader will have the benefit of knowing how the author of the reviewed paper arrived at his final conclusion and also upon which criteria the reviewer based his evaluation. The abbreviations used in the column "major criteria" are shown in Table IV.

TABLE IV

Abbreviations Used for Criteria in Assessment Tables (Chapters 4–7)

Method	Abbreviation
Acid chromogen	ACr
Adsorption chromatography	AC
Bioassay	Ba
Color tests	CT
Competitive protein binding assay	CPBA
Constant (C) isotope ratio	C ^{3}H/^{14}C; C ^{3}H/^{35}S, etc.
Constant isotope ratio of one derivative	C ^{3}H/^{14}C D
Constant isotope ratio through sequential derivations	C ^{3}H/^{14}C SD
Constant specific activity	CSA
Constant specific activity of one derivative	CSAD
Constant specific activity through sequential derivations	CSASD
Crystallization	Cry
Crystallization to constant isotope ratio	CryC ^{3}H/^{14}C
Crystallization to constant specific activity	CryCSA
Countercurrent distribution	Ccd
Derivatives (radioactive)	Der(r)
17,21-Dihydroxy-20-ketosteroids	17-OHCS
Double-isotope derivative assay	DIDA
Fluorescence (acid) (alkaline)	(Ac)Fl, (Alk)Fl
Gas–liquid chromatography	GLC
Gonadosomatic index	GSI
Infrared absorption spectra	IR
Isonicotinic acid hydrazide	INH
Isopolarity	Ip
Mass spectra	MS
Melting point	MP
Modified (radioactive) compound	m(r)C
Not applicable	NA
Nonmodified (radioactive) compound	nm(r)c
Nuclear magnetic resonance	NMR
Oxidation (enzymic)	(Enz)Ox
Oxidoreductase	OR
Paper chromatography	PC
Partition chromatography	PaC
Physical–chemical properties	PcP
Polarography	Po
Porter–Silber chromogens	PSCr
Reduction (enzymic)	(Enz)Re
Sequential derivatives	SD
Solvent partition	SPa
Steroid previously identified in species	SPIsp
Steroid not identified	SNI
Thin-layer chromatography	TLC
Ultraviolet absorption spectra	UV

III. Isolation and Quantification of Steroids

A. Brief Review of Methodology for Quantification

Any valid physicochemical method for the quantitative determination of a chemical substance should have the following attributes. (1) *Accuracy:* The method should be devised in such a way that the total amount of the substance to be detected is measured and compensation is made for losses incurred during manipulation. (2) *Precision:* The method must be reproducible. While it is very difficult to lay down exact norms, it is generally desirable that multiple determinations should agree within ±5%. (3) *Sensitivity:* The sensitivity of any physicochemical quantification should be such as to leave ample margin for the measurement of levels at least 10 times lower than the expected ones. Thus, no method can be called satisfactory in which measurement is performed by pushing the method to its extreme sensitivity limit. (4) *Specificity:* No quantitative method is acceptable without reasonable assurances that it will measure only the substance to be detected. In steroid biochemistry, the key to convincing measurement of naturally occurring steroids is the specificity of the quantification procedure. Ideally, any substance should be quantified only in pure form. Although this might not always be possible, certain acceptable compromises can be found which will result in chemically convincing data without rendering the methodology technically prohibitive.

In general, steroid substances can be quantified by one of the following methods: (1) ultraviolet and visible spectrophotometry, (2) fluorimetry, (3) gas–liquid chromatography, (4) double-isotope derivative assay, (5) competitive protein binding and radioimmunoassay. Gravimetry, the classic tool of organic and inorganic chemistry, has found little application in steroid biochemistry.

1. Steroids containing aromatic rings and polyene conjugated systems or α,β-unsaturated ketones exhibit characteristic absorption maxima between 220 and 300 mμ. These absorption patterns can aid in the identification of functional groups in unknown substances and can be used for quantitative measurements. Structural correlations with the position and intensity of the absorption peaks have been described by Dusza *et al.* (1963).

Steroids are colorless in solution in organic solvents or water. However, after treatment with strong mineral acids (e.g., sulfuric acid, phosphoric acid), steroids exhibit characteristic absorption spectra in the 200–600 mμ range (sulfuric acid: for a review, see Smith and Bernstein, 1963; phosphoric acid: Nowaczynski and Steyermark, 1955, 1956; Kalant, 1958a). These spectra can be utilized for quantification and for the identification and characterization of steroids. Addition of chromogenic substances to sulfuric acid may render the steroid–acid reaction more specific or may enhance the color development (phenylhydrazine: Porter and Silber, 1950; anthrone: Graff, 1952; methanol or water: Allen *et al.*, 1950; Kalant, 1958b; phenol: Kober, 1931; Bauld, 1954). Other spectrophotometric methods include formation of colored derivatives (2,4-dinitrophenylhydrazones: Gornall and MacDonald, 1953; isonicotinic acid hydrazones: Weichselbaum and Margraf, 1957; *m*-dinitrobenzene addition complex: Zimmermann, 1935; Callow *et al.*, 1938), formation of chromogens by oxidation (Norymberski *et al.*, 1953), formation of chromogens by reduction (phosphotungsto-molybdic acid: Heard and Sobel, 1946; formazan formation from blue tetrazolium: Mader and Buck, 1952; Nowaczynski *et al.*, 1955). It would be impossible to list all the reactions tried and published and we refer those interested to the excellent reviews published on this subject (Jayle, 1962; Dorfman, 1968).

2. Steroids normally do not exhibit fluorescence, but following exposure to strong acid or alkali, some species of steroid molecules will form fluorescent compounds. In general, fluorescence methods permit the detection of 10^{-1}–10^{-2} times the amount of material measured by ultraviolet or visible spectrophotometry. Fluorimetry, while very sensitive, has the drawback of errors caused by self-absorption and quenching. Modern spectrofluorimeters which allow the selection of the proper excitation and emission wavelengths improve the specificity of the method (for a review, see Goldzieher, 1963).

3. The introduction of gas–liquid chromatographic techniques for the separation and quantification of steroidal substances by Vandenheuvel *et al.* (1960) raised high hopes that this methodology would be the answer for the simultaneous isolation, identification, and quantification of microquantities of steroids originating from natural sources. An added attraction of gas–liquid chromatography (GLC) seemed to be that, as an instrumental technique, it lent itself to automation. In subsequent years, however it became clear that the potential of the method, at least as far as steroid analytical work was concerned, had been overestimated. Contrary to early claims, GLC cannot handle in a satisfactory manner crude solvent extracts of biological material. To obtain meaningful data from GLC, the steroid has to be submitted to fairly extensive purification prior to chromatography. Once the steroidal substance has been obtained in a more or less isolated form, the GLC technique can be used to its full advantage. This technique allows the quantification of steroids with a very high sensitivity (up to the 10^{-9} g range) and in some instances, GLC can also be used for the preliminary identification of a substance. However, only C_{18}-, C_{19}-, and C_{21}-deoxy compounds

chromatograph without decomposition. Corticosteroids with an α-ketol or dihydroxyacetone side chain are more or less heat labile. Methods used for the quantification of such compounds rely on preformation of stable oxidation products and more recently on the preparation of their methoxime–trimethylsilyl ethers (Bailey, 1968; Engel *et al.*, 1970). For details or steroid GLC, the reader is referred to the numerous reviews and monographs published on this subject in the last few years (Horning *et al.*, 1963; Patti and Stein, 1964; Lipsett, 1965; Wotiz and Clark, 1966; Grant, 1967; Polvani *et al.*, 1967; Eik-Nes and Horning, 1968).

4. The double-isotope derivative assay has been mentioned in Section II. When properly performed, this assay can serve as proof of identity of a compound in addition to its use as a quantitative method. Steroids can be measured in $10^{-7} - 10^{-10}$ g amounts, the amount dependent in part upon the specific activity of the derivatizing reagent. The derivatives most commonly prepared for steroid assays are ^{14}C- and ^{3}H-acetyl esters (e.g., Kliman and Peterson, 1960; Peterson, 1964; Coghlan and Scoggins, 1967) and ^{35}S-sulfonyl esters (Bojesen *et al.*, 1967). A method for α-ketolic corticosteroids using ^{14}C-blue tetrazolium was described by Vecsei *et al.* (1967).

5. The principle of competitive protein binding was described by Murphy *et al.* (1963) for the assay of plasma cortisol. The method takes advantage of the fact that vertebrate plasma contains a globulin fraction (transcortin or corticosteroid-binding globulin, CBG) which will bind steroid molecules in a more or less selective fashion. The steroid to be determined is extracted from the biological fluid and then mixed with a standard solution of CBG and a suitable ^{14}C- or tritium-labeled authentic steroid. The conditions are chosen so that the CBG of the solution is just saturated with the radioactive substance. Since the portion of the steroid pool bound to the CBG is in dynamic equilibrium with the unbound portion, the steroid in the sample will compete for binding sites with the radioactive standard and will displace a fraction of the latter and the measured percentage of tracer bound to the CBG will fall proportionally. By determining the amount of radioactivity either in the protein-bound or in the free fraction, one can quantify the displacement of the marker steroid.

Competitive protein binding assays have been developed for several plasmatic steroids, including the corticosteroids, progesterone, testosterone, and estradiol (Murphy, 1967, 1970). The assay for sex hormones is based on the presence of a sex-hormone-binding protein in blood plasma. Tissue proteins have been used for the assay of the estrogens (Korenman, 1968). Radioimmunoassays in which antibodies are used as binding proteins have been developed for estradiol (Ábrahám, 1969) and aldosterone (Mayes *et al.*, 1970). The great advantage of the method is its speed and simplicity. Sensitivity depends mainly upon the use of high specific activity tracer steroids and a low concentration of endogenous steroid in the protein binding solution. However, at present, the specificity of this methodology is not yet fully worked out. Problems have been encountered with interference from solvents and extracts of thin-layer and paper chromatograms. The attractiveness of all rapid methods decreases with time as limitations become apparent; protein binding is no exception and improved procedures now involve careful, preliminary purification of the steroid in question. For information on the theory and methodology of the competitive protein binding assay the reader is referred to Diczfalusy (1970).

B. Isolation of Steroids from Plasma

A few observations concerning the isolation of steroids from plasma may be helpful to those unfamiliar with steroid biochemistry. It is our experience that fish plasmas can be among the most difficult to process; we shall describe methods and precautions that we have adopted in the belief that most are equally applicable to plasma from other life forms.

1. Precautions with Glassware, Solvents, and Chromatography

Care in washing glassware is extremely important in order to avoid contamination and destruction of sensitive steroids. We avoid chromic acid cleaning solution except in the case of glassware used for fluorescence assays and radioactive samples. In general, we follow the recommendations of Bush (1961). Lipid and protein are removed from glassware before routine dishwashing. The glassware is then washed with detergent, hot water, acetic acid: methanol 1:4, distilled water, 0.1% Versene in 50% aqueous methanol, and finally methanol. In order to avoid creating active adsorptive sites the glassware is dried at room temperature.

Many elaborate procedures have been devised for the purification of paper for chromatography. One procedure involves extraction with hot acetic acid and then with methanol in a large Soxhlet. It is our experience that such procedures result in more, rather than less, extractable contaminants. We prefer to precut paper and wash it by descending chromatography overnight with distilled hexane followed by 24–48 hr with distilled methanol. The paper is dried at air temperature in a closed container.

Steroids can be eluted cleanly and quickly from paper, with very small volumes of solvent, by means of a prewashed fiberglass wick and descending chromatography (Bush, 1961). Mutliple thin-layer chromatography (TLC) can frequently lead to heavy losses of corticosteroids when methanol is used for elution of steroids from silica gel. The steroids can be protected by substituting dichloromethane:methanol (9:1) for methanol (Idler *et al.*, 1966; Idler and Horne, 1968).

The practice of storing solvents in plastic bottles can cause problems even though the plastic may be rated by the manufacturer as resistant to the solvent. It is common practice to quantify steroids with the Δ^4-3-ketone structure by measuring absorption at 220, 240, and 260 mμ and then applying Allen's formula to correct for baseline absorption. When we stored methanol in polyethylene for 0, 2, 4, and 6 weeks the readings at 220 mμ were 0.26, 0.43, 0.57, 0.72, respectively. When methanol was stored in Teflon or glass bottles there was no increase in ultraviolet (UV) absorption at 220 mμ with time.

2. Extraction and Processing of Steroids

All solvents used for the extraction and processing of steroids should be distilled before use. Ethyl acetate (and ethers) should be tested for peroxides with acidified potassium iodide (Burstein and Kimball, 1963). If peroxides are present they should be destroyed and the solvent distilled (Riddick and Toops, 1955).

We prefer dichloromethane for the extraction of nonconjugated steroids from plasma. This solvent is suitable for nonpolar as well as polar steroids such as cortisol and 1α-hydroxycorticosterone. It should be noted that some scientists prefer ethyl acetate; this solvent is less likely to produce emulsions and is more efficient in extraction of very polar metabolites of corticoids. However, unless such metabolites are the subject of interest, dichloromethane removes less nonsteroidal polar material from the plasma and thus yields cleaner extracts.

In order to avoid emulsions and destruction of steroids and to obtain the cleanest possible extracts we prefer (a) to work with fresh rather than frozen plasma, (b) to work at 2°–4°C, (c) to adjust the pH of the plasma to 9 with NaOH prior to extraction, (d) to extract as few times as possible (generally once) with a large volume of solvent (i.e., 5–10 volumes), (e) to mix thoroughly but not too vigorously, and (f) to wash the extract with successive 0.1 volumes of 5% sodium carbonate (or 0.05 N sodium hydroxide), 0.1 N acetic acid, and water.

The dichloromethane extract may be passed through a funnel containing glass wool to remove traces of water or emulsion. Large volumes of solvent are rapidly removed with a flash evaporator when the water bath is kept at 40°C and the receiver is chilled in dry ice–acetone. For small samples a stream of nitrogen will quickly remove the solvent at 40°C.

The lipid residue is partitioned between hexane and 70% methanol. For polar steroids such as cortisol the water content of the aqueous methanol can be increased and carbon tetrachloride substituted for hexane. In fact, with steroids of this polarity methanol may be omitted altogether and the extraneous lipid can be removed from water with benzene (Eik-Nes, 1957).

Most lipid extracts will now be ready for TLC. With extremely fatty plasma or tissue extracts, or in cases where very little steroid is present, further purifications may occasionally be desirable. It is beyond the scope of this book to discuss the many types of adsorption and partition chromatography and other techniques available, but a simple method that is frequently overlooked is dialysis. An excellent procedure which produces clean extracts suitable for paper chromatography involves dialysis against aqueous methanol (Axelrod and Zaffaroni, 1954; Kalant, 1958c). This technique provided a one-step purification of extracts of the corpuscles of Stannius of a teleost (Krishnamurthy, 1968). In our experience such extracts can be very difficult to clean up by more conventional methods.

A knowledge of partition coefficients of steroids among various solvents can be useful in the choice of purification procedures and chromatographic solvent systems (Engel and Carter, 1963). We have found TLC solvent systems used by Nandi and Bern (1965) very suitable for preliminary fractionation of steroidal extracts from fish plasma and tissues (for a recent review and tabulation of relative mobilities of steroidal compounds in TLC solvent systems, see Lisboa, 1969). In establishing isopolarity it is valuable to employ both typical and atypical solvent systems; with an atypical system the more polar steroid moves faster; e.g., cortisol moves faster than cortisone (Nienstedt, 1967).

Some steroids, such as testosterone and 1α-hydroxycorticosterone, are present in plasma of fish as glucuronosides, and the concentration may be equivalent to that of the free steroid. After the extraction of free steroids, protein is removed by ethanol precipitation. After removal of the ethanol by evaporation *in vacuo*, sufficient water is added to make the volume equal to the original volume of the plasma, and hydrolysis is effected with β-glucuronidase. If the enzyme is free of sulfatase activity the method can be made specific by incubation in the presence of glucosaccharo-1,4-lactone, a competitive inhibitor of β-glucuronidase (Levvy, 1952). The lactone occurs naturally in urine and makes the use of a large excess of enzyme necessary. We have not encountered any problem with fish plasma, although it is desirable to add additional enzyme after several hours of incubation. For additional information and references to hydrolysis of steroid conjugates the reader is referred to Bernstein *et al.* (1966) and Eik-Nes (1968). The steroids released from conjugates are extracted and processed as for the free steroid.

C. Pitfalls in the Quantification of Plasmatic Steroids

It is not our intention to discuss basic problems with the accuracy, specificity, or sensitivity of all methods of steroid assay but rather to outline problems which arise when a method is applied to tissues or fluids not previously the subject of intensive qualitative and quantitative studies.

As listed in Section III,A, the methods of quantification of steroids can be described by four general classifications. For several reasons methods based on spectrophotometry and fluorometry have been used most extensively in studies on nonmammalian vertebrates. These methods are convenient for the assay of the large numbers of samples required to study changes in steroid levels as a function of the physiological or pathological condition of the animal. Unfortunately, their relative simplicity, especially of abbreviated procedures, requires special precautions in their use, and data so obtained need careful assessment before being used as a basis for further studies.

Interference with the specificity of abbreviated methods for the determination of plasma steroids can occur in various ways. The interference may be from a plasmatic steroid other than that for which the method was designed to measure. Consider, for instance, a study on plasmatic steroids in humans where results from an abbreviated competitive protein binding assay (CPBA) for cortisol were in good agreement with those obtained by a double-isotope derivative method (DIDA) for some subjects, but the results from CPBA were three to six times higher than from DIDA in cases of adrenogenital syndrome (Iturzaeta *et al.*, 1970). This discrepancy was attributed to 21-hydroxylase deficiency and the occurrence in the plasma of steroids, other than cortisol, which competed for the binding sites on the protein. In salmon there are many examples of transient qualitative changes in plasma steroids, e.g., 11-ketotestosterone and testosterone with sexual maturation, in which abbreviated methods could result in difficulties with specificity. A second type of interference involves changes in specific nonsteroidal plasma components, e.g., lactic acid, which are measured by the abbreviated method. A third type of interference, which has qualitative as well as quantitative implications, is due to the frequently large and variable mass of nonsteroidal lipid relative to the mass of steroid. Finally, interference may result from some treatment of the experimental animal or plasma extract. Drugs, anesthetics, and anticoagulants fall into this category.

Abbreviated analytical methods have seldom been validated for the conditions under which they are subsequently employed. The abbreviated method is often validated by a comparison of the results so obtained with those found by a specific method on a specific group of animals. The method is then employed to determine the effect of stress, diet, sexual maturation, or other variables but without validation on samples from these animals. For example, in the rat it has been suggested that high-fat diets influence the concentration of plasmatic corticosterone as determined by a fluorometric assay of relatively crude lipid extracts. Surely, the possibility must be considered that the diet does not affect corticosterone but rather increases the amount of nonsteroidal fluorogen in the plasma.

For the determination of 17-hydroxycorticosteroids in small samples, use of the Porter–Silber reaction is limited by its lack of sensitivity. Specificity may also be a problem with an unfamiliar blood plasma. When plasma samples are scarce or difficult to obtain there is a natural reluctance to use such samples for the determination of specific blank values obtained by the omission of the reagent phenylhydrazine. If the response to the variable under investigation is very large, then low chromogen values for samples from control animals make it easier to detect the change. However, if such is not the case, the low steroid values for control animals may necessitate the use of larger samples and/or more sensitive methods.

Specificity rather than sensitivity is the more common problem when acid-induced fluorescence is used to measure corticosteroids in body fluids of many vertebrates. Fluorometric methods which depend upon the partition coefficients of steroids between carbon tetrachloride and aqueous alcohol should be applied only after the steroids in plasma samples have been identified. 1α-Hydroxycorticosterone, a steroid found in elasmobranch plasma, like cortisol is sufficiently polar to be concentrated in the aqueous fraction and is fluorescent in sulfuric acid:ethanol.

The sulfuric acid:ethanol reagent should be carefully chosen. High concentrations of sulfuric acid, i.e., 80% or over, destroy the steroid fluorogen and reduce the stability of the fluorescence and the sensitivity of the assay (Braunsberg and James, 1960). The rate of development of fluroescence provided by the plasma extract should be compared with that of the pure steroid. Nonspecific fluorescence tends to increase with time whereas fluorescence due to cortisol or corticosterone reaches a plateau with time. The reagent and reaction time should be chosen to minimize interference but should allow the intensity of the fluorescence to stabilize. Lower concentrations of acid, e.g., 65 or 70%, provide stable fluorescence of maximal intensity, but the development time is longer so that these conditions are most suitable for highly purified steroidal extracts.

Nonsteroidal but relatively polar lipid material interferes with the fluorometric assay of blood plasma extracts of fish, for example, especially if applied directly to the extract. When quantification by fluorescence is used, efforts should be made to keep the blank values as low as possible; otherwise it is difficult to determine changes which may be very significant as a fraction of the steroid but may not be significant as a fraction of the total fluorescence. Several workers have shown how serious this nonspecific fluorescence can be when simplified procedures which have not been validated for the plasma in question are employed. Thus, a simplified fluorescence procedure for determining cortisol in human plasma resulted in values 55% too high when compared with methods which specifically measure cortisol (James et al., 1967). Brief fluorometric methods, developed to measure corticosteroids in plasma of man and the laboratory rat, resulted in serious errors when applied to the measurement of corticosterone in avian plasma (Frankel et al., 1967). In this study, corticosterone was measured in avian adrenal plasma by six different methods: four abbreviated methods, an extended fluorometric method which included chromatographic isolation of corticosterone, and a double-isotope derivative assay. The values obtained by the extended fluorometric and double-isotope derivative assays were comparable (8.0 and 9.6 μg/100 ml, respectively) but the error of values obtained with the brief methods varied from 65 to 81.4%. Similarly, the abbreviated methods gave high values (5–22 μg/100 ml compared to 0.6 μg/100 ml) of corticosterone in plasma of Metopirone-treated adrenohypophysectomized cockerels. Thus, Frankel and his associates (1967) concluded that abbreviated fluorometric methods could not be used for the determination of corticosteroids in plasma or tissue of any nonmammalian vertebrate unless a rigorous validation procedure was carried out.

There is no doubt that abbreviated procedures have been valuable for clinical studies and are necessary for the solution of problems requring the analysis of many samples. However, in the development or modification of such methods for quantification of steroids in submammalian vertebrates recognition of interference by all or some of the factors previously mentioned must be made. Problems not normally encountered in studies on humans or the laboratory experimental animal must also be considered. The animals are often small, sometimes rare or at least difficult to capture in large numbers, of unknown history, and stressed from capture or maintenance in captivity.

One of the most serious problems in working with small animals has been the development of methods to measure specific steroids in small samples of blood. It has been claimed that samples as small as 1 ml containing less than 2 μg/100 ml of cortisol can be quantified by an abbreviated fluorometric procedure but only 10 fluorescence units are obtained when the plasma cortisol level is 4.5 μg/100 ml so that at lower levels the method is pushed to or beyond its sensitivity limit. However, used with proper precautions such methods have yielded relatively low "cortisol" levels and it has been shown that procedures known to depress blood steroid levels (i.e., hypophysectomy and dexamethasone treatment) have resulted in the expected decrease in "cortisol" levels.

Plasma samples from some species may contain relatively high levels of steroids, not normally found in the species, which could conceivably interfere with the assay of a specific steroid. For example, high levels of several steroids occur in the plasma of a Pacific salmon (*Oncorhynchus nerka*) at certain times in their life cycle (see Chapter 4). It is also likely that blood samples from the same species in differing physiological conditions will not contain equal amounts of extractable fluorogenic material which is nonsteroid in nature. Large amounts of lipid are extracted by organic solvents when blood of heavily feeding animals is extracted in contrast to the relatively cleaner extracts obtained from starved numbers of the same species. Even for isolated steroids, quantification can present serious problems since the chemical composition of the tissues and body fluids of species are dissimilar and vary within a species according to the physiological condition of the individual as determined by environmental factors, nutritional status, season, and/or reproductive stage. Difficulties in the application of a method can result from the amount of lipid which is extracted from plasma which has been frozen and refrozen or in frozen storage for some time compared to that extractable from fresh plasma. Another problem with methods based solely on solvent partition is that a nonsteroid metabolite in the plasma may be detected by the procedure and change in response to the same stimuli affecting the corticoids. An example is the interference of lactic acid in the Porter–Silber method for the determination of 17-hydroxycorticoids (Eik-Nes, 1957) and the known effect of stress on both.

Many procedures have been devised to validate simplified analytical methods. With some precaution, these procedures can be inexpensive, rapid, and suitable for simultaneous analysis of large number of samples. When sufficient steroid is present, such precaution may consist of little more than the addition of isotopically labeled steroid and one or two chromatograms.

To be sure, there are several reports that plasmatic steroids of nonmammalian vertebrates have been determined by more elaborate procedures, including chromatographic isolation, but here also the results have sometimes been less than satisfactory. For example, when fluorescence or some other procedure is carried out and the material eluted from a spot on a paper chromatogram the order of magnitude of the "blank" strips of paper immediately preceding and following the steroid should be measured and recorded. Strong fluorescence in these areas indicates that the material of interest is probably contaminated with a nonsteroidal fluorogen. While procedures involving chromatography add specificity, they also render reproducibility more difficult; it is therefore desirable to allow for recovery through the procedures for each sample. Recoveries have seldom been considered in studies on nonmammalian vertebrates except in *in vitro* studies involving radioisotopes. The simplest way of correcting for recovery is to add a small mass of the radioactive steroid prior to extraction of the sample. When the radioactive steroid is not available a radioactive steroid of similar but not identical polarity is probably acceptable. A known quantity of a radioinert, closely related, and separable steroid could be employed if the steroid was known not to occur in the sample.

For many quantitative procedures, true or total blank values are difficult to obtain. Water or preextracted plasma is sometimes used as a "blank" for plasma analyses, but can only serve as a nonspecific or reagent blank and does not indicate interference specific to the plasma under study.

Plasma collected from animals after ablation of the endocrine gland, e.g., adrenalectomy or gonadectomy, may be used to assess interference from plasma components other than steroids. Sometimes plasma is analyzed with and without the addition of the steroid being quantified. This procedure can be used to determine recovery although when possible this goal can be more easily achieved with the addition of the appropriate radioactive steroid. Also, the addition of known amounts of steroid and replicate analyses may be used to evaluate the precision of a method. When quantification is required for a steroid in blood from a little-investigated species it is necessary to purify the steroid extensively so that unknown plasmatic components do not contribute significantly to the blank values.

The above observations notwithstanding, there are excellent approaches to the quantification of steroids in small samples and this is particularly true if the steroid possesses some unique characteristic. Molecular transformation by either chemical reagents or enzyme reactions used in conjunction with chromatography can greatly improve the specificity of an assay methods. Cortisol fluorescence in ethanol:sulfuric acid is enhanced and sensitivity increased by prior treatment with alkali. The specificity of the reaction is also improved because fluorescence can be carried out before and after treatment with alkali; fluorescence due to corticosterone and 20-hydroxy derivatives of cortisol are not affected by the alkali treatment (Sobrinho, 1966). Reactions with steroid-specific enzymes can be used to advantage: Placental enzymes convert testosterone to estradiol and 20β-hydroxysteroid dehydrogenase is useful in the analysis of progesterone. Norymberski (1967) has discussed in more detail the potential use of selective agents in the analysis of steroidal compounds. The usefulness of techniques which increase specificity should be of particular interest to investigators of plasmatic corticosteroids in unfamiliar and different species.

The double-isotope derivative assay is particularly useful for quantification of steroids in extracts of unfamiliar blood plasma samples in that identification and quantification are combined and, by using high specific activity derivatives, small blood volumes can suffice. However, since it is a tedious and time-consuming assay it is probably most useful in the initial definition of the plasmatic steroid content of a species and in the validation of simpler, more practicable methods of analysis. Again the procedural steps described for the quantification of a particular steroid in human blood cannot be used for blood of another species without confirmation that the procedures are adequate. Plasma samples containing high concentrations of lipid not removed by solvent partition may require further purification by column or thin-layer chromatography before preparation of the radioactive derivative. Multiple chromatographic steps which isolate the radioactive derivative from all other contaminants, including other steroids, contained in the plasma of one species may not be adequate for plasma of another species. The effectiveness of a chromatographic solvent system as applied to the plasma extract under study should be determined. For example, in the isolation of aldosterone diacetate, a reverse-phase paper chromatography in mesitylene–aqueous methanol was critical to the success of the assay (Coghlan and Scoggins, 1967). Since there is little inherent specificity in the formation of the radioactive derivatives, purity of the final chromatographic eluate should be checked by preparation of further derivatives and/or recrystallization to constant isotope ratios. When ^{3}H-acetic anhydride of high specific activity is used, the extra precautions needed to obtain accurate results (e.g., redistillation of reagents, prevention of contamination, contribution of blank values) have been discussed by Coghlan *et al.* (1966), Coghlan and Scoggins (1967), and Brodie *et al.* (1967).

Competitive protein binding assays (CPBA) would appear to have great potential for use in studies of plasmatic steroids of nonmammalian vertebrates, especially in those cases where only small blood samples are possible. In its original form, the CPBA was quick and easy but, due to its lack of specificity, the procedures have had to be revised to include an isolative step. Isolation of the steroid from the body fluid by extraction and chromatographic fractionation of the extract provided greater specificity to the assay but introduced problems of high blank values and interference from solvents, plastic labware, silica gel and filter paper. In the past few years, considerable effort has been expended by investigators interested in CPBA for clinical studies and the problems and their alleviation or solution have been discussed elsewhere, e.g., Diczfalusy (1970). Since CPBA's have been used only to a limited extent to study steroids of nonmammalian vertebrates, we shall refrain from further comment at this time. However, it should be appreciated that CPBA's are not an easy solution to the difficult problem of measuring steroid content of biological materials. Before data so obtained are acceptable, the methods must be validated by reliable procedures (on larger samples, if necessary) and the precision and accuracy of the protein binding method should be established over the entire range of steroid concentration for which it is used (Nugent and Mayes, 1970).

Finally, there are technical problems which probably are recognized in laboratories where steroid research is extensive but which may not be widely appreciated in laboratories where interest in steroids is secondary to more general physiological studies of nonmammalian vertebrates. The adsorption of polar steroids to glass surfaces and of nonpolar steroids to certain plastics is a case in point. Thus, when radioactivity of polar steroids is measured in toluene cocktails using glass vials, adsorption on the glass can drastically alter the results. This is particularly serious when steroids of high purity and high specific activity are involved. For example, 1α-hydroxycorticosterone-^{3}H is completely adsorbed and the count is reduced by 50% (Idler and Truscott, 1967). This problem can easily be overcome (Kandel and Gornall, 1964) by the addition of small quantities of ethanol to the cocktail. During infusion of nonpolar steroids through plastic tubing, some steroids are adsorbed by the plastic and, again, the less the quantity and the greater the purity, the greater the problem; the most serious effects therefore occur with ^{3}H-labeled steroids. There may be several solutions to this problem but one which was used successfully on a fish involved infusion of radioactive steroid in dilute plasma (Fletcher *et al.*, 1969). Benzyl alcohol, sometimes incorporated in heparin solutions as a preservative, interferes with the fluorometric determination of corticosteroids (Werk *et al.*, 1967). When corticosteroids are eluted with methanol from silica gel after thin-layer chromatography and the eluate is evaporated to dryness under nitrogen the recovery of the steroid may be extremely low. Such destruction can be overcome by the use of dichloromethane:methanol 9:1 in place of methanol (Idler *et al.*, 1966; Idler and Horne, 1968).

While going through the literature it becomes quite obvious that steroid levels reported for the same species have undergone large changes as with the passing years more sophisticated methods became available. In early studies, the paper chromatographic methods employed were simply not able to cope with the large quantity of lipids in the extract and this resulted in insufficient purification prior to quantification. The situation has greatly improved since the widespread use of thin-layer chromatography. This improvement is going on steadily with the availability and acceptance of newer and more precise methodology.

IV. Methods for Study of Steroid Biosynthesis

A. *In Vivo* versus *in Vitro*

There are several experimental avenues open to the scientist wishing to study steroid patterns of an animal. The venous effluent blood of a hormone-secreting tissue can be analyzed and the steroids isolated and identified; in this event the qualitative and quantitative pattern is thought to reflect closely the situation under natural conditions, although surgical stress must be considered. Also, in many animals and tissues, the effluent is either contaminated by blood from other tissues or the venous effluent may not be representative of the total steroid output of the tissue. In animals without discrete endocrine glands, e.g., adrenal tissue of teleosts, collection of venous effluent may not be possible. A major advantage of working with venous effluent is that the steroid is in high concentration relative to peripheral blood. Conversely, the greatest difficulty in working with peripheral blood is the relatively low concentrations of most steroids. The main advantage of studying peripheral blood is that the hormones contained in it are those reaching the target organs. However, from a quantitative viewpoint, such factors as protein binding and its effect on biological activity must ultimately be taken into consideration. Unfortunately, nearly the entire literature on plasma steroid levels in nonmammalian vertebrates is based on steroids extractable by dichloromethane, chloroform, or ethyl acetate, and there is little information on chemically conjugated, let alone protein-bound, steroids. Another approach which has yielded much valuable information is organ perfusion *in situ* or in the isolated organ. This technique permits the ready treatment of the secretory tissue with a variety of stimulators and inhibitors of steroidogenesis. Perfusion may be conducted with or without the addition of exogenous steroid precursors. Steroids may also be studied by the analysis of excreta but catabolic and detoxication mechanisms frequently complicate the interpretation of results.

In vitro steroidal secretions may be examined by removal of endocrine tissue from the animal. Either the steroids are extracted and analyzed or the tissue is first incubated in a medium containing the necessary nutrients, cofactors, and, sometimes, steroid substrates. There is evidence that during the initial period of incubation without added cofactors (preincubate) the activity of the gland can be indicative of its performance *in vivo* (Idler and Truscott, 1969). Thus, an excised adrenal which had a good steroid output *in vivo* also produces well *in vitro*. Analysis of endocrine tissue without incubation frequently presents technical difficulties due to the small quantities of steroid and the large quantities of extractable lipid. Major disadvantages of tissue incubations are cell destruction, the accumulation of products in the medium, and the possible effects of these products on subsequent transformations, depletion of cofactors and substrates, and deterioration of enzyme systems. A continuous flow or superfusion technique may also be used to study steroid production *in vitro* (Orti *et al.*, 1965; Tait *et al.*, 1967). There are many potential advantages to this technique including removal of products and continuous replenishment of known cofactors and substrates, but leaching of enzymes and unknown cofactors conceivably could be a problem. Finally, tissue culture shows considerable promise but it will be some time before cell lines will be available for most nonmammalian vertebrates.

The results obtained by *in vivo* experiments have a much more general and immediate validity than those obtained by *in vitro* experimentation. Nevertheless, *in vitro* methodology offers greater flexibility and ease of manipulation, and for this reason most steroid biochemical work in nonmammalian vertebrates has been performed by this method. In addition, the study of steroid biosynthesis is almost impossible to achieve *in vivo* in those cases where the animals do not possess anatomically distinct endocrine glands. The *in vitro* technique is an extremely valuable one so long as the inherent difficulties are properly considered. While it is impossible to lay down general rules, it can be said that this methodology gives qualitatively valid results although the quantitative aspects of the experiments may not be extrapolated directly to reactions occurring in the intact animal.

B. Tissue Preparations

In general, living tissue taken from an organism for experimental purposes can be prepared in the following forms. It can be cut into slices, minced, or homogenized. Homogenates may be utilized as such (whole homogenate) or further fractionated by differential centrifugation.

Tissue slices, usually cut 0.5 mm thick, are thought to represent surviving organized tissue. Minces are intermediate between slices and homogenates, and contain a high percentage of partially damaged cells. In a properly prepared homogenate, the fraction of residual whole cells should be negligible.

In tissue slices, the reactions take place inside the cell. Exogenous substrates have to enter the slice by diffusion and the product of the reaction has to diffuse out again into the medium. It is generally believed that the inside of an adrenal cell is freely accessible to steroidal substances although diffusion phenomena have not been studied in detail. Thus, it is not known whether the chemical nature of the steroid influences its diffusion rate into and out of the cell. Recent experiments have shown that even whole, uncut rat adrenals are permeable to exogenous progesterone (Tsang and Stachenko, 1970). However, in slices, and even more so in mince preparations, some of the enzyme systems leak out into the incubation medium and thus some of the reactions are performed by enzymes outside the cell structure (Carballeira and Durnhofer, 1968). In consequence, results obtained from experiments using tissue slices or minces must be interpreted with caution.

In a homogenate the cells are ruptured and soluble enzyme systems and particulate cell components are evenly distributed in the homogenizing medium. The problems connected with membrane permeability are thereby obviated, although the geographical distribution of enzyme systems present in the intact cell are now destroyed and the orderly progression of sequential reactions possibly disrupted. As the availability of substrates to enzymes is facilitated, reactions proceed at a faster rate in homogenates than they do in sliced or minced preparations.

Recently, an increasing number of studies has been undertaken to determine the intracellular distribution of steroidogenic enzymes in vertebrate adrenals. Centrifugal fractionation of tissue homogenates in 0.25 M sucrose as described by Schneider and Hogeboom (1950) ("low-speed sediment" or "nuclear fraction," 700–750 g; "mitochondrial fraction," 6000–10,500 g; "microsomal fraction," 105,000 g sediment; "soluble fraction," 105,000 g supernatant), provides enriched enzyme fractions and thus facilitates their more detailed characterization. However, it should be kept in mind that even such intracellular particles as mitochondria have encasing membranes and homogenization of the endocrine tissue does not necessarily assure that, in experiments using multiple substrates, all the precursors will simultaneously come into contact with enzyme systems.

As mentioned earlier, many studies on the steroid biochemistry of nonmammalian vertebrates have been based on *in vitro* methodology. In the preceding discussion only a few of the inherent difficulties have been mentioned. Nevertheless, it is apparent that extrapolation of *in vitro* data to conditions existing in the intact animal is a delicate problem and requires the exercise of critical and sound judgment. A detailed discussion of the methods for tissue preparations has been presented by Umbreit *et al.* (1964).

C. CRITERIA FOR PRECURSOR–PRODUCT RELATIONSHIPS

Once the chemical nature of the steroid hormone secreted by an endocrine gland is known, the next logical step in the investigation is to find the chemical sequence by which these substances are synthesized by the secretory organ. *In vitro* methodology has been used extensively in studies of this nature, especially since the latest advances in tracer technique, and the availability of high specific activity tritiated and ^{14}C-labeled steroidal substrates. One limitation of this approach is that precursors may be selected which do not normally have access to the enzyme systems under test. For example, it has been shown that testicular tissue of a salmonid fish transforms adrenosterone to 11-ketotestosterone, but if adrenosterone does not occur in testicular tissue one can claim only identification of the necessary enzyme system. Similarly, dehydroepiandrosterone (DHA) is a major secretory product of the mammalian adrenal and if such tissue were incubated with radioactive DHA the transformation could be more easily interpreted than if fish interrenal tissue, which is not known to produce DHA, were incubated. Even if a substrate is present, the quantitative relationship may be such that other precursors would get first call on the enzyme.

If a substance is offered to an endocrine gland, either *in vivo* by perfusion or *in vitro*, the transformation product of this substrate will have been produced enzymically by the endocrine tissue. This very simple statement becomes complicated by the fact that, in most instances, the substrate will undergo multiple transformations and the metabolite isolated from the experiment may be the product of as many as six different consecutive enzymic reactions. Thus, the next step in the investigation is the establishment of the correct sequence of these multiple reactions by determining the appropriate precursor–product relationship between each and all intermediates. Several methods have been applied to problems of this nature. One method involves the transformation of a basic presumed precursor of steroid hormones, e.g., acetate or cholesterol, to steroidal end products by the endocrine tissue. In this case, in addition to end products, intermediates are isolated, although the latter may sometimes occur only in trace amounts. Once the probable list of intermediates is known, each of them may be offered in turn to the endocrine gland as substrate and the probable reaction sequence deduced from the metabolic transformation of these intermediates. This approach, although extremely fruitful, has the basic disadvantage that it is difficult to detect the transformation of one of the substrates into two metabolites simultaneously. Both metabolites will be present in the reaction mixture and moreover, both may be precursors of the next link in the metabolic chain.

A general solution of the definition of a precursor–product relationship was given by Zilversmit *et al.* (1943) for experiments using isotopically labeled substrates. They pointed out that the variation of specific activity with time in a series of compounds which become labeled with an isotope may indicate whether one compound is an immediate precursor of another compound in the series. In general terms, these specific-activity–time correlations can be described as follows. If the serial reaction under investigation is irreversible and no side reactions occur, the specific activity of the product will rise as long as it is inferior to that of the precursor; the two specific-activity–time curves will intersect at the point where the specific activity of the product is maximal; thereafter, both curves will fall, the curve of the product remaining higher than the curve of the precursor. (It is understood that, at the time of intersection, the specific activity of the precursor has already started to fall due to dilution from endogenously produced material.) Thus, in a reaction sequence consisting of several members, a family of interlocking specific-activity–time curves will be obtained, each subsequent member having a lower specific activity peak where the immediate precursor–product curves cross.

Another method for the determination of precursor–product relationships uses the classical theory of series first-order reactions. By determining the concentration–time relationship of all the intermediates and by measuring the velocity constants involved in the reaction sequence, it is sometimes possible to achieve a satisfactory description of the biosynthetic chain. Although the use of an isotopically labeled substrate does facilitate the performance of this type of experiment, in practice it is very difficult to measure all the necessary variables, especially mass determinations in the 10^{-7}–10^{-9} g range.

In the last decade, instrument technology for measuring the radioactivity of weak β emitters has advanced rapidly, culminating in the commercial availability of liquid scintillation spectrometers. With the aid of these instruments, the simultaneous and differential counting of radioactivity, originating from two different β emitter sources but contained in the same sample, became possible. This new counting technology permitted new experimental approaches for the formulation of criteria of precursor–product relationships. In one of these techniques two substrates are simultaneously offered to an endocrine gland, either *in vivo* or *in vitro*. These substrates are labeled with two different radioactive isotopes (usually with tritium and carbon-14) and are in a presumed precursor–product relationship. If steroid X, labeled with isotope A, and steroid Y, labeled with isotope B, are indeed a precursor –product pair, the following events should take place. Precursor ^{A}X will give rise to ^{A}Y, while the exogenous ^{B}Y will be further transformed, say, to ^{B}Z. However, after an initial lag period, the Y pool will be composed of molecules labeled with both isotopes and, in consequence, the resulting Z pool will also be doubly labeled. If all three compounds, X, Y, and Z, are in a strict sequential relationship, the isotope composition of the Z pool has to become identical, after a certain time, with the isotope composition of the Y pool. If Z is composed only of ^{A}Z molecules, then Y is not an intermediary. Conversely, if the Z pool is exclusively labeled with isotope B, X is excluded as a possible precursor. By following the changes in the isotope composition of the metabolites as a function of the time of the reaction, very useful information on steroidogenic pathways has been obtained in both mammalian and lower vertebrate steroid biochemistry.

Most of the above discussion refers to the use of isotopically labeled substrates. When radioactive substrates are used, it is implicitly understood that the substrates are added in *tracer* amounts and that they will mix intimately with any preexisting endogenous substrate pool. These conditions are not always easily fulfilled. The preexisting steroid pool in a steroid-producing tissue preparation is generally not known, and without this knowledge it is very difficult to determine what really constitutes *tracer* amounts. In general practice, the addition of about 20–50 nmoles of radioactive steroid to 100 mg tissue (substrate:tissue ratio of about $1:10^4$) is considered the upper limit of *tracer* amount, but this ratio has been arrived at by wholly empirical means.

Until recently, it was accepted without question that there is no separation between the endogenous steroid pool and the added tracer. This concept is now being reexamined as apparent differences have been noted between the metabolism of endogenous substrates and exogenous precursors (Vinson and Whitehouse, 1969a,b). There would also appear to be real differences in the metabolism of some exogenous precursors, e.g., Δ^5- and Δ^4-steroids as used in double-label experiments designed to determine preferential routes of steroid biosynthesis (Matsumoto and Samuels, 1969). For a more detailed discussion on problems associated with the interpretation of *in vitro* data, the reader is referred to Samuels *et al.* (1969). It should always be kept in mind that some of the biosynthetic schemes, although based upon irrefutable chemical evidence, may reflect only the biochemical transformation of the exogenous substrate and that, in reality, the gland synthesizes its own steroid hormones by quite different mechanisms.

REFERENCES

Ábrahám, G. E. (1969). *J. Clin. Endocrinol. Metab.* **29**, 866.

Allen, W. M., Hayward, S. J., and Pinto, A. (1950). *J. Clin. Endocrinol. Metabl.* **10**, 54.

Axelrod, L. R., and Zaffaroni, A. (1954). *Arch. Biochem. Biophys.* **50**, 347.

Bailey, E. (1968). *In* "Monographs on Endocrinology. Gas Phase Chromatography of Steroids" (K. B. Eik-Nes and E. C. Horning, eds.), Vol. 2, pp. 316–347. Springer-Verlag, Berlin and New York.

Bauld, W. S. (1954). *Biochem. J.* **56**, 426.

Bernstein, S., Cantrall, E. W., Dusza, J. P., and Joseph, J. P. (1966). "Steroid Conjugates, a Bibliography." Amer. Chem. Soc., Washington, D.C.

Bojesen, E., Buus, O., Svendsen, R., and Thuneberg, L. (1967). *In* "Steroid Hormone Analysis" (H. Carstensen, ed.), Vol. 1, pp. 1–53. Dekker, New York.

Braunsberg, H., and James, V. H. T. (1960). *Anal. Biochem.* **1**, 452.

Brodie, A. H., Shimizu, N., Tait, S. A. S., and Tait, J. F. (1967). *J. Clin. Endocrinol. Metab.* **27**, 997.

Burstein, S., and Kimball, H. L. (1963). *Steroids* **2**, 209.

Bush, I. E. (1961). "The Chromatography of Steroids." Pergamon, Oxford.

Callow, N. H., Callow, R. K., and Emmens, C. W. (1938). *Biochem. J.* **32**, 1312.

Carballeira, A., and Durnhofer, F. (1968). *Steroids* **11**, 513.

Chieffi, G., and Bern, H. A. (1966). *Gen. Comp. Endocrinol.* **7**, 203.

Coghlan, J. P., and Scoggins, B. A. (1967). *J. Clin. Endocrinol. Metab.* **27**, 1470.

Coghlan, J. P., Wintour, M., and Scoggins, B. A. (1966). *Aust. J. Exp. Biol. Med. Sci.* **44**, 639.

Diczfalusy, E., ed. (1970). "Steroid Assay by Protein Binding." *Acta Endocrinol. (Copenhagen) Suppl.* **147**.

Dorfman, R. I., ed. (1968). "Methods in Hormone Research. Chemical Determinations," 2nd ed., Vol. 1. Academic Press, New York.

Dusza, J. P., Heller, M., and Bernstein, S. (1963). *In* "Physical Properties of Steroid Hormones" (L. L. Engel, ed.), pp. 69–287. Macmillan, New York.

Eik-Nes, K. B. (1957). *J. Clin. Endocrinol. Metab.* **17**, 502.

Eik-Nes, K. B. (1968). *In* "Methods in Hormone Research. Chemical Determinations" (R. I. Dorfman, ed.), 2nd ed., Vol. 1, pp. 271–322. Academic Press, New York.

Eik-Nes, K. B., and Horning, E. C., eds. (1968). "Monographs on Endocrinology. Gas Phase Chromatography of Steroids," Vol. 2. Springer-Verlag, Berlin and New York.

Engel, L. L., and Carter, P. (1963). *In* "Physical Properties of the Steroid Hormones" (L. L. Engel, ed.), pp. 1–36. Macmillan, New York.

Engel, L. L., Neville, A. M., Orr, J. C., and Raggatt, P. R. (1970). *Steroids* **16**, 377.

Fletcher, G. L., Hardy, D. C., and Idler, D. R. (1969). *Endocrinology* **85**, 552.

Frankel, A. I., Cook, B., Graber, J. W., and Nalbandov, A. V. (1967). *Endocrinology* **80**, 181.

Goldzieher, J. W. ((1963). *In* "Physical Properties of the Steroid Hormones" (L. L. Engel, ed.), pp. 288–320. Macmillan, New York.

Gornall, A. G., and MacDonald, M. P. (1953). *J. Biol. Chem.* **201**, 279.

Graff, M. M. (1952). *J. Biol. Chem.* **197**, 741.

Grant, J. K., ed. (1967). "The Gas–Liquid Chromatography of Steroids," Memoirs of the Society for Endocrinology, No. 16. Cambridge Univ. Press, London and New York.

Greep, R. O. (1966). *Endocrinology* **79**, 823.

Heard, R. D. H., and Sobel, H. (1946). *J. Biol. Chem.* **165**, 687.

Horning, E. C., Luukkainen, T., Haahti, E. O. A., Creech, B. G., and Vandenheuvel, W. J. A. (1963). *Recent Progr. Horm. Res.* **19**, 57.

Idler, D. R., and Horne, D. A. (1968). *Steroids* **11**, 909.

Idler, D. R., and Trustcott, B. (1967). *Steroids* **9**, 457.

Idler, D. R., and Trustcott, B. (1969). *Gen. Comp. Endocrinol. Suppl.* **2**, 325.

Idler, D. R., Kimball, N. R., and Trustcott, B. (1966). *Steroids* **8**, 865.

Iturzaeta, N. F., Hillman, D. A., and Colle, E. (1970). *J. Clin. Endocrinol. Metab.* **30**, 185.

James, V. H. T., Townsend, J., and Fraser, R. (1967). *J. Endocrinol.* **37**, xxviii.

Jayle, M. F. (1962). "Analyse des Stéroides Hormonaux." Masson, Paris.

Kalant, H. (1958a). *Biochem. J.* **69**, 79.

Kalant, H. (1958b). *Biochem. J.* **69**, 93.

Kalant, H. (1958c). *Biochem. J.* **69**, 99.

Kandel, M., and Gornall, A. G. (1964). *Can. J. Biochem.* **42**, 1833.

Kliman, B., and Peterson, R. E. (1960). *J. Biol. Chem.* **235**, 1639.

Krishnamurthy, V. G. (1968). *Gen. Comp. Endocrinol.* **11**, 92.

Kober, S. (1931). *Biochem. Z.* **239**, 209.

Korenman, S. G. (1968). *J. Clin. Endocrinol. Metab.* **28**, 127.

Levvy, G. A. (1952). *Riochem. J.* **52**, 464.

Lipsett, M. B., ed. (1965). "Gas Chromatography of Steroids in Biological Fluids." Plenum, New York.

Lisboa, B. P. (1969). *In* "Methods in Enzymology. Steroids and Terpenoids" (R. B. Clayton, ed.), Vol. 15, pp. 3–158. Academic Press, New York.

Mader, W. J., and Buck, R. R. (1952). *Anal. Chem.* **24**, 666.

Matsumoto, K., and Samuels, L. T. (1969). *Endocrinology* **85**, 402.

Mayes, D., Furuyama, S., Kem, D. C., and Nugent, C. A. (1970). *J. Clin. Endocrinol. Metab.* **30**, 682.

Murphy, B. E. P. (1967). *J. Clin. Endocrinol. Metab.* **27**, 973.
Murphy, B. E. P. (1970). *In* "Steroid Assay by Protein Binding" (E. Diczfalusy, ed.), pp. 37–60. *Acta Endocrinol. (Copenhagen) Suppl.* **147**.
Murphy, B. E. P., Engelberg, W., and Pattee, C. J. (1963). *J. Clin. Endocrinol. Metab.* **23**, 293.
Nandi, J., and Bern, H. A. (1965). *Gen. Comp. Endocrinol.* **5**, 1.
Nienstedt, W. (1967). *Acta Endocrinol. (Copenhagen) Suppl.* **114**.
Norymberski, J. K. (1967). *Excerpta Med. Found. Int. Congr. Ser.* **132**, 16.
Norymberski, J. K., Stubbs, R. D., and West, H. F. (1953). *Lancet* **164**, 1276.
Nowaczynski, W. J., and Steyermark, P. R. (1955). *Arch. Biochem. Biophys.* **58**, 453.
Nowaczynski, W. J., and Steyermark, P. R. (1956). *Can. J. Biochem. Physiol.* **34**, 592.
Nowaczynski, W., Goldner, M., and Genest, J. (1955). *J. Lab. Clin. Med.* **45**, 818.
Nugent, C. A., and Mayes, D. (1970). *Acta Endocrinol. (Copenhagen) Suppl.* **147**, 257.
Orti, E., Baker, R. K., Lanman, J. T., and Brasch, H. (1965). *J. Lab. Clin. Med.* **66**, 973.
Patti, A., and Stein, A. A. (1964). "Steroid Analysis by Gas–Liquid Chromatography." Thomas, Springfield, Illinois.
Peterson, R. E. (1964). *In* "Aldosterone" (E. E. Baulieu and P. Robel. eds.), pp. 145–161. Blackwell, Oxford.
Polvani, F., Surace, M., and Luisi, M., eds. (1967). "Gas Chromatographic Determination of Hormonal Steroids." Academic Press, New York.
Porter, C. C., and Silber, R. H. (1950). *J. Biol. Chem.* **185**, 201.
Riddick, J. E., and Toops, E. (1955). "Techniques of Organic Chemistry. Organic Solvents" (A. Weissberger, ed.), 2nd ed., Vol. 7. Wiley (Interscience), New York.
Samuels, L. T., Matsumoto, K., Aoshima, Y., and Bedrak, E. (1969). *Excerpta Med. Found. Int. Congr. Ser.* **184**, 845.
Schneider, W. C., and Hogeboom, G. H. (1950). *J. Biol. Chem.* **183**, 123.
Smith, L. L., and Bernstein, S. (1963). *In* "Physical Properties of the Steroid Hormones" (L. L. Engel, ed.), pp. 321–448. Macmillan, New York.
Sobrinho, L. G. (1966). *Steroids* **7**, 289.
Tait, S. A. S., Tait, J. F., Okamoto, M., and Flood, C. (1967). *Endocrinology* **81**, 1213.
Tsang, C. P. W., and Stachenko, J. (1970). *Steroids* **16**, 707.
Umbreit, W. W., Burris, R. H., and Stauffer, J. F. (1964). "Manometric Techniques." Burgess, Minneapolis, Minnesota.
Vandenheuvel, W. J. A., Sweeley, C. C., and Horning, R. A. (1960). *J. Amer. Chem. Soc.* **82**, 3481.
Vecsei, P., Lommer, D., Steinacher, H. G., and Wolff, H. P. (1967), *J. Chromatogr.* **26**, 533.
Vinson, G. P., and Whitehouse, B. J. (1969a). *Acta Endocrinol. (Copenhagen)* **61**, 695.
Vinson, G. P., and Whitehouse, B. J. (1969b). *Acta Endocrinol. (Copenhagen)* **61**, 709.
Weichselbaum, T. E., and Margraf, H. W. (1957). *J. Clin. Endocrinol. Metab.* **17**, 959.
Werk, E. E., Jr., Theiss, K. E., Choi, Y. K., and Marnell, R. T. (1967). *J. Clin. Endocrinol. Metab.* **27**, 1350.
Wotiz, H. H., and Clark, S. J. (1966). "Gas Chromatography in the Analysis of Steroid Hormones." Plenum, New York.
Zilversmit, D. B., Entenman, C., and Fischler, M. C. (1943). *J. Gen. Physiol.* **26**, 325.
Zimmermann, W. (1935). *Z. Physiol. Chem.* **233**, 251.

Chapter 3

THE FUNCTIONAL MORPHOLOGY
OF STEROIDOGENIC TISSUES

BRIAN LOFTS and HOWARD A. BERN*

I. Introduction

The steroid-producing endocrine organs of the nonmammalian vertebrates are the male and female gonads and the adrenal cortex, or its homolog,

*Studies from my laboratory referred to herein have been aided by NIH grants AM-07896
and CA-05388.

the interrenal tissue of lower forms. These structures are linked by their common basic embryological origin from a thickening of the dorsal coelomic epithelium. Furthermore, they utilize essentially the same substrates for the synthesis of their respective steroid products and, to a certain extent, operate by similar mechanisms. Thus, the functional activities of the steroidogenic tissues of the mammalian testis, ovary, and adrenal gland are all regulated by the secretion of protein hormones from the anterior pituitary gland, and evidence is accumulating which suggests that this controlling mechanism spans the whole vertebrate series. The mammalian placenta is also an important transient source of steroidogenic hormones.

In mammals, it has been shown that the steroid-producing cells, whether adrenal, testicular, or ovarian, have certain features in common. At the ultrastructural level they all have a well-developed agranular endoplasmic reticulum, and their mitochondria differ from those in cells of nonsteroidogenic tissues in having tubular cristae (Belt and Pease, 1956; Christensen and Gillim, 1969). Generally, lipids are found in their cytoplasm which often react positively to tests for cholesterol and appear birefringent when viewed under polarized light. The majority of vertebrates are seasonal breeders, and the cyclic fluctuations in this cholesterol-positive sudanophilic (lipid) material are often a useful parameter of the functional activity of the tissue, although they are insufficient to implicate unequivocally a tissue as a steroid-producing structure.

It is now well established that the biosynthesis of almost all the active steroid hormones involves the Δ^5-3β-hydroxysteroid dehydrogenase (3β-HSDH) enzyme system which catalyzes the conversion of Δ^5-3β-hydroxysteroids, such as pregnenolone and dehydroepiandrosterone, to Δ^4-keto-steroids (progesterone, androstenedione). The recent development of methods for the visualization of this enzyme, particularly when taken in conjunction with the histochemical tests for lipids and cholesterol, has provided a much more reliable indication of steroid synthesis and has added significantly to the possibility for investigating the morphology and physiology of the steroidogenic endocrine tissues throughout the vertebrate series.

To date, many of the data regarding sources of steroids within the body have been derived largely from investigations on mammalian species. However, in the last decade our knowledge of steroid-producing structures in nonmammalian animals has been steadily increasing, and there is now an extensive literature concerning seasonal changes in the morphology of the steroidogenic endocrine organs of fishes, amphibians, reptiles, and birds. In this chapter we have confined ourselves almost exclusively to a consideration of the testis, ovary, interrenal tissue, and adnexa, such as Bidder's organ and the corpuscles of Stannius, of these nonmammalian vertebrate animals. This survey is not intended to be exhaustive, and only the later literature is partially cited. We have excluded any dissertation on other endocrine glands such as the pituitary gland and hypothalamic neurosecretory system with which they are intimately involved, but which themselves do not synthesize steroid hormones. For details of the latter organ complexes and other endocrine tissues, the reader is directed to the several excellent textbooks on comparative vertebrate endocrinology which are now available (Gorbman and Bern, 1962; Barrington, 1963; von Euler and Heller, 1963; Barrington and Jørgensen, 1968).

II. Testis

Generally, the male gonads are paired structures which in mammals are housed seasonally or permanently in an extraabdominal sac, the scrotum; in nonmammalians they are more usually located in the abdominal cavity, in close proximity to the kidneys. Some urodeles possess testes consisting of a series of separate lobes joined by narrow bridges of tissue, but in most other members of the gnathostome series the gonads are compact bodies drained by gonoducts (ducti deferentes) derived from embryonic mesonephric (Wolffian) ducts. Cyclostomes differ in possessing a single, medially placed testis without gonoducts, and spermatozoa in these animals are discharged directly into the coelom, from which they pass out of the body via abdominal pores.

Functionally, the vertebrate testes are responsible both for the proliferation of male gametes, the spermatozoa, and for the secretion of the male sex steroids, the androgens, on which the seasonal development and activity of the secondary sexual characters depend. Thus, both gametogenetic tissue and endocrine tissue occur in the same organ, unlike crustaceans where they are often anatomically separate. Commonly, throughout the whole vertebrate series, therefore, castration produces atrophy of the accessory sexual structures during the breeding season or, if performed during the nonbreeding phase, prevents their seasonal development. Conversely, injections of testicular extracts or androgenic steroids into castrated animals restore the functional activity of the atrophied structures. Biochemically, it has been established that the testicular tissues of fishes, amphibians, reptiles, and birds possess the capacity for manufacturing the steroids necessary for the maintenance of these secondary sexual features (see the later chapters). The steroids are usually synthesized by easily distinguishable interstitial cells located between the seminiferous tubules, but in some poikilotherms, the steroidogenic tissue appears to exist as circumtubular elements apparently derived from modified fibroblasts, just as are the normal interstitial cells (Figs. 1 and 2).

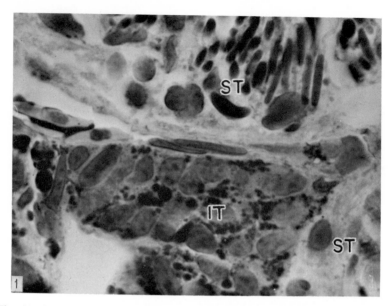

Fig. 1. Section of frog (*Rana esculenta*) testis showing interstitial cells (IT) located in the interstices between the seminiferous tubules (ST). Sudanophilic droplets are seen in the interstitial cells. Formol—calcium, frozen, sudan black; × 500.

In mammals the production of both spermatozoa and androgens is regulated by the secretion of two distinct gonadotropic hormones from the anterior pituitary gland. These are the follicle-stimulating hormone (FSH), primarily responsible for regulating the spermatogenetic activity of the germinal epithelium, and the interstitial-cell-stimulating hormone or luteinizing hormone (LH), which regulates the secretory activity of the interstitial tissue. With the exception of fishes, the exogenous administration of purified preparations of these mammalian gonadotropins produces similar responses in the testes of nonmammalian vertebrates, although a separation of distinct FSH-like and LH-like factors has so far been achieved only in mammals and, more recently, in birds (Stockell-Hartree and Cunningham 1969; Furr and Cunningham, 1970; Wentworth, 1971). Pituitary cytological data also indicate that testicular control in amphibians, reptiles, and birds may be similarly based on the secretory activity of two distinct gonadotropes. In fishes, the evidence is less clear-cut, and so far piscine testes have been reported to respond only to exogenous LH, injections of FSH being without apparent effect. Furthermore, purified gonadotropin from salmon pituitary stimulates both spermatogenesis and spermiation when administered to hypophysectomized male goldfish, and both vitellogenesis and ovulation are stimulated in hypophysectomized females (Yama-

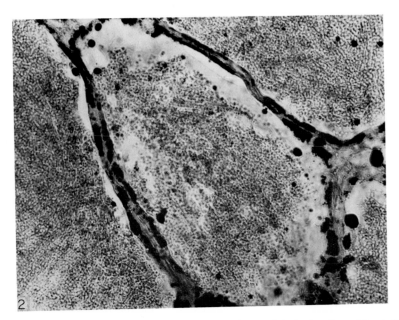

Fig. 2.   Section of pike (*Esox lucius*) testis showing perilobular location of the sudanophilic boundary cells. Formol—calcium, frozen, sudan black; × 500. (From Lofts and Marshall, 1957.)

zaki and Donaldson, 1968). In hypophysectomized catfish *Heteropneustes fossilis*, salmon gonadotropin has been reported to be ten times more potent than ovine LH in reinitiating spermatogenesis (Sundararaj *et al.*, 1971). There is a need, however, for much more research before firm conclusions can be drawn, since experimentation has been based on the effects produced by administration of purified mammalian gonadotropins, and it remains uncertain whether these are identical with nonmammalian gonadotropins.

Reproduction is a cyclical phenomenon, and most vertebrates are seasonal breeders with cycles synchronized by environmental stimuli to ensure the propagation of young at the most propitious time of year. Generally, only some domestic species, or animals occupying habitats with little seasonal variation in climatic conditions and food availability, produce spermatozoa continuously. More commonly, testes regress after the breeding season, and the production of spermatozoa is restricted to a relatively brief period of the year. These species exhibit considerable annual variation in the size of their gonads and show cyclical fluctuations of activity in both the exocrine and endocrine components. In mammals and birds, there is distinct evidence that the fluctuations are produced by the environmental stimuli exerting their influence through a central nervous control of gonadotropin release, mediated by hormones which are liberated from the median eminence of the neurohypophysis and transported by portal vessels to the pars distalis of the pituitary gland. Poikilotherms have not been so extensively investigated, but here too experimental data suggest that a similar mechanism also exists in reptiles, amphibians, and some fishes (see reviews by Jørgensen and Larsen, 1963; Dodd *et al.*, 1966; Green, 1966). Thus, fundamentally uniform gonad-controlling mechanisms appear to operate throughout the vertebrate series, and it is perhaps not surprising that the histophysiology of the testis also shows many similarities in the different vertebrate groups.

A. REPTILES AND BIRDS

The testes of both reptiles and birds have the basic mammalian structure of an ovoid encapsulated body surrounded by a thick fibrous outer covering, the tunica albuginea. Internally, each testis is composed primarily of a mass of convoluted seminiferous tubules which in birds, unlike mammals, are anastomotic and not restricted by septa. The boundary wall of the tubule is the tunica propria, a fibrous connective tissue layer which, together with the tunica albuginea, becomes seasonally stretched by the buildup of germinal products as the sexual season approaches. The avian testis in particular is subject to great annual variation, sometimes as much as 500-fold, and in the Japanese quail *Coturnix coturnix japonica*, for example, testis weight increases from 8 to 3000 mg. Such gross extremes impose a great strain on the

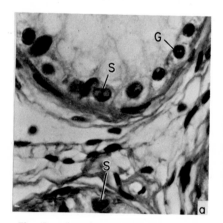 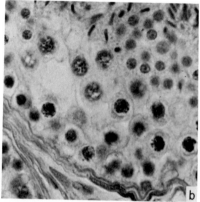

Fig. 3. Sections of cobra (*Naja naja*) testis showing (a) regressed condition with only sustentacular cells (S) and spermatogonia (G) in the germinal epithelium and (b) full breeding condition with the germinal epithelium several layers thick. Hematoxylin and eosin (H and E); × 700.

tunica albuginea, and it is replaced annually by a proliferation of new fibroblasts rebuilding the new capsule from beneath.

The seminiferous tubules are lined by the germinal epithelium consisting of developing germ cells and nongerminal sustentacular or Sertoli cells. During the period of sexual quiescence, only a single layer of stem spermatogonia and sustentacular cells lines the tubules (Fig. 3a), but with the seasonal recovery of spermatogenetic activity, the germinal epithelium soon becomes several cells thick (Fig. 3b) and the tubules consequently become greatly distended. The timing of this event differs in reptiles and birds. In Reptilia, spermatogenetic activity resumes in many species soon after the breeding season, and advanced germinal stages are produced in the tubules before the onset of winter. Spermatozoa may be stored for several months before the copulatory period. In birds, on the other hand, this never occurs and, after the breeding period, the testes collapse and remain in a sexually quiescent state until shortly before the succeeding breeding phase. Then, a period of intense spermatogenetic activity rapidly repopulates the tubules, and spermatozoa are produced only shortly before the onset of breeding.

The interstices between tubules are filled with tissue composed of blood capillaries, lymph spaces, and the steroid-producing component, the interstitial (Leydig) cells. In some species, great numbers of melanoblasts are also located in this tissue and impart a black or gray appearance to the organ. As the seminiferous tubules seasonally expand, the interstitial tissue becomes dispersed and compressed into tight wedges; consequently fewer interstitial cells appear in any given section (Fig. 4a). The interstitial tissue

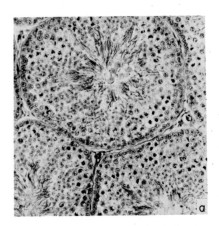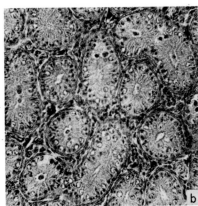

Fig. 4. Sections of house sparrow (*Passer domesticus*) testis in breeding (a) and winter condition (b). Note how the interstitial tissue becomes dispersed and compressed with the expansion of the seminiferous tubules (H and E; × 280).

of the sexually quiescent animal, on the other hand, is more conspicuous (Fig. 4b). As a result, an inverse relationship between sexuality and interstitial cell activity has sometimes been claimed. This of course is not true, and the biosynthetic capacity for androgen production is clearly established in mammals, where the interstitial tissue of the laboratory rat has been separated from the seminiferous tubules by microdissection (Christensen and Mason, 1965; Collins *et al.*, 1968). By incubating the isolated tissue with radioactive precursors such as progesterone-4-^{14}C, these workers have been able to demonstrate its capacity to produce testosterone and other androgenic steroids. Furthermore, the selective destruction of the germinal epithelium by X irradiation or artificial cryptorchidism (see Burrows, 1949, for a review of the earlier literature), which leaves the interstitium and the secondary sexual characteristics apparently unaffected, also indicates that the interstitial cells are the site of androgen biosynthesis. In both the avian testis (Botte and Rosati, 1964; Woods and Domm, 1966) and the reptilian testis (Arvy, 1962; Mesure, 1968), histochemical techniques have pinpointed the presence of 3β-HSDH in the interstitial tissue, thus confirming its involvement in steroid biosynthesis; this is also supported by the presence of large mitochondria characterized by tubular cristae and abundant agranular endoplasmic reticulum in the cellular cytoplasm (Porte and Weniger, 1961).

In birds and reptiles, the interstitial cells show well-marked seasonal secretory cycles. In winter months a gradual accumulation of small, cholesterol-positive lipid droplets occurs in these cells, and these build up as the sexual season approaches (Marshall, 1955). There is a rapid depletion of this material at the height of the breeding activity (Fig. 5a and b). Cholesterol is a known precursor of androgen biosynthesis and its depletion at this stage is probably indicative of its rapid utilization at a time of high androgen release. In birds, the interstitial cells next pass into a final vacuolated end phase, disintegrate, and are removed by macrophage activity. In reptiles, disintegration is more gradual; the cells first metamorphose into a densely lipoidal and strongly cholesterol-positive end stage before their final dispersal. Thus, an accumulation of precursor occurs with the decline of androgen release at the end of the sexual season. In *Lacerta vivipara*, interstitial cell 3β-HSDH activity has been shown to increase in February and becomes most intense at the height of the breeding phase in April–May. In *L. sicula* the seasonal changes in the ultrastructural appearance closely correlate with these histochemical observations (Della Corte *et al.*, 1969). Thus, during hibernation the endoplasmic reticulum of the interstitial tissue is poorly developed and the small mitochondria show laminar cristae, but during the mating period the cells display a very well formed agranular endoplasmic reticulum and the mitochondria are more numerous and large with prevailing tubular cristae. Then there is a rapid decline in the enzymic

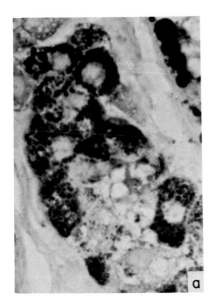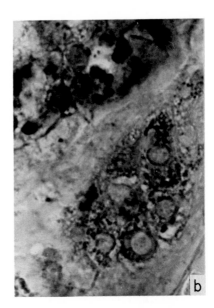

Fig. 5. Sections of cobra testis in December (a) and March (b). Note depletion of lipoidal material from the interstitial cells. Formol—saline, frozen, sudan black; × 890. (From Lofts *et al.*, 1966a).

activity which coincides with this densely lipoidal postnuptial phase (Mesure, 1968). In both birds and reptiles, rehabilitation of the exhausted interstitium now takes place; a new generation of juvenile interstitial cells replaces the old spent tissue (Fig. 6) and the cycle is repeated. In some reptilian species the androgen-dependent accessory sexual structures sometimes show their maximum development when the testes are apparently atrophic. Physiologically, however, the interstitium is secretory. This situation occurs, for example, in the chelonian *Clemmys caspica* in which the spermatozoa evacuate from the tubule lumina to become seasonally stored in the epididymidal canals for several months. During the copulatory period, females are fertilized by spermatozoa from the epididymidal reservoir, and the testes, although regressed and spermatogenetically inactive, contain interstitial cells at the peak of their secretory cycle, which maintain the androgen-dependent secondary sexual characteristics in a functional state (Lofts and Boswell, 1961). This rarely occurs in birds.

   The chemical analysis of the fluctuations in the biosynthetic capacity for androgen production in testicular tissue has so far been carried out on a seasonal basis in only one nonmammalian species, the cobra *Naja naja* (Tam, et al., 1967). In this snake, the testicular production of androgens under *in vitro* conditions closely parallels the histochemical events outlined above.

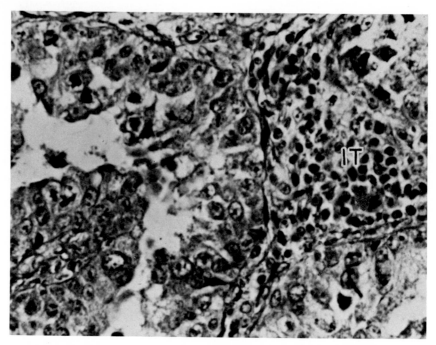

Fig. 6. Proliferation of interstitial cells (IT) in the regressed testis of the wood pigeon *Columba palumbus.* The adjacent seminiferous tubules are spermatogenetically inactive with some necrosis of the germinal epithelium (H and E; × 700).

Thus, the synthesis of androstenedione and testosterone from progesterone-4-^{14}C is at a minimum immediately after the breeding season when the interstitial cells are metamorphosing into their densely lipoidal state and accumulating precursor material. With the reestablishment of a new generation of interstitial cells, androgen production rapidly rises but declines when hibernation causes a suppression of the biosynthetic activity during the colder winter months. The interstitium becomes heavily lipoidal and cholesterol positive during this period (Lofts *et al.,* 1966a). With the return of warmer weather, there is a vernal increase in androgen synthesis and a concomitant depletion of cholesterol-positive lipids. A similar seasonal relationship between the interstitial lipid cycle and testicular androgen production also occurs in the Chinese teal *Anas crecca* (Lofts and Chan, 1971). In the domestic Pekin duck Garnier and Attal (1970) have correlated the seasonal variations in the plasma testosterone levels with the interstitial cell cycle.

As well as the interstitial cells, the sustentacular (Sertoli) cells of the seminiferous tubules may also be sites of steroid biosynthesis. In the past, there have been scattered references suggesting that these cells are the source of the female sex hormones produced by the testes of most vertebrates, but such claims have generally been based on cytological data from pathological tissue, mainly mammalian. More recently, however, it has been shown that the Sertoli cells of avian (Woods and Domm, 1966) and reptilian (Callard, 1967) species contain steroid dehydrogenases, and ultrastructurally they do have the characteristic agranular endoplasmic reticulum and tubular mito-chondrial cristae which Christensen (1965) and others associate with steroid-producing tissues and which are present in the interstitial cells. Furthermore, the sustentacular cells show a cyclic waxing and waning of cholesterol-positive lipoidal material similar to that observed in the interstitial tissue. It is therefore possible that here, too, the lipids may be indicative of seasonal fluctuations in steroid synthesis. Strong evidence of this endocrine function has recently been obtained in the snake *Naja* by microscopically dissecting free seminiferous tubules from the interstitial tissue. By incubating the tubules with labeled progesterone, it has been shown that they possess the capacity to produce 17α-hydroxyprogesterone, androstenedione, testoster-one, and estradiol-17β from this precursor (Lofts, 1968a, 1972). Similar results have also been obtained from both normal (Christensen and Mason, 1965; Bell *et al.*, 1968) and heat-treated rats (Lacy, 1967; Collins *et al.*, 1968; Lacy *et al.*, 1969).

The marked seasonal histochemical changes in these testicular steroid-producing tissues underline the great caution that must be taken when attempting to extrapolate androstenedione/testosterone relationships among vertebrates on the basis of steroid analyses of testicular incubations or plasma samples (Rivarola *et al.*, 1968). True correlations can be made only if cognizance is taken of the cycles to ensure that the endocrine tissues of animals under investigation are in a similar seasonal condition. In cobra, data from monthly incubations of testicular tubules currently being carried out at the Department of Zoology, University of Hong Kong, show that tubule steroid biosynthesis fluctuates very markedly on a seasonal basis (Lofts, 1972).

The role that such tubule steroid biosynthesis plays under *in vivo* con-ditions is not known. In avian and reptilian species the sustentacular cells rapidly fill with large masses of cholesterol-rich lipids at the end of the breed-ing season when all spermatogenetic activity in the germinal epithelium finishes (Lofts *et al.*, 1966a). As a consequence, the sectioned seminiferous tubules of the collapsed gonad appear to be filled with a dense amorphous mass when stained with dyes such as sudan black (Fig. 7a). This mass gives a strong cholesterol reaction. The tubules remain in this condition until the resumption of mitotic activity by the stem spermatogonia and then become rapidly cleared of their cholesterol material as spermatogenetic activity builds up (Fig. 7b and c). In wild birds the sustentacular cells remain lipoidal

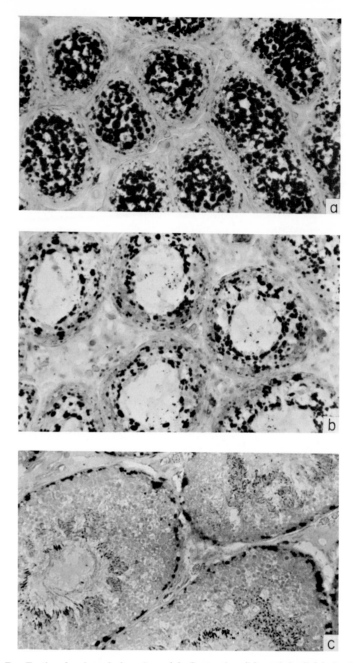

Fig. 7. Testis of cobra during June (a), September (b), and April (c). In June the seminiferous tubules are filled with dense sudanophilic masses, which subsequently disappear with the resumption of spermatogenetic activity. Formol—saline, frozen, sudan black; × 170. (From Lofts *et al.*, 1966a.)

for several months until spermatogenetic recrudescence in the following spring. A few reptilian species show a similar delay, but, more commonly, postnuptial lipids and cholesterol rapidly become cleared from the seminiferous tubules soon after testicular collapse, and spermatogenesis resumes within a few weeks.

In a chemical study of the cholesterol content of the testis of the Indian house lizard *Hemidactylus flaviviridis*, Sanyal and Prasad (1965) have shown that the free and esterified cholesterol contents are highest during the regressed state and then drop sharply in July, when there is an intense utilization of cholesterol with the resumption of spermatogenesis. This closely parallels the tubule lipid cycle. Hypophysectomy during the spermatogenetically active period leads to a premature buildup of the testicular neutral lipid content and cholesterol level, and a parallel reduction in the concentration of phospholipids (Reddy and Prasad, 1971). An inverse relationship, therefore, appears to exist between accumulation of cholesterol-rich lipoidal material in the sustentacular cytoplasm and the gametogenetic activity in the adjacent germinal epithelium. Androgenic steroids are known to stimulate spermatogenesis, and it may be that steroid synthesis by these cells is involved in the regulation of spermatogenetic activity.

The overall control of spermatogenesis is regulated by FSH, and exogenously administered FSH stimulates clearance of sustentacular cell lipids with a resumption of gametogenesis. Conversely, a suppression of FSH secretion, either by hypophysectomy or by estrogens, leads to an accumulation of cholesterol-rich lipids in these cells. It seems possible, therefore, that FSH may exert its spermatokinetic influence, either partially or wholly, through regulating the secretory activity of the sustentacular cells. Although this is speculative, such a mechanism is more in line with the known actions of other tropic pituitary hormones, such as LH and ACTH (adrenocorticotropic hormone), which stimulate the secretory activity of other steroid-producing tissues: the interstitial cells and the adrenocortical cells, respectively. Furthermore, since exogenous androgens stimulate spermatogenesis, the hypothesis that FSH acts on the germinal epithelium indirectly by stimulating the secretion of a steroid is more attractive than the supposition that a protein hormone on the one hand and a steroid on the other can mediate the same biological action.

B. Amphibians

Although many amphibians are terrestrial for the greater part of their lives, they are not completely emancipated from an aquatic medium, to which they return for breeding. Fertilization is external, as males and females synchronously extrude spermatozoa and eggs into the water. Relatively little is known about the Apoda, a small tropical group of blind snakelike amphibians, but the reproductive physiology of some members of the Urodela (newts and salamanders) and Anura (frogs and toads) has been extensively studied.

The reproductive cycles are mostly seasonal, but tropical species such as the Indian frogs *Rana erytrea* and *R. tigrina* or the South American toads *Bufo arenarum* and *B. paracmenis* are continuous breeders. Some temperate-zone frogs like *R. esculenta* also show continuous spermatogenesis in populations occupying more southernly, semitropical Mediterranean areas, but generally in most species, as in other poikilothermic vertebrates, spermatogenesis resumes soon after breeding and the seminiferous tubules fill with spermatozoa before the onset of hibernation. The mitotic activity of the spermatogonia is usually completed by early autumn and resumes only after the succeeding breeding season.

The spermatogenetic mechanism differs from that of the amniote vertebrates in that germ cells develop in coordinated clusters or cysts (Fig. 8a)

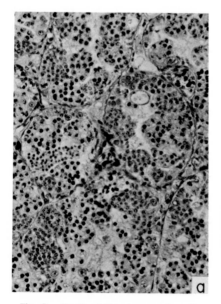 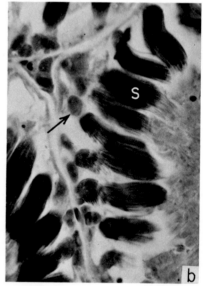

Fig. 8. Testis of the common frog *Rana temporaria* (a) at the peak of spermatogenetic activity (June) and (b) in December when the tubules are filled with bundles of spermatozoa (S) embedded in conspicuous sustentacular cells (arrow). Note the cystic type of spermatogenesis by which the germ cells develop in coordinated clusters within the seminiferous tubules (cf. Fig. 3a, b). H. and E; × 170, × 425.

contained within a membranous sheath (Lofts, 1968b). In close association with each spermatogonium, therefore, is the small nucleus of a cell forming the cyst wall. When the stem, or primary, spermatogonium regains its mitotic activity, it divides to form a cluster of secondary spermatogonia within this wall. All of the cells within a cyst are in the same stage of development and mature synchronously. The cyst thus changes into a primary spermatocyte cyst, then into a secondary spermatocyte cyst, and so on, until its wall eventually ruptures releasing the germinal contents. The cyst wall cells develop in conjunction with the dividing germinal cells; at first spindle shaped, they become glandular with a well-developed endoplasmic reticulum and numerous glycogen granules by the time the cyst is about to rupture. When this occurs, these cells transform into sustentacular cells adhering to the tunica propria, and the heads of the maturing spermatozoa embed in their cytoplasm. Thus, winter testes often show sectioned tubules or ampullae with radiating bundles of spermatozoa attached to conspicuous sustentacular cells (Fig. 8b), which ultrastructurally resemble steroid-producing elements (Brökelmann, 1964).

The testicular structure in the Anura is basically similar to amniotes in consisting of a mass of seminiferous tubules lined with a permanent germinal epithelium and interspersed in a conspicuous interstitial tissue. The Urodela, on the other hand, show a testicular structure closely similar to the piscine pattern. In many urodeles, as has been mentioned, each testis may consist of several well-marked lobes, the number varying from one species to another. The lobes are drained by efferent ductules leading to the mesonephric duct system, and seminiferous tubules are absent. Instead, germinal cysts are contained within ampullae with connective tissue walls. Each lobe is organized into two distinct zones with the spermatogonial ampullae concentrated in the cephalic region (Fig. 9). The ampullae migrate toward the caudal region as the contained spermatogonia propagate germinal cysts and expand the ampullae. When fully mature, each ampulla contains a mass of spermatozoa held together in bundles by sustentacular cells. As more and more spermatozoal ampullae accumulate in the caudal lobe it becomes distended and white and is easily distinguishable from the smaller, more translucent sector which contains the spermatogonial and spermatocytic cysts. During the breeding season the spermatozoa are discharged into the efferent ducts and the caudal region rapidly regresses. The discharged ampullae become compressed and eventually resorbed. Spermatogenesis is reestablished with the resumption of mitotic division by the residual germinal cells in the cephalic lobe.

The location of the amphibian steroid-producing tissue has, in the past, been the subject of a good deal of controversy, but modern histochemical techniques have clearly established the presence of secretory interstitial

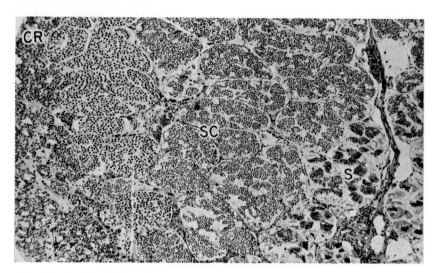

Fig. 9. Testis of *Trituroides honkongensis* showing the zonation of the seminiferous ampullae; the cephalic region (CR) contains proliferating spermatogonial ampullae. More caudally, the ampullae mature into spermatocytic (SC) and eventually spermatozoal (S) ampullae (H and E; × 68).

cells in the intertubular interstices of frogs and toads (Fig. 1), and a strongly positive response to 3β-HSDH tests has pinpointed these cells as sites of steroid biosynthesis in a number of species (Chieffi, 1967a). They are also similar in their ultrastructure to the mammalian interstitial cell (Doerr-Schott, 1964). They have a seasonal lipid cycle similar to reptilian interstitial cells and, as in the latter, there is a close correlation between this and the development of such secondary sexual structures as the thumb pads. During winter, interstitial cells contain relatively few sudanophilic droplets, but as the breeding period approaches, numerous small lipid droplets accumulate in the cytoplasm (Fig. 1) and give a faint cholesterol reaction. The cells react strongly to 3β-HSDH tests during this period; the cell nucleus also increases in size and becomes more rounded (Fig. 10a and b). A sudden depletion does not occur, but soon after the spermatozoa have been discharged, the cells become densely lipoidal and strongly cholesterol positive as in the amniote vertebrates. The reaction to 3β-HSDH tests now becomes negative. In the common frog *Rana temporaria* this condition is succeeded by the gradual weakening of the lipid and cholesterol reactions as the cells regress and become indistinguishable from ordinary connective tissue cells (Lofts and Boswell, 1960). However, in other species such as the edible frog *R. esculenta*, the

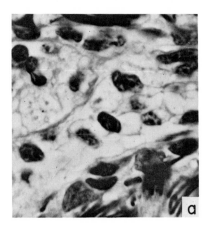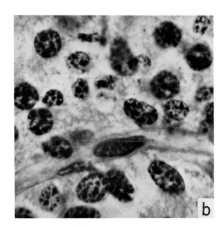

Fig. 10.   Interstitial tissue of the toad *Bufo bufo* showing the morphological differences in the interstitial cell nuclei of (a) a winter testis and (b) a testis during the breeding season. H and E; × 1000. (From Lofts, 1968b.)

interstitial cells remain densely lipoidal for some months and are distinguishable at all times (Lofts, 1964) but are negative to 3β-HSDH reactions (van Oordt and de Kort, 1969). As in amniotes, the sudden postspawning accumulation of cholesterol-positive lipids in these cells can be attributed to an interruption of androgen synthesis (Lofts, 1965). Thumb pads thus show evidence of accelerated growth and glandular development corresponding with vernal buildup of small, weakly cholesterol-positive lipid droplets and 3β-HSDH activity in the interstitial cells, they rapidly regress and enter a physiologically inactive phase coincident with the filling up of interstitial cell cytoplasm with large globules of lipid giving a strong cholesterol reaction and reacting negatively to 3β-HSDH tests. In *R. esculenta*, thumb pad recovery commences in the autumn as lipid depletion occurs in the interstitial tissue. A concomitant recrudescence of 3β-HSDH activity also occurs in these cells during this period (van Oordt and de Kort, 1969).

The situation in urodeles is less clear since interstitial cells of the anuran type are often absent. In these forms, connective tissue elements of the ampullar wall change into glandular cells. Few data are available about these cells in the Urodela, but they have been more extensively studied in fishes (Fig. 2), where they occur in some freshwater teleosts (see below). The name "boundary cells" has been given to these units, which are thought to be the source of the sex steroids in these animals (Marshall and Lofts, 1956; Lofts and Marshall, 1957). In the salamander *Taricha torosa*, small lipoidal granules start accumulating in these cells when the secondary sexual characters start to develop, and they become densely lipoidal and cholesterol positive when the characters atrophy after discharge of the spermatozoa (Miller and Robbins, 1954). A similar lipid cycle occurs in the boundary tissue of *Trituroides hongkongensis*, and a positive 3β-HSDH reaction is given by these cells during the September–November breeding period (Lofts and Tso, 1971). In the worm salamander *Batrachoseps*, electron microscopy has confirmed that ultrastructurally the cells are similar to other steroid-producing tissues (Fig. 11). Thus, although they at first appear to be distinct from the normal mammalian type of interstitial cell, boundary cells similarly contain agranular endoplasmic reticulum and undergo an identical histochemical cycle which, as in normal Leydig cells, closely correlates with the development and functional activity of the secondary sexual features. Furthermore, both the anuran interstitial cell and urodelan boundary cell appear to originate from fibrous connective tissue cells.

The phenomenon of a seasonal accumulation of large quantities of cholesterol-positive lipids in the spent tubules of reptiles and birds is also an integral part of the testicular cycle in Amphibia. Here, too, sustentacular cells become densely lipoidal after the breeding season and remain thus until there is a resumption of spermatogenesis. In *Taricha*, the lipoidal sustentacular cells of discharged ampullae become compressed to form the so-called "yellow gland" and are resorbed coincident with spermatogenetic recrudescence in the cephalic lobe. The enzyme 3β-HSDH has been located in the discharged and discharging ampullae of *Triturus cristatus* and *Pleurodeles waltlii* (Certain *et al.*, 1964; Ozon, 1967; Picheral, 1970), and incubation with labeled precursors has confirmed these areas to be the main location of steroid biosynthesis in these testes (Ozon, 1965, 1967). Picheral (1968) has demonstrated that the glandular tissue cells of *P. waltlii* possess all the general ultrastructural features associated with steroidogenic tissues and, more recently (Picheral, 1970), has shown that these features and also the 3β-HSDH activity persist for several months after hypophysectomy.

In frogs, the cycle is known in greater detail. Ultrastructurally and cytochemically, the sustentacular cells of the common frog *Rana temporaria* are similar to those of the amniotes. In winter they are generally without sudanophilic material (Fig. 12a), but as the breeding season approaches they elongate and some small, but as yet cholesterol-negative, lipoidal granules appear in the cytoplasm (Fig. 12b). The endoplasmic reticulum also becomes particularly well developed at this stage, and van Oordt and Brands (1970)

Fig. 11. An electron micrograph of a lobule boundary cell of *Batrachoseps* in June. Note mitochondria with tubular cristae and numerous lipid droplets. × 9,000. (From A. K. Christensen, Stanford University.)

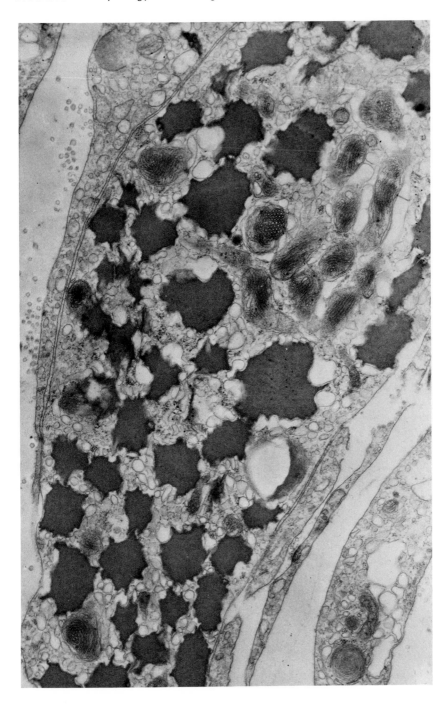

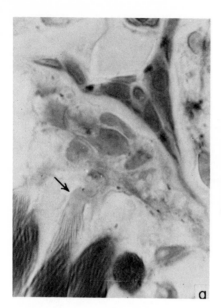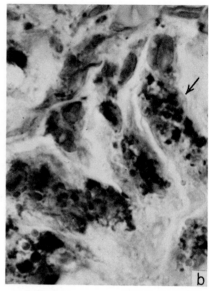

Fig. 12. Sustentacular (Sertoli) cells of *Rana temporaria*. In winter (a) the sustentacular cells (arrows) are generally without sudanophilic inclusions, but during the breeding period (b) they elongate and the cytoplasm becomes filled with sudanophilic droplets. Formol—saline, frozen, sudan black; × 750.

have reported that 3β-HSDH and glucose 6-phosphate dehydrogenase are detectable in the cells at this time. After the release of the sperm bundle (spermiation), usually in late February, the cells become densely lipoidal and give a strong cholesterol reaction; they then detach from the tubule wall and aggregate in the lumen. The 3β-HSDH reaction disappears but a strong acid phosphatase reaction develops (van Oordt and Brands, 1970). Thus, soon after the discharge of the spermatozoa, tubule lumina contain large quantities of cholesterol and lipid which gradually disappear several weeks later with the resumption of intense spermatogenetic activity. The chemical analysis of testicular cholesterol throughout the year closely parallels the histochemical data, showing a rapid rise during the period of tubule sudanophilia, mainly contributed by cholesterol esters, and a sharp decline with the disappearance of the lipoidal material and elevation of spermatogenetic activity (Lofts *et al.*, 1972).

The edible frog *R. esculenta* differs in that the spermatogonia never completely stop their mitotic activity, and even in winter the testes contain small germinal cysts interspersed among the sustentacular—sperm bundle systems.

Thus, the tubules contain sustentacular cells in different stages of development. There is a gradual accumulation of intratubular lipid as individual cells reach their end stage and detach from the boundary wall building up to a maximum in June, but there is not the synchronous release of an entire tubule generation of lipoidal cells as occurs in the common frog (Lofts, 1965).

The sustentacular cell cycle of Amphibia is similar to that of the amniotes, both histochemically and physiologically, in that FSH acts on these cells. As in birds, the exogenous introduction of this gonadotropin always produces a dispersal of the postnuptial tubule lipids and a resumption of spermatogenesis. Hypophysectomy in winter frogs (*R. temporaria*) results in a buildup of lipids in the sustentacular cell without affecting the release of the sperm bundles and without any apparent effect on the resting spermatogonia. However, injections of FSH into these animals cause the sustentacular cell lipids to disappear and germinal cysts start developing among the sperm bundles (Lofts, 1961). One basic difference between the amniote and amphibian sustentacular cell cycles is that in the latter, there is an annual replacement of the sustentacular cells by a new generation of cells transformed from cyst cells. In reptiles and birds, no such transformation occurs and sustentacular cells are permanently attached to the tunica propria.

C. FISHES

The testicular structure of most fishes differs from the tetrapod pattern in consisting of a mass of elongated branching tubules with thin fibrous walls lacking a permanent lining germinal epithelium. For this reason they are sometimes called lobules and not seminiferous tubules. In *Eucalia inconstans*, Ruby and McMillan (1970) have distinguished a series of primary, secondary, and tertiary tubules forming a network of anastomosing loops, but here too they are apparently devoid of a permanent germinal epithelium. In many species, there is a relatively brief annual spawning assembly where males and females extrude vast numbers of spermotozoa and eggs into the water and fertilization is external. The testicular lobules of such breeding males are filled almost exclusively with large masses of spermatozoa which become ejected during this period. Although several species of elasmobranchs and teleosts are viviparous or ovoviviparous, testicular structure shows little variation, and morphological refinements are confined to the accessory glands and ducts. Since the phenomenon of intersexuality, which commonly occurs in many species, is not considered in this chapter, the reader is directed to the excellent reviews by Reinboth (1970) and Chan (1970) for data on this aspect of gonadal morphology.

1. Gnathostome Fishes

As in the Amphibia, spermatogenesis in gnathostomes is cystic and usually resumes in the spent testis soon after breeding, although in some species it is continuous. In seasonal breeders, the means whereby the collapsed lobules become repopulated with germinal cysts is variable. A migration of primary germ cells through the lobule wall takes place in some teleosts, but in others migratory cells do not occur and the spermatogenetic wave arises from dormant spermatogonia. The latter may be concentrated in a precise zone (Lehri, 1967). For example, in the cyprinodont killifish *Fundulus heteroclitus*, the primary spermatogonia form a peripheral layer, and the lobules run radially from the surface of the testis toward a central core of efferent ducts. The germinal cysts formed from the spermatogonial zone mature as they move along the lobules toward the central duct area (Lofts, 1968b). In the spotted dogfish *Scyliorhinus caniculus*, on the other hand, the germinal zone of primary spermatogonia runs along the mesoventral region of the testis; ampullae of germinal cysts arise in this region and move away in a dorsolateral direction (Fratini, 1953; Chieffi, 1967b).

Sustentacular cells have been reported in some chondrichthyean species (Stanley, 1962) and also in the teleosts *Gasterosteus* (Craig-Bennet, 1931), *Lebistes* (Follenius, 1953), *Gobius* (Stanley *et al.*, 1965), *Fundulus* (Fig. 13) (Lofts *et al.*, 1966b), *Poecilia* (Grier, 1970), and *Cymatogaster* (Wiebe, 1968a) and probably in salmonids as "intralobular somatic cells" (see Hiroi and Yamamoto, 1970). In elasmobranchs, however, the Sertoli cells are well developed and easily distinguishable. As in the Amphibia, they are derived from the connective tissue cells surrounding the primary spermatogonia, and the nuclei apparently migrate to the central region of the germinal cyst during its early development. When the germinal contents transform to spermatids, the nuclei migrate peripherally and become reoriented as a cellular layer lining the ampullae to which the spermatozoa become attached (Fratini, 1953). This migration has not been observed in teleosts, but here too cyst cells become glandular with the maturation of the germinal content (Lofts *et al.*, 1966b). In the sea perch *Cymatogaster aggregata*, Wiebe (1968a, 1969a) described a seasonal transition from small Sertoli cells lying adjacent to the basement membrane in winter, to a large columnar layer of sudanophilic cells surrounding the sperm mass in the sexually mature gonad in summer.

In the pike *Esox lucius* (Lofts and Marshall, 1957) and the paddy field eel *Monopterus albus* (Chan, 1968), a postnuptial accumulation of large quantities of cholesterol-positive lipid occurs in the spent lobules. It rapidly disperses with the reestablishment of spermatogenetic activity in a manner basically similar to that in amphibians, reptiles, and birds. A small accumulation of lipid in the spent lobules of *Gobius paganellus* has also been reported

(Stanley *et al.*, 1965). This phenomenon, however, is not universal throughout the teleosts, as it appears to be in the tetrapod groups, and does not occur in the testicular cycles of many species. In elasmobranchs, the sustentacular cells become densely lipoidal and cholesterol positive after the discharge of spermatozoa and eventually become resorbed in a cycle very similar to the urodelan pattern. In two species, *Scyliorhinus caniculus* (Collenot and Ozon, 1964) and *Squalus acanthias* (Simpson and Wardle, 1967), steroid dehydrogenase activity has been located in these cells, thus implicating them as loci of steroid biosynthesis and conforming with similar data on higher vertebrates. In an electron microscope study of the testis in the latter species, Holstein (1969) noted the production of secretory products within the sustentacular cells which he considered might be involved in a steroidogenic function. These cells are probably responsible for the considerable concentrations of steroids reported in the semen of *Squalus* by Simpson and his co-workers (1963a, 1964), although the possibility that they are synthesized by the semen itself cannot be excluded since Ozon and Collenot (1955) have demonstrated the presence of 3β- and 17β-HSDH in the spermatozoa of *Scyliorhinus caniculus*. In *Cymatogaster* the sustentacular cells also give a strong 3β-HSDH reaction (Wiebe, 1968b, 1969a). A similar positive response has been recorded in the Sertoli calls of *Fundulus heteroclitus* (Bara, 1969). In *Monopterus*, chromatographic analysis of testicular extracts shows large concentrations of progesterone only when gonads contain sudanophilic lobules (Chan and Phillips, 1967) and provides confirmatory evidence of an earlier study by Lofts and Marshall (1959) in birds, in which testicular extracts of hypophysectomized pigeons with lipoidal sustentacular cells similarly showed progestogenic activity. Progesterone is a steroid occurring early in the biosynthetic chain of androgenic and estrogenic steroids, and its occurrence in the postnuptial testis is consistent with the hypothesis that the genesis of large quantities of cholesterol-positive lipids in sustentacular cells is representative of a disruption of steroid biosynthesis.

In *Squalus*, all of the positive steroid dehydrogenase response is confined to the germinal ampullae and none can be detected in an interlobular location (Simpson and Wardle, 1967), but in several other elasmobranchs and teleosts it occurs in cells located in the interstices between lobules in the typical mammalian manner (Chieffi, 1967a,b; Bara, 1969). These cells are cytologically (Fig. 13) and ultrastructurally similar to the mammalian interstitial cells (Follenius and Porte, 1960; Oota and Yamamoto, 1966). The seasonal fluctuations in their secretory activity are sometimes not easily observed since, in some species, they appear to be without sudanophilic inclusions for much of the year. In *Fundulus*, for example, small lipoidal droplets can be seen only at the height of sexual activity (Lofts *et al.*, 1966b). In other species, the interstitial cells are more

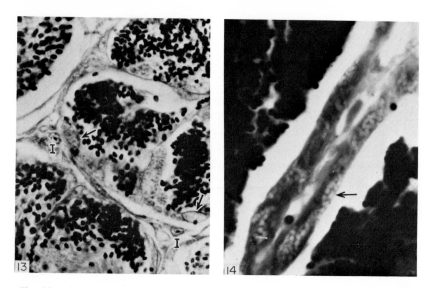

Fig. 13.   Sustentacular cells (arrows) of the killifish *Fundulus heteroclitus*. These cells enlarge when the contents of the germinal cysts mature into spermatozoa. Interstitial cells (I) can also be seen. Iron–hematoxylin and orange G; × 700. (From Lofts *et al.*, 1966b.)

Fig. 14.   Lobule boundary cells (arrow) in the testis of the pike *Esox lucius*. Note the vacuoles left in the cell cytoplasm as a result of the dissolution of the lipid during alcoholic dehydration. Iron–hematoxylin and orange G; × 910. (From Lofts and Marshall, 1957.)

sudanophilic and, as in higher vertebrates, seasonal accumulation and prenuptial depletion of cholesterol-positive lipids in Leydig cells are believed to be indicative of the elaboration of sex hormones which regulate the development of secondary sexual characters (Stoll, 1955; Wai and Hoar, 1963) and behavioral activities (Marshall, 1960; Hoar, 1962). In *Monopterus*, for example, the male prenuptial behavior of building nest burrows, formation of a foam mass, and guarding of territory, which is associated with high androgen titers, occurs concomitantly with the maximum accumulation and rapid depletion of cholesterol-positive lipids in the interstitial Leydig cells (Chan, 1968). In this species, too, a regeneration of interstitial cells, reminiscent of interstitial rehabilitation by juvenile cells of reptiles and birds, occurs during the postnuptial period of testicular inactivity. In *Cymatogaster*, even in midwinter the well-defined interstitial cells contain small sudanophilic droplets which accumulate as the animal approaches its breeding season. In *Gobius paganellus* Stanley *et al.*, (1965) found almost no difference in the intensity of 3β-HSDH reaction in the interstitial cells at different seasons of the year, but Wiebe (1969a) had demonstrated that 3β-HSDH activity in these cells closely parallels the lipid cycle in *Cymatogaster*, being undetectable in the winter gonad but becoming strongly positive with the buildup of sudanophilia. A weak reaction for 17β-HSDH was also given by these cells during the breeding phase. In *Lebistes reticulatus*, the young and active cells contain sudanophilic droplets and become densely lipoidal in the terminal stages before disintegration, similar to the interstitial cells of frogs and reptiles (Follenius and Porte, 1960). Degeneration involving extensive sudanophilia also occurs in some salmonid species.

In a few teleost species, such as *Gobius* and *Blennius*, there occurs a concentration of the interstitial tissue quite separate from the seminiferous area. Thus, in *Gobius paganellus*, Stanley *et al.* (1965) described a glandular mass adjacent to the mesorchium which is quite distinct from the seminiferous region of the testis, although a squamous epithelium commonly encloses both the glandular and seminiferous regions. The cells of this interstitial gland have all the cytochemical characteristics of normal Leydig cells, and tests for 3β-HSDH have shown it to be present exclusively in this gland and absent from the seminiferous zone. The cells are lipoidal and contain cholesterol which shows a seasonal fluctuation, being of greatest amount in December and becoming depleted by the end of the sexual season.

An interstitial distribution of endocrine cells is sometimes absent, and boundary cells develop in the lobule walls (Figs. 2 and 14). In the pike *Esox lucius*, they develop from modified fibroblasts and undergo a seasonal lipid cycle which is essentially similar to the normal events recorded in the reptilian interstitium. Thus, cholesterol-positive lipids accumulate in the cytoplasm during the winter and become rapidly depleted when the fishes are assembling for spawning. Similar cells have also been recorded in the testes of the char, rainbow trout, and lake chub. Henderson (1962) has reported that typical interstitial tissue is also absent from the testis of *Salvelinus fontinalis*, but that lobule boundary cells undergo seasonal cyclic changes and become highly vacuolated during the latter part of the breeding season, and a similar seasonal cycle has also been noted in the lobule boundary cells of *Belone belone*, where the cells become greatly hypertrophied and filled with diffuse lipoproteins (Upadhyay and Guraya, 1971). In the testis of *Tilapia mossambica*, Yaron (1966) has recorded a positive 3β-HSDH response, both in an interstitial location and in lobule boundary cells. Lobule boundary cells are also present in the Atlantic salmon *Salmo salar* and have been reported to be full of lipids just before and at the time of spawning (O'Halloran and Idler, 1970). Weakly positive 3β- and 3α-HSDH activity was observed in these cells, but no quantitative difference in the lipid material was apparent between prespawning and spawning fish although the plasma level of 11-ketosteroids in the testicular vein effluent increased significantly immediately prior to spawning. In some fishes, for example in *Esox lucius*, where testicular tissue has similarly been subjected to the histochemical tests for steroid dehydrogenase activity (Delrio *et al.*, 1968; Lupo di Prisco *et al.*, 1970) the lobule boundary cells have given negative responses. The interlobular areas in these species also failed to react, yet castration experiments have conclusively proved the relationship between the testes and secondary sexual character development. It is therefore premature to accept a negative result in these fishes until more histochemical evidence is forthcoming; as Arvy (1962) has noted, even among mammals there are marked species differences in the activity of this enzyme.

Evidence of a physiological homology between the interstitial cell and boundary cell has been shown in *Couesius* by Ahsan (1966), who has recorded a stimulation of the lobule boundary cells in hypophysectomized lake chub injected with LH. This hormone produces an intensification of the cholesterol reaction in these cells which cannot be produced by injections of FSH. In *Fundulus*, injections of LH stimulate interlobular Leydig cells and 3β-HSDH therein (Pickford *et al.*, 1972), and Wiebe (1969b) reported a similar effect on the interstitial tissue of *Cymatogaster*.

2. Cyclostome Fishes

The mature testis of cyclostomes consists of a number of lobules filled with germinal cysts which, when fully mature, rupture and liberate spermatozoa into the body cavity. Since the animal dies soon after the extrusion of the germinal products, individuals do not undergo annually recurring spermatogenetic cycles. In *Lampetra planeri* and *L. fluviatilis* (the common river lamprey of northern Europe) the ammocoete larva is a feeding stage which metamorphoses in the fourth year with a concomitant atrophy of the gut and ripening of the gonads. This is followed by a migration to the breeding grounds. In *L. fluviatilis*, the single testis is already filled with primary spermatocyte cysts by the time the lampreys start their anadromous migration. These cysts then gradually transform into spermatozoal masses, the final stages of spermatogenesis taking place in the early spring close to the time of spawning. Both species have well-defined secondary sexual characters (enlarged cloacal labia and an erectile papilla) which develop when sexual maturity is imminent. In *L. fluviatilis*, Evennett and Dodd (1963) have shown that these features do not develop in gonadectomized lampreys, so that the dependence of the secondary sexual characters on gonadal secretions, which is well established in other vertebrates, is also operative in cyclostomes.

The interstitial cells are easily distinguishable cytologically when the upstream migration begins. They consist of isolated units which increase in number and come to form compact acinar clusters of cells between the testicular lobules. They also accumulate cholesterol-positive lipids, and by the time the animals are assembling to spawn, these cells reach the terminal stages of their secretory cycle and are densely lipoidal. This is followed by the disintegration of the cell (Hardisty *et al.*, 1967). Interestingly, in the later stages of spermatogenesis, lipoidal lobule boundary cells also develop, and Larsen (1965) has shown a pituitary influence on these cells; there is a buildup of their cholesterol after hypophysectomy, whereas the cholesterol reaction of the interstitial tissue remains unaffected. Hardisty and Barnes (1968) have obtained a positive reaction for 3β-HSDH in an interstitial location in *L. fluviatilis*. Males treated in the October–December period, when the testis contains only spermatogonia or primary spermatocytes, gave only a weak reaction, but this intensified during February and March. In the hagfish *Myxine glutinosa*, interstitial cells are absent, but Schreiner (1955) has reported large secretory cells with abundant mitochondria and lipid inclusions in the lobules.

III. Ovary

The female gonad, like that of the male, has both gametogenetic and endocrine functions, producing ova as well as steroid hormones that regulate the secondary sexual features, the accessory sexual apparatus, and the behavioral activities associated with breeding. Similarly too, its functional activity is controlled by the gonadotropic hormones secreted by the pituitary gland. Thus, in mammals the follicle-stimulating hormone, as its name implies, causes follicular maturation with its consequent secretion of estrogenic hormones, and the luteinizing hormone induces ovulation and the formation of corpora lutea. In a few mammalian species, a third gonadotropin, luteotropin (LTH) or prolactin, may evoke the secretion of progesterone by the corpus luteum after its formation under the influence of LH. Although there is evidence that follicular maturation and concomitant estrogen secretion in nonmammalian vertebrates are similarly dependent on gonadotropic regulation, evidence of a luteinizing factor is more questionable, and the existence of three gonadotropins has so far been established only in the Mammalia, although a prolactin of some type is probably present throughout the Vertebrata (Bern and Nicoll, 1969).

In mammalian species reproduction is viviparous, but birds reproduce exclusively by oviparous mechanisms. In the fishes, amphibians, and reptiles, examples of oviparous, ovoviviparous, and viviparous forms of reproduction can be found; the phenomenon of viviparity has evolved independently several times within the vertebrate series. It is a matter of considerable interest as to whether viviparity in these lower vertebrate groups is controlled by the same glands and hormonal mechanisms that operate in mammals (see Browning, 1969).

Female reproductive activity, like that of the male, is characteristically cyclical, and the ovary presents a variety of morphological pictures depending on both the level of activity and the phase of the cycle reached. There is often considerable variation among the classes and even among members of the same group. Thus, there is far less uniformity in vertebrate ovarian morphology than that displayed in the testicular structure of the males.

Both ovaries and testes are derived from a pair of sexually undifferentiated primordia associated with the intermediate mesoderm (nephrotome). The primordial germ cells are generally assumed to arise from yolk-sac endoderm and to migrate into a stroma provided by these two presumptive gonads. In female amphibians, reptiles, and mammals, the primordia give rise to paired ovarian structures located in the peritoneal cavity in close proximity to the kidneys, near the dorsal wall. In the majority of avian groups, however, only the left gonadal rudiment develops and the contralateral partner remains regressed and nonfunctional. In cyclostomes there is only a single medially placed ovary, derived either from a fusion of the two primordia (in lampreys) or by a failure of one of the two primordia to complete its development, as in most birds (in myxinoids). The same situation arises also in some elasmobranch species and in some teleosts, although most gnathostome fishes possess paired ovaries.

Ovarian structural complexity derives from the fact that the ovary is not a single entity, but a composite structure of several organs. Thus, in addition to large numbers of follicles in various stages of development, an ovarian section also shows other structures derived from growing and discharged follicles, such as corpora atretica and corpora lutea. All of these contribute to the endocrine activity of the organ. Much work has been concentrated upon the localization of the cells responsible for steroid production in the mammalian ovary, and the follicular epithelium and its derivative structures, in particular, have aroused special interest dating from the discovery that the corpus luteum secretes progesterone. In the nonmammalian vertebrates, however, the sites of steroid biosynthesis are less certain.

The structure of the mammalian ovary, and the distribution of its steroidogenic endocrine tissue, are better understood than in nonmammalian forms, and for this reason we shall first define its components and use this information as a basis for comparison with the ovaries of the lower vertebrate groups.

A. The Mammalian Ovary

The typical mature mammalian ovary consists of several major components (Fig. 15). (a) A *germinal epithelium* covers the ovary and is continuous with the peritoneal membrane lining the abdominal cavity. It gives rise to two types of cells: the oogonia, which have the ability to accumulate food reserves and to undergo meiotic (reduction) division to form the mature ovum, and the granulosa (or follicle) cells, which surround the developing oocyte and give rise to the major components of the follicle wall. (b) The *follicle* (Graafian) is initially a primordial structure consisting of a single layer of flattened granulosa cells ensheathing the oocyte. It finally develops into a large mass of cells containing a fluid-filled cavity (the antrum) and is surrounded by external layers (the thecae). (c) The *corpus luteum* is generally derived from the follicle after the expulsion of the mature ovum (ovulation), mostly by the transformation of granulosa cells into pigmented lutein cells. (d) The *interstitial tissue* consists of epithelioid cells presumably equivalent to similar cells in the testis and related to the epithelioid theca interna of the follicle. It is often present as large masses of cells scattered through the ovary but sometimes appears as special groups of cells which may be con-

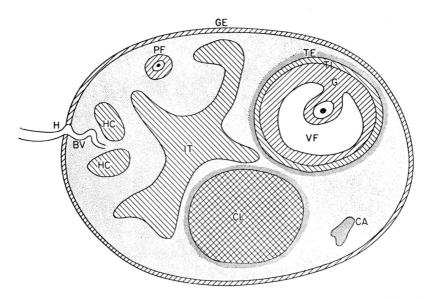

Fig. 15. Diagram of histogenetic relationships in mammalian ovary: BV, blood vessels; CA, corpus atreticum; CL, corpus luteum; G, granulosa cells (follicle cells); GE, germinal epithelium; H, hilum; HC, hilar cells; IT, interstitial tissue; PF, primary follicle; TE, theca externa; TI, theca interna; VF, antrum of vesicular follicle.

centrated in the hilar region (as in the human ovary). (e) The *connective tissue stroma* forms the basic supporting framework for the several organs described above. It gives rise also to the outermost fibrous wall of the follicle, the theca externa. (f) The *corpus albicans*, a scarlike connective tissue remnant, remains after the degeneration of a corpus luteum. (g) The *corpus atreticum* is formed by the fatty degeneration of an unovulated follicle. This is generally accompanied by hypertrophy of the theca interna, the cells of which infiltrate the atretic follicle.

Functionally, the ovarian cycle is divisible into two phases, both anatomically and hormonally. In the *follicular phase*, developing vesicular and preovulatory follicles can be distinguished. Not all the follicles ovulate; many undergo preovulatory degeneration to form the corpora atretica and hence are no longer of oogenic significance. In the *luteal phase*, the postovulatory follicle (initially recognizable as a "blutpunkt" on the surface of the ovary owing to the rupture of ovarian capillaries into the follicular cavity to produce a corpus hemorrhagicum) transforms into a corpus luteum. As indicated above, the granulosa cells provide the major source of lutein cells, but the cells of the theca interna also contribute to a greater or lesser extent. The respective contribution of these two cell lines is difficult to estimate. The corpus luteum is maintained for a variable period, depending on the species and the physiological state of the mammal; then, in the absence of fertilization, it degenerates leaving a corpus albicans to mark its position in the ovary. If mating does result in fertilization, the duration of corpus luteum activity is prolonged and may last for part, or all, of the period of pregnancy.

The main ovarian secretions during the follicular phase are the estrogenic hormones (female sex hormones) responsible for the maintenance of the accessory reproductive tract and the sexual behavior (during estrus) of the female. With the transition into the luteal phase after ovulation, the titer of estrogenic steroids declines concomitant with the increasing elaboration of progesterone by the newly formed corpus luteum. Progesterone and the other progestogenic steroids are responsible for promoting proliferation of the uterine endometrium in preparation for implantation and for preventing further ovulation during pregnancy. In many mammals, the placenta also becomes an important site of progesterone release during the later stages of pregnancy.

Current opinion generally credits the thecal cells with the secretion of estrogens, and a strong 3β-HSDH activity is concentrated in the theca interna during follicular development. Cholesterol-rich lipids with birefringent properties also accumulate in these hypertrophied cells during this period and become depleted at the height of estrus in a manner analogous to the cyclical events in the interstitial cells of the testis. *In vitro* incubation studies (Ryan and Short, 1965; Ryan and Smith, 1965; Savard,

1968) of isolated thecal tissue have confirmed this capacity for estrogen biosynthesis, and although isolated granulosa tissue can also produce estrogens under *in vitro* conditions, the thecal tissue is the major source. Studies of Channing and Grieves (1969), in which granulosa and thecal cell cultures were used to determine their respective steroidogenic capacities, endorse these results.

The corpus luteum is the main source of progesterone secretion, and this hormone has been isolated from corpora lutea extracts of a variety of mammals (Parkes and Deanesly, 1966). Experiments with corpus luteum slices incubated with radioactive precursors confirm that progesterone is the primary product of this tissue (Savard, 1967). The granulosa lutein cells are the probable site of hormone production, since a marked development of agranular endoplasmic reticulum takes place in these cells (Björkman 1962; Green and Maqueo, 1965) and is accompanied by an appearance of small birefringent sudanophilic droplets throughout the cytoplasm after luteinization. Furthermore, the tissue becomes strongly positive to histochemical tests showing 3β-HSDH activity (Galil and Deane, 1966). Deane *et al.* (1966) have shown that the decline in secretory activity of the ovine corpus luteum, measured by peripheral and glandular progesterone levels, closely correlates with the subsequent depletion of this lipid and 3β-HSDH activity. Thus, there is strong evidence that the granulosa lutein cells are the primary locus of progesterone production, and granulosa cells grown in tissue culture have been shown to manufacture progesterone (Channing, 1966; Channing and Grieves, 1969).

The role of the interstitial tissue has remained problematic. These large polyhedral cells show a great variation in their prominence in the ovaries of different mammals, being very plentiful in some (Insectivora, Chiroptera, Rodentia, and Carnivora) but much more difficult to locate in others (Cetacea, Artiodactyla, and Primates). They have the characteristics of other ovarian steroid-producing tissues: The cells contain cytoplasmic lipid droplets which autofluoresce and are birefringent, and they react positively to the Schultz cholesterol test and to the techniques which visualize the presence of the 3β-HSDH enzyme system (Jacoby, 1962). The development of a fluorescent antibody technique for the direct histological visualization of androgenic steroids has demonstrated that the interstitial cells of rat ovary are most likely the site of ovarian androgen production (Woods and Domm, 1966). This is further supported by incubation studies on the human ovary in which, after incubation of separate thecal, granulosa, and stromal tissue with radioactive steroid hormone precursors, androgens are found to be produced in extremely high yields by the stromal tissue, but not by the other two components (Ryan and Smith, 1961; Smith and Ryan, 1961; Rice *et al.*, 1964; Rice and Savard, 1966; Ryan and Petro, 1966).

B. Birds

There is a great paucity of information about the functional morphology of the ovary in wild birds, and data on the avian female gonad have almost all been derived from investigations on the domestic hen *Gallus domesticus* and, more recently, on the Japanese quail *Coturnix coturnix*. In most avian species only the left ovary and oviduct reach functional development, the right usually remaining undeveloped in an ambisexual state. Although birds with two functional gonads are occasionally found, particularly members of the Accipitrinae, Falconinae, and Cathartidae, a corresponding development of the associated right oviduct does not always occur. When the left ovary is removed, or when it becomes nonfunctional due to some pathological condition, a compensatory development of the rudimentary gonad may take place under the influence of the increased circulation of gonadotropin.

The functional left ovary of the breeding female is a relatively large structure attached to the body wall by a short mesovarium. The mature follicles are enormously distended due to the deposition of a large amount of yolk, and they bulge conspicuously from the surface of the ovary (Fig. 16), the largest follicles ultimately becoming suspended from the surface by a narrow isthmus of tissue (pedicle). In the continuously ovulating fowl, the ovary more or less retains this form throughout the year, but in seasonally breeding wild species, the gonad undergoes enormous fluctuations in size and morphological appearance. A regression occurs at the end of the breeding season

Fig. 16. Ovary of the fowl. Note the large follicles suspended from the ovarian surface by the pedicle (P). Atretic follicles (CA) and ovulated follicles (OF) can also be seen.

Fig. 17. Diagram of histogenetic relationships in the avian ovary: A, oogonium; B, developing follicle at time of the genesis and incorporation of its thecal gland cells; C, developing follicle at later stage; D, follicle showing faint beginnings of lipoidal atresia; E, younger follicle showing pronounced lipoidal atresia; F, follicle in total atresia; G, cholesterol-positive lipid cells (presumptive "ex-follicular" cells) that arise in atretic follicles; H, "ex-follicular" gland cells, free in the ovarian stroma; I, follicle that has undergone an essentially nonlipoidal atresia; J, as I, except that some cells are becoming lipoidal; K, sinusoidal blood vessel; L, a type of atresia in which an amorphous clot of fat is expressed into the follicle centre and isolated by a wall of fibroblasts; M, an atresia in which lipoidal cells nearest the central clot discharge their cholesterol and become pycnotic, with distorted nuclei; N, hyaline, sometimes lobate, mass of pycnotic cells that resemble the mammalian corpus albicans; O, restricted area of a hyaline scar that has become glandular; P, scars from a discharged follicle (these occasionally hold depot fat that does not contain cholesterol); behind is Q, a scar from a discharged follicle that has been invaded by fibroblasts; R, group of glandular cells that have arisen from connective tissue cells in the stroma and are therefore probably homologous with male interstitial (Leydig) cells. (From Marshall and Coombs, 1957.)

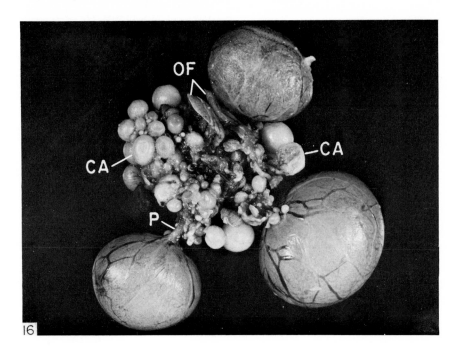

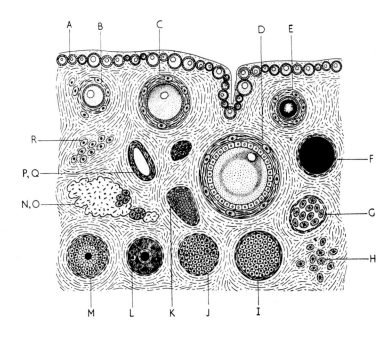

and the ovary reduces to a small, compact structure devoid of large pedunculate follicles.

The ovary consists essentially of an outer cortex containing the developing follicles, which surrounds a highly vascular medulla composed primarily of connective tissue. As in the mammalian ovary, the periphery of the cortex is covered by the germinal epithelium (Fig. 17). Gametogenesis begins in the embryonic state, and the ovary is already endowed with primary oocytes by the time the young are hatched. Of these, only a minute proportion matures sufficiently to undergo ovulation, and the majority become atretic while still in an early stage of follicular maturation.

The smallest follicles consist of an oocyte surrounded by a single layer of flattened lipid-free granulosa cells containing a granular endoplasmic reticulum, and, as they mature, a multilayered thecal tissue forms around the outside and becomes highly vascularized. The oocyte fills the developing follicle, so that no antrum or other internal organization is evident. During this growth, some cells of the theca interna become glandular and their nuclei increase in size. Cytoplasmic lipid droplets begin to accumulate in these cells and subsequently they become positive to tests for cholesterol and, in the hen at least, for 3β-HSDH activity (Chieffi and Botte, 1965, Boucek and Savard, 1970). In wild birds, with the approach of the breeding season, some of the follicles become atretic, but the large nonatretic follicles enter a phase of rapid growth, brought about mainly by the deposition of yolk, which causes them to bulge conspicuously from the surface. Ultrastructurally, the granulosa tissue now appears to undergo a reorganization and develops an abundant agranular endoplasmic reticulum and small sudanophilic granules which suggest a possible steroidogenic activity near the time of ovulation (Wyburn *et al.*, 1966; Dahl, 1971). At the same time, the theca interna becomes depleted of lipids and cholesterol. When ovulation occurs, the discharged follicle becomes deflated, and the constriction of spiral arteries which this produces prevents hemorrhage into the follicular cavity. Consequently, a "blutpunkt" does not develop. The granulosa cells become inflated with lipids and remain conspicuous in the hen for about 72 hr after ovulation (Wyburn *et al.*, 1966), but luteinization does not occur and no corpus luteum develops. The ruptured follicle rapidly regresses, disintegrates, and is cleared by phagocytic action within a few days in the chicken and the rook, but in pheasants and the mallard duck, the postovulatory structures may persist for as long as 3 months.

Atresia is first observable in sectioned material as a sudanophilic band around the periphery of the oocyte which then spreads inward until the whole interior of the follicle appears to be occluded by a dense mass of strongly cholesterol-positive lipoidal material (Fig. 17). In the rook, this fatty atresia is accompanied by a rapid proliferation of fibroblasts which invade the lipoidal mass. Some of these cells then apparently enlarge, becoming glandular and lipoidal, and are released into the general ovarian stroma with the disintegration of the follicle so that they may be scattered singly or in groups (Marshall and Coombs, 1957). Marshall and Coombs have called these cells "ex-follicular gland cells," and emphasize their distinction from the normal interstitial cells in the stroma, which develop from the ordinary connective tissue and are homologous with those of the mammalian ovary.

As with the gonad of female mammals, the avian ovary is also a source of androgenic, estrogenic, and progestogenic secretions. However, the intra-ovarian cellular locations for their respective biosyntheses are far more speculative due to the great lack of experimentation in this field of avian endocrinology. We have noted that thecal, granulosa, and interstitial tissues, as well as atretic follicles, all possess cholesterol-rich lipoidal material and have other glandular characteristics which might suggest an endocrine func-tion. This is confirmed by the fact that a positive reaction for 3β-HSDH activity has been recorded for all four tissues, indicating their steroidogenic capacity (Chieffi and Botte 1965; Woods and Domm, 1966; Sayler *et al.*, 1970). As in the mammalian ovary, the interestitial cells arising from the stromal tissue are regarded to be the most likely source of androgenic secretion (Benoit, 1950; Taber, 1951; Marshall and Coombs, 1957), and this has been confirmed by means of the fluorescent antibody technique (Woods and Domm, 1966). In the hen, Boucek and Savard (1970) have recorded an intense 17β-HSDH response both in these stromal cells and in the thecal tissue during the sexually inactive molting period.

The tremendous increase in size of the oviduct which is coincident with sexual maturity is an estrogen-dependent effect (Brant and Nalbandov, 1956) and indicates that in birds, as in mammals, estrogen secretion appears to be a consistent consequence of follicular development. Indeed, estrogen secre-tion must occur prior to the final phase of follicular maturation since vitel-logenesis is dependent on this hormone. In the rook, the accumulation of cholesterol and lipid in the glandular cells of the theca interna becomes depleted at the time of maximum follicular development in March and April when estrogen titers (as judged by accessory sexual development) are reach-ing a peak. The lipid disperses just before the culminating yolk-depositing phase, so that by the time yolk appears in the follicle only a faint sprinkling of lipid remains in the cytoplasm of the thecal gland cells. The granulosa cells, on the other hand, are without cholesterol and lipid throughout the follicular phase (Marshall and Coombs, 1957). These events might suggest the theca interna as the possible site of estrogen production, as in the mammalian ovary; incubated thecal tissue from growing follicles of the hen's ovary has been shown to have the capacity to convert cholesterol to estrogens (Botte *et al.*, 1966). However, the apparent limitation of 17β-HSDH to the granulosa tissue (Chieffi and Botte, 1965) has led Chieffi (1967a) to suggest that estrogen biosynthesis occurs at this site. Arvy and Hadjiisky (1970) have also shown that dehydrogenase activity is concentrated in this layer in both the hen and quail, although the adjacent theca interna is also a source of activity. The more recent studies of Boucek and Savard (1970) have confirmed Chieffi's earlier observations that 17β-HSDH is confined to the granulosa tissue and also that 3β-HSDH activity is most intense in these cells in laying hens. When the hen enters its molting stage, however, the intensity of the 3β-HSDH reaction diminishes; the 17β-HSDH reaction disappears altogether from this tissue but shows up very strongly in the thecal and stromal cells. Electron microscope observations, on the other hand, do not support this suggestion, since granulosa cells start developing abundant agranular endoplasmic reticulum, mitochondria with tubular cristae, cholesterol, and sudanophilic granules only when the follicles are ready to ovulate, thus suggesting that their steroidogenic activity is relatively slight up to this time.

Although birds do not possess postovulatory corpora lutea, there is ample evidence that the gonad produces progesterone, and it is believed by some investigators that the postovulatory follicle is the likely source. As has been pointed out, however, in many species these structures are transient and disappear within a few days. Furthermore, Fraps and his associates reported that high levels of progesterone occur in hens during ovulation and not during the postovulatory period (Fraps, 1955). Nevertheless, it may perhaps be premature to dismiss the postovulatory follicle as having no endocrine role, since Wyburn and co-workers (1966) have recorded the extensive development of the agranular endoplasmic reticulum which occurs in the granulosa cells at this time, together with an increase in sudanophilia and cholesterol content, and Botte and co-workers (1966) have shown the steroid-biosynthesis capacity of isolated postovulatory follicles of hen *in vitro*. Again the experimental removal of recently ruptured follicles has been shown to influence the retention time of eggs in the oviduct (Rothchild and Fraps, 1944a,b; Conner and Fraps, 1954). Furr (1969) and Furr and Pope (1970) have established by gas–liquid chromatographic procedures that the highest level of progesterone in the hen ovary is found in the growing follicles but is also present in the postovulatory follicle. Marshall and Coombs (1957) have suggested that the atretic follicles are involved in progesterone production, and certainly the presence of cholesterol and 3β-HSDH (Woods and Domm, 1966) in these structures indicates a possible role in steroid biosynthesis. Great numbers of follicles undergo such lipoidal atresia, and this phenomenon builds up a considerable reservoir of ovarian cholesterol by the time of ovulation. It is evident, however, that there is a need for much more information before the precise locus of any of the ovarian steroids can be established with certainty.

C. Reptiles

The paired reptilian ovaries may be elongate fusiform bodies (e.g., as in *Leiolopisma rhomboidalis* and snakes) or ovoid structures (e.g., as in *Xantusia vigilis*) or may consist of two loose membranous organs which spread laterally and ventrally over the kidneys and posterior part of the lungs as they do in the turtle *Emys blandingii* (Nicholson and Risley, 1940). They differ structurally from the ovaries of birds and mammals in containing a fluid-filled central cavity, or series of cavities, lined with squamous epithelium. Stromal tissue is sparse, and the bulk of the ovary consists of a narrow cortex surrounding the central cavity, with a thin, covering germinal epithelium in which can clearly be seen numerous follicles in varying degrees of maturity. Gametogenesis generally continues throughout the life of the animal, and the production of primary oocytes from oogonia in the germinal epithelium occurs in the adult organ, thus differing from the avian situation in which the ovary is already in possession of its finite complement of primary oocytes before hatching. Reptiles also differ from birds in developing true corpora lutea at certain times of the year. Corpora atretica are also common in the cortical tissue.

During the breeding period the enlarged follicles bulge out from the surface and into the central cavity. In reptiles living in warmer climates, follicular development may occur fairly rapidly and ova grow to maturity within a few months, but in north-temperate species this process may become protracted over two, three, or even four years (Rahn, 1942; Cieslak, 1945; Miller, 1948). Generally, during the period of breeding activity, the numbers of follicles which reach an enlarged size at any one time are relatively few, and each ovary may contain only one fully mature follicle and ovulate only one mature ovum at a time, as in *Leiolopisma rhomboidalis*. In some lizards, comparatively few are ovulated in a season, and in extreme cases, such as in the geckos, only one ovum is discharged annually from each gonad (Boyd, 1940).

With the exception of the few continuously breeding tropical species such as the skink *Emoia cyanura*, which lives in the remarkably unvarying climate of Espiritu Santo, most reptiles have well-marked breeding seasons, and the development of large ovulating follicles is confined to a few months of the year. Even in some tropical forms, like the Australian lizard *Leiolopisma rhomboidalis*, the female is markedly seasonal although the males show no parallel cessation of sperm production (Wilhoft, 1963). The same is also true of the equatorial East African lizard *Agama agama* (Marshall and Hook, 1960).

The ovum is always macrolecithal, and as follicular development proceeds the ova become surrounded by a fibrous theca externa and a glandular theca interna separated from the granulosa layer by the membrana propria (Fig. 18a). In the sparse stroma, interstitial cells are not very evident and there seems to be little evidence of androgen secretion. These cells have been claimed to be absent from the reptilian ovary by some (Fraenkel *et al.*, 1940; Betz, 1963), but Dutta (1944) has reported their presence in *Hemidactylus flaviviridis* and Guraya (1965) has suggested they may be formed from the disruption of the thecal cells in the atretic follicles of the snakes *Naja tripudians* and *Bungarus coeruleus*. However, the vernal recrudescence of follicular development is, as in birds and mammals, always accompanied by a parallel estrogen-dependent development of the oviducts. Similarly, too, the histrochemical reactions of the thecal cells during this period suggest that they are the most probable locus of estrogen secretion; thus during estrus the theca interna of the developing follicles becomes hypertrophied

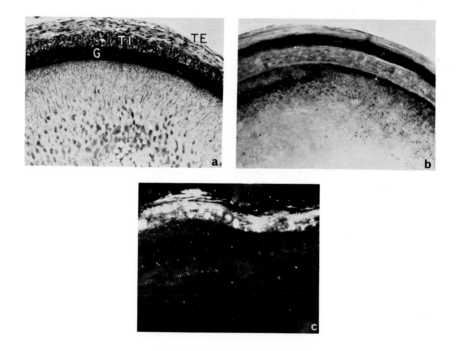

Fig. 18. Follicle of *Vipera aspis* showing the thecal and granulosa layers. (a) Developing follicle with a fibrous theca externa (TE), a glandular theca interna (TI), and a very chromophilic granulosa layer (G). Trichrome. (b) Shows heavily sudanophilic theca interna of the developing follicle, whereas the granulosa layer is lipid free. Formalin, frozen, BZL. (c) Shows abundance of birefringent lipids in the theca interna when viewed under polarized light. × 70. (From Gabe and Saint Girons, 1962.)

(Fig. 18b) and the cells become filled with numerous cytoplasmic cholesterol-positive lipid droplets. There is also a strong 3β-HSDH activity in these cells during this period. In sectioned ovarian material viewd with polarized light, the cellular content is strongly birefringent, whereas the adjacent granulosa tissue shows very little birefringence (Fig. 18c). In their histochemical study on the ovary of *Lacerta sicula*, Botte and Delrio (1965) reported a positive 3β-HSDH reaction in both the granulosa and theca interna in the developing follicle, but here too (as judged by their published photographs) the reaction is much more extensive in the thecal cells. During anestrus, on the other hand, the thecal cells of the resting follicles show few or no sudanophilic inclusions and are nonbirefringent.

The above-mentioned histochemical manifestations of increasing secretory activity in the theca interna during the follicular phase of the breeding cycle are closely paralleled by the development of the secondary sexual characters and are also associated with an increasing secretory activity of the β cells (FSH gonadotropes) in the adenohypophysis in *Vipera aspis* (Gabe and Saint Girons, 1962) and *Cerastes cerastes* (Saint Girons, 1962). In the viviparous snake *V. aspis*, which has both a spring and autumn period of sexual activity, the thecal cells of the developing follicles enlarge and become filled with birefringent lipids that are rapidly depleted during the preovulatory period of the first breeding phase. If fertilization fails to occur, these cells become involuted until they enter their subsequent autumnal sexual phase when sudanophilia and birefringency once again return (Gabe and Saint Girons, 1962). Estrogen titers in this snake, as indicated by the heights of the oviducal and cloacal epithelium, fluctuate with the histochemical cycles. Thus, both tissues increase in height as the sudanophilic thecal cells increase their birefringent properties in the spring, reaching maximum size at the time of rapid lipid depletion, then sharply regressing in the postovulatory period, only to become elevated again in the autumn.

At the approach of ovulation, granulosa cells start to accumulate cholesterol-rich lipoidal material; then, with the ejection of the ovum, they become luteinized and proliferate to transform the discharged follicle into a corpus luteum. The majority of reptiles (including all Crocodilia and Chelonia) are oviparous, but some lizards and snakes are ovoviviparous or viviparous. All, however, develop true postovulatory corpora lutea. In the majority of cases these are derived mainly from the granulosa lutein cells, but the thecal elements may also form a connective tissue envelope surrounding the mass of granulosa cells and, in some cases, give rise to connective tissue trabeculae which penetrate the central mass of lipoidal tissue to form a supporting framework. The corpus luteum usually becomes well vascularized, and its cells not only become heavily sudanophilic, cholesterol positive, and birefringent, but are also markedly positive to tests for 3β-

HSDH and therefore bear a close resemblance to the mammalian corpus luteum. In oviparous species, the corpus luteum usually persists until the end of egg laying, but in the ovoviviparous and viviparous forms it remains for much of the period of gestation and, in some cases (for example, in the viviparous sea snake *Hydrophis* or the ovoviviparous garter snake *Thamnophis*), it may persist until after the birth of the young, before final degeneration sets in (Cieslak, 1945; Harrison Matthews, 1955).

It is difficult to evaluate the functional activity of the reptilian corpus luteum, and its role in the control and maintenance of gestation is still far from clear. In a number of viviparous snakes it appears to be necessary for embryonic survival in early pregnancy, and deluteinization is followed by resorption of embryos (Clausen, 1935, 1940; Fraenkel *et al.*, 1940), but in *Thamnophis sirtalis*, *Natrix sipedon*, and the ovoviviparous lizard *Zootoca vivipara*, ovariectomy of pregnant animals has no effect on gestation, although an inhibition of parturition is produced (Bragdon, 1951; Panigel, 1956). That some progestogenic type of hormone is secreted by the ovary or placenta of some viviparous snakes is suggested by the biochemical investigations of Callard and Leathem (1965), which shows an increase in progesterone synthesis by the ovaries of pregnant snakes as compared with nonpregnant females and the ability of the ovaries of ovoviviparous forms (*Natrix sipedon, N. taxispilota*) to synthesize more progesterone than oviparous species (*Coluber c. constrictor*). In *Vipera aspis*, the sudanophilia and birefringency of the newly formed corpus luteum diminish as the gestation period proceeds, suggesting a possible utilization of precursor material which would agree with the findings outlined above.

As in the avian ovary, follicular atresia is also a common occurrence in the gonad of female reptiles. When a follicle becomes atretic, a proliferation of fibroblastlike cells arising from the thecal tissue invade and phagocytize the yolk and progressively become more lipoidal and cholesterol positive as atresia progresses (Guraya, 1965). In the sectioned ovary, atretic follicles show varying degrees of sudanophilia, and Miller (1959) has suggested these structures as a possible source of estrogens. In contrast to the avian situation, however, no 3β-HSDH has so far been shown in these bodies (data summarized in Nandi, 1967).

D. AMPHIBIANS

The ovaries of amphibians are hollow saclike structures, the walls of which are thrown into folds and consist of a narrow cortical region covered by the germinal epithelium. The inner lining is formed from cells derived from the embryonic gonadal medullary tissue. The Amphibia are predominantly oviparous, the eggs being released into the body cavity and extruded via the genital (Mullerian) ducts into the water where fertilization takes place externally. True viviparity does not occur, but ovoviviparity, associated with internal fertilization, occurs in a few apodan and urodelan species. In the latter, the duration of gestation in the oviducts is dependent on the species and is generally only a few months long, but in extreme cases, such as in *Salamandra atra*, it can last up to 4 years. In the two anuran genera, *Pipa* and *Nototrema*, the frogs exhibit a curious pseudoplacentation. The eggs of these species are not retained in the reproductive tract but are transferred to pouches on the back of the female where gestation takes place. When the eggs are deposited in this site, the skin of the back proliferates between the eggs, which thus become enclosed in a highly vascularized cutaneous pouch.

The oogonia of the germinal epithelium give rise to successive generations of oocytes which are surrounded by a single layer of flattened granulosa cells. The follicular epithelium remains a single layer of cells throughout the whole period of maturation, and this differs from the multicellular granulosa tissue which is seen in the higher vertebrates. During the postnuptial period, it is possible to distinguish three populations of follicles in the cortical tissue of the regressed ovary: (a) young follicles from which succeeding generations of eggs for the next spawning period will develop, (b) numerous cell nests which will replace the latter and provide eggs for the subsequent spawning, and (c) the primary germ cells from which the cell nests become replenished. In *Rana temporaria*, the eggs take 3 years to mature. Thus, during the winter of the first year, the primary germ cells divide repeatedly to produce the cell nests from which the young follicles develop in the following summer. These then mature and are ovulated in the succeeding breeding season (Smith, 1955).

A thecal layer becomes associated with the developing follicle. Although in some species it is not easily distinguishable by light microscopy, electron microscopy confirms its presence and, in *Bufo bufo*, indicates that it is essentially acellular (Fig. 19). Generally, the thecal layer is moderately sudanophilic during the follicular phase, and a positive response to 3β-HSDH has been recorded in *Triturus cristatus* (Della Corte *et al.*, 1962), *Rana esculenta* (Chieffi and Botte, 1963; Botte, 1964), and *Bufo bufo* (Nicholls, 1969). Ozon (1967) reported 3β-HSDH activity in the follicular cells of the newt *Pleurodeles waltii*, and Botte and Cottino (1964) were able to confirm its presence in both thecal and granulosa cells, but not in the interstitial tissue, of *R. esculenta* and *T. cristatus*. A similar localization of 3β-HSDH in both thecal and granulosa cells has also been found in the viviparous anuran *Nectophrynoides occidentalis* (Xavier *et al.*, 1970). In *Bufo* both 3β- and 17β-HSDH have been located in the follicular region (Follett *et al.*, 1968). In *Xenopus laevis* the synthesis of steroid hormones appears to be restricted to the follicular layers, as judged by histochemical incubations, and 17β-, 17α-, 3β-, and

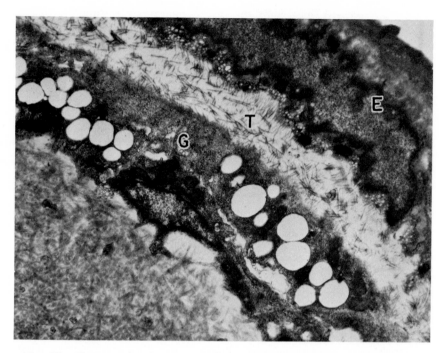

Fig. 19. Electron micrograph of follicle of the toad *Bufo bufo*. The granulosa (follicle) cells (G) are filled with clear vacuoles which are left by the dissolution of the lipid material. The outermost layer (E) is comprised of epithelial cells with characteristics much like those of the capillary endothelium. The thecal layer (T) appears to be acellular with numerous collagen fibrils. × 7500. (From V. F. Thornton, Leeds University.)

3α-HSDH systems have all been found in these cells in vitellogenic or mature oocytes. (Redshaw and Nicholls, 1971). Furthermore, this dehydrogenase activity is increased in *Xenopus* injected with pregnant mare serum gonadotropin.

After the ejection of the eggs, the granulosa cells hypertrophy and cholesterol-positive lipoidal material accumulates in the cytoplasm. Then, with the collapse of the evacuated follicle, the follicular lumen disappears and the proliferating granulosa tissue becomes compressed into a central core of lipoidal cells (Fig. 20) surrounded by a fibrous thecal capsule. Guraya (1968) reported that this metamorphosis of the postovulatory follicle in the bullfrog *R. catesbeiana* is accompanied by the synthesis of diffuse lipoproteins throughout the cytoplasm of the granulosa tissue, a phenomenon which he interprets as being indicative of active hormone secretion. However, in the majority of oviparous amphibian species, this simple postovulatory follicle is a very transient structure, with its nuclei soon becoming pycnotic and the

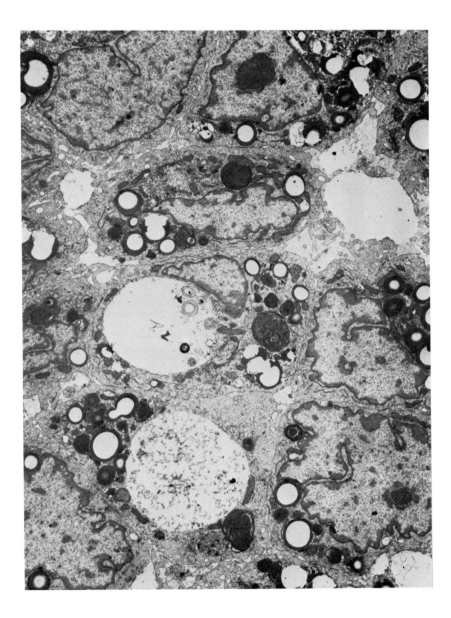

Fig. 20. Electron micrograph of postovulatory follicle of *Bufo bufo*. Lipid accumulates in the granulosa cells after spawning. Note the myelin figures and inactive mitochondria. × 3800. (From V. F. Thornton.)

organ being resorbed soon after its formation. In *Taricha torosa*, Miller and Robbins (1954) reported that this resorption of corpora lutea is complete 6–8 weeks after ovulation, when they then appear as blackish specks on the ovarian surface.

Evidence that these structures have a steroid-secreting role in oviparous forms is tenuous, although a positive response to 3β-HSDH has been reported in *Triturus cristatus* (Botte and Cottino, 1964) and *R. esculanta* (Chieffi and Botte, 1963). Galli-Mainini (1950) has suggested that the postovulatory follicles may be the source of a hormone which induces the secretion by the oviducal glands in *B. arenarum*, but there is now experimental evidence, in *Bufo bufo* at least, that the source of the hormone causing jelly release and meiosis in the oocyte prior to ovulation is the preovulatory follicle (Thornton and Evennett, 1969). The secretion of the oviducts in this toad and many other amphibians forms the jellylike coat which the eggs acquire in their passage along the oviducts to the exterior.

In the ovoviviparous urodelan species, and the anuran species showing cutaneous gestation pouches such as *Pipa pipa*, *Gastrotheca marsupiata*, and *Nectophrynoides occidentalis*, the postovulatory corpora lutea are more persistent and a high 3β-HSDH activity is located in the cells of the corpora lutea of the latter species (Xavier *et al.*, 1970). These structures remain (as judged by histochemical and histological criteria) in a functional condition during the whole gestation period, degenerating only after the young have been born (Lamotte and Rey, 1954), and this activity has been confirmed by recent *in vitro* incubation studies which have shown that the ovarian tissue retains the capacity to convert radioactive pregnenolone exclusively to progesterone throughout this peroid (Xavier and Ozon, 1971). In *N. occidentalis*, there is a distinct correlation between the decrease of corpora lutea and the growth of a new batch of eggs, suggesting an inhibition of follicular development by the functional corpora lutea (Lamotte and Rey, 1954); in *Taricha torosa*, too, the resumption of oogenesis and follicular development is deferred until resorption of the corpora lutea is complete (Miller and Robbins, 1954). In the ovoviviparous *Salamandra salamandra*, the granulosa lutein cells contain both birefringent lipids and 3β-HSDH and show all the ultrastructural characteristics of an active steroid-secreting tissue (Joly *et al.*, 1969). In *S. atra*, where the gestation period is of 4 years' duration, Vilter and Vilter (1964) have recorded that 30 or more corpora lutea persist in each ovary of the gravid female for the first 2 years of gestation, although gradually fewer remain as full term approaches. Their mean diameter also declines during this period, so that by the fourth year they are only a quarter of their original size.

The seasonal development and enlargement of the oviducts are dependent upon estrogenic steroids. Thus, atrophy of the oviducts consequent upon ovariectomy can be prevented and even reversed by the exogenous administration of estrogens. Estrogens also cause hypertrophy of the accessory sexual structures when administered to intact frogs (March, 1937; Galli-Mainini, 1950). During the anestrous period, the oviducts are generally thin collapsed tubules which become markedly hypertrophied with the recrudescence of the succeeding follicular phase. The precise site of estrogen secretion during this period is unknown, but the corpora atretica have been suggested as a likely source. These structures are a consistent feature of the ovarian cortex. They may be formed either from unovulated mature oocytes left in the ovary after termination of the spawning season, or from primary oocytes during their secondary growth phase.

Atresia involves, as it does in the vertebrate groups already considered, the invasion and resorption of the disintegrating oocyte by the proliferation of cells from the wall of the follicle. But, whereas in the reptiles and birds it is the cells of the thecal layer which invade the follicular lumen and the contained egg, in amphibians it is a proliferation and hypertrophy of the granulosa layer that leads to the formation of the corpora atretica (Smith, 1955). Practically all ova above a critical size degenerate in this way after hypophysectomy. The term "preovulatory corpora lutea" has been applied to these structures in amphibians and also in fishes (Bretschneider and de Wit, 1947). The suggestion that they may be involved in estrogen biosynthesis is speculative, since there is as yet no evidence other than the glandular appearance of the cells; in the limited numbers of amphibian species so far tested histochemically for 3β-HSDH activity, none has shown a positive response in atretic follicles. In *Bufo bufo*, atretic follicles contain only follicle cells which phagocytize the yolk and become filled with the pigmented breakdown products (Fig. 21). Although Joly (1965) has found that the corpora atretica of *Salamandra salamandra* react positively, he has also shown that a similar result can be obtained even when the ovarian tissue is incubated without substrate. It is evident, therefore, that there is a need for much more experimentation before one can attribute any steroidogenic capacity to the amphibian corpora atretica. The follicle cells, on the other hand, are both histochemically and ultrastructurally characteristic of steroid-producing tissue and in *Bufo bufo* undergo a well-defined lipid cycle. Thus lipid accumulates in the cell cytoplasm during winter, reaching a peak just before spawning. Lipid depletion then occurs, and the cells become filled with whorled membranous inclusions (Fig. 22) reminiscent of the multilaminate structures present in mammalian lutein cells (Thornton, 1969).

In the Bufonidae, both sexes possess paired rounded structures anterior to the gonads. These are Bidder's organs, which are rudimentary ovaries formed from the cortical remnants of the embryonic germinal ridge. Histologically, each organ consists of a compact mass of small oocytes (Fig. 23) which

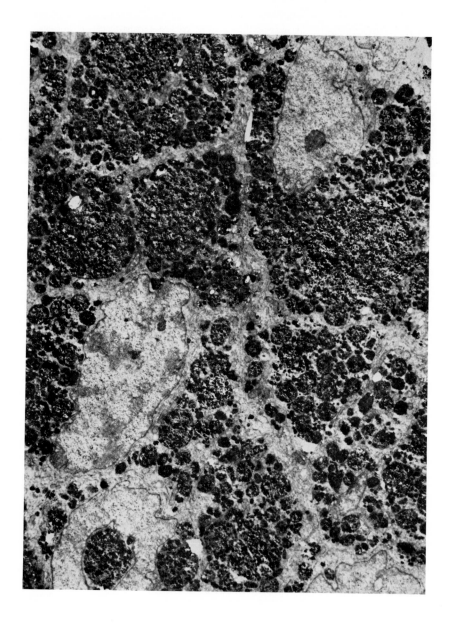

Fig. 21. Electron micrograph of atretic follicle of *Bufo bufo*. The granulosa cells are filled with vacuoles containing pigmented material, probably the breakdown products of yolk. x 3800. (From V. F. Thornton.)

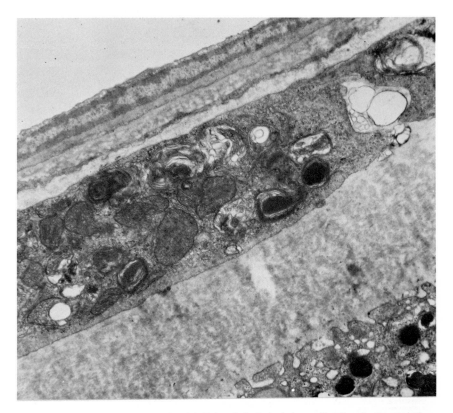

Fig. 22. Electron micrograph of follicle of *Bufo bufo* immediately prior to ovulation. Lipid depletion has occurred in the granulosa cells (cf. Fig. 19) and the cytoplasm is now filled with whorled membranous inclusions. Note the enlarged and apparently active mitochondria. × 15,000. (From V. F. Thornton.)

remain in an immature state but which can be induced to hypertrophy by the removal of the gonads. Chieffi and Lupo (1961) have reported that these structures have the capacity of biosynthesizing steroids from added precursors *in vitro*, and the steroids isolated are the same as those found in the ovarian tissue of the same species. Whether, however, Bidder's organ plays any significant role in steroid production *in vivo* is not known but would seem unlikely. Histochemical data about this organ are lacking.

E. FISHES

It is not possible to write a complete section on the "fish" ovary. The variation among the several classes of fishes is at least as great as that among the

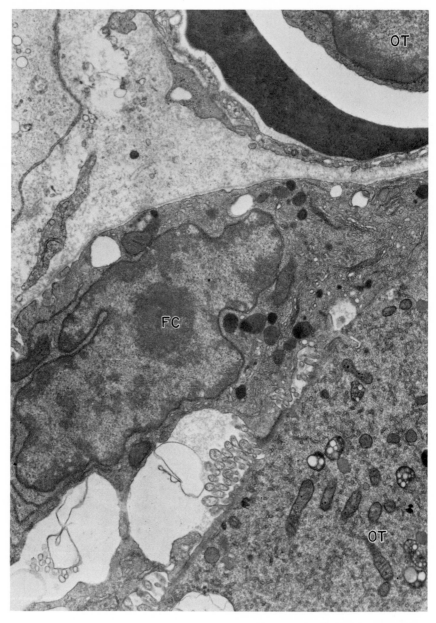

Fig. 23. Electron micrograph of Bidder's organ of *Bufo bufo*. The oocyte (OT) is similar to the previtellogenic oocyte of the ovary, except for the presence of the vesicular inclusions. The follicle cell (FC) has an extensive Golgi apparatus. × 9,750. (From V. F. Thornton.)

classes of tetrapods. Furthermore, the diversity of morphological form resulting from the radiation of just one superorder, the Teleostei, is as great, if not greater, than that encountered within any class of tetrapods. The most primitive and predominant form of reproduction is oviparity, and in many species the sexes associate for a relatively brief spawning period each year and shed their eggs into the water. Ovoviviparity and viviparity, however, are also common phenomena, and the latter has evolved repeatedly and independently in several actinopterygian and elasmobranchian species.

1. Actinopterygii

The Actinopterygii comprise by far the largest class of vertebrates, and the reproductive mechanisms found in this group present examples of almost every vertebrate type. Most of our knowledge of ovarian morphology and physiology is derived from studies of teleost species and relatively little information is available regarding ovarian structure and function in other groups of bony fishes. Essentially, the ovary is a fusiform body extending through the greater part of the body cavity and is suspended along its length by a mesovarium through which the vascular elements pass. It consists of a mass of follicles embedded in a rather sparse connective tissue stroma, and it can be either a solid structure, as in most Dipnoi, Chondrostei, and a few teleosts, or a hollow structure incorporating an internal coelomic cavity, as in the majority of teleost species. The gonad is derived exclusively from the embryonic cortical tissue (Franchi, 1962). In many species possessing the compact type of ovary, such as the ganoid fish *Amia calva*, the eggs are ovulated directly into the body cavity and pass to the exterior via oviducts which have free internal openings; in fishes with hollow ovaries, the gonadal lumen is continuous with the cavity of the oviduct.

The majority of bony fishes show well-marked reproductive rhythms with a restricted breeding season, and even species which are sexually active throughout the year (e.g., *Xiphophorus helleri*) generally have a period of maximum activity. The gonads undergo gross fluctuations, often regressing in the spent animal to thin threadlike organs consisting mainly of immature oocytes and a few stromal cells. Generally in oviparous forms, fertilization is external, but in the internally fertilized ovoviviparous and viviparous teleosts, the spermatozoa swim into the ovarian cavity and fertilize the eggs as they are released into the lumen (e.g., *Zoarces viviparus*) or, as is the case in *Hollienisia latipinna*, *Xyphosphorus helleri*, and *Lebistes reticulatus*, fertilization may actually occur within the ovarian follicle where the subsequent gestation takes place (Fig. 24).

In its early development, each oocyte is surrounded by follicle (granulosa) cells, which during the subsequent growth phases multiply to preserve a con-

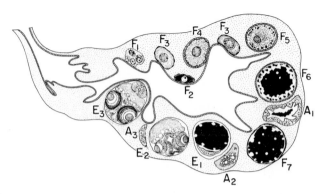

24

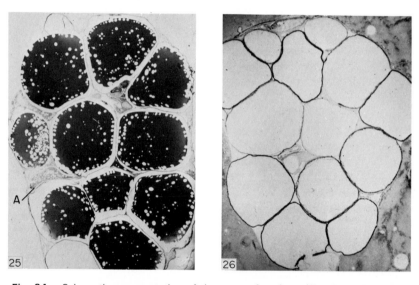

Fig. 24. Schematic representation of the ovary of a teleost (*Poecilia reticulata*). The ovary is a sacculate organ and the development of oocytes and embryos (E_1 — E3′) takes place in the wall. The various stages of follicle growth (F_1 — F_7) and follicle atresia (A_1 — A_3) have been combined into one picture—they do not actually occur simultaneously. (From J. G. D. Lambert, De Rijksuniversiteit, Utrecht.)

Fig. 25. Section of the ovary in *Poecilia reticulata*, 8 days after parturition. Note a few atretic follicles (A) between the fertilized oocytes. H and E; × 7.8. (From J. G. D. Lambert.)

Fig. 26. Section of the ovary in *Platypoecilus* sp. showing Δ^5-3β-hydroxysteroid dehydrogenase activity in the granulosa cells surrounding the oocytes. × 7.8. (From J. G. D. Lambert.)

tinuous layer around the oocyte (Fig. 25). The stromal connective tissue also becomes organized to form a distinct theca surrounding the granulosa cells. The subsequent fate of the follicular membranes remaining behind after ovulation is variable. In many oviparous teleosts there is a rapid post-ovulatory disintegration of the follicular structure, but in many ovovivi-parous and viviparous species hypertrophy of the follicular cells produces a structure morphologically similar to the mammalian corpus luteum. As in the latter, the cells of the fish corpus luteum are densely lipoidal, and Bara (1965a, b) has reported slight 3β-HSDH activity in some of its cellular components in *Scomber scomber*. This has led her to suggest a possible steroid-biosynthesis capacity in the corpus luteum, but others regard these structures in teleosts as being of doubtful endocrinological significance (Hoar, 1955; Pickford and Atz, 1957). In the viviparous species with intrafollicular gestation, a corpus luteum often does not develop.

Corpora atretica are a very conspicuous feature in the piscine ovary, and in most teleosts many of the developing follicles undergo atretic changes involving a proliferation of the granulosa cells with resorption of the oocyte. During this process, the granulosa cells become densely lipoidal and strongly cholesterol positive. The atretic follicles thus resemble a postovulatory corpus luteum, and while many investigators have simply regarded them as degenerate structures, others ascribe an endocrine function to them (pre-ovulatory corpus luteum). It has been suggested (Ball, 1960) that the number of ovarian corpora atretica increases toward the spawning season, but there is little precise quantitative information on this point; Pickford and Atz (1957), in reviewing the literature, concluded that the evidence for ascribing steroid activity to these structures was equivocal. Furthermore, the more recent development of histochemical methods which better indicate the steroid-producing capacities of tissues has so far failed to produce a positive 3β-HSDH response in the teleost atretic structures.

That the ovary of bony fishes undoubtedly has endocrine functions has been proved by surgical removal and replacement therapy, and ovarian incubations with radioactive precursors have clearly indicated its capacity for estrogen production. Tests for 3β-HSDH activity have produced varying results. In the viviparous guppy *Poecilia reticulata*, Lambert and van Oordt (1965) failed to obtain a positive response for this enzyme in corpora atretica, but instead found these structures to be rich in nonspecific esterases and acid phosphatases, and Yaron (1971) has found a similar situation in *Tilapia nilotica* and *Acanthobrama terrae-sanctae*. Lambert (1966) inter-prets this, as well as the dense sudanophilia and cholesterol in these structures, as being indicative of a degenerating steroid-producing tissue. This is supported by the fact that strong 3β-HSDH activity and glucose 6-phosphate dehydrogenase are found in the granulosa cells of the

developing follicle (Fig. 26). Since these cells eventually become the lutein cells of the corpus atreticum, it appears likely that they lose their
capacity for steroid biosynthesis after metamorphosing into atretic follicles. The glucose 6-phosphate dehydrogenase is involved in the hexose
monophosphate shunt, known to be a necessary process in the synthesis
of steroid hormones, and its presence in the follicle granulosa cells confirms the steroid-synthesizing activity of this tissue. In the guppy, 17β-
HSDH activity can also be readily demonstrated in these cells, strongly
suggesting that they are the most likely site of estrogen production in this
fish (Lambert, 1970). Lambert also found 17β-HSDH and 3α-HSDH in
the peripheral plasma of the older yolk-loaded oocytes, and suggested that
steroids synthesized in the granulosa cells may also be transported to the
oocyte.

In contrast to the events in the *Poecilia* ovary, the investigations of Bara
(1965a) on the distribution of 3β-HSDH in the ovary of the mackerel *Scomber
scomber* at different stages of the reproductive cycle have shown that in this
species the activity is greatest in some of the theca cells and not in the
granulosa tissue. The activity is strongest at the beginning of vitellogenesis
and reduces in intensity as the follicle matures. The distribution of glucose
6-phosphate dehydrogenase follows that of the 3β-HSDH, except that in
addition it is also found at a low level in the granulosa cells (Bara 1965b). In
the zebra fish *Brachydanio rerio*, 3β-HSDH activity is also similarly confined
to the thecal layer where it occurs in enlarged cells that are clearly distinguishable from the remaining thecal cells by their fine structure (Yamamoto and Onozato, 1968). In the latter species, these investigators also
found small mesenchymal cells in the stroma of the immature ovary which
gave a positive 3β-HSDH reaction and contained the ultrastructural organelles associated with steroid-producing tissues. They suggested that these
cells are the source of the glandular cells found in the theca interna of maturing and mature follicles. In *Tilapia nilotica* 3β-HSDH activity is found in both
granulosa and thecal cells (Yaron, 1971).

Thus, on the basis of limited evidence in bony fishes, it appears that the
follicular membranes of the growing oocyte may be involved in steroid biosynthesis, although there is conflicting information as to which layer is
involved.

2. Elasmobranchii

The elasmobranchs possess many more features in common with higher
vertebrates than do the teleosts. Like the latter, they can be oviparous,
ovoviviparous, or viviparous, but fertilization is always internal and the

ova are larger than those of bony fishes due to the more extensive deposition of yolk. They differ from teleosts in possessing well-developed sexual ducts and ovaries which consist of both a cortical and a medullary component. The primordial gonads are paired, but in the early development of a number of species the left gonad atrophies and only the right develops into the functional adult organ. It is suspended from the dorsal body wall by the mesovarium and consists of a loose stroma filled with large numbers of follicles. There is generally no ovarian cavity, although in some forms (e.g., *Scyliorhinus caniculus*) traces of a saclike structure are retained.

In the sexually mature female, the ovary usually contains 10–20 large yolk-ladened eggs, large numbers of maturing follicles in different stages of vitellogenesis, and primary oocytes. Numerous corpora lutea have also been described in the ovaries of several species. Each follicle has a distinct granulosa layer and a two-layered theca. The granulosa tissue is composed of a single layer of uniform columnar cells in *Squalus acanthias* (Fig. 27a), *Spinax niger*, *Chiloscyllium griseum*, and *Scyliorhinus stellaris*, but in others, such as *Rhinobatus granulatus*, *Torpedo marmorata*, and *Raja* sp., the granulosa is composed of two cell types, a large yolk-secreting cell with a reticular nucleus and abundant cytoplasm and a small columnar cell with a densely staining nucleus (Chieffi, 1961). The granulosa cytoplasm contains numerous small lipoidal droplets which become more numerous during follicular maturation, and it has all the appearances of glandular activity (Fig. 27b). In *Squalus acanthias*, 3β-HSDH activity is concentrated in the granulosa cells (Fig. 27c), which also react to tests for the revelation of glucose 6-phosphate dehydrogenase (Lance 1968, 1971). Furthermore, the activity of both enzyme systems increases with follicular development, suggesting the granulosa layer to be the probable site of estrogen biosynthesis. This hypothesis is strengthened by the extraction studies of Simpson *et al.* (1963b), which show that in *Squalus acanthias* ovarian tissues with mature follicles contain much higher concentrations of estrogenic hormones than does tissue from ovaries with immature follicles.

In an incubation study, Simpson *et al.* (1968) separated the component tissues of the ovaries of *Scyliorhinus caniculus* into mature follicles, regressed follicles, corpora lutea, and residual ovarian stroma containing many tiny follicles. Their results confirmed that estrogen synthesis is centered in the follicular membranes of the mature follicles, whereas the contribution of the other components is less significant.

The theca interna appears to be largely composed of connective tissue fibers, among which a few small connective tissue cells are interspersed. It is apparently without any great steroid dehydrogenase activity.

The histology and histochemistry of the elasmobranch corpus luteum present a somewhat confusing picture. In most of the species so far studied,

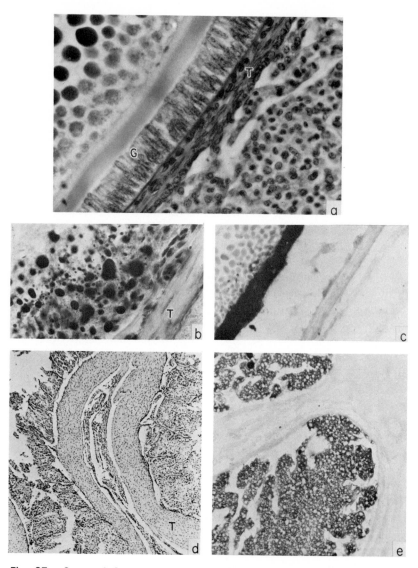

Fig. 27. Ovary of *Squalus acanthias*. (a) Developing follicle with a well-defined thecal layer (T) and a granulosa layer (G) composed of a single layer of columnar cells. The granulosa cells contain sudanophilic droplets (b) and are strongly positive for Δ^5-3β-hydroxysteroid dehydrogenase (c). The postovulatory corpus luteum (d) is formed by a proliferation of the granulosa tissue surrounded by a fibrous thecal layer and becomes strongly positive to Δ^5-3β-hydroxysteroid dehydrogenase activity (e). (From Lance and Callard, 1969.)

the postovulatory follicle develops into a solid glandlike structure (Fig. 27d), which is densely lipoidal and cholesterol positive. In *Squalus* it is formed by a hypertrophy of the granulosa cells, and the thecal layer forms a distinct and separate sheath surrounding the central lipoidal mass. In *Rhinobatos*, however, the thecal cells also contribute to the lutein tissue (Samuel, 1943), and the same is also true of *Scyliorhinus stellaris* and several species of the genus *Raia* (Chieffi, 1967b). *Squalus acanthias* is an ovoviviparous species, and in this fish the corpora lutea persist in the ovary for much of the gestation period. The oviducts during this time undergo considerable modification, and it seems possible that a hormone of follicular or luteal origin might be responsible. In this species, in the oviparous *Scyliorhinus stellaris* (Lupo *et al.*, 1965), and in several species of *Raja* (Botte, 1963), a positive 3β-HSDH activity occurs in the corpus luteum (Fig. 27e), thus suggesting that the granulosa lutein tissue might retain a capacity for synthesizing steroids although perhaps to a lesser extent than the granulosa cells of the developing follicle. Lance (1968) has reported that the 3β-HSDH activity in *Squalus* is confined almost specifically to the granulosa lutein cells of the corpus luteum, although occasionally weak responses are also given by the outer thecal cells. The intensity of the reaction diminishes as gestation proceeds. The results of Callard and Leathem (1965) support these histochemical data and show that the ovarian tissue of *Squalus acanthias* synthesizes twice as much progesterone *in vitro* when the fishes are pregnant than when it is taken from nonpregnant animals.

Follicular atresia in the elasmobranch ovary is as common an event as it is in the ovaries of the bony fishes and, as in the latter, often results in the production of a structure similar to the corpus luteum. In *Squalus*, the "preovulatory corpora lutea" are distinct from the postovulatory structures, since cells from the theca interna migrate into the follicle. Furthermore, they are distinguishable in that although they are densely lipoidal (as are the corpora lutea), they are negative to both histochemical tests for cholesterol and 3β-HSDH (Lance, 1968, 1971). In *Torpedo marmorata* and *T. ocellata*, on the other hand, the reverse is true; it is the granulosa cells that develop into the corpora atretica, while the corpus luteum undergoes an early sclerosis and is negative to both tests for cholesterol and 3β-HSDH (Chieffi and Gualà, 1959; Chieffi, 1961; Lupo *et al.*, 1965). Postovulatory follicles of *T. marmorata* separated from the main ovarian mass and tested for their biosynthetic capacity produce no progesterone but can synthesize estrogens since they are not subjected to the luteinizing process, whereas the corpora lutea of *Scyliorhinus stellaris* yield progesterone and no estrogens under identical conditions (Lupo di Prisco, 1968). Chieffi (1961) has noted in *T. marmorata* that the preovulatory structures show the positive 3β-HSDH response and that they increase in number during pregnancy. Thus, in this species it appears on histochemical grounds that the corpora atretica may have a steroid-biosynthesizing capacity. This has been confirmed by the *in vitro* incubation of isolated atretic follicles (Lupo di Prisco, 1968).

3. Cyclostomata

Information about the detailed ovarian morphology and cytology of the cyclostome ovary is relatively sparse. As in the male, the female gonad is a single elongate structure covered by a thin germinal epithelium, and it consists of masses of small follicles with a rather sparse interfollicular stroma. The eggs are located within sacs of peritoneal epithelium with the vegetative poles resting on the epithelium (Busson-Mabillot, 1967). They are released into the body cavity by the rupture of the ovary wall and are extruded through abdominal pores. The eggs of the lampreys are small, but in the hagfishes they are contained in an elaborate egg case which is secreted by the ovary. In *Lampetra fluviatilis*, the ovary consists of oocytes in which vitellogenesis has already started by the time the lamprey starts its migration in the autumn (Larsen, 1965); maturation of the follicles proceeds slowly throughout winter and accelerates only with the rise in water temperature in spring. Follicles are fully mature by April. The follicular epithelium remains a single granular layer of cells covering the vegetative pole (Fig. 28a and b) in close contact with the oocyte, and in *L. fluviatilis*, they grow to a maximal height in March. Immediately before ovulation, they disintegrate (Larsen, 1970). Although a thecal layer is difficult to distinguish by light microscopy, the electron microscope shows a distinct thecal layer organized around the primordial follicles.

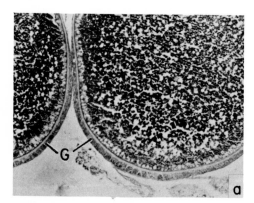 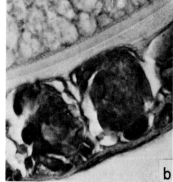

Fig. 28. Follicle of *Lampetra fluviatilis*. (a) The granulosa cells (G) cover the vegetative pole; (b) these cells at a higher magnification. (From L. O. Larsen (1970), University of Copenhagen.)

Lyngnes (1936) has reported that well-developed corpora lutea are formed in both the atretic and ruptured follicles of *Myxine*, but nothing is known concerning their functional activity. More recently, Hardisty and Barnes (1968) have recorded 3β-HSDH in the granulosa cells in *L. fluviatilis* caught during the autumn; this activity becomes more marked in specimens examined in February and early March.

IV. Adrenocortical (Interrenal) Tissue

Adrenocortical (interrenal) tissue is present in all vertebrate groups. Although much of our knowledge of its functional morphology is derived from mammalian studies, there is an increasing accumulation of information on the distribution of this tissue among other vertebrates. This section is intended to provide a morphological basis for the considerations of adrenal steroid biochemistry and physiology which follow in subsequent chapters. References can be made to standard textbooks and recent reviews (Hartman and Brownell, 1949; Chester Jones, 1957; Hoar, 1957; Deane, 1962; deRoos, 1963; Fontaine, 1963; Bern and Nandi, 1964; Gabe *et al.*, 1964; Barr, 1965; Matty, 1966; Bern, 1967a; Chester Jones *et al.*, 1969) for earlier bibliographic information.

A verbal sketch of the mammalian adrenal gland is desirable as a basis for understanding the differences in adrenal structure among other vertebrate groups and as a point of departure for histophysiological interpretations in nonmammalian vertebrates. The mammalian adrenal gland is unique in its organization of steroidogenic interrenal tissue into a cortex surrounding major masses of catecholamine-secreting chromaffin tissue forming a distinct medulla. The cortex–medulla relationship is not always so discrete as is pictured in textbooks (see Gorbman and Bern, 1962), however, and cortical nodules and ectopic cortical masses are not uncommon. In monotremes, envelopment of the medulla by the cortex is incomplete.

The mammalian adrenal cortex is characterized by its obvious zonation. Classically, these zones are a narrow external zona glomerulosa, an extensive middle zona fasciculata, and a variable internal (generally juxtamedullary) zona reticularis. However, the characteristic zonation is often difficult to recognize and may vary with functional state, reproductive condition, and age of the animal. In some species, or under some conditions of hypo- and hyperactivity, one or two zones may be unidentifiable. In other species, or at some stages in the life cycle, additional zones may be present. In some mammals, cortical tissue (presumably zona reticularis) may penetrate and even form islands in the medulla. An important point to be made about the comparative histology of the mammalian adrenal cortex is that exceptions and abnormalities may be more frequent than is suggested by the so-called normal picture.

In view of the cortex–medulla relationship and zonal organization, the structural features described above represent distinctly mammalian specializations, and there will be little evidence in the discussion of nonmammalian adrenals, which forecasts the evolutionary emergence of the mammalian pattern (Fig. 29). Functionally in mammals, the zona glomerulosa is considered to be involved with mineralocorticoid (aldosterone) secretion, the zona fasciculata largely with glucocorticoid (cortisol and/or corticosterone) secretion, and the zona reticularis with glucocorticoid and possibly sex steroid secretion.

A. ANATOMY AND HISTOLOGY

1. Fishes

a. General. The adrenocortical homolog (interrenal tissue) is still not so well defined in fishes as cursory examination of the literature may first indicate. In teleosts, the interrenal tissue is generally found embedded in the remains of the anterior portion of the kidney; in chondrichthyeans the tissue is generally organized into a large gland between the posterior ends of the kidneys in a location topographically almost the converse of its site in teleosts. The morphology of the adrenocortical system of the remaining fish groups is much less well documented, and one cannot extrapolate from either the chondrichthyeans or the teleosts to the cyclostomes, ganoids, coelacanths, and lungfishes (Fig. 29).

There are obviously gross differences in the location and organization of the interrenal (adrenocortical) tissue between teleosts and chondrichthyeans, which alone would make it impossible to present any generalized "piscine" picture. Further differences emerge from examination of the relationship between chromaffin (adrenomedullary, catecholamine-secreting) tissues and the interrenal (adrenocortical, steroid-secreting) cells. In teleosts, a highly variable picture is encountered, with chromaffin cells sometimes intermingled diffusely with the interrenal cells, sometimes organized into an internal band in contact with the lining of the postcardinal vein, sometimes organized as an external covering of the interrenal cells, and sometimes totally absent from the interrenal sites and indeed conceivably from the anterior kidney itself (Nandi, 1961, 1962). In elasmobranchs, the chromaffin tissue is organized into segmentally arranged, bilaterally located islets associated with branches of the dorsal aorta. An additional complication arises from the early suggestion of Giacomini, still

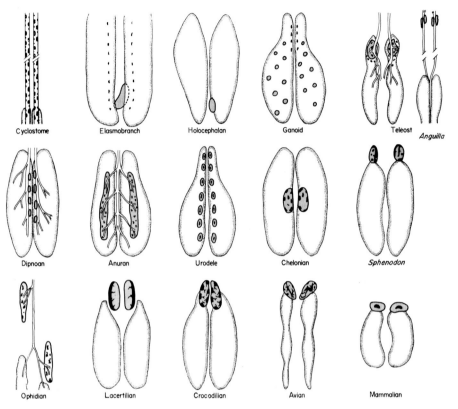

Fig. 29. Diagrams showing distribution of interrenal (dense stipple) and chromaffin (black) tissues in association with kidney (outlined by light stipple) in various vertebrate groups. Some ophidian species show a partial "cortex" of chromaffin tissue as in *Sphenodon* and lacertilians. (Compiled from diagrams of H. A. Bern and I. Chester Jones.)

occasionally resuscitated despite his own later rejection of the idea (Gia-comini, 1933), that the corpuscles of Stannius of actinopterygian fishes (holostean and telostean) should also be considered as part of the adreno-cortical system (as "posterior interrenals"). At least their topography and ontogeny may qualify them for such consideration. Their location in teleosts is reminiscent of the similarly posterior interrenal of chondrichthyeans rather than the anterior interrenal tissue; however, they are generally intrarenal rather than interrenal glands. In the freshwater teleost *Notopterus notopterus*, Nagalakshmi (1970) claims that interrenal tissue surrounds the corpuscles in the anteriormost end of the trunk kidney.

b. Cyclostomes. Among cyclostomes, the adrenocortical homolog has not been definitively established. In the lamprey, supposed interrenal cells in small groups are located above the pronephric funnels and in the walls of the large dorsal vessels (Sterba, 1955, 1962). Recently, these cells have been shown to have steroidogenic features (Hardisty and Baines, 1971). However, not even this much can be said with certainty for the hagfish (Chester Jones, 1963); although cells similar in appearance and location to those in the lamprey have been located in *Myxine*, corticosteroidogenesis has not been demonstrated. Corticosteroid synthesis by appropriate areas of the lamprey has also not been shown, but Sterba (1955) has demonstrated cell hypertrophy consequent to ACTH administration. If these cell islands are truly adreno-cortical homologs, the primitive condition of the agnathan is evident. Chromaffin cells are completely separate from these small interrenal islets, and there is no organized structure that can be referred to as a gland.

c. *Chondrichthyeans*. The chondrichthyean adrenocortical homolog, located interrenally and posteriorly, is organized into a distinct, encapsulated gland, which may be rod-shaped or asymmetrically U-shaped and relatively easily dissected intact. In many species, islands of interrenal tissue are often found extending anteriorly. The two chondrichthyean subclasses, elasmo-branchs and holocephalans, which show such major differences in other endocrine systems, are similar in their interrenal morphology. The tissue is organized into cords and lobules and usually consists of a single cell type (Fig. 30).

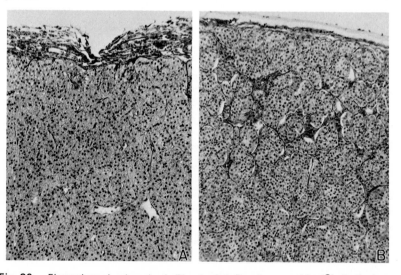

Fig. 30.   Elasmobranch adrenals. A, The dogfish *Squalus acanthias* (♀); B, the bat ray *Holorhinus californicus* (♀). Note islands of smaller, more eosinophilic interrenal cells of unknown significance in B. H, and E; × 75).

It is of interest to note that almost no recent histophysiological, histoen-zymological, or cytological studies of the chondrichthyean interrenal tissue have been published. These prominent masses of steroidogenic tissue seem to repel modern investigation, although the advantages of working with "pure" interrenal tissues (devoid of chromaffin tissue) have long been recognized. However, Chieffi (1965) demonstrated the presence of 3β-HSDH both biochemically and histochemically in interrenal cells of *Torpedo marmorata*, *T. ocellata*, *Scyliorhinus stellaris*, and *S. caniculus*.

d. Lower Actinopterygians. Whereas much information is available in regard to interrenal morphology in the teleostean radiation, almost no data exist in regard to the lower actinopterygians: the ganoids and polypterines. In these fishes, the interrenal tissue is scattered throughout the kidneys, a situation intermediate between that of chondrichthyeans and teleosts. It is particularly abundant and prominent in *Polypterus* (de Smet, 1970). Interrenal tissue of the sturgeon *Acipenser oxyrhynchus* Mitchill has been identified by histological and histochemical methods (Idler and O'Halloran, 1970). Yellow bodies were found scattered throughout the kidney and along the posterior cardinal veins to their point of entry into the heart. Some of the yellow bodies were deeply embedded in the kidney; others, encapsulated and distinct from kidney tissue, were lying on the dorsal surface of each kidney. Their histology resembled that of interrenal tissue rather than that of corpuscles of Stannius. Positive 3β-HSDH activity was obtained using dehydroepiandrosterone and pregnenolone as substrates. Definite proof of their adrenocortical nature was provided by isolation and identification of corticosteroids after incubation with labeled precursors (Idler and Sangalang, 1970).

Both the typical chondrichthyean arrangement and the typical teleost location may represent alternative evolutionary end points for the interrenal tissues derived embryologically from the coelomic epithelium adjacent to the intermediate mesoderm. However, the identification of interrenal tissue in holosteans (including *Amia* and *Lepisosteus*) is complicated by the presence of large numbers of corpuscles of Stannius and of "tubule corpuscles" resembling the Stannius corpuscles (cf. De Smet, 1962). Many more studies of the interrenal organization in nonteleostean bony fishes are needed to allow precise anatomical, let alone functional, descriptions to be made.

e. Teleosts. In teleosts generally, the steroidogenic adrenocortical tissue is found in association with the postcardinal veins (Fig. 31). When embedded in the anteriormost part of the kidney, the surrounding tissue is often entirely nonrenal in function and is instead an organized mass of hemo-poietic tissue (lymphoid, myeloid, or both). The anterior or "head" kidney

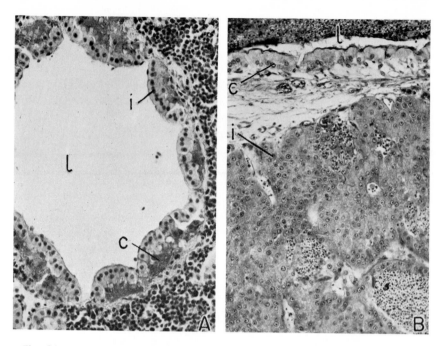

Fig. 31. Teleost head kidneys showing interrenal (i) and chromaffin (c) tissues. A, *Cheilinus rhodochrous* (Labridae) showing interrenal cells nearest lumen (subendothelially) and chromaffin cells (chromates stained) externally. Orth's; hematoxylin and eosin; × 330. B, *Chaetodon lineolatus* (Chaetodontidae) showing chromaffin cells bordering lumen (l) of branch of postcardinal vein, separated by connective tissue from masses of interrenal cells. Bouin's; hematoxylin and phloxin; × 225. (From J. Nandi, 1962; Reprinted by permission of the Regents of the University of California.)

is sometimes dissociated entirely from the functional abdominal kidney. In a few instances, as in congrid and muraenid eels and in some acanthurids (Nandi, 1962), the interrenal cells form a partial collar around the post-cardinal vein and are visible as a pair of large masses, entirely extrarenal in location. In anguillids, interrenal islands are in the wall of the vein, but are still associated with head kidney (Chester Jones *et al.*, 1964). In species which do not have a definable head kidney, the interrenal cords are found anteriorly in the trunk kidney, from which they also extend posteriorly (Ogawa, 1962).

Comparative studies of adrenal histology in teleosts reveal a variety of types based upon distribution of the interrenal and chromaffin cells in the head kidney and upon their relationship to blood vessels (van Overbeeke, 1960; Oguri, 1960a; Nandi, 1961, 1962; Banerji and Ghosh, 1965). Nandi (1962) has recognized four major patterns of distribution of interrenal tissue

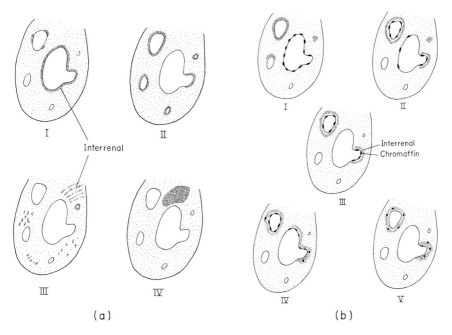

Fig. 32. Types of adrenal tissue patterns in teleost head or anterior kidney. (a) Interrenal cell distribution; (b) chromaffin cell distribution. Open spaces represent postcardinal vein and major branches; light stippling, kidney; dense stippling, interrenal; black, chromaffin. (From J. Nandi, 1962; Reprinted by permission of the Regents of the University of California.)

and five major patterns of distribution of chromaffin tissue (Fig. 32). There is little taxonomic value that can be associated with these distribution patterns, and indeed physiological activation or inactivation can be expected to change appreciably the microanatomic arrangements (Robertson and Wexler, 1959, 1960; Robertson *et al.*, 1961; Hane *et al.*, 1966). According to Olivereau (1967), activation of the eel interrenal results in a follicular organization of the tissue. Sometimes closely related species show considerable differences in their interrenal histology (Nandi, 1965).

f. Corpuscles of Stannius and Steroid Transformation. The corpuscles of Stannius are particularly numerous in holosteans and are present in some form in all teleosteans. De Smet (1962, 1963) suggested an evolutionary line that leads from multiple small corpuscles in the holosteans to reduction in number and increase in size in the teleosts (Fig. 33). Krishnamurthy and Bern (1969) describe four types of corpuscles in teleosts, based on degree of subdivision and lobulation by connective tissue septa, but could

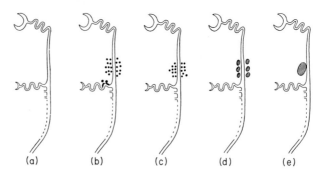

Fig. 33. Morphological series representing possible evolution of Stannius corpuscles in actinopterygians. (a) Polypteriformes, Chondrostei; (b) Holostei, *(Amia)*; (c) Holostei *(Lepisosteus)*; (d) primitive Teleostei; (e) more advanced Teleostei. (From De Smet, 1962.)

find no relation between histological pattern and taxonomical position, (These articles can be referred to for citation of the earlier and later literature on the corpuscles.) In at least some species, the corpuscles appear to have a notable innervation (Krishnamurthy and Bern, 1971).

The cytology of the corpuscles of Stannius in no way suggests that they could be steroidogenic (in the sense of the adrenal cortex). The cells are equipped with an elaborate protein-synthetic apparatus and are often highly granular. Their typical mitochondria, stacks of granular endoplasmic reticulum, and Golgi membranes associated with electron-dense material are all in contradistinction to the image of a steroidogenic cell (p. 38). At best, the corpuscle cell may be a steroid-transforming unit (Idler and Free-man, 1966); however, critical examination of the most recently available data makes it difficult to ascribe to them a role of this kind that may have even minimal physiological significance. The corpuscles of some species possess more than one cell type (Fig. 34); in *Salmo gairdnerii*, electron microscopy revealed secretory granules in both types (Krishnamurthy and Bern, 1969).

The special problem raised by the corpuscles of Stannius concerns the significance of steroid transformation (see Bern, 1967b). It has become increasingly evident that a variety of vertebrate (and invertebrate) tissues can transform steroids, i.e., transform a steroid precursor into a hormone, or a relatively inactive compound into an active hormonelike principal. This ability may reside in target organs but also in organs which are not them-selves directly affected by either the entering or the departing steroid.

Fig. 34. Corpuscles of Stannius showing two types of cells: granular and agranular (arrows in A). A, *Salmo gairdnerii*, × 950. B, *Gymnothorax flavimarginatus*; × 750; aldehyde fuchsin trichrome. (From Krishnamurthy and Bern, 1969.)

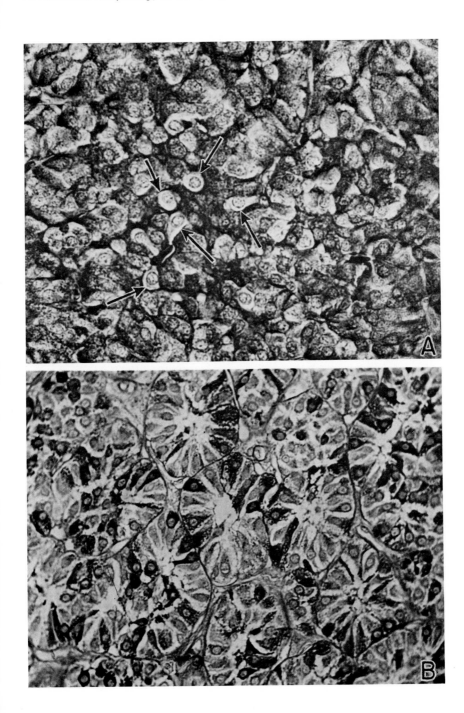

"Cooperative steroidogenesis" may yield important amounts of a biologically active principal, but the transformation step may confer no special distinction upon the organ or tissue performing it—no more distinction than
is conferred upon other tissues that transform active steroids into inactive
catabolites (with the steroid nucleus intact).

Hydroxylases and dehydrogenases may be relatively nonspecific, and
modification of the steroid structure would appear to be a feature common
to many tissues (the adrenomedullary tissue, for example, has been shown
to have a remarkable ability to modify steroids). Whereas true steroidogenic cells may show characteristic organellar features (see p. 38) and Fig.
11), steroid-transforming cells may not be cytologically distinctive. Nandi
(1968) and Colombo *et al.* (1970) have demonstrated greater steroid transformation by the body kidney of *Tilapia* than by the Stannius corpuscles; neither
tissue has steroidogenic activity like that of the interrenal-containing head
kidney (cf. Chester Jones *et al.*, 1969; Arai *et al.*, 1969). Accordingly, the
endocrine significance that could be derived even from incontrovertible proof
of steroid transformation by the corpuscles of Stannius is questionable (cf.
Nandi, 1967; Bern, 1967b). It would seem more profitable to extend the
findings of the Chester Jones group (1966) regarding the relation of the
corpuscles to blood pressure regulation (the renin mechanism?).

   g. Lungfishes. After much controversy, the localization of the interrenal
tissue in a lungfish (*Protopterus*) has been accomplished by a combination of
biochemical (steroidogenic capacity) and histochemical (lipid, cholesterol,
Δ^5-3β-hydroxysteroid dehydrogenase activity) methods (Gérard, 1951;
Janssens, 1964; Janssens *et al.*, 1965). Small cords of sudanophilic cells are
located between the renal and perirenal tissues adjacent to branches of the
postcardinal veins and resemble the interrenal tissue of adult urodeles
(Fig. 35).

2. Amphibians

   Amphibian adrenals are extrarenal in location and variable in distribution. They may be irregular nodular structures organized into a pair of glands
(as in anurans), or they may be islands of tissue scattered on the ventral
surface of the kidneys (as in urodeles and apodans). Histological examination reveals that chromaffin and interrenal cells are inseparably intermingled
(Fig. 36) and that this close association is an almost constant feature in the
Amphibia. However, in *Xenopus laevis* the adrenal tissue is composed of
interrenal islets to whose margins groups of two to three chromaffin cells
are attached (Rapola, 1962). Here, as in most species, there is considerably
more interrenal than chromaffin tissue. In *Rana hexadactyla*, however, there
is more chromaffin than interrenal tissue (Lakshman, 1964).

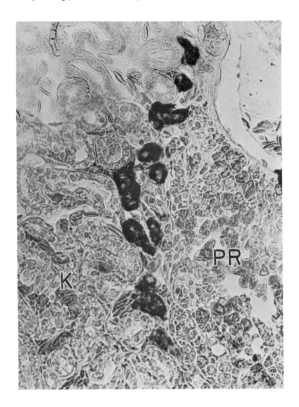

Fig. 35. Islands of presumed interrenal (adrenocortical) cells in the African lungfish (*Protopterus* sp.). These sudanophilic cells are located between the kidney (K) and the perirenal tissue (PR). Formol–calcium, frozen, sudan black; × 140. (From Janssens *et al.*, 1965.)

In some anuran species (ranids) a third cell type, the summer (or Stilling) cells, may also be located in the tissue mass (cf. Burgos, 1959). This third type of eosinophilic cell resembles mast cells. They may occur only seasonally in the species where they are found, and their significance remains enigmatic. They show signs of atrophy after hypophysectomy and exposure to salt water (Scheer and Wise, 1969). Like the cells of many Stannius corpuscles, the summer cells are heavily granule laden, but no other resemblance has been noted, and their isolated occurrence, suggesting an invation of motile cells, is not consonant with the high degree of organization shown by Stannius corpuscle tissue. The chromophilic cells of other ranids are presumably of similar (albeit unknown) significance, and apparently both can transform into interrenal cells (van Kemenade *et al.*, 1968). Yoshimura and Harumiya (1968) referred to an "intermediary cell between lipid cell and summer cell"

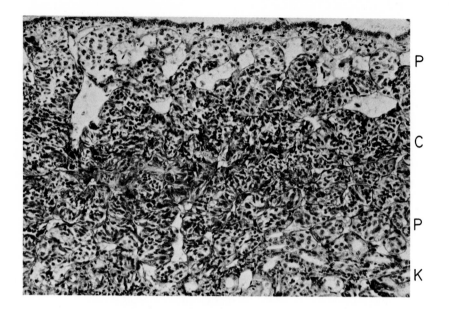

Fig. 36. Section of adrenal gland of *Rana temporaria* (collected in October) to show evidence of zonation: active peripheral regions (P) and inactive central region (C). Chromaffin cells are intermingled with interrenal cells in the central region (K, kidney). × 135. (Prepared by W. Hanke, University of Frankfurt.)

in the bullfrog interrenal. Moorhouse (1963) emphasized the presence of still a fourth type of cell, comprising the lymphoid tissue in the adrenal gland.

Two types of chromaffin cells are present in randomly distributed clusters among the interrenal cords in anurans (Piezzi, 1965, 1967; Benedeczky, 1967).

3. Reptiles

A generalized picture of the adrenals of reptiles is not possible. However, following the excellent survey by Gabe and his colleagues (1964), one can divide the general adrenal picture in reptiles into two major structural varieties (Fig. 37); that seen in chelonians, crocodilians, and some snakes, and that seen in most squamates and *Sphenodon*.

In the former group, the chromaffin tissue is present in a manner somewhat like that seen in birds, but to varying degrees. In turtles (Gabe and Martoja, 1962), much of the chromaffin tissue (with two types of cells according to Khiruvathukal, 1967) is located at the periphery of the gland, with only a few cords extending internally. In crocodilians, there is a discontinuous superficial chromaffin layer with considerable penetration of the interrenal tissue by chromaffin tissue (Gabe and Rancurel, 1964). Unlike the chelonians, and like the birds, in crocodilians the chromaffin cords are regularly interspersed among the interrenal cords.

In the second group, lizards characteristically show a partial encapsulation of the interrenal gland mass by chromaffin tissue on the craniodorsal surface. Strands of chromaffin tissue also occur among the interrenal cords. In some snakes (Lofts and Phillips, 1965), there is a dorsal superficial band of chromaffin tissue, again with penetration of the cells; in *Naja* this band may occupy 25% of the gland width and is spatially separated from the chromaffin islets scattered among the adrenocortical cords. However, the majority of snakes appear to lack this dorsal concentration and thus more resemble the chelonian–crododilian–avian arrangement. In *Sphenodon*, chromaffin tissue surrounds the entire dorsal aspect of the adrenal, with some islands of cells also occurring more centrally (Gabe and Saint Girons, 1964).

In snakes with a dorsal superficial band there appears to be a complete separation (and separate functional control) of the chromaffin cells secreting noradrenaline and those secreting adrenaline (Wassermann and Tramezzani, 1961, 1963; Houssay *et al.*, 1962; Lofts and Phillips, 1965). The superficial cells contain noradrenaline, and the deeper cells, intermingled with the interrenal cells, contain adrenaline.

4. Birds

Among birds, the adrenal gland is located suprarenally as in mammals, and, in external appearance as well as topography, the adrenals in the two homeothermic classes are similar. However, the microanatomy is distinctly different, and the birds show an intermingling of cortical (interrenal) and medullary (chromaffin) components reminiscent of that seen in some reptilian subclasses (Figs. 37K, L and 38), including the crocodilians (a generalized sauropsid picture thus emerges with the exception of *Sphenodon*, the lizards, and some snakes). The relative amounts of interrenal tissue and chromaffin tissue vary in different groups of birds. In most species the former is more abundant; in others the latter may predominate, with islets of interrenal tissue appearing to be embedded in the larger mass of chromaffin tissue (see Ghosh, 1962; Ghosh and Ghosh, 1962).

B. Histophysiology

1. Functional Cytology and Cytochemistry

In all nonmammalian vertebrates so far examined, the interrenal cell shows an ultrastructure characteristic of steroid production and resembles

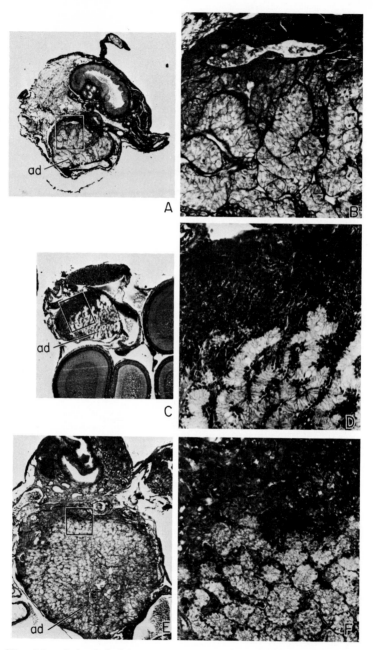

Fig. 37. Adrenal glands (ad) from sauropsid vertebrates. Right photographs (× 135) are enlargements of boxed areas of left photographs (× 19.2). A, B, *Sphenodon punctatus* (Rhynchocephalia); C, D, *Lacerta muralis* (Lacertilia); E, F, *Python regius* (Ophidia). In A—F, note dorsal "encapsulation" of interrenal mass (light) by chromaffin cells (dark). G, H,

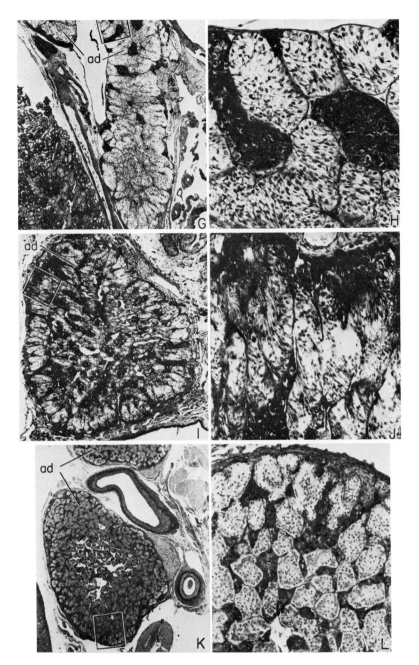

Clemmys leprosa (Chelonia). In G—H, note projection of chromaffin masses to surface of gland. I. J, *Crocodylus niloticus* (Crocodilia); K,L, *Gallus gallus* (Aves). In I—L, note interspersion of chromaffin islands among interrenal cords. Bouin's; one-step trichrome (Gabe and Martoja). (Prepared by M. Gabe, University of Paris.)

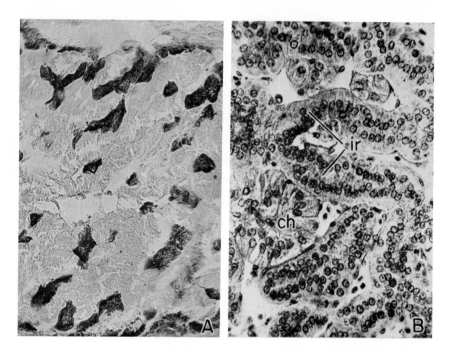

Fig. 38. Adrenal gland of pigeon showing intermingling of interrenal (adrenocortical) and chromaffin (adrenomedullary) components characteristic of birds. A, Chromaffin reaction (with dichromate) showing masses of reactive cells among interrenal cords; × 105. B, Cords of interrenal tissues (ir) with islands of chromaffin cells (ch) Masson's; × 340. (From A. Ghosh, University of Calcutta.)

the active cell of the zona fasciculata of the mammalian adrenal cortex (cf. Idelman, 1970). Agranular endoplasmic reticulum and mitochondria with tubular cristae (Fig. 39) and often with osmiophilic inclusions are present in interrenal cells from cyclostomes (Hardisty and Baines, 1971), teleosts (Yamamoto and Onozato, 1965; Ogawa, 1967), amphibians (Burgos, 1959; Sheridan and Belt, 1964; Pehlemann *et al.*, 1967; Berchtold, 1968a, 1969a, 1970; Pehlemann and Hanke, 1968; Piezzi and Burgos, 1968; Ábrahám, 1969; Picheral, 1969, 1970), reptiles (Sheridan, 1963; Harrison, 1966; Varano and Della Corte, 1969; Dufaure, 1970), and birds (Fujita *et al.*, 1963; Sheridan *et al.*, 1963; Belt *et al.*, 1965; Kondics and Kjaerheim, 1966; Harrison, 1966; Kjaerheim, 1968a,b,c,d).

As in mammals, both microsomes and mitochondria are concerned with corticosteroid elaboration. Figure 40 summarizes the relationship between steroidogenic enzymes and cell organelles, as exemplified in an anuran amphibian (see Pehlemann and Hanke, 1968). Active and inactive cells are

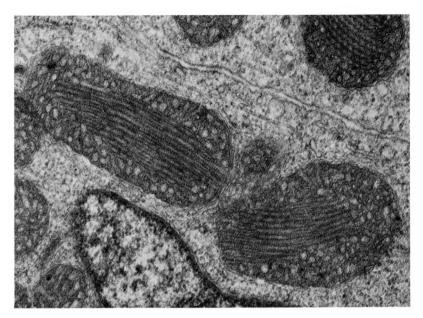

Fig. 39.   Mitochondria from slightly active interrenal cell of *Rana temporaria*. Note tubular cristae and dense mitochondrial matrix. × 24,000 (From Pehlemann and Hanke, 1968.)

present in the normal frog interrenal (Fig. 36) and their ultrastructure is clearly distinguishable by the reduced cytoplasm, abundance of clear lipid droplets, and decrease in size and increase in density of the mitochondria in the inactive cells (Fig. 41A and B). Administration of ACTH intensifies the pictures of activity (Fig. 41C) and hypophysectomy that of inactivity (Fig. 41D). The activated cells show larger nuclei, nucleoli, mitochondria, and Golgi apparatuses. Smooth endoplasmic reticulum envelops the mitochondria, and rough reticulum is found around electron-dense lipid droplets. Similar responses occur in urodeles (Berchtold, 1969b). Administration of ACTH also stimulates amitotic cell division in *Rana temporaria*, and a beautiful study of this dramatic response has been published by Pehlemann (1968).

The histochemical properties of nonmammalian interrenal tissue are essentially similar to those of mammalian vertebrates [see, as examples, in teleosts: Oguri (1960b), Chavin and Kovacevic (1961), Mahon *et al.*(1962), Chavin (1966), Bara (1968); in anurans: Chieffi and Botte (1963), Rapola (1963), Hanke and Weber (1964), Gallien *et al.* (1964), Mukherji (1968), Pehlemann and Hanke (1968), Piezzi and Burgos (1968); in urodeles: Berchtold (1967, 1968b), Berchtold and Hugon (1971), Peyrot and Vellano

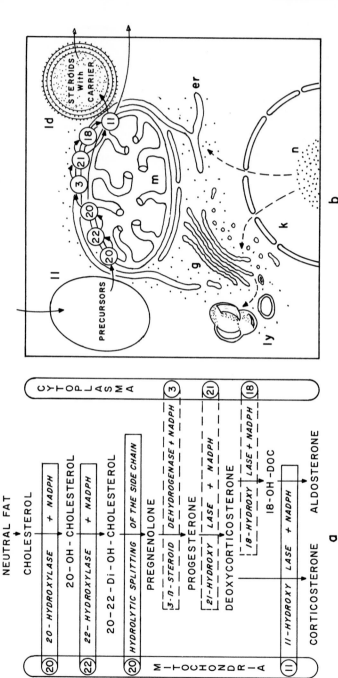

Fig. 40. Relationship between steroid synthesis (a) and cell organelles (b) in frog interrenal cell, according to Pehlemann and Hanke (1968). Corticosterone may also be the precursor of aldosterone (through 18-OH-corticosterone), and 18-hydroxylase may be a mitochondrial rather than a microsomal enzyme, at least in some species. In vertebrates other than amphibians, reptiles, and birds (wherein cortisol apparently is not synthesized), an additional microsomal enzyme would be present, namely, 17α-hydroxylase, active on progesterone and leading to 17α-OH-progesterone, deoxycortisol, cortisol, and cortisone (er, smooth endoplasmic reticulum; g, Golgi apparatus; k, nucleus; ld, electron-dense lipid droplet; ll, electron–lucent lipid droplet; ly, lysosomes; m, mitochondrion with tubular cristae; n, nucleolus). Solid arrows indicate pathways of steroid synthesis from precursors to steroid bound to carrier; broken arrows indicate cellular responses activated by ACTH (increased activity of membrane systems, production of synthetic organelles and lysosomes).

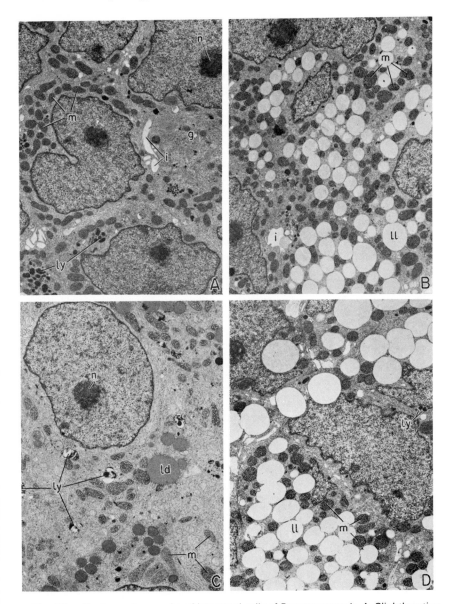

Fig. 41. Electron micrographs of interrenal cells of *Rana temporaria*. A, Slightly active cells from peripheral zone of normal interrenal; B, Inactive cells from central zone of normal interrenal; C, hyperactive cell after ACTH treatment; D, Inactive cell 3 weeks after hypophysectomy (g, Golgi apparatus; i, intercellular space; ld, electron-dense lipid droplet; ll, electron-lucent lipid droplet; ly, lysosomes; m, mitochondria; n, nucleolus). × 4680. (From F. W. Pehlemann, See Pehlemann and Hanke, 1968.)

(1968); in reptiles: Arvy (1962), Morat (1969): in birds: Ghosh (1962), Arvy (1962), Sinha and Ghosh (1964), Bhattacharyya *et al.* (1967)]. Activated cells show an increase in cytoplasmic basophilia (RNA) and steroid dehydrogenases and a decrease in lipids, cholesterol, and ascorbic acid. However, the extent of transport of ascorbic acid into the adrenal varies with the species and this is reflected in normal concentration values and in degree of depletion with interrenal activation (de Nicola *et al.*, 1968).

2. Functional Zonation

Adrenocortical zonation is generally considered to be a mammalian characteristic, and indeed functionally speaking this may prove to be unreservedly correct. However, a clear suggestion of interrenal zonation is reported for some birds (see Chester Jones, 1957; Sivaram, 1965; Kondics and Kjaerheim, 1966), the looping peripheral cords being distinguishable from the more central cords, and in some snakes. In the cobra (Lofts and Phillips, 1965), for example, the outer subcapsular cortical zone is clearly distinguishable from the inner cortical tissue throughout the year. Kondics (1963) claims that the external interrenal cells in the pigeon secrete mineralocorticoids; however, Bhattacharjee and Ghosh (1964) do not support any functional zonation in this species. Moens and Coessens (1970) report a differential seasonal response of central and peripheral interrenal cells in the sparrow (*Passer domesticus*). There is evidence in some avian species for a differential response to hypophysectomy, which may reveal zonal differences more clearly. In view of the constant occurence of aldosterone-secreting ability in all tetrapods, and the relegation of this capacity primarily to the zona glomerulosa in mammals, it would not be surprising if a meaningful zonation, or at least the existence of two types of interrenal cell populations, were ultimately demonstrable in tetrapods generally.

On histometric grounds, Gaudray (1967) has distinguished between an external zone of smaller cells (and nuclei) and an internal (renal) zone of larger cells in the interrenal tissue of *Rana esculenta*, a distinction which persists even after ACTH stimulation. After metopirone injections, the renal zone is particularly stimulated, suggesting a functional significance of the zonation (Gaudray, 1968). Evidence for zonation was also given by Hanke and Weber (1965) and van Kemenade and van Dongen (1965) in *R. temporaria*, but they noted its disappearance after stimulation of the tissue. In any case, the latter observations indicate that the larger cells are external (on both subcapsular and renal sides), whereas the central cells in the less stimulated animal are smaller in this species (Fig. 36). Accordingly, there may be no real functional zonation in this species but merely differences in secretory activity of a single cell type (van Kemenade *et al.*, 1968). In *R.*

adspersa, Moorhouse (1963) found no evidence of zonation. A sophisticated ultracytophysiological analysis of the interrenal tissue in *Rana catesbeiana* by Varma (1971) indicates the presence of two cell types, one possibly concerned with aldosterone secretion and the other with "glucocorticoid" secretion. At present, one can only note with interest the morphological indications of functional differentiation in those few species where such has been reported and await critical comparisons of steroidogenic capacity of different regions (parallel to the studies of catecholamine-secreting cells in reptiles—see Section IV,A,3).

3. Seasonal Variation

The interrenal tissue undergoes seasonal changes in morphology and may vary considerably in different individuals of the same species depending upon other physiological correlates. Adrenal gland weights are generally greater in the summer than in the winter. An adrenal–gonad relationship has long been recognized in mammals; it appears to be of similar significance in nonmammalian vertebrates as well—at least in elasmobranchs (e.g., Fancello, 1937), teleosts (e.g., Honma, 1959), amphibians, and reptiles. In general, the peak of seasonal activity, as judged histologically, would seem to correspond to the end of the reproductive period. In the anadromous spawning migration of salmonids, for example, a dramatic hyperplasia of interrenal tissue occurs. Whether this is physiologically activated tissue at this time, or a pathological response (in terms of pituitary basophilism or Selyean stress), remains a debatable point (e.g., Robertson and Wexler, 1959, 1960; Oguri, 1960c,d; Honma, 1960; Robertson *et al.*, 1961; McBride and van Overbeeke, 1969), but Hane *et al.* (1966) have found that the terminal hyperplasia is accompanied by decreased steroidogenic response to ACTH. Less prominent changes correlative with gonadal function are seen in other teleost species (Honma and Tamura, 1963; Honma, 1966; Chambolle, 1967; Yaron, 1970; Yadav *et al.*, 1970) although interrenal stimulation consequent to thyroid activation remains a possibility (cf. Chavin, 1966). Temporary interrenal hypertrophy may also occur in the catadromous migration (smoltification) of *Salmo salar* (Olivereau, 1960, 1962), although again "stress" may be the significant factor. In general, transfer of teleosts (Olivereau, 1966a; Hanke *et al.*, 1969) or birds (Péczely, 1964) to different salinities may result in histological evidence of interrenal activation. However, caution requires that conclusions regarding physiological hypercorticism not be based solely on histological responses.

In winter, the toad *Bufo arenarum* shows fewer signs of physiological activity than in summer. The former cells show more lipid, glycogen, and lysosomes; the latter show more Δ^5-3β-HSDH activity, smooth endoplasmic reticulum ribonucleoprotein particles, and dense mitochondria (Piezzi and Burgos, 1968). In *Rana temporaria*, high interrenal secretory activity and weak cholesterol histochemical reaction are related to the peak of reproductive activity (van Kemenade *et al.*, 1968). In *Triturus alpestris*, the smooth endoplasmic reticulum of the interrenal cell is much better developed in the aquatic phase than in the terrestrial phase (Picheral, 1969).

In the Australian lizard *Leiolopisma rhomboidalis*, interrenal "activity" is greatest in males during the hot, wet season and correlates to some extent with reproductive activity (Wilhoft, 1964). In general, Grignon and Grignon (1964) have indicated a direct correlation between sexual activity and interrenal secretion. However, in the cobra, as in *Vipera berus* (Saint Girons and Martoja, 1963), Tam *et al.* (1969) found no correlation between reproduction and the cycle of interrenal activity, and instead related the spring surge of activity with increased social behavior (arousal). "Stress" causes interrenal hypertrophy in *Natrix rhombifera* (Fickess, 1962).

In the cobra, a clearly defined seasonal cycle can be distinguished by histological and histochemical criteria (Lofts *et al.*, 1971). The winter phase from about late October to January is marked by cortical cells showing little signs of activity. They are densely sudanophilic and strongly cholesterol positive, and some cellular necrosis is apparent during this time. This quiescent phase is succeeded by a period of high activity in the spring, and cellular hypertrophy together with a depletion of lipids and cholesterol takes place at this time. The adrenal weight continues to rise after the copulatory period in April; then in June a sharp reduction in cellular size sets in, paralleled by an increase in the cytoplasmic lipid content and cholesterol reaction. This stage persists until September. Before the approach of winter, there is a short but well-defined period of activity marked by a temporary increase in cortical cell size and number and adrenal weight, which probably reflects a recrudescence of pituitary function since it also coincides with the seasonal start of the spermatogenetic cycle. These events are summarized in Fig. 42 (Lofts *et al.*, 1971). The biosynthetic capacity for corticosterone production from labeled precursors closely parallels the above events, being greatest during the spring period (Tam *et al.*, 1969).

Lorenzen and Farner (1964) found distinct seasonal changes in the white-crowned sparrow (*Zonotrichia leucophrys gambelii*) adrenal, where the amount of interrenal (cortical) tissue and sudanophilia are highest in winter and spring and lowest in summer. Inasmuch as hyperplasia is interpreted as implying activity and lipid storage inactivity, it is not possible to reconcile (and interpret) these findings functionally. Minimal interrenal tissue is evident when thyroid activity is lowest and testicular activity is highest. In the European blackbird, however, increased thyroid activity just precedes maximal interrenal tissue, and both are at a minimum simultaneously

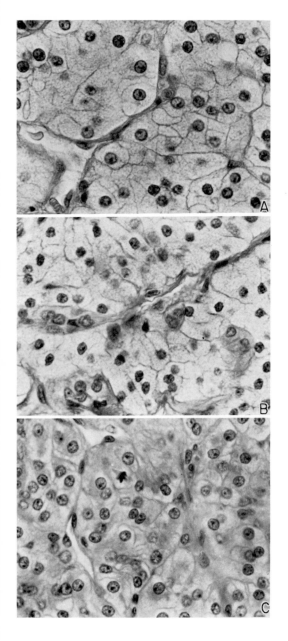

Fig. 42. Seasonal changes in cobra (*Naja naja*) interrenal cells. A, April; nuclear and cellular hypertrophy (accompanied by lipid and cholesterol depletion). B, June; atrophy (accompanied by increased cytoplasmic lipid and cholesterol). C. September; hyperplasia (note mitotic figure); small cells with large spherical nuclei. (Lofts *et al.*, 1971).

(Fromme-Bouman, 1962). Hall (1968) found a correlation between maximal amount of interrenal tissue with maturation of the gonads and onset of breeding in the Eastern rosella *Platycercus eximuis*, unlike the situation in *Zonotrichia*. The experimental analysis of responses of the pigeon adrenal to gonadectomy and gonadal steroids indicates similarities to mammalian responses, with no consistent correlation evident between gonadal state and adrenal weight and histology (Bhattacharyya, 1968). Soulé and Assenmacher (1966) found an inverse correlation between plasma corticosterone levels and the testis cycle in the duck. There would appear to be important species differences, and one must question whether a positive correlation, when observed, really represents any functional relation.

4. Functional Control

The mammalian control systems involving ACTH stimulation of gluco-corticoid secretion and angiotensin II stimulation of aldosterone secretion are both found in nonmammalian vertebrates, although the latter has been established only in birds (deRoos and deRoos, 1963). Adrenocortical cel-lular responses after ACTH stimulation and after hypophysectomy seem well established in representatives of all vertebrate groups in which they have been studied, and negative feedback responses are also evident when glucocorticoids are injected [see, as examples, in cyclostomes: Sterba (1955), Chester Jones (1963); in teleosts: Mahon *et al.* (1962), Handin *et al.* (1964), Olivereau (1965, 1966b), Basu *et al.* (1965), Ball and Olivereau (1966), Donaldson and McBride (1967), Hanke *et al.* (1967), Sundararaj and Gos-wami (1968), Butler *et al.* (1969), Dixit (1970), Fleming *et al.* (1971); in lungfish: Janssens *et al.* (1965); in amphibians: Piper and de Roos (1967), Suzuki (1968), van Kemenade (1968a,b), Gaudray (1968), Leist *et al.* (1969), Hanke and Pehlemann (1969); in reptiles: Ramaswami (1966); in birds: Sinha and Ghosh (1964), Bhattacharyya *et al.* (1967), Boissin (1967), Kjaer-heim (1968b,c,d)].

However, there are some discrepancies in regard to the ability of ACTH to stimulate steroidogenesis by poikilothermic interrenals, and Gist and deRoos (1966) have suggested a distinction between two tropic consequen-ces of ACTH: stimulation of steroidogenic pathways and stimulation of cell growth and anabolism ("histological" responses). The latter effect may be the more important in at least some poikilotherms (see also Hanke, 1966; Macchi, 1966; Sekiguchi, 1968; Leloup-Hatey, 1968; Mialhe and Koch, 1969). Frankel and Nalbandov (1966) emphasized the relative pituitary independence of the cockerel adrenal compared with that of mammals.

REFERENCES

Ábrahám, A. (1969). *Gen. Comp. Endocrinol.* **13**, 489.
Ahsan, S. N. (1966). *Can. J. Zool.* **44**, 703.
Arai, R., Tajima, H., and Tamaoki, B. (1969). *Gen. Comp. Endocrinol.* **12**, 99.
Arvy, L. (1962). *C.R. Acad. Sci.* **255**, 1803.
Arvy, L., and Hadjiisky, P. (1970). *C.R. Ass. Anat.* **54**, 50.
Ball, J. N. (1960). *Symp. Zool. Soc. (London)* **1**, 105.
Ball, J. N., and Olivereau, M. (1966). *Gen. Comp. Endocrinol.* **6**, 5.
Banerji, T. K., and Ghosh, A. (1965). "Proceedings of the Zoological Seminar 1965, Ujjain, M.P., India," pp. 61–68.
Bara, G. (1965a). *Gen. Comp. Endocrinol.* **5**, 284.
Bara, G. (1965b). *Experientia* **21**, 638.
Bara, G. (1968). *Gen. Comp. Endocrinol.* **10**, 126.
Bara, G. (1969). *Gen. Comp. Endocrinol.* **13**, 189.
Barr, W. A. (1965). *In* "Oceanography and Marine Biology. An Annual Review" (H. Barnes, ed.), Vol. III, pp. 257–298. Allen & Unwin, London.
Barrington, E. J. W. (1963). "An Introduction to General and Comparative Anatomy." Oxford Univ. Press (Clarendon), London and New York.
Barrington, E. J. W., and Jørgensen, C. B. (1968). "Perspectives in Endocrinology: Hormones in the Lives of Lower Vertebrates." Academic Press, New York.
Basu, J., Nandi, J., and Bern, H. A. (1965). *J. Exp. Zool.* **159**, 347.
Bell, J. B. G., Vinson, G. P., Hopkin, D. J., and Lacy, D. (1968). *Biochim. Biophys. Acta* **164**, 412.
Belt, W. D., and Pease, D. C. (1956). *J. Biophys. Biochem. Cytol.* **2**, 369.
Belt, W. D., Sheridan, M. N., Knouff, R. A., and Hartman, F. A. (1965). *Z. Zellforsch. Mikrosk. Anat.* **68**, 864.
Benedeczky, I. (1967). *Acta Morphol.* **15**, 271.
Benoit, J. (1950). *In* "Traité de Zoologie" (P. P. Grassé, ed.), Vol. 15, pp. 384–478. Masson, Paris.
Berchtold, J. P. (1967). *Ann. Endocrinol.* **28**, 299.
Berchtold, J. P. (1968a). *C.R. Acad. Sci.* **266**, 155.
Berchtold, J. P. (1968b). *C.R. Acad. Sci.* **266**, 2345.
Berchtold, J. P. (1969a). *Gen. Comp. Endocrinol.* **13**, 493.
Berchtold, J. P. (1969b). *Z. Zellforsch. Mikrosk. Anat.* **102**, 357.
Berchtold, J. P. (1970). *Z. Zellforsch. Mikrosk. Anat.* **110**, 517.
Berchtold, J. P., and Hugon, J. S. (1971). *Histochemie* **26**, 258.
Bern, H. A. (1967a). *Science* **158**, 455.
Bern, H. A. (1967b). *Amer. Zool.* **7**, 815.
Bern, H. A., and Nandi, J. (1964). *In* "The Hormones" (G. Pincus, K. V. Thimann, and E. B. Astwood, eds.), Vol. IV, pp. 199–298. Academic Press, New York.
Bern, H. A., and Nicoll, C. S. (1969). *Excerpta Med. Found. Int. Congr. Ser.* **184**, 433.
Betz, T. W. (1963). *J. Morphol.* **113**, 245.
Bhattacharjee, D., and Ghosh, A. (1964). *Endokrinologie* **46**, 262.
Bhattacharyya, T. K. (1968). *Zool. Anz.* **180**, 155.
Bhattacharyya, T. K., Sarkar, A. K., Ghosh, A., and Ganguli, A. (1967). *J. Exp. Zool.* **165**, 301.
Björkman, N. (1962). *Acta Anat.* **51**, 125.
Boissin, J. (1967). *J. Physiol. (Paris)* **59**, 423.
Botte, V. (1963). *Acta Med. Romana* **1**, 1.
Botte, V. (1964). *Atti Soc. Peloritana Sci. Fis. Mat. Natur.* **10**, 521.

Botte, V., and Cottino, E. (1964). *Boll. Zool.* **31**, 491.
Botte, V., and Delrio, G. (1965). *Boll. Zool.* **32**, 191.
Botte, V., and Rosati, P. (1964). *Acta Med. Vet.* **10**, 1.
Botte, V., Delrio, G., and Lupo di Prisco, P. (1966). *Excerpta Med. Found. Int. Congr. Ser.* **111**, 370.
Boucek, R. J., and Savard, K. (1970). *Gen. Comp. Endocrinol.* **15**, 6.
Boyd, M. M. M. (1940). *Quart. J. Microsc. Sci.* **82**, 337.
Bragdon, D. E. (1951). *J. Exp. Zool.* **118**, 419.
Brant, J. W. A., and Nalbandov, A. V. (1956). *Poultry Sci.* **35**, 692.
Bretschneider, L. H., and de Wit, J. J. D. (1947). "Sexual Endocrinology of Non-mammalian Vertebrates." Elsevier, Amsterdam.
Brökelmann, J. (1964). *Z. Zellforsch. Mikrosk. Anat.* **64**, 429.
Browning, H. C. (1969). *Gen. Comp. Endocrinol. Suppl.* **2**, 42.
Burgos, M. H. (1959). *Anat. Rec.* **133**, 163.
Burrows, H. (1949). "Biological Actions of Sex Hormones." Cambridge Univ. Press, London and New York.
Busson-Mabillot, S. (1967). *J. Microsc. (Paris)* **6**, 807.
Butler, D. G., Donaldson, E. M., and Clarke, W. C. (1969). *Gen. Comp. Endocrinol.* **12**, 173.
Callard, I. P. (1967). *J. Endocrinol.* **37**, 105.
Callard, I. P., and Leathem, J. H. (1965). *Arch. Anat. Microsc. Morphol. Exp.* **54**, 35.
Certain, P., Collenot, G., Collenot, A., and Ozon, R. (1964). *C.R. Soc. Biol.* **158**, 1040.
Chambolle, P. (1967). *C.R. Acad. Sci.* **265**, 1514.
Chan, S. T. H. (1968). "The Endocrinology of Sex-reversal in the Ricefield Eel, *Monopterus albus* (Zuiew)." Thesis, University of Hong Kong.
Chan, S. T. H. (1970). *Phil. Trans. Roy. Soc. Lond. B.* **259**, 59.
Chan, S. T. H., and Phillips, J. G. (1967). *J. Zool.* **152**, 31.
Channing, C. P. (1966). *Nature (London)* **210**, 1266.
Channing, C. P., and Grieves, S. A. (1969). *J. Endocrinol.* **43**, 391.
Chavin, W. (1966). *Gen. Comp. Endocrinol.* **6**, 183.
Chavin, W., and Kovacevic, A. (1961). *Gen. Comp. Endocrinol.* **1**, 264.
Chester Jones, I. (1957). "The Adrenal Cortex." Cambridge Univ. Press, London and New York.
Chester Jones, I. (1963). *In* "Biology of Myxine" (A. Brodal and R. Fange, eds.), pp. 488–502. Oslo Univ. Press, Oslo.
Chester Jones, I., Henderson, I. W., and Mosley, W. (1964). *J. Endocrinol.* **30**, 155.
Chester Jones, I., Henderson, I. W., Chan, D. K. O., and Rankin, J. C. (1966). *Excerpta Med. Found. Int. Congr. Ser.* **132**, 136.
Chester Jones, I., Chan, D. K. O., Henderson, I. W., and Ball, J. N. (1969). *In* "Fish Physiology" (W. S. Hoar and D. J. Randall, eds.), Vol. 2, pp. 321–376. Academic Press, New York.
Chieffi, G. (1961). *Pubbl. Sta. Zool. Napoli* **32**, 145.
Chieffi, G. (1965). *Riv. Biol.* **58**, 285.
Chieffi, G. (1967a). *Excerpta Med. Found. Int. Congr. Ser.* **132**, 1047.
Chieffi, G. (1967b). *In* "Sharks, Skates and Rays" (P. W. Gilbert, R. F. Mathewson, and D. P. Rall, eds.), pp. 553–580, Johns Hopkins Press, Baltimore, Maryland.
Chieffi, G., and Botte, V. (1963). *Riv. Istochim. Norm. Patol.* **9**, 172.
Chieffi, G., and Botte, V. (1965). *Experientia* **21**, 16.
Chieffi, G., and Gualà, L., (1959). *Boll. Zool.* **26**, 121.
Chieffi, G., and Lupo, C. (1961). *Atti Accad. Naz. Lincei Cl. Sci. Fis. Mat. Natur. Rend.* **30**, 399.

Christensen, A. K. (1965). *J. Cell Biol.* **26**, 911.
Christensen, A. K., and Mason, N. R. (1965). *Endocrinology* **76**, 646.
Christensen, A. K., and Gillim, S. W. (1969). *In* "The Gonads" (K. W. McKerns, ed.), pp. 415–488. North-Holland Publ., Amsterdam.
Cieslak, E. S. (1945). *Physiol. Zool.* **18**, 299.
Clausen, H. J. (1935). *Anat. Rec.* **64**, 88.
Clausen, H. J. (1940). *Endocrinology*, **27**, 700.
Collenot, G., and Ozon, R. (1964). *Bull. Soc. Zool. Fr.* **89**, 577.
Collins, P. M., Bell, J. B. G., and Vinson, G. P. (1968). *Proc. VI Congr. Int. Reprod. Anim. Insem. Artif.* **1**, 261.
Colombo, L., Bern, H. A., and Pieprzyk, J. (1970). *Gen. Comp. Endocrinol.* **16**, 74.
Conner, M. H., and Fraps, R. M. (1954). *Poultry Sci.* **33**, 1051.
Craig-Bennett, A. (1931). *Phil. Trans. Roy. Soc. London Ser.* B **219**, 197.
Dahl, E. (1971). *Z. Zellforsch. Mikrosk. Anat.* **119**, 58.
Deane, H. W. (1962). *In* "The Adrenocortical Hormones: Their Origin, Chemistry, Physiology and Pharmacology" (H. W. Deane, ed.), Part 1, pp. 1–185. Springer-Verlag, Berlin and New York.
Deane, H. W., Hay, M. F., Moor, R. M., Ronson, L. E. A., and Short, R. V. (1966). *Acta Endocrinol. (Copenhagen)* **51**, 245.
Della Corte, F., Galgano, M., and Cosenza, L. (1962). *Arch. Zool. Ital.* **47**, 353.
Della Corte, F., Galgano, M., and Varano, L. (1969). *Z. Zellforsch. Mikrosk. Anat.* **98**, 561.
Delrio, G., Botte, V., and Chieffi, G. (1968). *In* "Enzyme Histochemistry." Simp. Antonio Baselli, May 1967.
de Nicola, A. F., Clayman, M., and Johnstone, R. M. (1968). *Gen. Comp. Endocrinol.* **11**, 332.
deRoos, R. (1963). *Proc. XIII Int. Ornithol. Congr.* **2**, 1041.
deRoos, R., and deRoos, C. C. (1963). *Science* **141**, 1284.
De Smet, W. (1962). *Acta Zool. (Stockholm)* **43**, 201.
De Smet, W. (1963). *Acta Zool. (Stockholm)* **44**, 269.
De Smet, W. (1970). *Anat. Anz.* **126**, 391.
Dixit, V. P. (1970). *Acta anat.* **77**, 310.
Dodd, J. M., Perks, A. M., and Dodd, M. H. I. (1966). *In* "The Pituitary Gland" (G. W. Harris and B. T. Donovan, eds.), Vol. 3, pp. 578–623. Univ. of California Press, Berkeley.
Doerr-Schott, J. (1964). *C.R. Acad. Sci.* **258**, 2896.
Donaldson, E. M., and McBride, J. R. (1967). *Gen. Comp. Endocrinol.* **9**, 93.
Dufaure, J.- P. (1970). *J. Microsc. (Paris)* **9**, 89.
Dutta, S. K. (1944). *Allahabad Univ. Stud. Zool. Sec.* **57**, 153.
Evennett, P. J., and Dodd, J. M. (1963). *Nature (London)* **197**, 715.
Fancello, O. (1937). *Pubbl. Sta. Zool. Napoli* **16**, 80.
Fickess, D. R. (1962). *Herpetologica* **18**, 250.
Fleming, W. R., Ball, J. N., and Conaway, C. H. (1971). *Z. vergl. Physiol.* **74**, 121.
Follenius, E. (1953). *Bull. Biol. Fr. Belg.* **87**, 68.
Follenius, E., and Porte, A. (1960). *Experientia* **16**, 190.
Follett, B. K., Nicholls, T. J., and Redshaw, M. R. (1968). *J. Cell. Physiol.* **72**, Suppl. 1, 91.
Fontaine, M. (1963). *Proc. XVI Int. Congr. Zool.* **3**, 25.
Fraenkel, L., Martins, T., and Mello, R. F. (1940). *Endocrinology* **27**, 836.
Franchi, L. L. (1962). *In* "The Ovary" (S. Zuckerman, ed.), pp. 121–142. Academic Press, New York.
Frankel, A. I., and Nalbandov, A. V. (1966). *Excerpta Med. Found. Int. Congr. Ser.* **111**, 106.
Fraps, R. M. (1955). *Mem. Soc. Endocrinol.* **4**, 205.

Fratini, L. (1953). *Pubbl. Sta. Zool. Napoli* **24**, 201.
Fromme-Bouman, H. (1962). *Vogelwarte* **21**, 188.
Fujita, H., Manchino, M., and Tokura, T. (1963). *Arch. Histol. (Japan)* **24**, 77.
Furr, B. J. A. (1969). *Gen. Comp. Endocrinol.* **13**, Abstracts 56 and 57.
Furr, B. J. A., and Cunningham, F. J. (1970). *Brit. Poult. Sci.* **11**, 7.
Furr, B. J. A., and Pope, G. S. (1970). *Steroids* **16**, 471.
Gabe, M., and Martoja, M. (1962). *Arch. Anat. Microsc. Morphol. Exp.* **51**, 107.
Gabe, M., and Rancurel, R. (1964). *Arch. Anat. Microsc. Morphol. Exp.* **53**, 225.
Gabe, M., and Saint Girons, H. (1962). *Acta Anat.* **50**, 22.
Gabe, M., and Saint Girons, H. (1964). *C.R. Acad. Sci.* **258**, 3559.
Gabe, M., Martoja, M., and Saint Girons, H. (1964). *Ann. Biol.* **3**, 304.
Galil, A. K. A., and Deane, H. W. (1966). *J. Reprod. Fert.* **11**, 333.
Gallien, L., Certain, P., and Ozon, R. (1964). *C.R. Acad. Sci.* **258**, 5729.
Galli-Mainini, C. (1950). *Rev. Soc. Argent. Biol.* **26**, 166.
Garnier, D. H., and Attal, J. (1970). *C. R. Acad. Sci.* **270**, 2472.
Gaudray, A. (1967). *C.R. Soc. Biol.* **161**, 2360.
Gaudray, A. (1968). *C.R. Soc. Biol.* **162**, 381.
Gérard, P. (1951). *Arch. Biol.* **62**, 371.
Ghosh, A. (1962). *Gen. Comp. Endocrinol. Suppl.* **1**, 75.
Ghosh, I., and Ghosh, A. (1962). *Proc. Zool. Soc. Calcutta* **15**, 135.
Giacomini, E. (1933). *Boll. Soc. Ital. Biol. Sper.* **8**, 1215.
Gist, D. H., and deRoos, R. (1966). *Gen. Comp. Endocrinol.* **7**, 304.
Gorbman, A., and Bern, H. A. (1962). "A Textbook of Comparative Endocrinology," pp. 297–339. Wiley, New York.
Green, J. A., and Maqueo, M. (1965). *Amer. J. Obstet. Gynecol.* **92**, 946.
Green, J. D. (1966). *In* "The Pituitary Gland" (G. W. Harris and B. T. Donovan, eds.), Vol. 1, pp. 127–146. Univ. of California Press, Berkeley.
Grier, H. J. (1970). *Am. Zool.* **10**, 498.
Grignon, G., and Grignon, M. (1964). *Excerpta Med. Found. Int. Congr. Ser.* **83**, 106.
Guraya, S. S. (1965). *J. Morphol.* **117**, 151.
Guraya, S. S. (1968). *Gen. Comp. Endocrinol.* **10**, 138.
Hall, B. K. (1968). *Aust. J. Zool.* **16**, 609.
Handin, R. I., Nandi, J., and Bern, H. A. (1964). *J. Exp. Zool.* **157**, 339.
Hane, S., Robertson, O. H., Wexler, B. C., and Krupp, M. A. (1966). *Endocrinology* **78**, 791.
Hanke, W. (1966). *Excerpta Med. Found. Int. Congr. Ser.* **111**, 104.
Hanke, W., and Pehlemann, F. W. (1969). *Gen. Comp. Endocrinol.* **13**, 509.
Hanke, W., and Weber, K. (1964). *Gen. Comp. Endocrinol.* **4**, 662.
Hanke, W., and Weber, K. (1965). *Gen. Comp. Endocrinol.* **5**, 144.
Hanke, W., Bergerhoff, K., and Chan, D. K. O. (1967). *Gen. Comp. Endocrinol.* **9**, 64.
Hanke, W., Bergerhoff, K., and Chan, D. K. O. (1969). *Gen. Comp. Endocrinol. Suppl.* **2**, 331.
Hardisty, M. W., and Baines, M. E. (1971). *Experientia* **27**, 1072.
Hardisty, M. W., and Barnes, K. (1968). *Nature (London)* **218**, 880.
Hardisty, M. W., Rothwell, B., and Steele, K. (1967). *J. Zool.* **152**, 9.
Harrison, G. A. (1966). *J. Ultrastruct. Res.* **14**, 158.
Harrison Matthews, L. (1955). *Mem. Soc. Endocrinol.* **4**, 129.
Hartman, F. A., and Brownell, K. A. (1949). "The Adrenal Gland." Lea & Febiger, Philadelphia.
Henderson, N. E. (1962). *Can. J. Zool.* **40**, 631.
Hiroi, O., and Yamamoto, K. (1970). *Bull. Fac. Fish. Hokkaido Univ.* **20**, 252.
Hoar, W. S. (1955). *Mem. Soc. Endocrinol.* **4**, 5.

Hoar, W. S. (1957). *In* "The Physiology of Fishes" (M. E. Brown, ed.), Vol. 1, pp. 245–286. Academic Press, New York.

Hoar, W. S. (1962). *Gen. Comp. Endocrinol. Suppl.* **1**, 206.

Holstein, A. F. (1969). *Z. Zellforsch. Mikrosk. Anat.* **93**, 265.

Honma, Y. (1959). *J. Fac. Sci. Niigata Univ. Ser. 11.* **2**, 225.

Honma, Y. (1960). *Annot. Zool. Jap.* **33**, 234.

Honma, Y. (1966). *La Mer* **4**, 27.

Honma, Y., and Tamura, E. (1963). *Zoologica (New York)* **48**, 25.

Houssay, B. A., Wassermann, G. F., and Tramezzani, J. H. (1962). *Arch. Int. Pharmacodyn. Ther.* **140**, 84.

Idelman, S. (1970). *Int. Rev. Cytol.* **27**, 181.

Idler, D. R., and Freeman, H. C. (1966). *J. Fish. Res. Bd. Can.* **23**, 1249.

Idler, D. R., and O'Halloran, M. J. (1970). *J. Endocrinol.* **48**, 621.

Idler, D. R., and Sangalang, G. B. (1970). *J. Endocrinol.* **48**, 627.

Jacoby, F. (1962). *In* "The Ovary" (S. Zuckerman, ed.), pp. 189–245. Academic Press, New York.

Janssens, P. A. (1964). *Excerpta Med. Found. Int. Congr. Ser.* **83**, 95.

Janssens, P. A., Vinson, G. P., Chester Jones, I., and Mosley, W. (1965). *J. Endocrinol.* **32**, 373.

Joly, J. (1965). *C.R. Acad. Sci.* **261**, 1569.

Joly, J., Picheral, B., and Boisseau, C. (1969). *Gen. Comp. Endocrinol.* **13**, 510.

Jørgensen, C. B., and Larsen, L. O. (1963). *Symp. Zool. Soc. (London)* **9**, 59.

Khiruvathukal, K. V. (1967). *Amer. Zool.* **7**, 809.

Kjaerheim, A. (1968a). *Z. Zellforsch. Mikrosk. Anat.* **91**, 429.

Kjaerheim, A. (1968b). *Z. Zellforsch. Mikrosk. Anat.* **91**, 456.

Kjaerheim, A. (1968c). *J. Microsc. (Paris)* **7**, 715.

Kjaerheim, A. (1968d). *J. Microsc. (Paris)* **7**, 739.

Kondics, L. (1963). *Acta Biol. (Budapest)* **13**, 48.

Kondics, L., and Kjaerheim, A. (1966). *Z. Zellforsch. Mikrosk. Anat.* **70**, 81.

Krishnamurthy, V. G., and Bern, H. A. (1969). *Gen. Comp. Endocrinol.* **13**, 313.

Krishnamurthy, V. G., and Bern, H. A. (1971). *Gen. Comp. Endorcinol.* **16**, 162.

Lacy, D. (1967). *Endeavour* **26**, 101.

Lacy, D., Vinson, G. P., Collins, P., Bell, J., Fyson, P., Pudney, J., and Pettitt, A. J. (1969). *Excerpta. Med. Found. Int. Congr. Ser.* **184**, 1019.

Lakshman, A. B. (1964). *Endocrinol. Jap.* **11**, 169.

Lambert, J. G. D. (1966). *Experientia* **22**, 476.

Lambert, J. G. D. (1970). *Gen. Comp. Endocrinol.* **15**, 464.

Lambert, J. G. D., and van Oordt, P. G. W. J. (1965). *Gen. Comp. Endocrinol.* **5**, 693.

Lamotte, M., and Rey, P. (1954). *C.R. Acad. Sci.* **238**, 393.

Lance, V. A. (1971). Unpublished results.

Lance, V. A. (1968). "Ovarian Functions in the Ovoviviparous Elasmobranch *Squalus acanthias:* A Histological and Histochemical Study." M.Sc. thesis, College of William and Mary, Williamsburg, Virginia.

Lance, V., and Callard, I. P. (1969). *Gen. Comp. Endocrinol.* **13**, 255.

Larsen, L. O. (1965). *Gen. Comp. Endocrinol.* **5**, 16.

Larsen, L. O. (1970). *Biol. Reprod.* **2**, 37.

Lehri, G. K. (1967). *Acta Anat.* **67**, 135.

Leist, K. H., Bergerhoff, K., Pehlemann, F. W., and Hanke, W. (1969). *Z. Zellforsch. Mikrosk. Anat.* **93**, 105.

Leloup-Hatey, J. (1968). *Comp. Biochem. Physiol.* **26**, 997.

Lofts, B. (1961). *Gen. Comp. Endocrinol.* **1**, 179.
Lofts, B. (1964). *Gen. Comp. Endocrinol.* **4**, 550.
Lofts, B. (1965). *Excerpta Med. Found. Int. Congr. Ser.* **83**, 100.
Lofts, B. (1968a). *Gen. Comp. Endocrinol. Suppl.* **2**, 147.
Lofts, B. (1968b). *In* "Perspectives in Endocrinology: Hormones in the Lives of Lower Vertebrates" (E. J. W. Barrington and C. B. Jørgensen, eds.), pp. 239–304. Academic Press, New York.
Lofts, B. (1972). *Gen. Comp. Endocrinol. Suppl.* **3**, In press.
Lofts, B., and Boswell, C. (1960). *Nature (London)* **187**, 708.
Lofts, B., and Boswell, C. (1961). *Proc. Zool. Soc. London* **136**, 581.
Lofts, B., and Chan, M. B. (1971). Unpublished results.
Lofts, B., and Marshall, A. J. (1957). *Quart. J. Microsc. Sci.* **98**, 79.
Lofts, B., and Marshall, A. J. (1959). *J. Endocrinol.* **19**, 16.
Lofts, B., and Phillips, J. G. (1965). *J. Endocrinol.* **33**, 327.
Lofts, B., and Tso, E. (1971). Unpublished results.
Lofts, B., Phillips, J. G., and Tam, W. H. (1966a). *Gen. Comp. Endocrinol.* **6**, 466.
Lofts, B., Pickford, G. E., and Atz, J. W. (1966b). *Gen. Comp. Endocrinol.* **6**, 74.
Lofts, B., Phillips, J. G., and Tam, W. H. (1971). *Gen. Comp. Endocrinol.* **16**, 121.
Lofts, B., Wellen, J., and Benraad, T. (1972). *Gen. Comp. Endocrinol.* In press.
Lorenzen, L. C., and Farner, D. S. (1964). *Gen. Comp. Endocrinol.* **4**, 253.
Lupo, C., Botte, V., and Chieffi, G. (1965). *Boll. Zool.* **32**, 185.
Lupo di Prisco. C. (1968). *Riv. Biol.* **61**, 113.
Lupo di Prisco, C., Materazzi, G., and Chieffi, G. (1970). *Gen. Comp. Endocrinol.* **14**, 595.
Lyngnes, R. (1936). *Skr. Norske VidenskAkad., Oslo, I. Mat. Naturv. Kl.* **4**, 1.
McBride, J. R., and van Overbeeke, A. P. (1969). *J. Fish Res. Bd. Can.* **29**, 2975.
Macchi, I. A. (1966). *Excerpta Med. Found. Int. Congr. Ser.* **111**, 105.
Mahon, E. F., Hoar, W. S., and Tabata, S. (1962). *Can. J. Zool.* **40**, 449.
March, F. (1937). *Proc. Zool. Soc. London* **107**, 603.
Marshall, A. J. (1955). *Mem. Soc. Endocrinol.* **4**, 75.
Marshall, A. J. (1960). *Symp. Zool. Soc. (London)* **1**, 137.
Marshall, A. J., and Coombs, C. J. F. (1957). *Proc. Zool. Soc. London* **128**, 545.
Marshall, A. J., and Hook, R. (1960). *Proc. Zool. Soc. London* **134**, 197.
Marshall, A. J., and Lofts, B. (1956). *Nature (London)* **177**, 704.
Matty, A. J. (1966). *In* "International Review of General and Experimental Zoology" (W. J. L. Felts and R. J. Harrison, eds.), Vol. 2, pp. 43–138. Academic Press, New York.
Mesure, M. (1968). *C.R. Soc. Biol.* **162**, 422.
Mialhe, C., and Koch, B. (1969). *In* "La Spécificité Zoologique des Hormones Hypophysaires et de Leurs Activités," pp. 103–134. CNRS, Paris.
Miller, M. R. (1948). *Univ. Calif. Publ. Zool.* **47**, 197.
Miller, M. R. (1959). *In* "Comparative Endocrinology" (A. Gorbman, ed.), pp. 499–516. Wiley, New York.
Miller, M. R., and Robbins, M. E. (1954). *J. Exp. Zool.* **125**, 415.
Moens, L., and Coessens, R. (1970). *Gen. Comp. Endocrinol.* **15**, 95.
Moorhouse, D. E. (1963). *Quart. J. Microsc. Sci.* **104**, 51.
Morat, M. (1969). *Gen. Comp. Endocrinol.* **13**, 521.
Mukherji, M. (1968). *Acta Histochem.* **29**, 297.
Nagalakshmi, C. M. (1970). Personal communication.
Nandi, J. (1961). *Science* **134**, 389.
Nandi, J. (1962). *Univ. Calif. Publ. Zool.* **65**, 129.
Nandi, J. (1965). *Proc. Zool. Soc. Calcutta* **18**, 1.
Nandi, J. (1967). *Amer. Zool.* **7**, 115.

Nandi, J. (1968). Unpublished observations.
Nicholls, T. J. (1969). Unpublished results.
Nicholson, F. A., and Risley, P. L. (1940). *Proc. Iowa Acad. Sci.* **47**, 343.
Ogawa, M. (1962). *Sci. Rep. Saitama Univ. Ser. B* **4**, 107.
Ogawa, M. (1967). *Z. Zellforsch. Mikrosk. Anat.* **81**, 174.
Oguri, M. (1960a). *Bull. Jap. Soc. Sci. Fish.* **26**, 443.
Oguri, M. (1960b). *Bull. Jap. Soc. Sci. Fish.* **26**, 448.
Oguri, M. (1960c). *Bull. Jap. Soc. Sci. Fish.* **26**, 476.
Oguri, M. (1960d). *Bull. Jap. Soc. Sci. Fish.* **26**, 981.
O'Halloran, M. J., and Idler, D. R. (1970). *Gen. Comp. Endocrinol.* **15**, 361.
Olivereau, M. (1960). *Acta Endocrinol. (Copenhagen)* **33**, 142.
Olivereau, M. (1962). *Gen. Comp. Endocrinol.* **2**, 565.
Olivereau, M. (1965). *Gen. Comp. Endocrinol.* **5**, 109.
Olivereau, M. (1966a). *Ann. Endocrinol.* **27**, 549.
Olivereau, M. (1966b). *Ann. Endocrinol.* **27**, 665.
Olivereau, M. (1967). *Gen. Comp. Endocrinol.* **9**, 478.
Oota, I., and Yamamoto, K. (1966). *Annot. Zool. Jap.* **39**, 142.
Ozon, R. (1965). *Gen. Comp. Endocrinol.* **5**, 704.
Ozon, R. (1967). *Gen. Comp. Endocrinol.* **8**, 214.
Ozon. R., and Collenot, G. (1955). *C.R. Soc. Biol.* **261**, 3204.
Panigel, M. (1956). *Ann. Sci. Natur. (Zool.)* **18**, 569.
Parkes, A. S., and Deanesly, R. (1966). *In* "Marshall's Physiology of Reproduction" (A. S. Parkes, ed.), pp. 570–828. Longmans, Green, New York.
Péczely, P. (1964). *Acta Biol. (Budapest)* **15**, 171.
Pehlemann, F. W. (1968). *Z. Zellforsch. Mikrosk. Anat.* **84**, 516.
Pehlemann, F. W., and Hanke, W. (1968). *Z. Zellforsch. Mikrosk. Anat.* **89**, 281.
Pehlemann, F. W., Hanke, W., and Bergerhoff, K. (1967). *Zool. Anz.* **31**, Suppl., 216.
Peyrot, A., and Vellano, C. (1968). *In* "Enzyme Histochemistry." Simp. Antonio Baselli, May 1967. Succ. Fusi, Pavia.
Picheral, B. (1968). *J. Microsc. (Paris)* **7**, 115.
Picheral, B. (1969). *Gen. Comp. Endocrinol.* **31**, 526.
Picheral, B. (1970). *Z. Zellforsch. Microsc. Anat.* **107**, 68.
Pickford, G. E., and Atz, J. W. (1957). "The Physiology of the Pituitary Gland of Fishes." New York Zoological Society, New York.
Pickford, G. E., Lofts, B., Bara, G., and Atz, J. W. (1972). *Biol. Reprod.* in press.
Piezzi, R. S. (1965). *Acta Physiol. Lat. Amer.* **15**, 96.
Piezzi, R. S. (1967). *Gen. Comp. Endocrinol.* **9**, 143.
Piezzi, R. S., and Burgos, M. H. (1968). *Gen. Comp. Endocrinol.* **10**, 344.
Piper, G. D., and deRoos, R. (1967). *Gen. Comp. Endocrinol.* **8**, 134.
Porte, A., and Weniger, J. P. (1961). *C.R. Soc. Biol.* **155**, 2181.
Rahn, H. (1942). *Copeia* **1942**, 231.
Ramaswami, L. S. (1966). *Excerpta Med. Found. Int. Congr. Ser.* **111**, 104.
Rapola, J. (1962). *Ann. Acad. Sci. Fenn. Ser. A4* **64**, 1.
Rapola, J. (1963). *Gen. Comp. Endocrinol.* **3**, 412.
Reddy, P. R. K., and Prasad, M. R. N. (1971). *Gen. Comp. Endocrinol.* **16**, 288.
Redshaw, M. R., and Nicholls, T. J. (1971). *Gen. Comp. Endocrinol.* **61**, 85.
Reinboth, R. (1970). *Mem. Soc. Endocrinol.* **18**, 515.
Rice, B. F., and Savard, K. (1966). *J. Clin. Endocrinol. Metab.* **26**, 593.
Rice, B. F., Hammerstein, J., and Savard, K. (1964). *Steroids* **4**, 199.
Rivarola, M. A., Snipes, C. A., and Migeon, C. J. (1968). *Endocrinology* **82**, 115.
Robertson, O. H., and Wexler, B. C. (1959). *Endocrinology* **65**, 225.

Robertson, O. H., and Wexler, B. C. (1960). *Endocrinology* **66**, 222.
Robertson, O. H., Krupp, M. A., Thomas, S. F., Favour, C. B., Hane, S., and Wexler, B. C. (1961). *Gen. Comp. Endocrinol.* **1**, 473.
Rothchild, I., and Fraps, R. M. (1944a). *Proc. Soc. Exp. Biol. Med.* **56**, 79.
Rothchild, I., and Fraps, R. M. (1944b). *Endocrinology*, **35**, 355.
Ruby, S. M., and McMillan, D. B. (1970). *J. Morphol.* **131**, 447.
Ryan, K. J., and Petro, Z. (1966). *J. Clin. Endocrinol. Metab.* **26**, 46.
Ryan, K. J., and Short, R. V. (1965). *Endocrinology*, **76**, 108.
Ryan, K. J., and Smith, O. W. (1961). *J. Biol. Chem.* **236**, 2207.
Ryan, K. J., and Smith, O. W. (1965). *Recent Progr. Horm. Res.* **21**, 367.
Saint Girons, H. (1962). *Bull. Soc. Zool. Fr.* **87**, 41.
Saint Girons, H., and Martoja, M. (1963). *C.R. Soc. Biol.* **157**, 1928.
Samuel, M. (1943). *Proc. Indian Acad. Sci. Sect. B* **18**, 133.
Sanyal, M. K., and Prasad, M. R. N. (1965). *Steroids* **6**, 313.
Savard, K. (1967). *Excerpta Med. Found. Int. Congr. Ser.* **132**, 837.
Sayler, A., Dowd, A. J., and Wolfson, A. (1970). *Gen. Comp. Endocrinol.* **15**, 30.
Scheer, B. T., and Wise, P. T. (1969). *Gen. Comp. Endocrinol.* **13**, 474.
Schreiner, K. E. (1955). *Univ. Bergen Arb.* **8**, 1.
Sekiguchi, T. (1968). *Endocrinol. Jap.* **15**, 70.
Sheridan, M. N. (1963). *Anat. Rec.* **145**, 285.
Sheridan, M. N., and Belt, W. D. (1964). *Anat. Rec.* **148**, 402.
Sheridan, M. N., Belt, W. D., and Hartman, F. A. (1963). *Acta Anat.* **53**, 55.
Simpson. T. H., and Wardle, C. S. (1967). *J. Mar. Biol. Ass. U.K.* **47**, 699.
Simpson, T. H., Wright, R. S., and Gottfried, H. (1963a). *J. Endocrinol.* **26**, 489.
Simpson, T. H., Wright, R. S., and Hunt, S. V. (1963b). *J. Endocrinol.* **26**, 499.
Simpson, T. H., Wright, R. S., and Renfrew, J. (1964). *J. Endocrinol.* **31**, 11.
Simpson, T. H., Wright, R. S., and Hunt, S. V. (1968). *J. Endocrinol.* **42**, 519.
Sinha, D., and Ghosh, A. (1964). *Acta Histochem.* **17**, 222.
Sivaram, S. (1965). *Can. J. Zool.* **43**, 1021.
Smith, C. L. (1955). *Mem. Soc. Endocrinol.* **4**, 39.
Smith, O. W., and Ryan, K. J. (1961). *Endocrinology* **69**, 970.
Soulé, J., and Assenmacher, I. (1966). *C.R. Acad. Sci.* **263**, 983.
Stanley, H. P. (1962). *Amer. Zool.* **2**, 561.
Stanley, H. P., Chieffi, G., and Botte, V. (1965). *Z. Zellforsch Mikrosk. Anat.* **65**, 350.
Sterba, G. (1955). *Zool. Anz.* **155**, 151.
Sterba, G. (1962). *Handbuch der Binnenrifischerei Mitteleuropas* **3**, 263.
Stockell-Hartree, A., and Cunningham, F. J. (1969). *J. Endocrinol.* **43**, 609.
Stoll, L. M. (1955). *Zoologica (New York)* **40**, 125.
Sundararaj, B. I., and Goswami, S. V. (1968). *J. Exp. Zool.* **168**, 85.
Sundararaj, B. I., Nayyar, S. K., Amand, T. C. and Donaldson, E. M. (1971) *Gen. Comp. Endocrinol.* **17**, 73.
Suzuki, N. (1968). *Endocrinol. Jap.* **15**, 82.
Taber, E. (1951). *Endocrinology* **48**, 6.
Tam, W. H., Phillips, J. G., and Lofts, B. (1967). *Proc. Asia Oceania Congr. Endocrinol., 3rd, 1967,* 369.
Tam, W. H., Phillips, J. G., and Lofts, B. (1969). *J. Endocrinol.* **43**, 111.
Thornton, V. F. (1971). Unpublished results.
Thornton, V. F., and Evennett, P. J. (1969). *Gen. Comp. Endocrinol.* **13**, 268.
Upadhyay, S. N., and Guraya, S. S. (1971). *Gen. Comp. Endocrinol.* **16**, 504.
van Kemenade, J. A. M. (1968a). *Z. Zellforsch. Mikrosk. Anat.* **92**, 549.

van Kemenade, J. A. M. (1968b). *Z. Zellforsch. Mikrosk. Anat.* **92**, 567.

van Kemenade, J. A. M., and van Dongen, W. J. (1965). *Nature (London)* **205**, 4967.

van Kemenade, J. A. M., van Dongen, W. J., and van Oordt, P. G. W. J. (1968). *Z. Zellforsch. Mikrosk. Anat.* **91**, 96.

van Oordt, P. G. W. J., and Brands, F. (1970). *J. Endocrinol.* **48**, Abstract (p.1).

van Oordt, P. G. W. J., and de Korte, E. J. M. (1969). *Colloq. Int. Cent. Nat. Rech. Sci.* **177**, 345.

van Overbeeke, A. P. (1960). "Histological Studies on the Interrenal and the Phaeochromic Tissue in Teleostei." Van Munster's, Amsterdam.

Varano, L., and Della Corte, F. (1969). *Gen. Comp. Endocrinol.* **13**, 536.

Varma, M. M. (1971). *Am. Zool.* **11**, 655.

Vilter, V., and Vilter, A. (1964). *C.R. Soc. Riol.* **158**, 457.

von Euler, U. S., and Heller, H. (1963). "Comparative Endocrinology." Academic Press, New York.

Wai, E. H., and Hoar, W. S. (1963). *Can. J. Zool.* **41**, 611.

Wassermann, G. F., and Tramezzani, J. H. (1961). *Acta Physiol. Lat. Amer.* **11**, 148.

Wassermann, G. F., and Tramezzani, J. H. (1963). *Gen. Comp. Endocrinol.* **3**, 480.

Wentworth, B. C. (1971). *Biol. Reprod.* **5**, 107.

Wiebe, J. P. (1968a). *Can. J. Zool.* **46**, 751.

Wiebe, J. P. (1968b). *Can. J. Zool.* **46**, 1221.

Wiebe, J. P. (1969a). *Gen. Comp. Endocrinol.* **12**, 256.

Wiebe, J. P. (1969b). *Gen. Comp. Endocrinol.* **12**, 267.

Wilhoft, D. C. (1963). *Amer. Midl. Natur.* **70**, 442.

Wilhoft, D. C. (1964). *Gen. Comp. Endocrinol.* **4**, 42.

Woods, J. W., and Domm, L. V. (1966). *Gen. Comp. Endocrinol.* **7**, 559.

Wyburn, G. M., Johnston, H. S., and Aitken, R. N. C. (1966). *Z. Zellforsch. Mikrosk. Anat.* **72**, 53.

Xavier, F., and Ozon, R. (1971). *Gen. Comp. Endocrinol.* **16**, 30.

Xavier, F., Zuber-Vogeli, M., and Le Quang Trong, Y. (1970). *Gen Comp. Endocrinol.* **15**, 425.

Yadav, B. N., Singh, B. R., and Munshi, J. S. D. (1970). *Mikroskopie* **25**, 41.

Yamamoto, K., and Onozato, H. (1965). *Annot. Zool. Jap.* **38**, 140.

Yamamoto, K., and Onozato, H. (1968). *Annot. Zool. Jap.* **41**, 119.

Yamazaki, F., and Donaldson, E. M. (1968). *Gen. Comp. Endocrinol.* **10**, 383.

Yaron, Z. (1966). *J. Endocrinol.* **34**, 127.

Yaron, Z. (1970). *Gen. Comp. Endocrinol.* **14**, 542.

Yaron, Z. (1971). *Gen. Comp. Endocrinol.* **17**, 247.

Yoshimura, F., and Harumiya, K. (1968). *Endocrinol. Jap.* **15**, 94.

Chapter 4

CORTICOSTEROIDS IN FISH

D. R. IDLER and B. TRUSCOTT

I. Introduction

The list of corticosteroids that have been reported in fish (Tables A.I–A. XI) may suggest that more is known about these steroids than is actually the case. Thus, the list of probable identifications is relatively small (Table A.XI). To bring the picture into perspective with the mammalian literature, the pioneering nature of the early investigations to demonstrate the presence of corticosteroids in fish plasma should be emphasized. In 1953, cortisol was identified as the principal 17-hydroxycorticosteroid in human plasma (Bush and Sandberg, 1953) and in the following year the first report of 17-hydroxy-corticosteroids in fish plasma was made from Fontaine's laboratory (Fontaine and Hatey, 1954). These authors noted that the concentration of Porter–Silber chromogens in the plasma of the Atlantic salmon *Salmo salar* was generally higher than that found in human plasma, especially in samples collected from migratory salmon smolts. A bioassay based on the stimulatory action of corticosteroids on the deposition of glycogen in the liver of adrena-lectomized mice (Venning *et al.*, 1946) confirmed the presence of adreno-cortical compounds in the blood of the salmon (Hatey, 1954).

No attempts were made to identify the corticosteroids in fish plasma until 1957 when Bondy *et al.* isolated a compound from the plasma of the carp *Cyprinus carpio* and the flounder *Pseudopleuronectes americanus* which behaved chromatographically on paper as cortisol, exhibited alkali fluorescence, and was blue tetrazolium positive. Similar methods were employed to study the plasmatic steroids of several species of fish and other non-mammalian vertebrates. Quantities of steroid were estimated in most samples by visual examination of color tests. The results of this original survey suggested that cortisol and/or corticosterone were common to all vertebrate classes (Phillips and Chester Jones, 1957; Phillips, 1959; Chester Jones *et al.*, 1959). Subsequently, cortisone and cortisol were isolated from the plasma of the Pacific sockeye salmon *Oncorhynchus nerka* and their identity established by chemical and physical properties, including infrared spectra (Idler *et al.*, 1959a). The plasma of postspawned and therefore moribund Pacific salmon proved to be a rich source of several C_{21} steroids (Table A.VIII) although not all would necessarily be secretory products of the interrenal gland. Improvements in methodology for the isolation and quantification of corticosteroids in biological extracts have made it necessary to amend qualitatively and quantitatively the more general conclusions of some of the early investigations.

In the Elasmobranchii there is now considerable evidence that a C_{21} steroid, 1α-hydroxycorticosterone, not previously known from any source, is a major product of the interrenal tissue and a principal component of the plasmatic steroids (Idler and Truscott, 1966a; Truscott and Idler, 1968a).

Whether significant 17-hydroxylation of corticosteroids occurs in interrenal tissue of any species of this subclass is an open question.

From a quantitative viewpoint the use of more specific methods of analysis indicates that the levels of corticosteroids in the blood of several species are considerably lower than originally reported and, especially in the teleosts, are subject to the physiological condition of the fish at the time of blood collection.

There also has been a considerable amount of work done with *in vitro* techniques, i.e., incubation of fish interrenal tissues with steroidal (radioactive) precursors. Certain limitations of tissue incubations for the study of corticosteroidogenesis are discussed in Chapter 2 but other factors particularly pertinent to fish have to be considered. A number of investigations of the synthesis of corticosteriods *in vitro* by fish interrenal tissue have failed to acknowledge the source of the enzyme systems under study, the source being an aquatic poikilothermic vertebrate. Experimental conditions, e.g., chemical composition of incubation media and incubation temperatures, used to study steroid synthesis in mammalian adrenocortical tissue have been applied without modification to fish tissues. To our knowledge there is no evidence to suggest that the use of mammalian Ringer solutions rather than specially consitituted solutions (e.g., Lockwood, 1961) has influenced the results, at least in a qualitative sense. There is, however, reason to be concerned about the use of unphysiological temperatures. The corticosteroid $l\alpha$-hydroxylase enzyme system of interrenal tissue of elasmobranchs was irreversibly inhibited at 37°C (Idler and Truscott, 1967b); enzyme systems of tissues other than interrenal, e.g., liver microsomes, in marine vertebrates were reported to be thermolabile and less active at 37°C than at lower temperatures (Adamson, 1967); and, conversely, in the rat adrenal corticosteroid 21-hydroxylase was partially impaired at 37°C compared to its activity at 21°C (Tsang and Stachenko, 1970). In studies designed to determine pathways of corticosteroidogenesis involving more than one enzyme system unphysiological temperatures can adversely affect one enzyme more than another and lead to erroneous conclusions. In poikilotherms the increase in substrate affinity, which frequently occurs at low temperatures, can offset the decrease expected in catalytic velocity at the lower temperature. Some isoenzyme systems in fact may not function at physiological substrate concentrations at temperatures near the upper tolerance limit for the poikilotherm (Hochachka and Somero, 1968; Somero and Hochachka, 1969).

Thus, studies of steroid production or transformation *in vitro* have been most useful in the definition of steroidogenic enzyme systems present in fish interrenal tissue and have also served to corroborate and sometimes to question results obtained from *in vivo* studies.

The text of this chapter is primarily concerned with the identity and factors affecting the quantity of corticosteroids in the body fluids and tissues of the three classes of vertebrates commonly and collectively known as fish. Results obtained by studies of corticosteroidogenesis *in vitro* are tabulated and discussed separately from *in vivo* data, partly for the sake of simplicity of presentation but also to avoid the temptation of using *in vitro* data to describe the situation as it occurs *in vivo*. No attempt has been to interpret or discuss all investigations concerned with corticosteroids as reported in the literature.

Tables A.I–A.XI are arranged alphabetically according to species. Within a species, studies are referred to in chronological order. Abbreviations are listed in Chapter 2, Tables II–IV. In some instances data are not recorded; this applies particularly to studies in which identification or quantification are not the principal subject of the investigation. Some selection of data has been necessary where several variables have been studied but where all are not essential to illustrate the principal results. The rating system used in Tables A.I–A.X is described in Chapter 2, Tables I–III.

II. Fish as Experimental Animals

Fish are receiving increasing recognition as useful experimental animals for studies on steroids (Idler, 1969). They may present some transport, holding, and sampling problems to people who are more familiar with handling other nonmammalian vertebrates or mammals and a few comments may be helpful.

Transport tanks for fish should have nonabrasive surfaces; smoothly finished fiberglass is excellent. The tank should be equipped with a water-circulating pump and aerator. For transport of cold-water species in warm weather a chilling unit or ice in plastic bags should be used to keep the temperature down (5°–10°C is usually satisfactory) but sudden temperature changes must be avoided at all times. A light anesthetic, e.g., tricaine methanesulfonate (10–20 ppm) or 2-phenoxyethanol (100 ppm), some salt in the water, chloromycetin palmitate (5 ppm), and tris buffer to control pH at 7.0 in fresh water and 8.4 in seawater (McFarland and Norris, 1958) are useful additives (Idler *et al.*, 1961a). Pacific salmon, 1 kg fish/18 liters water, have been transported for several hundred miles without mortality when these precautions, except the buffer, were used. Live fish can be transported great distances by air when appropriate precautions are taken.

Before the collection of blood samples fish may be stunned by a blow on the head or anesthetized (for a review of anesthetics see Bell, 1964). When large blood samples are required many species may be bled by severing the tail. To exclude slime and excreta, the tail is wrapped in paper towelling and the anus closed with a forceps. This method works well for many larger actinopterygians but is generally unsatisfactory for other fish. Heart punctures work well in fish with a rapid pumping rate, e.g., salmonids, but poorly for various reasons with elasmobranchs. In the latter case a canula in the conus arteriosus, leading from the heart, is very successful. For small samples, many teleosts may be bled by syringe from the dorsal aorta, either from the tail or the mouth (Shiffman, 1959); similarly, serial blood samples may be taken from the caudal circulatory system of elasmobranchs. A convenient method for the collection of blood from myxinoids (the hagfish) was described by Germain and Gagnon (1968); neither caudal section nor syringes are very satisfactory for these fish.

For holding fish in the laboratory care should be taken to exclude from the water even trace quantities of heavy metals (plastic water lines), chlorine (charcoal filters), and supersaturation from sucking air into water intakes (vigorous aeration will usually remedy this). Ozone seems to have potential application for destroying toxic organic substances. Fish should not be handled with bare hands and each tank should be supplied with a net to avoid spread of disease. Chloromycetin palmitate and seawater baths are useful for keeping some diseases under control. Access to the sea is not always essential for work on "saltwater species" since many can tolerate relatively low salinity and seawater salt mixtures can be purchased or prepared.

III. Identification and Quantification of Corticosteroids

A. AGNATHA

The current status of corticosteroids in cyclostomes is summarized in Table A.I. Phillips (1959) and Chester Jones and Phillips (1960) reported 14 μg of corticosterone and 10 μg cortisol per 100 ml plasma in the Pacific hagfish *Polistotrema stoutii* and 47 μg cortisol and 4 μg corticosterone in the sea lamprey *Petromyzon marinus*. Phillips et al. (1962) found 27 μg corticosterone and 11 μg cortisol per 100 ml serum in the Atlantic hagfish *Myxine glutinosa*. These preliminary identifications of corticosteroids in hagfish and lamprey blood followed the method of Bush and Ferguson (1953) as outlined by Phillips et al. (1962). The specificity of this method, which involved the spraying of paper chromatograms with triphenyltetrazolium chloride and observation of the resulting reduced formazans as pink spots under ultraviolet light, was questioned by Bush and Ferguson (1953). Leloup-Hatey (1964b) reported 23 μg of total 17-hydroxycorticosteroids in female and 2.2

μg/100 ml plasma of male *Petromyzon marinus*. However, Weisbart and Idler (1970), using a double-isotope assay and crystallization according to Axelrod *et al.* (1965), were unable to corroborate the high levels of corticosteroids reported by the Sheffield group for the Atlantic hagfish and the sea lamprey. There was evidence for the presence of nanogram quantities of cortisol, cortisone, or corticosterone in the plasma of these two cyclostomes but the results were not conclusive. Nevertheless, the assays did establish that if cortisol, cortisone, or corticosterone were present in these fish, plasma concentrations were very low.

In an attempt to obtain sufficiently elevated serum corticosteroid levels in hagfish to permit identification by crystallization of steroid acetates to constant specific activity, a group of 51 fish was treated with adrenocorticotropic hormone (ACTH); all animals were anesthetized with tricaine methanesulfonate before injection and bleeding (Idler *et al.*, 1971). The ^{3}H: ^{14}C ratios for the final crystals and mother liquors were cortisol, 2.15(2.18); cortisone, 31.5 (31.2); corticosterone, 9.81 (9.45); and 11-deoxycortisol, 7.25 (7.09). The serum contained 0.09 μg cortisol, 1.38 μg cortisone, 0.37 μg corticosterone, and 0.34 μg 11-deoxycortisol per 100 ml. The experiment was repeated with another group of ACTH-treated hagfish and saline-treated controls. Each fish was injected with 60 IU porcine ACTH in saline (or saline alone) in three equal doses on days 1, 3, and 7 and were bled on the tenth day. The results are summarized in Table A.I. There was no difficulty in confirming the elevated levels of cortisol, cortisone, and 11-deoxycortisol following ACTH treatment. It is of interest that very little corticosterone was present before ACTH treatment and there was no elevation with ACTH. It is not known why corticosterone was present in readily detectable concentration in one group of hagfish but not in the other; a similar situation has occasionally been observed in Atlantic salmon (Leloup-Hatey, 1964b). An explanation may be forthcoming when factors affecting the now well documented 17α-hydroxylation of 21-hydroxycorticoids by fish interrenal tissue are better understood (Sandor *et al.*, 1966, 1970; Idler *et al.*, 1969). In any event, the principal corticoid of hagfish seems to be cortisol but cortisone predominates after prolonged treatment with ACTH. It is interesting to speculate that the relatively greater accumulation of cortisone relative to cortisol following prolonged ACTH treatment reflects a protective mechanism against hypercorticism; this reasoning assumes that cortisol is the more biologically active steroid in fish as it is believed to be in mammals. The accumulation of 11-deoxycortisol following prolonged ACTH treatment reflects inhibition of 11β-hydroxylase or a limited activity of 11β-hydroxylase relative to the stimulation of other steroidogenic enzyme systems and could provide a second mechanism for controlling plasma cortisol levels.

The extremely low levels of plasma corticosteroids in hagfish considered along with the difficulties which have been experienced in demonstrating steroidogenesis by presumed interrenal tissue suggest that such tissue is very limited in quantity and difficult to obtain in a reasonably pure state. Presumed adrenocortical tissue of hagfish failed to convert progesterone to any known steroids (Chester Jones *et al.*, 1962). Weisbart and Idler (1970) incubated presumptive adrenocortical tissue of Atlantic hagfish with corticosterone-4-^{14}C and 17α-hydroxyprogesterone-4-^{14}C and failed to obtain transformation to known corticosteroids. Incubations of presumptive adrenocortical tissue of another cyclostome, the sea lamprey, with progesterone-4-^{14}C, 17α-hydroxyprogesterone-4-^{14}C, pregnenolone-4-^{14}C, and 11-deoxycortisol-4-^{14}C also failed to produce corticosteroids. However, Weisbart and Idler (1970) did definitively identify 17α-hydroxyprogesterone-4-^{14}C following the incubation of presumed adrenocortical tissue of lamprey with progesterone-4-^{14}C; no evidence was found for the presence of 17α-hydroxyprogesterone in the plasma.

The source of corticosteroids in cyclostome plasma is not known with any certainty. Seiler *et al.* (1970) could not find Δ^5-3β-hydroxysteroid dehydrogenase in so-called interrenal cells of *Lampetra planeri* and *Petromyzon marinus*; these authors concluded from histochemical reactions that the presumed interrenal cells of lamprey more closely resemble corpuscles of Stannius found in teleosts than they do interrenal cells of higher vertebrates. Limited attempts in this laboratory to locate adrenocortical tissue of Atlantic hagfish by histochemical methods have not been conclusive; at least one other worker has been unsuccessful (Chavin, 1967).

B. CHONDRICHTHYES

1. Introduction

Until recent years surprisingly little work was done on the identification of corticosteroids in the interrenal gland of Chondrichthyes; surprising when one considers that in 1934 extracts of interrenal tissue from *Raja* sp. were used to maintain life in adrenalectomized animals (Grollman *et al.*, 1934) and conversely that symptoms of interrenalectomy in two species of *Torpedo* were shown to be alleviated by commercial preparations of mammalian adrenocortical hormones (Dittus, 1941). Furthermore, the interrenal tissue is a discrete body of cortical tissue free of chromaffin tissue and is in many ways very suitable for *in vitro* studies. The only real problem with extracts or incubates of this tissue is the high fat and lipid content, complete with solvent-extractable and relatively polar fluorogenic material. Thus the concentrated extracts tend to be bulky and require extra preliminary purification in order to be examined successfully for steroidal content by chromatographic methods. Polar steroids are particularly difficult to isolate and detect by conventional methods and this feature more than any other probably led to the doubtful conclusion that the steroidogenic potential of chondrichthyean interrenal tissue is limited (Bern, 1967). The development of thin-layer chromatography provided a simple method of fractionation of such extracts, and with this technique a polar steroid, 1α-hydroxycorticosterone, not previously known, was identified as a major product of interrenal tissue of many species belonging to the subclass Elasmobranchii (Idler and Truscott, 1966a; Truscott and Idler, 1968a).

Evidence to date indicates that there is a basic qualitative difference in the corticosteroid patterns of the two subclasses of Chondrichthyes. No corticosteroid 1α-hydroxylase could be demonstrated *in vitro* in interrenal tissue of a holocephalan, the Pacific ratfish. Exogenous precursors were converted in high yields to their 17α-hydroxylated derivatives (Idler *et al.*, 1969). In the Elasmobranchii, 17α-hydroxylase activity in interrenal tissue appears to be weak or perhaps absent.

The cellular locations of the enzyme systems involved in corticosteroidogenesis in chondrichthyean interrenal tissue has not been investigated but the inhibition of corticosteroid 1α-hydroxylase by metyrapone CIBA suggests that it is of mitochondrial origin (Idler and Truscott, 1967b). There have been no reports of experiments designed specifically to study optimal conditions *in vitro* and cofactor requirements of the interrenal enzyme systems. Presumably the cofactor requirements are the same as those of mammalian adrenal enzyme systems. With tissue previously frozen for convenience of collection and storage, the addition of a NADP-generating system to the incubation medium was necessary in order to obtain satisfactory conversion of precursor to product (Simpson and Wright, 1970). With freshly excised tissue, the production rate of 1α-hydroxycorticosterone from endogenous precursors without addition of cofactors compared favorably with corticosteroid production in adrenal tissue of other vertebrates (Idler and Truscott, 1969).

Although the effect of temperature on steroid production by interrenal tissue of elasmobranchs has not been examined in detail, the 1α-hydroxylase enzyme appears to be thermolabile. Interrenal tissue of a cold-water skate, *Raja radiata*, converted corticosterone to 1α-hydroxycorticosterone *in vitro* at temperatures between 4° and 30°C but the corticosteroid 1α-hydroxylase was irreversibly inactivated at 37°C (Idler and Truscott, 1967b). The effect of the higher temperature on 21- and 11β-hydroxylase systems was not investigated. Total steroid production from endogenous precursors was more efficient at low temperatures; when aliquots of homogeneous interrenal tissue of *R. radiata* were incubated at 2° and 24°C, production at 24°C was higher for the first hour but at the lower temperature the production rate was maintained in the second and third hour so that the total production over 3 hr was greater at 2° than at 24°C (Idler and Truscott, 1967c).

There have been no intensive studies of corticosteroids in the circulating blood of the chondrichthyeans although reviews of this subject record cortisol and corticosterone as the principal plasmatic corticosteroids of the elasmobranchs. A critical look at the original literature reveals that in fact very little is known about the plasmatic steroids of elasmobranchs and nothing of those in holocephalans.

In many ways the elasmobranchs are very suitable for endocrinological investigations which require blood analyses. Although the larger man-eating sharks may not be one's first choice as an experimental animal, other species are small enough to maintain in aquaria but large enough to permit repeated blood sampling. Larger blood samples can be collected without hemolysis by cannulation of the conus arteriosus and smaller blood samples can be easily obtained from the caudal artery. Methods of hypophysectomy, partial or complete, have been published (Dodd *et al.*, 1960; Idler *et al.*, 1970) and some species of batoids can be successfully interrenalectomized (Dittus, 1941; Hartman *et al.*, 1944; Idler and Szeplaki, 1968). At the present time the principal drawbacks to the use of blood analyses for the study of the role of corticosteroids in elasmobranchs are the lack of information on the nature of the plasmatic corticosteroids and the application of methods sufficiently sensitive and specific to measure them quantitatively.

2. Elasmobranchii

a. Corticosteroid Synthesis in Vitro. Papers describing *in vitro* studies on corticosteroidogenesis in elasmobranchs are summarized in Table A.II. Macchi and Rizzo (1962) reported the production *in vitro* by interrenal tissue from *Raja erinacea* of compounds which absorbed ultraviolet light at 240 mμ and reduced blue tetrazolium but they did not further identify these products. In the same year, Bern *et al.* (1962) published the results of experiments with two species of elasmobranch, a selachian (*Squalus acanthias*) and a batoid (*Raja rhina*). Chromatographic fractionation of extracts of interrenal tissue of *S. acanthias* permitted the identification of corticosterone by color test and the spectrum of its sulfuric acid chromogens. With the double-isotope derivative assay of Kliman and Peterson (1960) aldosterone and corticosterone were identified and quantified for both *S. acanthias* and *R. rhina* and cortisol was also found in interrenal incubates of *R. rhina*. Unfortunately, the application of the assay to the elasmobranch interrenal extracts is not described in detail so that the specificity of the assay for these samples cannot be judged.

Without extensive chromatographic purification and demonstration of the purity of the isolated radioactive steroid acetate, the quantitative results must be considered as maximal values. Nonspecific blank values or radioactivity associated with contaminants could account for the radioactivity attributed to the presence of submicrogram amounts of cortisol and aldosterone.

More recent studies have shown that interrenal tissue of elasmobranchs contains a 1α-corticosteroid hydroxylase, an enzyme system not previously found in adrenal tissue of other vertebrates. A very polar steroid first detected in the blood of *R. radiata* was shown to be the principal product of interrenal tissue *in vitro* and a biosynthetic product of exogenous corticosterone (Idler and Truscott, 1966a). Since 1α-hydroxycorticosterone had not been described previously and was not available as a product of microbial or chemical synthesis, sufficient quantities to define its physical and chemical characteristics were prepared by *in vitro* incubation of corticosterone with interrenal tissue of two species of *Raja* (Idler and Truscott, 1967a). Tissue from all species of elasmobranchs which have been examined contained the 1α-hydroxylating enzyme system, and 1α-hydroxycorticosterone was the principal corticosteroid produced *in vitro* from endogenous precursors. Smaller amounts of corticosterone were isolated and identified from incubates of interrenal tissue of some selachians. 11-Deoxycorticosterone was also identified as an incubation product of endogenous precursors in frozen interrenal tissue of the blue shark *Prionace glauca* (Truscott and Idler, 1968a). A corticosteroid 1α-hydroxylase has now been demonstrated in 18 species of Elasmobranchii; five species, including a *Torpedo* sp. and a freshwater stingray (*Potamotrygon* sp.), have been studied since 1968 and are listed in Table A.II (Truscott and Idler, 1970). Simpson and Wright (1970) used radioactive pregnenolone and progesterone to study the biosynthesis of corticosteroids in three species of selachian elasmobranchs. With homogenates of frozen interrenal tissue as the source of enzyme, pregnenolone was transformed to progesterone, 11-deoxycorticosterone, and corticosterone. Freshly excised interrenal tissue of *Scyliorhynus caniculus* produced 11-deoxycorticosterone, corticosterone, and in lesser amount 1α-hydroxycorticosterone from exogenous progesterone. In all cases, 11-deoxycorticosterone and corticosterone were the major products formed from exogenous pregnenolone and progesterone, whereas Truscott and Idler (1968a) reported 1α-hydroxycorticosterone to be the major product of endogenous precursors. This difference in results may be due to the different experimental conditions used for tissue incubation but may also represent a real difference in the metabolism *in vitro* of exogenous and endogenous precursors (Vinson and Whitehouse, 1969). Another enzyme system found in elasmobranch interrenal is 11β-dehydrogenase. Bern *et al.* (1962) observed a compound with the chromatographic mobility of 11-dehydrocorticosterone in extracts of interrenal tissue of *Squalus acanthias* and a metabolite of exogenous corticosterone produced by interrenal tissue of several species was presumptively identified as 11-dehydrocorticosterone (Truscott and Idler, 1968a).

Simpson and Wright (1970) were unable to obtain any evidence of 18-hydroxylase or 17α-hydroxylase activity in selachian interrenal tissue. Neither 17-hydroxylated C_{21} steroids (cortisol, cortisone, 11-deoxycortisol, and 17α-hydroxyprogesterone) nor the androgenic C_{19} steroids (testosterone, androstenedione, and adrenosterone) could be detected as transformation products of pregnenolone and progesterone. Similarly, neither cortisol nor aldosterone were identified as products of endogenous precursors in interrenal incubates of either the batoid or selachian elasmobranch; nor was aldosterone a transformation product of corticosterone (Idler and Truscott, 1966a, 1967a; Truscott and Idler, 1968a). Although highly sensitive methods were not applied in these studies relatively large amounts of interrenal tissue were used so that even minor products should have been detected. At this time, there would appear to be insufficient evidence to assume that 17α- and 18-hydroxylated steroids are elaborated by the elasmobranch interrenal gland, and if their presence is suspected in an interrenal extract, experimental confirmation would be in order. Whether aldosterone is a product of the elasmobranch interrenal remains an interesting question, especially since a renin–angiotensin system appears to be absent in this class of vertebrates (Sokabe, 1968; Nishimura *et al.*, 1970).

Although evidence to date suggests little or no 17α-hydroxylase activity in the interrenal tissue, 17α-hydroxylation and 21-hydroxylation do occur in the gonadal tissue of at least one elasmobranch. 11-Deoxycorticosterone in high concentration was isolated and identified in the semen of the dogfish *Squalus acanthias* and, *in vitro*, cholesterol was converted to 11-deoxycorticosterone through pregnenolone and progesterone (Simpson *et al.*, 1963a; 1964a). 11-Deoxycorticosterone was a major, and 11-deoxycortisol a minor, transformation product of progesterone when testicular tissue of mature *S. acanthias* was used as the source of enzyme; thus, consecutive hydroxylations at C-17 and C-21 were demonstrated (Simpson *et al.*, 1964b). The authors pointed out that spermatozoa were present in the tissue and may have been the source of the 21-hydroxylase but until further experiments are done, 21-hydroxylation by elasmobranch testicular tissue must be considered possible. Despite the source of steroid and enzyme, the identification of these C_{21} steroids is included in Table A.II since 11-deoxycorticosterone and 11-deoxycortisol are usually considered as products of adrenal tissue.

a. Plasmatic Corticosteroids. Corticosteroids reported to occur in the blood of elasmobranchs are listed in Table A.III. In a survey of lower vertebrates, cortisol or corticosterone or both were tentatively identified in the peripheral plasma of both batoids and selachians (Phillips and Chester Jones, 1957; Phillips, 1959; Chester Jones *et al.*, 1959). In the assessment of these experiments one must appreciate that they were pioneer studies when the presence of corticosteroids of any structure had not previously been demonstrated in the blood of lower vertebrates. The identity of a specific compound was based solely on its polarity as determined by paper chromatography since the other tests used, absorption of ultraviolet light at 240 mμ, the reduction of blue tetrazolium, and alkali fluorescence, are characteristic of several corticosteroids. For some samples (Phillips, 1959) the alkali fluorescence method of Bondy and Upton (1957) was used to identify and quantify the corticosteroids; this method employs limited purification of blood extracts and depends upon paper chromatography to isolate and separate the corticosteroids. The validity of a quantitative method needs to be verified when applied to samples of different origin and it is possible that the fluorescence measured here, and attributed to cortisol and corticosterone, was nonspecific because elasmobranch plasma does contain high levels of polar nonsteroidal fluorogens which "streak" on paper chromatograms. There are still insufficient data on elasmobranch plasma to refute these results but the methods used were almost certainly inadequate for some species included in the survey. For example, cortisol was identified in plasma of amphibians and reptiles but the 17-deoxycorticosteroids are now considered to predominate in these classes of vertebrate (see Chapter 5).

Plasma samples from two species of *Raja, R. radiata* and *R. ocellata*, were reported to contain approximately 0.1 μg/100 ml of cortisol and corticosterone as determined by double-isotope derivative assay (Idler and Truscott, 1966a). Again, without demonstration of the specificity of the method to the type of sample being analyzed, the presence of cortisol and corticosterone cannot be considered established; rather the quantities are the maximum possible. The double-isotope derivative assay used for the samples was a commercial assay developed for the measurement of cortisol and corticosterone in human blood and thus not necessarily adequate for the blood of other species (unpublished confession!).

In a study of steroid hormones in the plasma of female *Torpedo marmorata* at four stages of the sexual cycle, Lupo di Prisco *et al.* (1967) identified cortisol, cortisone, corticosterone, and 11-deoxycorticosterone as well as progesterone, estrogens, and testosterone by a method combining thin-layer and gas chromatography. The final steroid as measured represented not only free steroids extractable with ethyl acetate but also conjugated steroids released by hydrolysis with β-glucuronidase. Gas–liquid chromatography can be very useful in the identification and quantification of steroids in biological extracts but certain conditions must be met in order to make legitimate claims of identity and quantity. Biological extracts should be highly purified before gas chromatography (Eik-Nes, 1968) and from data reported by Lupo di Prisco *et al.* (1967) the thin-layer chromatography used for this purpose was not very efficient; cortisol and cortisone, for example, were reportedly spread through three thin-layer fractions. The thin-layer fractions were subjected to gas chromatographic analysis without further purification or preparation of derivatives. Thermal degradation is a well-known property of unsubstituted corticosteroids and the nonquantitative aspect of this transformation further complicates the interpretation of gas chromatographic data obtained with impure extracts. Even under the best conditions, column retention time can hardly be accepted as the sole criterion of identity. The use of gas–liquid chromatography for the identification and quantification of steroids in biological fluids was a subject of discussion after a symposium held a few years ago in Glasgow (Grant, 1967). The plasma corticosteroids of *T. marmorata* may in fact include cortisol, cortisone, corticosterone, and 11-deoxycorticosterone but more specific methods will be required to confirm their presence.

Sufficient 1α-hydroxycorticosterone was isolated from the blood of the thorny skate *Raja radiata* to establish its identity with biosynthetic 1α-hydroxycorticosterone, the structure of which was established by its chemical and physical properties (Idler and Truscott, 1967a). 1α-Hydroxycorticosterone has also been tentatively identified and quantified in the plasma of *R. ocellata*, *R. laevis*, *R. erinacea*, and *R. clavata* (Idler and Truscott, 1969).

Treatment of the blood plasma of *R. radiata* with β-glucuronidase released a substance which was presumed to be 1α-hydroxycorticosterone (Idler and Truscott, 1968). Conjugated steroids in the blood of the elasmobranchs could be an interesting study; chromatographic examination of extracts of the glucuronide and "sulfate" fractions of a blood sample from *R. radiata* provided exploratory evidence for several compounds which absorbed ultraviolet light at 240 mμ or reduced blue tetrazolium or both or reacted with the Zimmermann reagent (Idler and Truscott, 1966c). Conjugation of steroids with glucuronic acid may show species differences; testosterone glucuronide was identified in the blood of *R. radiata* but could not be detected in the plasma of *R. ocellata* (Idler and Truscott, 1966b). The interpretation of gas chromatographic data obtained with plasma extracts of *Torpedo marmorata* (Lupo di Prisco *et al.*, 1967) may have been complicated by the inclusion of compounds released by β-glucuronidase with the free steroid fraction.

1α-Hydroxycorticosterone was isolated and presumptively identified in the perivisceral fluid of *Raja radiata* at a concentration of 5–50 μg/100 ml, i.e., approximately 10 times higher than the concentration usually found in the blood plasma (Idler and Truscott, 1968). This steroid was also concentrated in the pericardial fluid, but in the cranial fluid the concentration did not differ from that found in plasma. Recent experiments have shown that periviscereal 1α-hydroxycorticosterone is slowly transferred to the blood stream and can maintain, for ∼ 2–3 weeks, nanogram levels of steroid in the peripheral blood of interrenalectomized fish (Idler, 1971). How the steroid is concentrated in the periviscereal and pericardial fluids of *R. radiata* has not been determined. Individual fish of other species of Atlantic elasmobranchs (*R. ocellata, R. erinacea, R. laevis,* and *Squalus acanthias*) have been examined but there was no evidence of a concentration of 1α-hydroxycorticosterone in the periviscereal fluids (Idler and Truscott, 1970).

11-Deoxycorticosterone was isolated from the semen of *S. acanthias* (Simpson *et al.*, 1963a), although not from semen of some other elasmobranchs (Simpson *et al.*, 1963b). Testes of *Scyliorhinus caniculus* were shown to contain a 17-hydroxylase but not a 21-hydroxylase; 17α-hydroxyprogesterone and its 20β-dihydro derivative were identified in the blood plasma of this species (Simpson *et al.*, 1969). Thus, in some species or under certain physiological conditions, there exists the possibility that 21-hydroxy- and 17,21-dihydroxy steroids are secretory products of the gonad, and if found in the blood plasma their source should not be assumed to be interrenal tissue.

3. Holocephali

One holocephalan, the Pacific ratfish *Hydrolagus colliei*, is the most prevalent species of this primitive order and the only species examined for corticosteroids. The results are summarized in Table A.IV. As in the other subclass Elasmobranchii the interrenal is a distinct encapsulated gland of cortical tissue free of chromaffin cells.

In 1962, Bern *et al.* identified cortisol as the principal corticosteroid with lesser amounts of aldosterone in extracts and incubated interrenal tissue of *H. colliei*. With the demonstration of 1α-hydroxycorticosterone as a major product of interrenal tissue of the elasmobranchs, Idler *et al.* (1969) examined interrenal tissue of the same species for a corticosteroid 1α-hydroxylase. Neither progesterone nor corticosterone, the immediate precursor of 1α-hydroxycorticosterone in elasmobranchs, was hydroxylated in the 1 position. Cortisol was tentatively identified as a product of endogenous precursors. Transformation products of progesterone-^{14}C demonstrated the presence of a strong 17α-hydroxylase, 21-hydroxylase, and 11β-hydroxylase; 17-deoxysteroids did not accumulate in the incubation medium. Cortisol-^{14}C was the principal transformation product (32%) of corticosterone-[14]C. Unchanged corticosterone-^{14}C, an unidentified polar transformation product, and a compound isopolar with 11-dehydrocorticosterone accounted for the remainder of the radioactive precursor. In contrast to mammalian adrenal tissue, 17-hydroxylation of a 21-hydroxycorticosteroid has also been demonstrated *in vitro* in teleost interrenal tissue but in comparatively lower yields. Whether this reaction can or does occur *in vivo* in the ratfish has not yet been investigated. It would be interesting to further characterize the 17α-hydroxylase system of holocephalan interrenal tissue, e.g., cellular location and effect of inhibitors, for comparison with the 17α-hydroxylase of mammalian adrenocortical tissue.

In the experiments described by Idler *et al.* (1969), the transformation products of both progesterone-^{14}C and corticosterone-^{14}C were analyzed for aldosterone-^{14}C but none could be detected. Bern *et al.* (1962) reported aldosterone to be a product of endogenous precursors in *H. colliei* interrenal incubates as measured by double-isotope assay. There are several possible explanations for the discrepancy in the results: (a) the fact that the glands used by Idler *et al.* (1969) were held in ice for 20 hr before incubation and the activity of the 18-hydroxylating enzyme system may have been destroyed or markedly reduced, (b) a difference in the physiological condition or history of the fish, (c) mistaken identity of nonspecific radioactivity in the double-isotope assay.

There are no records of studies on the metabolism of cholesterol or pregnenolone in interrenal tissue of a holocephalan, and whether progesterone is an obligatory intermediate cannot be decided at this time.

4. Summary

In the subclass Elasmobranchii, the presence of the following enzyme systems in the interrenal tissue has been established: Δ^5-3β-ol dehydrogenase and $\Delta^5 \longrightarrow \Delta^4$-isomerase, 21-hydroxylase, 11β-hydroxylase, 1α-hydroxylase, and 11β-dehydrogenase. There is less evidence that enzyme systems necessary for hydroxylation at C-17 and C-18 are present. Consideration of all published data indicates that the sequence of corticosteroidogenic reactions in the interrenal of Elasmobranchii is as follows: pregnenolone $\longrightarrow$ progesterone $\longrightarrow$ 11-deoxycorticosterone $\longrightarrow$ corticosterone $\longrightarrow$ 1α-hydroxycorticosterone or 11-dehydrocorticosterone. Presumably pregnenolone is formed from cholesterol but this reaction has not received particular attention.

On the basis of studies *in vitro* as well as *in vivo*, our conclusions regarding corticosteroids in the body fluids of Elasmobranchii are as follows. (a) The chances are high that 1α-hydroxycorticosterone occurs in the blood of most or all species. (b) Deoxycorticosterone and corticosterone might be expected to occur, generally in small amounts, because of their positions as intermediates in the biosynthesis of 1α-hydroxycorticosterone. (c) There is no solid evidence for cortisol or other 17-hydroxycorticosteroids but the possibility of species differences cannot be ignored.

With regard to the concentration of corticosteroids in the plasma of elasmobranchs we would have to conclude, mainly from our own observations and experience, that the levels are low, i.e., in the range of less than 1–5 μg/100 ml, and in many cases higher levels reported in the literature resulted from the methods used for quantification. Again, this is a general conclusion and of course need not apply to all species at all stages of their life cycle.

In Holocephali, incubation of interrenal tissue *in vitro* has demonstrated the presence of 17α-hydroxylase, 21-hydroxylase, and 11β-hydroxylase. No 1α-hydroxylase could be demonstrated, and although 18-hydroxylation has been reported this reaction needs further confirmation. A quantitative comparison of transformation products of progesterone indicated the sequence of reactions to be 17α-hydroxylation, then 21-hydroxylation, and finally 11β-hydroxylation. No studies on corticosteroids in blood of Holocephali species have been reported.

C. OSTEICHTHYES

1. Introduction

Corticosteroids have been identified in the plasma of a representative species of each order of the bony fishes Osteichthyes. In the chondrosteans and holosteans studies have been confined to one species only and even among the teleosts relatively few of the thousands of species have been examined. Corticosteroids have been identified in the blood of the South American lungfish and corticosteroidogenic enzymes were used to aid in the identification of adrenocortical tissue of the African lungfish. Experiments conducted on species of Osteichthyes are summarized in Tables A.V–A.X.

Among teleosts, the salmonids *Oncorhynchus* sp. and *Salmo* sp. and the eels *Anguilla* sp. have received the most attention. Interest in the endocrinology of salmon is based in part on their commercial value as a wild species and the management of the fishery as well as the potential value of salmon and trout farming. The life cycle and the role of corticosteroids in the migratory and reproductive phases of this cycle make the salmon interesting subjects for their own sake. Species of trout are useful as experimental animals for physiological studies since they can be bred and maintained in captivity and are of sufficient size to permit serial blood analyses.

The European eel *A. anguilla* has been a favorite experimental animal for endocrinological studies both *in vivo* and *in vitro*. The eel is catadromous (descends to sea to spawn) and can be adapted in captivity to a freshwater or marine environment. Like many fishes, the eel can be hypophysectomized (see Pickford, 1957) but, unlike most teleosts, interrenalectomy is also possible (Chester Jones *et al.*, 1964). Thus, the role of the interrenal in electrolyte and carbohydrate metabolism can be studied *in vivo*. The interrenal tissue is concentrated in the walls of the cardinal veins and thus lends itself to studies on corticosteroidogenesis *in vitro*. For reproductive endocrinology the eel is less suitable than the salmonids, or catfish, since sexually mature adults are not available from natural waters and the eel does not breed in captivity, although Fontaine and his co-workers have successfully induced sexual maturation of the eel in captivity (Fontaine, 1936; Fontaine *et al.*, 1964).

The anatomy of the interrenal cells in Osteichthyes precludes the use of perfusion techniques or collection of interrenal venous blood for corticosteroid analyses. Information concerning the nature of corticosteroids in the bony fishes has been obtained from qualitative and quantitative analyses of peripheral plasma and from incubation *in vitro* of interrenal tissues. Among the fishes studied by *in vitro* techniques, except for the Atlantic sturgeon, a chondrostean, more or less extraneous head kidney or cardinal vein tissue has had to be included with interrenal tissue; relatively pure interrenal tissue can be obtained from the walls of the posterior cardinal vein of the eel (Leloup-Hatey, 1964b). Results obtained by this technique are included in the discussions of each order and consideration of problems arising from incubation of heterogeneous tissue is outlined in Section III,C,4,a on the Teleostei.

Plasmatic corticosteroid analyses present no similar specific problems but, in common with those performed on blood of many nonmammalian vertebrates, assays developed for the analysis of corticosteroids in human plasma or even for another species of fish must be proven adequate for the plasma under investigation. The physiological condition of the fish may determine the actual concentration of plasmatic corticosteroids and in some cases qualitative changes have been reported. This factor has received considerable attention for the teleosts and may be true of the other orders as well, although there are insufficient data available to determine if such is the case.

2. Chondrostei

Among the chondrosteans, one species only, the Atlantic sturgeon *Acipenser oxyrhynchus*, has been examined for corticosteroidogenic tissue and for plasmatic steroids. The results are summarized in Table A.V. The interrenal tissue of the sturgeon occurs as discrete, small, yellow bodies throughout the kidney and posterior cardinal veins (Idler and O'Halloran,

1970) and thus for *in vitro* incubations relatively pure tissue can be obtained (cf. teleosts). Cortisol was the principal transformation product of cholesterol, pregnenolone, and progesterone (Idler and Sangalang, 1970). Cortisone was also produced from both precursors. Thus, the following enzyme systems were demonstrated to be present in interrenal tissues of a chondrostean: cholesterol desmolase, Δ^5-3β-hydroxysteroid dehydrogenase, $\Delta^5 \longrightarrow$ Δ^4-isomerase, 17α-hydroxylase, 21-hydroxylase, 11β-hydroxylase, and 11β-dehydrogenase. No evidence was found for a corticosteroid 1α-hydroxylase, 18-hydroxylase, or 18-ol dehydrogenase. On the basis of isotope ratios as measured in the products of double-label precursors, pregnenolone and progesterone, a biosynthetic pathway bypassing progesterone was proposed, i.e., pregnenolone$\longrightarrow$17α-hydroxypregnenolone$\longrightarrow$17α-hydroxyprogesterone $\longrightarrow$ 11-deoxycortisol $\longrightarrow$ cortisol. Similar experiments indicate that such a pathway may also be the favored route with teleost interrenal tissue (see Section III,C,4,a). 17-Deoxycorticosteroids were minor transformation products of precursor *in vitro*; corticosterone was presumptively identified but 11-deoxycorticosterone and aldosterone could not be detected.

Analysis of sturgeon plasma further demonstrated the predominant role of cortisol in this species (Sangalang *et al.*, 1971). Corticosteroids identified and quantified in plasma of this species are included in Table A.V. The plasmatic corticosteroids are similar to those found in other bony fishes but the concentrations are extremely low in comparison to those reported for many teleosts. Further studies on this species as well as other chondrosteans, e.g., the paddlefish, are required to determine if low levels of 17-hydroxycorticosteroids are typical of this group.

3. Holostei

Two species of holosteans, the garpike *Lepisosteus* sp. and the bowfin *Amia* sp., exist in North American freshwater lakes and rivers. There is no information concerning corticosteroids of the garpikes and a very limited amount is known about the bowfin.

In an effort to determine the distribution of a corticosteroid 1α-hydroxylase as found in the elasmobranchs, we performed a series of incubations of interrenal tissues with radioactive corticosterone. Head kidney tissue of the bowfin was included in this survey. Neither 1α-hydroxycorticosterone nor aldosterone could be detected as transformation products. Corticosterone was chosen as substrate for the demonstration of 1α- and 18-hydroxylation but its use precluded a search for other hydroxylases (Idler and Truscott, 1967c).

Corticosteroid analyses of the blood plasma of the bowfin have provided limited data, which are recorded in Table A.VI (Idler *et al.*, 1971). Cortisol was identified by a double-isotope derivative assay in 25 ml plasma collected from four male fish. There was some evidence of corticosterone but the identification has to be considered as tentative. The double-isotope assay is useful for the identification and quantification of selected compounds but does not accommodate the possibility of other unexpected steroids which may be present. Further studies with more or perhaps larger plasma samples are in order to confirm that cortisol is the principal plasmatic corticosteroid in holosteans as in other orders of Osteichthyes.

4. Teleostei

a. Corticosteroid Synthesis in Vitro. The interrenal tissue is not a discrete organ but consists of islets of cells associated with the head kidney and the walls of the cardinal veins (Chapter 3 and Nandi, 1962). The potential of the interrenal cells to produce corticosteroids and the presence of the necessary enzyme systems has been demonstrated in a few species by incubation of head kidney and cardinal vein tissue. Nandi and Bern (1960) discussed some of the factors which complicate the interpretation of results obtained from incubation of such tissue: (a) the presence of several tissue types, e.g., chromaffin, hemopoietic, and renal tubules, (b) a variation in the amounts, particularly of renal elements, in head kidney of different species, and (c) steroid binding and steroid catabolism by surrounding tissues.

Quantitative assessment of teleost corticosteroidogenesis *in vitro* is particularly difficult; incubates contain an unknown weight of interrenal tissue with more or less amounts of extraneous tissue. Thus, with tissue slices quantitative results among individual animals are not directly comparable, and sufficient numbers have to be analyzed to allow statistical analysis. For some purposes, e.g., fate of steroid intermediates, aliquots of homogenates are probably more suitable than tissue slices. Problems of absorption of steroids by extraneous tissue should be considered in experiments in which the tissue is removed from the aqueous medium before its extraction with organic solvents. Recovery of total radioactivity and of isolated transformation products of radioactive precursor are relatively low from incubates of tissue slices. Steroid products are absorbed by the tissue in unequal proportions so that an extract of the aqueous medium is not necessarily representative of the total incubate. After incubation of head kidney tissue of the Atlantic salmon *Salmo salar* with progesterone-^{14}C, only 31% of the total radioactivity was recovered in the aqueous medium whereas 60% was associated with the tissue (Lucis, 1966). Serial fractionation of the two extracts by paper chromatography demonstrated that polar compounds such as cortisol were more concentrated in the aqueous medium and the nonpolar metabolites were concentrated in the tissue. Better recovery of steroids is achieved from homogenates when the total homogenate is extracted with solvent. The percent transformation of precursor to product is also higher because of the disruption of tissue and cell wall barriers. Sandor et al., (1967a) compared tissue slices with homogenates of interrenal preparations of the European eel *Anguilla anguilla* as a source of steroidogenic enzyme systems. Although it is a difficult comparison since the weight of interrenal tissue is only proportional to the weight of kidney–vein tissue, these authors concluded that the homogenates were 100 times more efficient in substrate utilization.

General conclusions and comparisons of results from different species are further complicated by the conditions of incubations used by different groups of investigators. The effect of the chemical composition of the incubation medium on corticosteroidogenesis in teleost interrenal tissue *in vitro* has not been studied in detail. Roy (1964) reported that a medium with a doubled concentration of KCl resulted in an increase in steroid production by tissue from *Ophiocephalus punctatus* but did not report sufficient data to allow a critical evaluation of the results. Leloup-Hatey (1966b) adjusted the $Na^+:K^+$ concentration (in equivalents) from 20.5 to 2.8 in the incubation medium of European eel tissue with progesterone-^{14}C; the author concluded that the transformation of progesterone to cortisol was less efficient and the higher specific activity of the product, cortisol-^{14}C, indicated a decrease in endogenous production. Leloup-Hatey (1970) examined the effect of calcium ions, *in vitro*, on the production of cortisol from endogenous precursors and the transformation of progesterone by interrenal tissue of *Anguilla anguilla*. In tissue from intact eels, no effect of an increase in Ca^{2+}, from 0 to 12 mM, could be demonstrated. In low-activity interrenal tissue from hypophysectomized eels the higher concentrations of Ca^{2+} caused a decrease in endogenous production of cortisol but did not affect enzymic hydroxylations of progesterone. Adrenocorticotropic hormone stimulated corticosteroidogenesis *in vitro* only in glandular tissue from hypophysectomized eels (Leloup-Hatey, 1968), but in the absence of Ca^{2+}, cortisol production was not increased by ACTH. Maximal stimulation by ACTH was produced by the addition of 3 mM Ca^{2+} to the incubation medium. The effect of Ca^{2+} on corticosteroidogenesis in the eel is of particular interest since ablation of the corpuscles of Stannius resulted in an increase in Ca^{2+} levels in the blood and a decrease in the secretory activity of the interrenal (Leloup-Hatey, 1966a, 1970). The effect of incubation temperature on corticosteroid production or transformation by teleost interrenal tissue has received little attention; temperatures used for *in vitro* experiments reported in the literature vary from 15° to 37°C, with very few done at temperatures isothermal with those of the waters in which the fish live. Results obtained with eel interrenal tissue incubated at 5°, 15°, and 30°C were inconclusive and perhaps due to individual variations (Leloup-Hatey, 1968). There was, however, some indication that the production of cortisol from endogenous precursors was more efficient at 5°C than at the higher temperatures but the conversion of progesterone to cortisol was less at 5°C than at 15° or 30°C.

In all teleosts studied, 17-hydroxylated C_{21} steroids are the principal products of the interrenal tissue *in vitro*. Corticosteroidogenesis in the European eel has received the most attention and is the only species in which incubation products of tissue slices, homogenates, and cellular fractions have been compared (Sandor *et al.*, 1966, 1967a,b). The production of C_{21} corticosteroids from endogenous precursors has been examined in several teleosts but only in the eel has it been demonstrated that cholesterol is converted to corticosteroids *in vitro* (Sandor *et al.*, 1967a).

Table A.VII is a summary of corticosteroids isolated from *in vitro* incubations of teleost interrenal (kidney–cardinal vein) preparations with added radioactive precursors as well as steroids produced from endogenous precursors. The identification of steroids has been assessed as described in Chapter 2; when possible, quantities of steroids produced or percent conversion of precursor have been included. Although androgenic steroids (C_{19} steroids) are produced from exogenous precursors by interrenal tissue of teleosts, they are not included in Table A.VII (See Chapter 6). The following text is complementary to this table and for convenience of discussion is divided according to topic as follows: steroidogenesis through cholesterol to pregnenolone, biosynthetic pathways to 17-hydroxycorticosteroids, biosynthesis of 17-deoxycorticosteroids, and catabolic reactions.

Although the conversion of acetate-^{14}C to cortisol-^{14}C has been demonstrated *in vitro* in mammalian adrenal tissue (see Dorfman and Ungar, 1965) there are no records of such conversion by interrenal preparations of a teleost. Sandor *et al.* (1966) incubated tissue of European eel with radioactive sodium acetate with and without exogenous ACTH but could not detect corticosteroids as products. These authors reported the isolation of cholesterol from their preparation but doubted the significance of this result and did not confirm the identity of the sterol. Since negative results are inconclusive it is not possible at this time to say whether the interrenal tissue of teleosts is capable of synthesizing corticosteroids from acetate via cholesterol or depends upon plasma cholesterol as substrate.

The conversion of cholesterol to pregnenolone has not been studied extensively; there is only one well-documented report in the literature. From homogenates of European eel interrenal tissue incubated with cholesterol-^{3}H, Sandor *et al.* (1967a) were able to isolate and identify tritiated cortisol as well as a substance presumptively identified as pregnenolone-^{3}H. The proposed intermediates from cholesterol to pregnenolone, i.e., 20α-hydroxycholesterol and 20α,22-dihydroxycholesterol, have not been isolated or used as precursors in teleost interrenal preparations. Studies with a mitochondrial preparation from bovine adrenal cortex indicate that hydroxylated cholesterol intermediates do not accumulate and the conversion of cholesterol to pregnenolone is a one-step reaction in which "the steroid molecule is bound to the enzyme along with oxygen in a transition-state complex until the side chain is liberated" (Boyd and Simpson, 1968). A second pathway from cholesterol to 17-hydroxypregnenolone via 17α,20α-dihydroxycholesterol, which has been shown (*in vitro*) to be possible in human fetal adrenals (Shimizu *et al*., 1965), has not been investigated in tissues of lower vertebrates but in view of the lower substrate specificity of teleost 17α-hydroxylase this second pathway could be considered as a distinct possibility in the teleosts.

Interrenal tissue of all teleosts examined have shown the presence of a strong 17-hydroxylating enzyme system and 17-hydroxycorticosteroids were the principal products of endogenous precursors (Table A.VII). By means of exogenous radioactive precursors the competition between pregnenolone and progesterone for 17-hydroxylation has been examined in three species, the European eel (Sandor *et al*., 1966, 1967a), the Atlantic herring *Clupea harengus* (Idler, 1969), and the Atlantic salmon (Idler and Sangalang, 1971). With due regard to the problems of interpretation of results obtained by double-isotope incubation techniques, the results of all three investigations indicated that the principal pathway to cortisol was through 17α-hydroxypregnenolone to 17α-hydroxyprogesterone rather than pregnenolone $\longrightarrow$ progesterone $\longrightarrow$ 17α-hydroxyprogesterone. Indirectly, studies with adrenal tissue of the rainbow trout *Salmo gairdnerii* (Arai, 1967a; Arai *et al*., 1969) suggest that 17-hydroxylation in this species also occurs before the dehydrogenation and isomerization of pregnenolone. Homogenates of head kidney tissue incubated with pregnenolone-^{14}C resulted in its conversion to radioactive 17α-hydroxypregnenolone, 11-deoxycortisol, and cortisol, but radioactive 17-deoxysteroids, if detected, were not reported. Homogenates of the same tissue incubated with progesterone-^{14}C gave 11-deoxycorticosterone-^{14}C and probably corticosterone-^{14}C as well as radioactive 11-deoxycortisol and cortisol. It would seem that in teleost interrenal tissue progesterone is not an obligatory intermediate in the biosynthesis of cortisol, and pregnenolone is metabolized in a manner comparable to that of some mammals, e.g., human (Whitehouse and Vinson, 1968), rather than other submammalian vertebrates, e.g., birds, reptiles, or amphibians (Chapter 5). Only with exogenous progesterone as precursor have 17-deoxycorticosteroids been identified as major products of the teleost interrenal *in vitro*.

With teleost interrenal preparations, 17-hydroxylation of exogenous precursors can occur in a sequence not normally found in adrenal glands of mammals. It is generally accepted that hydroxylation at C-21 or C-11 precludes hydroxylation at C-17. Corticosterone was hydroxylated at C-17 to form cortisol in interrenal incubates of the European eel (Sandor *et al.*, 1966). In interrenal incubates of herring and salmon, 11-deoxycorticosterone, 21-deoxycortisol, and corticosterone could be converted to cortisol although none of these hydroxylations was as efficient as the conversion of 11-deoxycortisol to cortisol (Idler, 1969; Idler and Sangalang, 1971).

In teleosts as in mammals the second hydroxylation in the principal pathway between pregnenolone and cortisol involves C-21 hydroxylation. 11-Deoxycortisol has been isolated as a transformation product of exogenous precursors from interrenal incubates of several species (Table A.VII). In homogenized cardinal vein preparations of European eel 11-deoxycortisol was isolated as a transformation product of pregnenolone and/or progesterone in quantities equal to cortisol, the normal end product of corticosteroidogenesis in teleosts (Sandor *et al.*, 1967a). Whether C-21 hydroxylation can occur before dehydrogenation and isomerization at C-3 so that 21-hydroxyor 17α,21-dihydroxy derivatives of pregnenolone play a role in the biosynthesis of corticosteroids in teleost interrenal is not known. Such an alternative pathway has been demonstrated to be possible in adrenal tissue of some other vertebrates (Berliner *et al.*, 1962; Pasqualini *et al.*, 1964).

The presence of an 11β-steroid hydroxylase and dehydrogenase has been amply demonstrated in interrenal tissue of teleosts. In marine, euryhaline, and freshwater species, cortisol has been isolated as the principal corticosteroid produced *in vitro* from endogenous precursors and in most instances is the principal transformation product of exogenous pregnenolone and/or progesterone (Table A. VII). Cortisone usually accompanies cortisol in the products of minced or homogenized tissue incubates. There are no reports of cortisone only being produced by interrenal tissue; a preliminary report of cortisone as the sole product of interrenal tissue of *Tilapia mossambica* (Nandi and Bern, 1960) was later amended and the earlier failure to detect cortisol was attributed to inadequate methods for polar steroids (Nandi and Bern, 1965). As discussed earlier, quantification of steroid production *in vitro* in teleost interrenal preparations has little meaning in an absolute sense and few investigators have applied rigorous assay methods to the determination of cortisol and cortisone production from endogenous precursors. However, in general the ratio cortisol: cortisone favors cortisol (Leloup-Hatey, 1961, 1964b; Nandi and Bern, 1965). With radioactive pregnenolone or progesterone as precursor more cortisol than cortisone was produced by European eel interrenal (Leloup-Hatey, 1966b, 1968; Sandor *et al.*, 1966). Whether cortisone is a product of the interrenal or an artifact of incubation techniques has not been established. The enzyme 11-dehydrogenase occurs in rat kidney tissue (Mahesh and Ulrich, 1959) and conceivably could also occur in fish kidney tissue, which is always more or less present in teleost interrenal preparations. However, both cortisol and cortisone have been isolated from the plasma of several teleosts and may be the sum of peripheral conversion of cortisol $\longleftrightarrow$ cortisone and interrenal secretion of the two steroids.

The enzymes required for the biosynthesis of 11-deoxycorticosterone and corticosterone are present in the interrenal tissue of teleosts as outlined above. The question is whether, in the presence of a strong 17α-hydroxylase, the 17-deoxysteroids accumulate and are secreted by the interrenal cells. Experiments *in vitro* do not provide a positive, indisputable answer but rather seem to indicate that the production of 17-deoxysteroids may be governed by the conditions of the incubation and/or the physiological condition of the fish. Species differences are always a possibility. In general, 11-deoxycorticosterone and corticosterone are minor products of the teleost interrenal and as such have not in many cases been positively identified. Two compounds, one identified as 11-deoxycorticosterone and the other as cortisol, were extracted from the head kidney tissue and from incubated slices of the same tissue of a sexually mature catfish, *Heteropneustes fossilis* (Sundararaj and Goswami, 1969). Although the methods used to identify 11-deoxycorticosterone do not exclude all other possibilities, the chromatographic behavior and chemical reactions of this interrenal product suggest that the identification may be correct. 11-Deoxycorticosterone has not been reported as a product of endogenous precursors in other species. With the aid of radioactive precursors, Arai (1967a) identified 11-deoxycorticosterone as a transformation product of progesterone in homogenates of the head kidney of the freshwater rainbow trout. Since 11-deoxycorticosterone was not reported to be a transformation product of pregnenolone in head kidney homogenates of the same species (Arai *et al.*, 1969) its accumulation in the first instance may have been due to the choice of precursor, i.e., 17α-hydroxylation of progesterone is less efficient, relative to C-21 hydroxylation, than 17α-hydroxylation of pregnenolone.

Corticosterone has been tentatively identified as a minor product of steroidogenesis in several species: freshwater rainbow trout and the marine species *Bodianus bilinulatus* (Nandi and Bern, 1965) and four species of freshwater Indian fishes including the air-breathing *Ophiocephalus punctatus* (Roy, 1964). Identification of steroids in *O. punctatus* was based on chromatographic behavior, color tests, and sulfuric acid spectra. Production of corticosteroids *in vitro* from endogenous precursors can be quantitatively low and require sensitive methods of detection. Corticosteroids from endogenous incubates of the head kidney of Atlantic herring were identified and quantified by a double-isotope derivative assay which included recrystallization to constant specific activity; in 1 hr, 1 g of tissue produced only 6 ng corticosterone but synthesized 750 ng cortisol and 180 ng cortisone (Idler and Truscott, 1970). With radioactive precursors, corticosterone has been isolated as a transformation product of progesterone and 11-deoxycorticosterone (Leloup-Hatey, 1966b; Arai et al., 1969).

Experiments with the interrenal tissue of the European eel illustrate the desirability of positive identification of steroid products. Sandor et al. (1966, 1967a) were unable to isolate 17-deoxysteroids from incubates of European eel tissue with radioactive progesterone or pregnenolone; cortisol and 11-deoxycortisol were the principal products. From interrenal incubates of the same species Leloup-Hatey (1966b) reported the isolation of cortisol, cortisone, and corticosterone but not 11-deoxycortisol as transformation products of progesterone-^{14}C. Since the chromatographic behavior of corticosterone and 11-deoxycortisol can be similar, it has been suggested that the different results may be a case of mistaken identity (Sandor et al., 1967a). These conflicting results may also be caused by different techniques of incubation or by differences in the tissues themselves. 11-Dehydrocorticosterone has not been identified as a product of interrenal tissue in vitro. Since corticosterone is a relatively minor product, sensitive methods would be required to detect the 11-dehydrogenated derivative but the cortisol $\longleftrightarrow$ cortisone conversion is evidence of the necessary enzyme system.

The presence of an 18-hydroxylase has been demonstrated in interrenal tissue of a freshwater species, the trout (Arai and Tamaoki, 1967); three Atlantic marine species, herring (Truscott and Idler, 1968b), cod, and haddock (Sandor et al., 1970): and European eel adapted to fresh or salt water (Sandor et al., 1970). All three experiments were done with radioactive precursors and involved hydroxylation of 11-deoxycorticosterone or corticosterone; only in the herring incubation was 18-hydroxycorticosterone dehydrogenated to yield aldosterone (Truscott and Idler, 1968b). In earlier studies of eel incubates and homogenates, Sandor et al. (1966, 1967a) and Leloup-Hatey (1966b) could not isolate aldosterone as a transformation product of added precursors. However, with a mitochondrial fraction of posterior cardinal vein, Sandor et al. (1970) proved the existence of a low-activity 18-hydroxylating system for this species. A study by Phillips and Mulrow (1959b) with interrenal tissue of the killifish Fundulus heteroclitus deserves special mention; it was the first application of in vitro incubation methods to tissues from fishes. The experiment was well designed, with control tissue as well as interrenal tissue being incubated with radioactive progesterone. Cortisol was the principal transformation product of the interrenal tissue. A minor transformation product of both control and interrenal tissue was identified as aldosterone; the conclusions were described as tentative since the control tissue was less efficient in the transformation of progesterone to cortisol than was the interrenal tissue but was more efficient in the production of aldosterone. More recent studies have indicated that extensive chromatography is required to separate minute quantities of aldosterone from other steroidal products. Aldosterone has not been isolated as a product *in vitro* of endogenous precursors; interrenal tissue of the Atlantic herring did not produce aldosterone in detectable amounts when the products of the incubation were assayed by a double-isotope method capable of measuring aldosterone at a production rate of 2 ng/g hr (Idler and Truscott, 1970). In conclusion, the results of *in vitro* studies indicate that interrenal tissue of teleosts contain a weak 18-hydroxylating enzyme system. The failure in most cases to demonstrate further dehydrogenation to aldosterone may be the result of unfavorable experimental conditions during incubation or a lack of the necessary 18-ol dehydrogenase in some species.

There are no reports of conjugated C_{21} steroids isolated from incubates of fish interrenal tissue. Catabolic changes in C_{21} steroids, e.g., reduction at C-3 or C-20 during incubation, have received little attention. Interest in these compounds is no doubt minimal because they are considered to be biologically inactive. With body kidney, as opposed to head kidney, of the rainbow trout as a source of enzyme (Arai *et al.*, 1969), progesterone-^{14}C, though not transformed to corticosteroids, was hydrogenated to 5α- and 5β-pregnanedione, 3α- and 3β-hydroxy-5α-pregnan-20-one, and 3α- and 3β-hydroxy-5β-pregnan-20-one. Although the body kidney was shown to lack the enzyme systems necessary to hydroxylate progesterone, it is not clear from the published account whether the head kidney tissue lacked completely the enzymes necessary to reduce ring A or if their activity was low compared to the activity of the hydroxylases. Another metabolic reaction which could be expected to occur is reduction at the C-20 position. There are no reports of the isolation and identification of steroids reduced at C-20 as products of teleost interrenal tissue *in vitro* although there are several reports, especially in experiments with radioactive precursors, of unidentified metabolites. With no comprehensive study of the catabolism of corticosteroids by teleost interrenal–kidney tissue *in vitro* to serve as a guide, the possibility that products of an incubation may be contaminated with such reduced derivatives should be considered. This possibility is especially important in experiments with tracer amounts of radioactive precursors in which chemical tests for specific molecular configurations, e.g., α-ketol or Δ^4-3-keto groups, are not applicable.

b. Plasmatic Corticosteroids. Corticosteroids identified in the plasma of teleosts are listed in Table A.VIII. Quantitative measurements are included in the table; if the original publication was concerned with the effects of several experimental procedures, the information in the table is necessarily limited to a partial summary of the original publication. Changes in concentration of corticosteroids in plasma of fish as a function of physiological conditions (e.g., exercise, stress, and sexual maturity) or of experimental procedures (e.g., hypophysectomy or injections of physiologically active compounds) are discussed in Section IV. Since the concentration of plasmatic corticosteroids is dependent on these factors no attempt has been made to list *normal* values in the blood of individual species of teleosts. With some exceptions, e.g., hatchery-bred trout or aquaria-bred tropicals and goldfish, it is difficult if not impossible to maintain fish in captivity for any length of time under conditions comparable to their natural environment. Of necessity the movement of wild species is restricted and the water pressures, currents, and temperatures of their natural environment are not duplicated.

Cortisol and cortisone are the major corticosteroids identified in the peripheral plasma of all teleosts so far examined. In many investigations cortisol and cortisone have not been identified as such but rather 17,21-dihydroxy-20-ketosteroids (17-OHCS) were measured by the Porter–Silber reaction with phenylhydrazine. Relatively few of the thousands of species of teleosts have been studied even superficially but there is no evidence to date of a new or distinctive corticosteroid typical of this order (cf. subclass Elasmobranchii). The conclusion that cortisol is the principal plasmatic corticosteroid of teleosts is actually based on very few studies. Many investigations have been concerned with the effect of various physiological factors on the concentration of cortisol or 17-OHCS in the blood. Such investigations require the analysis of many samples so that methods which would detect other corticosteroids in the plasma are not practicable. However, cortisol has been identified in the blood of those teleosts which have been studied most intensively including the Pacific salmon *Oncorhynchus* sp., the Atlantic salmon and trout *Salmo* sp., and the eels *Anguilla* sp. (Table A. VIII).

Cortisone has been separated and identified in the blood of a few species and especially in fish where the total 17-OHCS levels are high, e.g., *Oncorhynchus* sp. after spawning and *Salmo* sp. during migratory phases of their life cycle. Whether cortisone is a product of the interrenal or a peripheral catabolite of cortisol has not been positively established; *in vitro* cortisone often appears as a product of the interrenal but may be a result of 11-dehydrogenase activity in the kidney tissue. Cortisol-^{14}C was rapidly converted to cortisone-^{14}C in the circulating blood of mature sockeye salmon (*O. nerka*) (Idler *et al.*, 1963) but cortisone-^{14}C was not reduced to cortisol-[14]C (Donaldson and Fagerlund, 1968). In the earlier study in which cortisone-^{14}C acetate was shown to be readily hydrolyzed to cortisone-^{14}C *in vivo* in Atlantic salmon (*S. salar*) Idler *et al.* (1963) reported a further conversion of less than 9% to cortisol-^{14}C but, although radioactivity was associated with the cortisol fraction, the conversion of cortisone to cortisol was not irrefutably established. There are at least two interrelated factors which may contribute to the accumulation of cortisone in the blood of some teleosts: equilibrium constants of the reaction cortisol $\longleftrightarrow$ cortisone and the metabolic clearance rate of cortisone relative to cortisol (see Sections V and VI).

Corticosterone has been reported to occur in the peripheral plasma of several species of teleosts (Table A.VIII), particularly freshwater or anadromous species during their migration from the sea into fresh water, but in no case has its identity been rigorously established. Rather its identity has been assumed on the basis of polarity in one or more chromatographic solvent systems, absorption of ultraviolet light at 240 mμ, color tests, and acid or alkali fluorescence. However, since the last three criteria are characteristic of reactive groups in the steroid molecule, only the polarity serves to distinguish one steroid from another. Steroid mixtures may not be sufficiently resolved and this may be of particular importance for steroids less polar than cortisone. Corticosterone and 11-deoxycortisol are not readily separated from one another, especially on paper chromatograms when aqueous alcohol is used as the stationary phase. Further, oxygenated C_{19} steroids are sufficiently polar not to separate easily from the less polar C_{21} corticosteroids, e.g., 11-ketotestosterone and corticosterone. Thus, if an ultraviolet-absorbing area on a chromatogram were also blue tetrazolium positive and then quantified by alkali fluorescence (a reaction typical of Δ^4-3-keto group) the quantity could be a measure of a C_{19} as well as the C_{21} steroid. Since the biosynthesis of corticosterone does not require any enzyme system not involved with the biosynthesis of cortisol, the teleost interrenal has the potential to secrete corticosterone and there is some evidence that under certain physiological conditions, corticosterone can accumulate in the peripheral plasma. It was reported to be present in the blood of carp (*Cyprinus carpio*) only after prolonged exercise and in Atlantic salmon only at the beginning of their upstream spawning migration (Leloup-Hatey, 1961, 1964b). Unfortunately, its identification was not established beyond doubt. If we assume that the identification was indeed correct, it would imply that under certain conditions either the 17-hydroxylase enzyme system was inhibited or the activity of the Δ^5-3β-hydroxysteroid delydrogenase–isomerase enzyme system was increased. This latter explanation is based on *in vitro* studies of steroid biosynthesis in interrenal tissue of Atlantic salmon where 17-hydroxylation of pregnenolone rather than progesterone was the preferential route to the principal product, cortisol; corticosterone was formed from progesterone rather than pregnenolone (Idler and Sangalang, 1971). Similarly studies on the European eel *Anguilla anguilla* (Sandor *et al.*, 1966, 1967a) indicated that 17-hydroxylation of pregnenolone precluded the accumulation of 17-deoxysteroids in the interrenal tissues.

Although 11-deoxycortisol has been identified as a major transformation product of exogenous precursors by teleost interrenal *in vitro* (Table A.VII), it has been reported (Idler *et al.*, 1960b), but not presumptively identified, only in the blood of postspawned Pacific sockeye salmon. Except for the possibility that in some instances 11-deoxycortisol may have been mistaken for corticosterone, there is no evidence that 11-deoxycortisol, although a precursor of cortisol, accumulates in the peripheral blood of teleosts.

Other C_{21} steroids, namely 17α-hydroxyprogesterone, 17α,20β-dihydroxyprogesterone, and 20β-dihydrocortisone, were isolated from the blood of postspawned sockeye salmon (Idler *et al.*, 1959b, 1960a, 1962). Since these fish die after spawning the 20β-hydroxy compounds may represent catabolic products which accumulate in the blood because of impaired metabolism and conjugation. The hydroxylated progesterone derivatives could be products of gonadal rather than interrenal tissue.

The major mineralocorticoid in mammals is aldosterone and its role as a salt-retaining hormone has been studied chiefly in humans, the rat, and sheep. Methods of assay and physiological and pathological variations in the adrenal secretion of aldosterone in mammals were reviewed by Coghlan and Blair-West (1967). For fish there is no information on the physiological activity of aldosterone, and with the demonstration of a mineral-regulating role for cortisol in the European eel (Mayer *et al.*, 1967) even the need of teleostean interrenal tissue to synthesize 18-hydroxylated steroids might be questioned. Since one of the principal controlling mechanisms of aldosterone secretion in mammals is the variation in "total body sodium status," theoretically it could be expected to play a critical role for anadromous species, e.g., *Oncorhynchus* or *Salmo* sp., during their migrations from salt to fresh water.

Recent studies have demonstrated the enzyme systems necessary to synthesize aldosterone, an 18-corticosteroid hydroxylase and an 18-ol dehydrogenase, in interrenal tissue of a marine fish, the Atlantic herring *Clupea harengus* (Truscott and Idler, 1968b). Attempts to demonstrate the production of aldosterone in other species have not been successful, although an 18-hydroxylase has been demonstrated in several (Table A.VII). Results with *in vitro* techniques are unpredictable and not always reproducible. This may also be true of aldosterone in the blood of teleosts; i.e., there is sometimes, but not always, sufficient aldosterone in the plasma to permit detection. In one of the earlier investigations Phillips *et al.* (1959) isolated a corticosteroid with the chromatographic mobility of aldosterone from a large volume of plasma from postspawned sockeye salmon but did not further confirm their identification. In a similar study of plasma from the same species Idler *et al.* (1959b) isolated a compound which, although isopolar with aldosterone, could not chemically be so identified (see Bern *et al.*, 1962) nor did it exhibit mineral-regulating activity in the rat bioassay. In the light of more recent evidence of unpredictable corticosteroid 18-hydroxylase activity in teleosts, the conclusions from these two studies of aldosterone in postspawned sockeye salmon may not necessarily be contradictory but rather reflect a real difference in corticosteroid metabolism due to physiological condition of the fish at the time of bleeding. However, it does underline the need for definitive identification of corticosteroids if we hope to understand their role in the physiology of fish.

No further studies with the more precise and sensitive assays now available for the determination of aldosterone in peripheral plasma of animal species (e.g., Brodie *et al.*, 1967; Coghlan and Scoggins, 1967) have been done on Pacific salmon either before or after their spawning migration into fresh water. However, aldosterone has recently been rigorously identified in three out of ten blood samples from Atlantic herring; identification was based on acetylation of the unknown with tritiated acetic anhydride, extensive chromatographic purification of the diacetate and derivatives, as well as recrystallization of the tritiated lactone derivative with authentic aldosterone 11,18-lactone 21-monoacetate (Truscott and Idler, 1969; Idler, 1971). In seven other samples of herring plasma, as well as plasma from the cod *Gadus morrhua*, the anadromous alewife *Alosa pseudoharengus* on its migration into fresh water, and postspawned Atlantic salmon, aldosterone could not be detected. The sensitivity of the method and blood volumes used would permit the detection of 2 ng/100 ml. Resting levels of aldosterone in the blood of teleosts may be in subnanogram amounts and only under certain physiological or pathological conditions does the concentration in the plasma increase sufficiently to allow detection by current methods.

There are no reports of corticosteroids or their catabolites conjugated with glucuronic or sulfuric acid in the blood of teleosts, although testosterone glucoronide was identified in the blood and testes of sockeye salmon (Grajcer and Idler, 1963).

c. *Corticosteroids of Corpuscles of Stannius.* The corpuscles of Stannius in teleosts were first described in 1839, but in spite of many investigations since that time their function is still in doubt. There is a phylogenetic progression from 40 to 50 corpuscles in the Holostei to a single pair in the more specialized teleosts (Garrett, 1942). Their ductless nature, excellent vascular supply, and changes in structure accompanied by cytological differences are evidence that corpuscles are endocrine glands.

For many years there has been a controversy concerning the possible adrenocortical function of these corpuscles; at one time they were called the "posterior interrenals" because of their morphological position on the surface of the kidney and because they showed histological characteristics normally associated with endocrine function. On the basis of a histophysiological investigation of the corpuscles of a freshwater teleost, *Astyanax mexicanus*, Rasquin (1956) suggested an osmoregulatory function, a role usually associated with steroids produced by the adrenal gland. Histological studies on other teleosts have confirmed the conclusion that the corpuscles of Stannius are in some way connected with the control of electrolyte and water metabolism. Ogawa (1963) observed hypertrophy of the corpuscles of Stannius in the Japanese goldfish *Carassius auratus* when the fish were kept in one-third seawater. Olivereau (1964) concluded from her histological studies on the European eel *Anguilla anguilla* that the corpuscles of Stannius of the eel are associated with electrolyte metabolism. Hanke *et al.* (1967) observed histological changes in the pituitary ACTH cells, adrenal cortex, and corpuscles of Stannius of the European eel after adrenalectomy, hypophysectomy, ACTH, and cortisol treatment. The changes in the corpuscles of Stannius were found to be variable; the only consistent effect was nuclear enlargement after ACTH or cortisol injections. In seawater yellow eels, in particular, adrenalectomy stimulated the cells of the corpuscles while the removal of the corpuscles had a stimulatory effect on the adrenocortical cells. It was concluded that the interrelationships between the corpuscles of Stannius and the pituitary, or the corpuscles of Stannius and the adrenal cortex, are still obscure but that the corpuscles of Stannius certainly play an important role in the maintenance of electrolyte balance of the body. In a study of the histology and cytology of these organs in the Atlantic salmon *Salmo salar*, Lopez (1969) found evidence for a correlation between the fresh- and saltwater phases of the life cycle and the functional activity of the corpuscles. The corpuscles appeared to be very active in the true smolts, completely inactive in adult, sexually immature, anadromous salmon, and very active in the reproductive adults, especially the male fish. In a rather similar study, Heyl (1970) reported that, although there were exceptions, histological changes in the corpuscles of Stannius of the Atlantic salmon during their spawning migration appeared to be associated with the length of time spent in fresh water rather than with gonadal development.

The biological action attributable to the corpuscles of Stannius in teleosts, including electrolyte metabolism, is discussed in Chapter 8. Further attention here is restricted to investigations of the corpuscles as steroid-secreting organs. Their steroidogenic capacity or potential has been studied by essentially two methods: (a) a search, using histochemical or biochemical techniques, for the enzyme systems necessary to produce steroids or (b) a quantitative determination of endogenous steroid content.

Histochemical investigations (Chieffi and Botte, 1963; Botte *et al.*, 1964; A. S. Grimm, cited by Idler and Freeman, 1966; Bara, 1968) have failed to demonstrate the presence of 3β-hydroxysteroid dehydrogenase in corpuscles of Stannius. This enzyme, which is responsible for the transformation of pregnenolone to progesterone, was shown to be present only in steroid-secreting glands of vertebrates (Chieffi and Botte, 1963). Bara (1968) was unable to demonstrate histochemically 3β-, 3α-, 11β-, and 17β-hydroxysteroid dehydrogenase activities in the corpuscles of Stannius of *Fundulus heteroclitus* although adrenocortical tissue under similar experimental conditions exhibited activity in every case. These incubations were usually performed at 37°C although parallel sections from the corpuscles of Stannius were in some instances incubated at room temperature. It is of interest to note that Grimm could not demonstrate 3β-hydroxysteroid dehydrogenase activity histochemically in corpuscles of Stannius from the Atlantic cod *Gadus morrhua*, although this activity was demonstrated biochemically (Idler and Freeman, 1966) in the same species. In his histochemical studies, Grimm used pregnenolone, pregnenolone sulfate, dehydroepiandrosterone, and dehydroepiandrosterone sulfate as substrates and nitro blue tetrazolium, tetranitro blue tetrazolium, blue tetrazolium, and neotetrazolium chloride as hydrogen acceptors. The discrepancy in the results of the histochemical and biochemical methods carried out on the same species may be explained by the greater sensitivity of the biochemical–isotope method; thus it seems that failure to demonstrate enzymes by histochemical methods should be treated with some reservations.

Biochemical methods designed to demonstrate the presence of corticosteroids or of enzyme systems necessary for the elaboration of corticosteroids have failed to provide consistent results when applied to corpuscles of Stannius of several teleosts. Results so obtained are summarized in Table A.IX.

Ford (1959) failed to detect corticosteroids in extracts of corpuscles of Stannius from the sockeye salmon *Oncorhynchus nerka*, although he found an appreciable quantity of cortisol in the plasma from the same fish. Phillips and Mulrow (1959a) did not detect cortisol, cortisone, corticosterone, or aldosterone when 105 mg of corpuscles from the winter flounder *Pseudopleuronectes americanus* were incubated at 37°C with progesterone. They concluded that, within the limitations of the techniques employed, the corpuscles of Stannius were not concerned with the production of adrenocorticosteroids. More recently, Chester Jones *et al.* (1965) reported the failure of *in vitro* incubations of corpuscles of Stannius of the European eel to transform pregnenolone and progesterone to 11-deoxycorticosterone, 17α-hydroxyprogesterone, 11-deoxycortisol, corticosterone, cortisone, cortisol, and aldosterone but reported a slight transformation of added precursors to unidentified products. It was concluded that the corpuscles of Stannius of the freshwater eel do not synthesize corticosteroids in amounts that could be detected by the methods employed. Arai *et al.* (1969) compared the steroidogenic potential of head kidney, body kidney, and corpuscles of Stannius of the rainbow trout *Salmo gairdnerii* by *in vitro* incubation at 37°C of homogenates of these tissues with radioactive steroidal precursors. All the enzymes necessary for the elaboration of adrenal steroids from pregnenolone or progesterone were present in the head kidney. However, pregnene $5\alpha,5\beta$-hydrogenase activities were predominant in the corpuscles of Stannius as well as the body kidney, and 3α- and 3β-hydroxysteroid dehydrogenase activities were also observed in the body kidney but not in the corpuscles of Stannius. When radioactive progesterone or 11-deoxycorticosterone were incubated with 1.5 g homogenates of corpuscles of Stannius of rainbow trout, no corticosteroids were detected as metabolites.

Investigations, similar to those described above, of other teleosts have yielded positive results. Fontaine and Leloup-Hatey (1959) reported that in the Atlantic salmon during spawning migration the corpuscles of Stannius as well as the head kidney contained corticosteroids but that the head kidney was richer in the hormones when the relative amount of endocrine cells was considered. Their results are given in Table I.

Other authors have reported corticosteroids in extracts of corpuscles of teleosts. Nandi and Pieprzyk (cited by Bern, 1967) found evidence of 11-deoxycorticosterone in corpuscles of Stannius of trout. Krishnamurthy (1968) obtained two UV-absorbing, tetrazolium-positive substances when extracts of 3.1 g of corpuscles of Stannius from *Colisa lalia* were run on paper chromatograms. These compounds with the chromatographic

TABLE I

Cortisol and Corticosterone in the Corpuscles of Stannius (CS) and Head Kidney (HK) of the Atlantic Salmon *Salmo salar*

Sex	No. of fish	Maturity	Cortisol[a]		Corticosterone[a]	
			CS	HK	CS	HK
M	13	Immature[b]	436	112	ND[c]	1
M	21	Mature[d]	39	62	ND	17
F	38	Immature	187	134	20	3
F	22	Mature	40	155	ND	9

[a]Quantity of steroid in micrograms per 100 g of tissue.
[b]In the spring at the beginning of the anadromous migration.
[c]Denotes not detected.
[d]Spawning salmon (in the winter).

mobility of cortisol and 11-deoxycortisol had sulfuric acid chromogens with maxima comparable to those of authentic cortisol and 11-deoxycortisol; the absorption spectra also indicated the presence of contaminants. The quantities of steroid in the extract were not reported but the sensitivity of the methods used indicated that 3 g of corpuscles of Stannius contained microgram quantities of steroids. The corpuscles of Stannius of *C. lalia* also contained an abundance of lipids, cholesterol, and ascorbic acid. Krishnamurthy proposed that these compounds together with the substances which showed the characteristics of cortisol and deoxycortisol indicated that the corpuscles resemble adrenocortical tissue. He suggested that the occurrence of significant protein-synthesis activity in such a tissue possibly results from the products of enzymes necessary for the synthesis of steroid hormones, or, alternatively, the presence of steroids in the corpuscles of Stannius may indicate storage and/or metabolism of circulating hormones by this tissue (Krishnamurthy, 1968).

Positive results have also been obtained by *in vitro* incubation techniques used to determine the capacity of corpuscles of Stannius to metabolize either endogenous or added precursors. Ogawa (1963) obtained a spot positive to triphenyltetrazolium chloride in the "deoxycorticosterone zone" of paper chromatograms of extracts prepared from incubations of corpuscles of Stannius from the Japanese goldfish *Carassius auratus*. Idler and Freeman (1966) found conversion of pregnenolone to progesterone (yield 1.02%) and progesterone to 11-deoxycorticosterone (yield 0.032%) by *in vitro* incubations at 20°–25°C of Atlantic cod corpuscles of Stannius. In another experiment 55 μg of a compound tentatively identified as cortisol (not corrected for losses that occurred during extraction and quantification) per 100 g of tissue was detected after incubation without added precursors of 550 mg of corpuscles of Stannius obtained from 25 mature Atlantic cod of mixed sex; the temperature of the incubation was 25°C. The cod were taken at sea in February 1967 and transported to the laboratory alive, where they arrived in poor condition. On arrival the fish were sacrificed and corpuscles of Stannius were removed and incubated immediately. "Cortisol" was quantified by fluorescence in sulfuric acid: ethanol (65:35) after purification by chromatography using two thin-layer silica gel systems followed by a benzene plus 50% methanol paper system. The areas immediately above and below "cortisol" on the paper chromatogram gave blank fluorescent values. We cannot say that there was not a similar amount of cortisol in an equal quantity of body kidney tissue as control kidney tissue was not incubated for comparison (Freeman and Idler, 1969).

The experimental conditions used for incubation of corpuscles of Stannius may be responsible, at least in part, for the conflicting results obtained by this technique. Incubation temperatures of 37°C may be ideal for mammalian tissues but may have an inhibitory effect on tissues of a poikilotherm. Co-factor requirements of corpuscle tissue have not been studied. Species difference is also a possibility; conflicting results have not been reported for the same species.

Corpuscles may carry out specific transformations on steroids formed elsewhere in the body but may not be capable of total steroid synthesis; their excellent blood supply would suit them to this role. This situation would be somewhat analogous to that which exists in bovine medullary tissue, where the enzyme systems necessary for hydroxylation are present but enzymes necessary to convert cholesterol to pregnenolone are not demonstrable *in vitro* (Carballeira *et al.*, 1965).

It is possible that the corpuscles of Stannius have more than one function and/or the variable results reported may be valid and associated with seasonal variations in fish, species differences, and other unidentified factors. One conclusion appears reasonably certain: It is unlikely that corpuscles of Stannius play a prominent role in the endogenous synthesis of steroids.

5. Dipnoi

Corticosteroidogenesis and plasmatic corticosteroids have been investigated in two species of Dipnoi. The results are summarized in Table A.X. The African lungfish *Protopterus* sp. was the subject of a study designed to identify the interrenal cells of Dipnoi (Janssens *et al.*, 1965). The corticosteroidogenic potential of the cells suspected to be interrenal was measured by incubation of these cells with progesterone-^{14}C. Tissue containing kidney tubules and perirenal tissue was used as a control. Corticosterone-^{14}C but not cortisol-^{14}C was identified as a product of the interrenal but not of the control tissue. Corticosterone-^{14}C was identified by the addition of authentic corticosterone-^{3}H and demonstration of a constant isotope ratio through sequential derivatives. In the published paper the initial ratio ^{3}H:^{14}C is given as 1:237 but it should be 237:1 (Chester Jones, 1969). The production of corticosterone is interesting since 17-deoxysteroids are typical of amphibians (Chapter 5) whereas the principal corticosteroids of the bony fish are 17-hydroxylated. In this experiment the transformation of progesterone to corticosterone served as corroborative evidence of the interrenal nature of the cells under examination. From the vantage point of hindsight, pregnenolone rather than progesterone would have been a better choice to determine whether the steroid produced by the lungfish was typical of amphibians or teleosts since in teleosts the principal pathway of corticosteroidogenesis appears to be 17-hydroxylation of pregnenolone and progesterone is not an obligatory intermediate.

In a comparative study of steroids in the blood of lower vertebrates, the

African lungfish *Protopterus annectens* was included (Phillips and Chester Jones, 1957). Cortisol only was tentatively identified as present in the peripheral blood. In peripheral plasma of the free-living aquatic form of the same species, the level of 17-hydroxycorticosteroids was 12.0 μg/100 ml (Leloup-Hatey, 1964b). The Porter–Silber chromogens were estimated from a plasma extract that was purified by chromatography on a florisil column (Eik-Nes *et al.*, 1953). Thus, the results obtained *in vivo* show a basic difference from those obtained *in vitro* (as outlined above) where 17α-hydroxylation could not be demonstrated (Janssens *et al.*, 1965). In the latter study the fish were in the aestivating state and collection of blood was not practicable (Janssens, 1965). Is the pattern of corticosteroidogenesis in the free-living phase different than that in the aestivating phase of the lungfish? This is an intriguing problem and these tentative experiments should be followed up utilizing more rigorous methodology.

The plasma of the free-living South American lungfish *Lepidosiren paradoxa* was examined for the presence of certain corticosteroids by double-isotope derivative assays and recrystallizations to constant isotope ratios (Idler *et al.*, 1972). Samples of plasma from four female South American lungfish were pooled to give a total volume of 39 ml for analysis. ^{14}C-Labeled corticosteroids were added to the plasma before solvent extraction and initial separation of steroid fractions by thin-layer chromatography. Plasma samples containing the ^{14}C-labeled tracer steroids and reference samples containing only the ^{14}C-labeled tracers were acetylated with tritiated acetic anhydride. The resulting double-labeled acetates were purified by sequential thin-layer and paper chromatography until isopolarity with the corresponding radioninert carrier steroid acetates was established. The acetates were then recrystallized to constant isotope ratios. Aldosterone was identified by conversion of the diacetate derivative to the 11,18-lactone 21-acetate and recrystallization of this final derivative to constant isotope ratio. The results of this experiment are included in Table A.X. Aldosterone, cortisol, corticosterone, and 11-deoxycortisol were identified in the plasma of *L. paradoxa*. Quantitatively, aldosterone and cortisol were the major plasmatic corticosteroids ($\sim$0.6 μg/100 ml) with less but significant amounts of corticosterone (0.16 μg/100 ml) and trace quantities of 11-deoxycortisol. Cortisone, 11-deoxycorticosterone, and 11-dehydrocorticosterone could not be detected. Thus, the plasmatic corticosteroids of this species of lungfish resemble both those of the bony ray-finned fishes (cortisol) and those of the amphibians (corticosterone and aldosterone). Further definitive studies will be required to determine if there is a change in the nature of corticosteroid secretion during aestivation and if the interrenal of other species of lungfish, in particular the more aquatic Australian lungfish, elaborates both 17-hydroxy- and 17-deoxycorticosteroids.

6. Summary

General conclusions regarding corticosteroids and corticosteroidogenesis in a group as large and diverse as Osteichthyes are difficult to draw and exceptions are to be expected. The following statements are based on data available from analyses of blood samples and interrenal tissues of a very few species.

Cortisol and cortisone have been identified in the blood and/or as a product of interrenal tissue *in vitro* of species representative of all orders of Actinopterygii. In teleosts, the total concentration of 17-hydroxycorticosteroids appears to depend upon various physiological and pathological factors; resting or basal levels are low compared to those recorded in fish subjected to stressful situations, either natural or artificial. The concentration of cortisone in the blood is usually lower than that of cortisol but exceptions have been recorded, e.g., in salmonids during the migratory or reproductive phases of their life cycle. There is insufficient evidence to conclude that cortisone is a secretory product of the interrenal gland; 11β-dehydrogenase activity has been demonstrated in interrenal tissue *in vitro* but could represent a catabolic reaction. The peripheral conversion of cortisol to cortisone has been demonstrated *in vivo* in teleosts, but the reverse reaction occurs only to a limited extent in a Pacific salmon.

The 17-deoxycorticosteroids, corticosterone, and 11-deoxycorticosterone have been identified in the blood of a few species but usually occur in trace quantities relative to 17-hydroxycorticosteroids. Again, exceptions have been recorded and further studies are required to determine if the secretion of 17-deoxycorticosteroids has any physiological significance.

Aldosterone was identified in the blood of a South American lungfish (subclass Sarcopterygii) at a concentration equal to that of cortisol. In the other subclass, Actinopterygii, aldosterone if present at all would seem to occur at extremely low levels, although it has been identified in the blood of one species of teleost.

The enzyme systems necessary for the conversion of cholesterol to cortisol or corticosterone (i.e., a cholesterol desmolase, Δ^5-3β-hydroxysteroid dehydrogenase, $\Delta^5 \longrightarrow \Delta^4$-isomerase, 17α-hydroxylase, 21-hydroxylase, and 11β-hydroxylase) have been demonstrated *in vitro* in interrenal tissue of Chondrostei and Teleostei. On the basis of results obtained with radioactive precursors the following biosynthetic pathways to cortisol and corticosterone have been proposed for both Chondrostei and Teleostei: cholesterol $\longrightarrow$ pregnenolone $\longrightarrow$ 17α-hydroxypregnenolone $\longrightarrow$ 17α-hydroxyprogesterone $\longrightarrow$ 11-deoxycortisol $\longrightarrow$ cortisol, and pregnenolone $\longrightarrow$ progesterone $\longrightarrow$ 11-deoxycorticosterone $\longrightarrow$ corticosterone. In both orders cortisol was the principal product of exogenous precursors *in vitro*.

Evidence for the presence of the enzyme systems necessary for the production of aldosterone has been difficult to obtain by *in vitro* methods. A low-activity 18-hydroxylase has been demonstrated in interrenal tissue of Teleostei but only in one species has an 18-ol dehydrogenase also been reported. In teleost interrenal preparations 17-hydroxylation is very efficient; *in vivo*, additional interrenal factors may influence the secretion of 17-deoxycorticosteroids including aldosterone.

IV. Factors Affecting Corticosteroidogenesis

A. Introduction

The importance of the pituitary–adrenal axis with respect to plasma corticoid levels is well documented for certain mammals. Numerous stressors stimulate the output of adrenocorticotropin (ACTH) from the anterior pituitary, which, in turn, stimulates the adrenal cortex to produce corticoids.

The effect of changes in water salinity on interrenal function has been studied chiefly, but not exclusively (carp being an exception), in species whose spawning migration is associated with a change in salinity of the environment. Many such studies are necessarily complicated by the maturation of the gonads at this time, and changes in concentration of plasmatic steroids may be influenced by the combined effects of sexual maturation and change of habitat. In this section the role of the hypophysis and neuroendocrine systems, thyroid and gonadal hormones in migratory patterns of fish will not be considered although this role is no doubt a basic one. Koch (1968) discussed the physiological and endocrinological aspects of migratory behavior of vertebrates. A review of hormones in fish in relation to migration, which includes a section on interrenal function, was published by Nomura (1962a,b) and studies on the influence of migration on the interrenal of two species of teleost, the Atlantic salmon *Salmo salar* and the European eel *Anguilla anguilla*, were compiled by Leloup-Hatey (1964b). The interest in interrenal steroid products during anadromous and catadromous migrations is naturally founded upon the mineralocorticoid activity of adrenal secretions in mammals, although in lower vertebrates a mineralocorticoid activity distinct from glucocorticoid activity may not be a valid distinction. The activity of corticosteroids in ionic regulation and osmoregulation in lower vertebrates is discussed in Chapter 8. A comprehensive review of salt and water metabolism in lower vertebrates has been published by Maetz (1968).

This discussion will *not* be concerned with the role of corticosteroids but rather with interrenal function as measured by the concentration of corticosteroids in the plasma of fish. Experiments designed to distinguish among the effects of natural environmental or physiological factors and unnatural factors, such as the struggle during capture, captivity, pollutants, surgery, and anesthesia, are discussed.

In the following account of factors affecting steroidogenesis in fish, the degree of sophistication of methodology should be borne in mind. Cortisone, a steroid found in peripheral blood, especially of salmonids, and a contributor to total Porter–Silber chromogens but not to fluorescence, has not generally been measured independently; factors that may influence the ratio of cortisol:cortisone have not been defined. Total 17-hydroxycorticosteroids (17-OHCS) as measured by earlier methods (Porter and Silber, 1950; Nelson and Samuels, 1952) were later modified to correct for problems of specificity. One nonsteroidal compound, lactic acid, which is chloroform extractable and is eluted from florisil columns, produced a typical Porter–Silber reaction (Eik-Nes, 1957). These authors suggested the use of benzene:water partition to further purify extracts before reaction with phenylhydrazine. Lactic acid can accumulate rapidly in fish after exercise; in the rainbow trout *Salmo gairdnerii* after 15 min of rigorous exercise, blood lactate increased from 16 to 100 mg/100 ml plasma and during 2 hr of subsequent recovery it increased further to 170 mg/100 ml plasma; lactate returned to control levels only after 4–6 hr (Black, 1957a). Similar results were obtained with the sockeye salmon *Oncorhynchus nerka* (Black, 1957b). Although the quantities of lactic acid in the plasma do not approach the 100 mg/10 ml plasma used by Eik-Nes (1957) to demonstrate interference, a part of the increase in Porter–Silber chromogens measured by earlier methods in exercised and fatigued fish may have been due to lactic acid. Few investigators have checked blank values with samples containing all reagents except phenylhydrazine when measuring plasma 17-OHCS with the Porter–Silber method. These and other examples (see Chapter 2) illustrate the need for caution in the application of methods to plasma samples taken from animals in different physiological states.

B. Osmotic Shock and Motor Activity

Histological studies have clearly demonstrated that a transfer of certain teleost fishes from fresh water to seawater results in a stimulation of the anterior interrenal which persists for various periods of time depending on the species (e.g., Pickford and Atz, 1957; Olivereau, 1962) and stimulation does not occur in hypophysectomized goldfish, *Carassius auratus* (Chavin,

1956). Unfortunately, these and many similar excellent investigations are outside the scope of this chapter.

1. Carp

Leloup-Hatey (1964a) reported a series of experiments designed to test the hypothesis that observed histological changes were a reaction against osmotic shock. Carp (*Cyprinus carpio* L.), which die within hours in salt water, were transferred by net from fresh water to seawater (Δ: $-2°C$) and plasma 17-OHCS levels were determined on groups of fish at timed intervals up to 2.5 hr. 17-Hydroxycorticoid levels increased substantially in the first 0.5 hr after transfer (from 2 to 21 $\mu g/100$ ml, $p = 0.001$), were still significantly elevated at 1 hr (8 $\mu g/100$ ml, $p = 0.01$), and had returned to normal at 2.5 hr. The author interpreted these data to indicate a temporary stimulation of the interrenal followed by a return to near normal activity when the gland was exhausted (Sayers and Sayers, 1948). When carp were subjected to the same salinity shock (Δ: $-2°C$, 0.5 hr) without the added stress of transfer by net, i.e., salt was introduced into the freshwater aquarium, plasma 17-OHCS again increased substantially: 27 $\mu g/100$ ml ($p = 0.001$) in fish which were transferred and 19 $\mu g/100$ ml ($p = 0.001$) in fish which were not transferred. The levels of plasma 17-OHCS of the two groups in salt water were not statistically different. Carp were next anesthetized with urethane or ether prior to transfer to seawater to eliminate motor activity. In this case there was no elevation of plasma 17-OHCS levels. The author pointed out that there is a negligible action of ether on the hypothalmic–hypophyseal connections (Guillemin *et al.*, 1959) and, presumably, there is no effect on steroidogenesis. It might be noted that ether rapidly elevates plasma corticosterone levels in the rat (e.g., Grimm and Kendall, 1968), while urethane has been shown to inhibit steroid output of the calf adrenal *in vitro* at concentrations comparable to those which were used to induce anesthesia in carp (Rosenfeld and Bascom, 1956). Since plasma 17-OHCS levels were the criteria of saltwater stimulation, the author recognized that production of mineralocorticoids such as aldosterone or 11-deoxycorticosterone would go undetected. The foregoing studies strongly suggested that motor activity rather than osmotic shock was a primary cause of elevated plasma 17-OHCS levels in carp.

In other experiments, Leloup-Hatey (1958, 1960, 1964a) studied the effects of muscular activity by transferring carp from one freshwater tank to another; there appeared to be a slight increase in 17-OHCS levels 0.5 hr after the transfer but the results were not statistically significant. However, when carp were transported a greater distance by net, prior to this test, plasma corticoid levels were significantly elevated (9 ± 3 $\mu g/100$ ml) compared with the controls (2 μg/100 ml). Elevated hormone levels (26 μg/100 ml) were also induced by stirring the water with a stick, thereby compelling the carp to swim for periods up to 2 hr. Plasma corticoid levels in carp which had been forced to swim for 0.5 hr had not decreased after a 6 hr rest period but were nearly normal again after 24 hr. Carp, unlike some teleosts, are not normally accustomed to vigorous activity in their natural environment and this lack of conditioning probably explains interrenal responsiveness and exhaustion in this species.

It is of great interest that plasma from two out of three groups of carp forced to swim for 0.5 hr contained high levels (11 and 26 μg/100 ml) of corticosterone whereas this steroid was not detected in other samples by the methods employed (Leloup-Hatey, 1964a). Corticosterone was isolated by paper chromatography, detected by absorption at 240 mμ, reduction of blue tetrazolium, and soda fluorescence, and quantified by acid fluorescence (Leloup-Hatey, 1960). Quantification by acid fluorescence would seem to rule out the possibility of interference by 11-deoxycortisol or 11-ketotestosterone, both of which conceivably would not be separated by the paper chromatographic systems used for isolation of corticosterone. High plasma levels of corticosterone have been found occasionally in Atlantic salmon (see Section III,C,4b). There are several possible explanations of this phenomenon. First, there may be two distinct 17α-hydroxylases in fish, one acting on corticosterone and the other on pregnenolone and progesterone. The relative amounts of these enzymes would then determine the product. Second, corticosterone is formed via the progesterone pathway and cortisol is formed primarily via the Δ^5 pathway. The pathway to corticosterone would then be favored by a stimulation of the conversion of pregnenolone to progesterone. Some of the corticosterone would subsequently be converted to cortisol, but *in vitro* studies suggest that this transformation is not competitive with those from 11-deoxycortisol and 21-deoxycortisol in the teleosts studied to date (see Section III,C,4a). Finally, inhibition of a single or multiple 17α-hydroxylase must be considered a possibility.

2. Ophiocephalus punctatus

Ophiocephalus punctatus is a freshwater teleost which is able to respire from the atmosphere and with its accessory respiratory organs can exist out of water for long periods. Roy (1964) found that forced swimming or surgical procedures (sham hypophysectomy) resulted in an increase in plasmatic 17-OHCS (Silber and Porter, 1954); a threefold increase was measured 3 hr after stimulus and again, as in the carp, 24 hr had elapsed before the 17-OHCS concentration had decreased to control levels. The dramatic elevation of plasma 17-OHCS levels and the long period required for return to normalcy were similar to the effects found for carp by Leloup-Hatey (1964a).

3. Eel

The silver European eel, unlike the carp, showed little activity when transferred from fresh water to seawater and there was no change in weight of interrenal tissue within several hours after transfer (Leloup-Hatey, 1964a). Similarly, there was no significant increase in plasma 17-OHCS within 2 hr when eels were placed in seawater (Δ: $-2°C$). Neither was there an effect when they were moved to hypertonic seawater (Δ: $-6°C$) even though they were unable to survive for any length of time in this salinity. These results are somewhat surprising in view of the fact that extremely small doses of mammalian ACTH, 0.05 USP units (U) per 100 g body weight (bw) resulted in increased levels of 17-OHCS in this species (Leloup-Hatey, 1961, 1964b). It would seem that under the conditions of the experiment the stress of a hypertonic environment either did not stimulate the production of ACTH in the silver eel or the duration of the stress (2 hr) was insufficient to produce detectable changes in the interrenal tissue and influence steroid-production rates. Leloup-Hatey (1964b) discussed the effect of season of the year, temperature, and gonadal development on the response of the interrenal of the eel to hypophysectomy and corticotropic stimulation.

Hirano (1969) reported that the transfer of intact cultured Japanese eels (*Anguilla japonica*) from fresh water to seawater resulted in a significant ($p <$ 0.02) increase in plasma cortisol but transfer from seawater to fresh water had no effect. A fluorescence procedure, which included a solvent partition step with carbon tetrachloride, was used to measure plasmatic cortisol, and the published data would indicate that the assay was probably adequate to measure relative changes in plasma cortisol.

4. Salmonids

In contrast to the carp, Atlantic salmon smolt are well adapted to prolonged activity and survive indefinitely when they are transferred to seawater. The results of experiments performed over a 3 year period to study effects of osmotic change were equivocal since the data do not suggest that seawater had any *consistent effect* on interrenal activity of smolt during a period varying from a few minutes to several days (Leloup-Hatey, 1964b). Plasma 17-OHCS levels for all groups of fish were high (24–120 μg/100 ml). The high levels of 17-OHCS suggest that either the salmon smolt were quite stimulated and unable to respond further, or nonsteroidal chromogens were present in the plasma. In the former case, it is possible that the high levels could not further be increased by response to salinity and exercise because the gland lacked the capacity (e.g., exhaustion of substrates?) to respond and not because the stimulus (ACTH?) was lacking. If non specific chromogens were present, a significant response might be masked (see Chapter 2).

Rainbow trout (*Salmo gairdnerii*) are also relatively active fish and well adjusted for sustained activity. The level of 17-OHCS in resting fish was modest (5 μg/100 ml) and there was no significant increase when the fish were exercised for periods up to 24 hr (Leloup-Hatey, 1964b). However, when they were exercised for 14–15 hr/day for periods of 9–20 days, there was a very significant increase in plasma 17-OHCS (16 μg/100 ml, $p = 0.001$). Leloup-Hatey concluded that the endocrine system was stimulated when muscular requirements exceeded the muscular glycogenic potential and that the threshold was related to the energy requirements of the fish in its biotope.

Hill and Fromm (1968) forced rainbow trout to swim at 0.40–0.65 meters/ sec. This performance is near the upper limit for this species and an electric shock was used to discourage the fish from falling back. There was a modest but significant elevation of plasma "cortisol" levels in the fish after 4 hr of forced swimming (64 μg/100 ml), but not after 2 hr (61 μg/100 ml), as compared to the controls (54 μg/100 ml). When the fish were exercised for 0.5 hr twice daily, for 1 and 2 weeks, and then rested for 24 hr the exercised fish had significantly lower "cortisol" levels (47 μg/100 ml) than did the controls (55 μg/100 ml). Thus, no chronic elevation of "cortisol" due to exercise was detected. The authors offered no explanation for the significant *decrease* in "cortisol" levels following prolonged exercise. It is conceivable that the exercised fish had less nonsteroidal fluorogenic lipid in the blood. The relatively lower "cortisol" levels obtained for control fish during periods of warm water (July, October) compared to December, January and February seem to be consistent with this suggestion.

The Pacific sockeye salmon *Oncorhynchus nerka*, when fighting very turbulent waters in the natural environment, has plasma cortisol levels (10–15 μg/100 ml) in both males and females in excess of those encountered elsewhere in resting fish (Fagerlund, 1967). By contrast, fish of the same race, caught in the same manner while fighting less turbulent waters, have relatively low cortisol levels (Schmidt and Idler, 1962).

Adult sockeye salmon held in captivity in a resting state had low cortisol plasma levels as determined fluorometrically (males, 2.1 $\pm$ 1.3 and females, 2.5 $\pm$ 1.7 μg/100 ml). Moderate swimming exercise for periods of up to 16 days did not significantly elevate the plasma steroid levels (Fagerlund, 1967). The difference between the results with rainbow trout (Leloup-Hatey, 1964a) and salmon probably reflects a difference in experimental condition (e.g., water velocity). To the writers' knowledge, no comparative studies have been reported.

In conclusion, salmonids, which are well adapted to exercise, seem able to put forth considerable effort without substantial elevation of plasma corticoid levels. However, when the exertion is very vigorous or sustained for long periods corticoid levels rise. There has not yet been sufficient control of variables to permit quantitative comparisons between stressors or closely related species. It would seem desirable if studies could be done on fish in a more natural environment, and "endless fish ladder" facilities exist for this purpose; in such a facility the fish swim under conditions which mimic the freshwater phase of their spawning migration and their capture, without undue struggle, is facilitated.

5. Elasmobranchs

With so little information available concerning the identity and concentration of corticosteroids in the blood of elasmobranchs, there are few clues to the role of corticosteroids in osmoregulation and carbohydrate metabolism. Some species of elasmobranchs are known to intrude brackish or fresh water and the ionic composition of the blood serum adjusts accordingly (Smith, 1931; Thorson, 1967; Urist and Van de Putte, 1967), but there seems to be no information regarding interrenal function during such migrations. Similarly there have been no reported experiments specifically designed to measure changes in corticosteroid levels as a result of muscular activity or experimental procedures.

Chuiko (1968a) compared the plasmatic concentration of 11-hydroxy-corticosteroids (11-OHCS), as measured by an abbreviated fluorometric procedure, in active pelagic fish with those of less active, littoral benthic species. Both teleosts and elasmobranchs were included in the survey; corticosteroid concentrations were expressed as cortisol equivalents in teleosts and as corticosterone equivalents in elasmobranchs. In teleosts, the concentration of plasmatic corticosteroids was significantly higher ($> 50 \mu g/$ 100 ml) in the active species ($n = 4$) than in the less active species ($< 25 \mu g/$ 100 ml, $n = 4$). In the elasmobranchs the results were inconclusive since only three species, two benthic (*Raja* and *Dasyatis*) and one pelagic (*Squalus*), were examined. Corticosteroid concentrations ranged from 5 to 14 $\mu g/100$ ml for the rays and averaged 24 $\mu g/100$ ml in the dogfish *Squalus acanthias*; in our experience with the plasma of several elasmobranchs these values are probably overestimated. It is unfortunate that more specific methods were not used for this survey since the conclusions now depend upon two assumptions: first, that either there was no contribution to the total fluorescence by plasmatic lipids, e.g., cholesterol esters (Stenlake *et al.*, 1970), or such components were of constant quantity in all species; and second, that composition of the plasmatic steroids was uniform. The author states that the fluorometric method was not applicable to plasma of haddock or the round goby *Gobius melanostomus* because of fluorogenic impurities in the plasma so that the problem of nonspecificity may have been one of degree rather than all or nothing. Doubts about the validity of the second assumption arise since not all plasmatic corticosteroids display the same degree of fluorescence. For example, in elasmobranchs, a part, probably the major portion, of the fluorogenic steroid in the plasma could be expected to be 1α-hydroxycorticosterone, which is considerably less fluorogenic in ethanol–sulfuric acid mixtures than is corticosterone. Thus, only if the ratio of corticosterone to 1α-hydroxycorticosterone remained constant would a higher value for total fluorescence necessarily mean a higher concentration of total corticosteroid.

From available information it seems justified to conclude that littoral benthic species generally do have low corticoid levels relative to their more active pelagic counterparts and the differences can be even greater than suggested by Chuiko's study.

C. CAPTIVITY, ANESTHESIA, AND TRANSPORT

1. Salmon

Pacific king (spring, chinook) salmon (*Oncorhynchus tshawytscha*) with infantile gonads were taken at sea by hook and line (Hane *et al*., 1966). The fish were exhausted when landed aboard ship and were immediately placed in running seawater. The state of exhaustion was indicated by the fact that the fish could be bled without anesthetic. The average 17-OHCS plasma level of 12 such fish was a moderate 11.8 μg/100 ml and there was no increase during the first hour in captivity. From this point on, there was a progressive increase in plasma 17-OHCS levels, and in the period from 3 to 48 hr the level was fourfold that of the freshly caught salmon. Histologically, the interrenal of the fish which had been held in captivity showed pronounced hyperplasia, but this was not evident when the fish were first landed on deck. The authors attributed these effects to the stress of restraining the salmon in a confined space. It seems equally possible that the interrenal was stimulated during capture but sufficient time had not elapsed for this to be reflected histologically or in maximal 17-OHCS levels when the fish were landed on deck. Response may have also been adversely affected by exhaustion of the fish. Impaired steroid metabolism associated with a moribund condition seems less likely because mortality was not high during a period of 24–48 hr. King salmon nearing the end of a 285 mile river migration were trapped without struggle at the top of a short fish ladder. Although these fish were of a silver color and in excellent condition, the 17-OHCS levels prior to ACTH injection were high (66 μg/100 ml, 11 fish). This dramatic effect of captivity on "wild" salmon was confirmed and extended when sockeye which were trapped at the top of a short fish ladder were shown to have plasma cortisol levels ranging from 33 to 60 μg/100 ml, while 2 months later more mature fish resting in pools nearby had very low levels (1.7 ± 1.2 μg/100 ml) (Fagerlund,

1967). The effect of captivity is transitory, however, as evidenced by the extremely low cortisol levels of sockeye held in captivity for long periods. It should be noted that fish are frequently crowded in traps and while they are free to swim they are in contact with all the disturbances of the environment. The effect of such captivity may be quite different from confinement in a large tank. Fagerlund (1967) reported that transportation of sockeye salmon "slightly anesthetized" with 2-phenoxyethanol resulted in a manyfold elevation of the cortisol levels of resting female fish (2.5 ± 1.7 to 46.6 ± 8.6 μg/100 ml); there were 25 fish (~ 50 kg) in 380 liters of water. It would seem difficult to separate the relative contributions of crowding and anesthetic. During another transport in 2-phenoxyethanol a group of males showed substantial, but less, elevation of plasma cortisol levels (14.1 ± 6.7 μg/100 ml); a single female had 40 μg/100 ml. After 1 day's rest the cortisol levels in most of the fish had returned to normal resting values. Light anesthesia is a useful tool for fish transport and an investigation of its effect independent of other variables would be of interest.

Adult sockeye trapped in a hand net for 2.5 min exhibited no increase in plasma cortisol levels (Fagerlund, 1967). When the fish were trapped in a hand net for 30 min, the cortisol concentration increased significantly in both male and female fish (14.7 ± 3.6 and 28.4 ± 10.5 μg/100 ml) (Fagerlund, 1967). Similar stress was observed in salmon when they were held in reduced water levels insufficient for normal swimming. It is of interest that when salmon were annoyed for a period of 15 min by a moving net the males did not respond to the stress while the female showed a fivefold elevation of cortisol levels. Generally plasma corticoid levels are greater in female than in male fish taken at the same location and under the same conditions (see Table A. VIII). These findings could be explained by a greater responsiveness of the female adrenal to stimulation (ACTH ?). An attempt to demonstrate a difference in the responsiveness to ACTH of male and female king salmon was only partially successful (Hane *et al.*, 1966). It had been established that estradiol renders the human more responsive to ACTH (Wallace *et al.*, 1957). Support for this possibility is provided by the demonstration that estradiol is present in ovaries (Botticelli and Hisaw, 1964) but not in testes of salmon (see Hane *et al.*, 1966). There is, however, no direct evidence that estrogens enhance the responsiveness of salmonids to ACTH. Estrogen also elevates the levels of cortisol-binding globulin (transcortin) in humans. If this occurred during spawning migration of salmonids the diminished catabolism of protein-bound corticoids would offer an alternate explanation. Two findings predicate against this argument; transcortin type of binding appears to be low or absent in salmonids and protein binding decreases during spawning migration (see Section V, B).

Sockeye salmon which were allowed to spawn in captivity had cortisol levels somewhat higher than those of resting fish in captivity but generally less than 8 μg/100 ml (Fagerlund, 1967). Spawning and spent sockeye salmon which were taken with very little struggle showed a wide variableness in cortisol concentrations. Some of the levels were comparable to those of resting salmon in captivity while others were extremely elevated. It should be noted that these determinations (Fagerlund, 1967) applied to cortisol and would not include cortisone, which can be a major component of the blood of salmon at this stage of their life cycle in the natural environment (Schmidt and Idler, 1962).

In conclusion, captivity and experimental procedures can result in such a profound elevation of plasma corticosteroid levels in many teleosts that great care must be exercised to separate such factors from the variable under investigation.

2. Sea Perch

Chuiko (1968b) measured 11-OHCS, as cortisol equivalents, in plasma of the sea perch *Scorpena porcus* by an acid fluorescence method immediately after capture, 3 hr after capture, and after 1 week in captivity. The concentration of 11-OHCS increased threefold 3 hr after capture but after 1 week in captivity the concentration had returned to the level measured immediately after capture (16 μg/100 ml). The method used for assay depended upon extraction with light hydrocarbons to remove nonsteroidal contaminants so that the reported 11-OHCS values are probably high. However, it is probably safe to assume that in the sea perch, like the salmon, plasmatic corticosteroid concentration is elevated by the stress of capture and restraint. The sea perch is a marine species of sedentary habits which lives in a stable environment and does not migrate (Chuiko, 1968b).

D. SURGERY

1. Teleosts

Plasma 17-OHCS levels were determined in the plasma of *Ophiocephalus punctatus* prior to and 1, 3, 5, 12, and 24 hr after sham hypophysectomy (Roy, 1964). The concentration was three times normal and maximal at 3 hr. Quantitatively the elevation was comparable to that following forced swimming or ACTH treatment. Plasma 17-OHCS levels returned to normal 24 hr after surgery.

2. Elasmobranchs

In an experiment to measure metabolic clearance rates of 1α-hydroxy-corticosterone, blood samples from the thorny skate *Raja radiata* were assayed for 1α-hydroxycorticosterone after minor surgical procedures and collection of blood samples over 2–3 hr. The concentration of plasmatic steroid measured by fluorescence after chromatographic isolation at the end of the experiment (4.1 μg/100 ml, 12 fish) was not significantly higher than that of animals of the same species when bled with a minimum of handling (4.3 μg/100 ml, 7 fish) (Idler and Truscott, 1969). However, these results do not necessarily mean that interrenal secretion of the thorny skate does not respond to the stress of capture and handling since all animals had been held captive in laboratory aquaria, an unnatural environment for a species usually found in water depths of 10 fathoms or more. Slow recovery from the initial stimulation of capture could explain the failure of the gland to respond to a further stimulation by surgical and blood-sampling procedures. Also, it should be noted that the response of the thorny skate to capture is not typical of fish; it does not attempt to flee or escape but rather "plays possum," curling up into an inert, thorny, and uncooperative ball.

E. METAL IONS

Exposure of rainbow trout to 0.02 and 0.20 mg/liter of hexavalent chromium for 1 week resulted in a significant increase of plasma "cortisol" (Hill and Fromm, 1968). The elevation was not noted at 2 or 3 weeks. Fish exposed to 20 mg/liter Cr^{6+} for 3 days had greatly elevated plasma "cortisol" (57 versus 38 μg/100 ml) levels, but fish exposed for 6 and 7 days did not differ from the controls. There was no trend which would suggest a response to stress followed by an exhaustion of the gland. It also seems unlikely that the fish would develop a tolerance to the higher levels of Cr^{6+}, but this explanation is consistent with the data.

F. BIOLOGICALLY ACTIVE SUBSTANCES OTHER THAN ACTH

The effects of "pitressin" and histamine on plasma 17-OHCS levels have been studied in *Ophiocephalus punctatus* (Roy, 1964). The effects were almost identical to those observed for ACTH. Quantitatively "pitressin" evoked a far greater response than histamine and somewhat greater than ACTH (see Section IV, G, 2, b). Caudal neurosecretory and diencephalic extracts prepared from *O. punctatus* and *Labeo rohita* produced about the same elevation of plasma 17-OHCS in *O. punctatus* as did ACTH; the pituitary was essential to the response, which did not occur in hypophysectomized fish.

Metyrapone inhibits 11β-hydroxylation and stimulates ACTH release in mammals. When the drug was injected into female castrated salmonids there was a decrease in plasma cortisol, a marked hypertrophy of interrenal cells, and hyperplasia of the pituitary (Fagerlund *et al.*, 1968). Hypertrophy of the interrenal following metyrapone was interpreted to indicate increased activity (corticoid secretion?). It would be of interest to attempt to obtain direct evidence for a cortisol negative feedback by determining if 11-deoxy-cortisol replaced cortisol in the blood.

Dexamethasone, a synthetic steroid (9-fluoro-11β,17,21-trihydroxy-16α-methylpregna-1,4-diene-3,20-dione), when administered to rainbow trout resulted in low plasmatic cortisol levels comparable to those of hypophysectomized trout (Donaldson and McBride, 1967). Injection of a single dose of dexamethasone, 1 mg/kg bw, inhibited the increase in plasmatic cortisol concentration as a response to the stress of handling and blood sampling in adult sockeye salmon (Fagerlund and McBride, 1969). The inhibitory effect on cortisol secretion persisted for more than 6 days in most animals. There was not, however, a complete blockage of cortisol production as observed in mammals; the authors suggested that the fluorescence measured in the blood of dexamethasone-treated fish was due to cortisol and not to "residual" fluorescence, since lower values had been recorded in "numerous salmon with the same analytical procedure." The fact remains, however, that they were not the *same* salmon and the true nature of the fluorescence, which was equivalent to basal levels of cortisol in resting fish, is unknown. It would be of interest to determine, by employing a method with the required specificity, sensitivity, and reproducibility, if dexamethasone completely blocks cortisol formation in salmon. The authors noted that in some diseased fish cortisol secretion was poorly blocked by dexamethasone; cortisol concentration in the blood was elevated within 1 hr by the stress of handling and bleeding. Histological examination of pituitary and interrenal tissue in these fish showed no abnormalities and a fourfold increase in the dosage of dexamethasone was effective in blocking cortisol production.

Injection of 4 mg/kg bw of dexamethasone significantly lowered, in 24 hr, the concentration of cortisol in peripheral plasma of the freshwater North American eel *Anguilla rostrata* (Butler *et al.*, 1969a). A second injection of dexamethasone, 2 mg/kg bw, caused a further decrease in cortisol concentration after a total of 48 hr. In the eel, as in the salmon, cortisol was still detectable in the blood of the injected fish. However, the assay, an abbreviated fluorometric procedure, was not sufficiently sensitive to measure differences in concentrations at the lower levels. Fluorescence measured in plasma 48 hr after dexamethasone treatment was slightly higher (1.1 μg/100 ml) than that of hypophysectomized fish (0.8 μg/100 ml) and may have represented residual cortisol or the blank value of the method. Bradshaw and Fontaine-Bertrand (1968) reported that dexamethasone injection reduced plasma cortisol levels in the European eel to 6% of normal after 24 hr and cortisol could not be detected after 48 hr; no data were given.

Triamcinolone (9-fluoro-11β, 16α,17,21-tetrahydroxypregna-1,4-diene-3,

20-dione) reduced the concentration of 11-OHCS (cortisol equivalents) in the plasma of sea perch from a control value of 22 μg/100 ml to 8 μg/100 ml. Bovine ACTH increased 11-OHCS concentration to 45 μg/100 ml in the control fish but the levels in triamcinolone-treated fish remained at 8 μg/100 ml after ACTH treatment (Chuiko, 1968b).

G. HYPOPHYSECTOMY AND ACTH

1. Activity of ACTH in Fish Pituitaries

a. Teleosts. Adrenocorticotropin activity has been demonstrated in the pituitary tissue of teleosts by studying the effects of hypophysectomy on the interrenal tissue or its secretion. In a few species attempts have been made to quantify and identify the corticotropic factor in fish pituitary with mammalian ACTH. Pituitary extracts of the bonito *Katsuwonus vagans* and the tuna *Thynnus orientalis* exhibited ACTH activity in the Sayers rat ascorbic acid depletion assay (Ito *et al.*, 1952). Lyophilized pituitary glands of the chum salmon *Oncorhynchus keta* were assayed for ACTH activity by the adrenal ascorbic acid depletion assay using hypophysectomized rats. The preparation had about 20 mU/mg of ACTH activity as compared with USP standard corticotropin (Rinfret and Hane, 1955). By the same assay another teleost, the Arctic cod *Gadus morrhua* L., was found to contain 3.5 mU of ACTH activity per milligram of whole pituitary (Woodhead, 1960). The author pointed out that this may not represent a quantitative difference between the species but rather may be due to the postmortem age of the fish when the pituitaries were collected. It would be of interest to determine if the pituitaries or blood of the more active marine teleosts (e.g., herring) contain more ACTH than do groundfish (e.g., cod) or other relatively inactive fish such as skates. A method for the assay of ACTH based on the stimulation of corticosteroidogenesis in the mouse adrenal *in vitro* (Purrott and Sage, 1969) was used to demonstrate the presence of approximately 44 mU ACTH/mg in homogenates of goldfish pituitary. The ACTH activity was concentrated in the anterior pituitary and was distinct from melanophore-stimulating hormone activity, which was released from the posterior portion of the gland (Sage and Purrott, 1969).

b. Chondrichthyeans. Acid extracts of the interrenal of three species of chondrichthyeans, the dogfish *Squalus acanthias*, the skate *Raja rhina*, and the ratfish *Hydrolagus colliei*, were reported to stimulate steroidogenesis in chick adrenal tissue *in vitro*. Most of the activity was confined to the rostral pars distalis and the nuerointermediate lobe (deRoos and deRoos, 1967). Although the ACTH content of the chondrichthyean pituitaries was not measured quantitatively, the authors reported that, on the basis of earlier studies with chicken and alligator adenohypophyses, the amount of ACTH activity extracted from chondrichthyean pituitaries was comparable to that of these vertebrates.

2. Effects of Hypophysectomy and ACTH in Vivo

a. *Eels*. The effect of hypophysectomy on plasmatic corticosteroids has been studied in three species of *Anguilla*: the European eel, the North American eel, and the Japanese eel.

Leloup-Hatey (1961) reported the effect of hypophysectomy on plasma 17-OHCS levels as measured with Porter–Silber reagent after column chromatography (Nelson and Samuels, 1952; Eik-Nes *et al.*, 1953) in the European eel. The experiments were described later in greater detail (Leloup-Hatey, 1964b). Sham-operated eels bled in autumn (water 10°–12°C) contained 5.2 μg/100 ml plasma (5 samples, 30 fish). Following hypophysectomy, there was no significant change in plasma 17-OHCS during the first day (4.0 μg/100 ml, 2 samples, 6 fish) but the average value of samples taken at 6, 12, and 27 days was 1.0 μg/100 ml (6 samples, 17 fish); the decrease was very significant ($p < 0.001$). When hypophysectomized eels were held at 16°C for 28 days in autumn the level of plasma 17-OHCS was very low (0.6 μg/100 ml, 2 samples, 6 fish); injection of mammalian ACTH, 12.5 U/100 g bw, into the perivisceral cavity resulted in a marked increase in 17-OHCS levels between 0.5 and 3 hr (9.6 μg/100 ml, 3 samples, 6 fish). The plasma corticosteroid levels had returned to normal within 6 hr after the injection (0.8 μg/100 ml, 1 sample, 2 fish).

The 17-OHCS level of intact eels held at 16°C in summer was 10 ± 2 μg/100 ml (19 fish). Sham-operated eels contained 15 μg/100 ml (2 samples, 6 fish) immediately after surgery and there was no demonstrable effect of hypophysectomy with these animals after 12 days (10 μg/100 ml, 2 samples, 6 fish). Following the injection of 12.5 USP U ACTH/100 g into the perivisceral cavity, there was an increase between 15 min and 24 hr to an average level of 24 μg/100 ml (11 samples, 33 fish). There was no noticeable diminution of the effect up to 24 hr in contrast with the fish injected in the fall. Although there were limited data for the effect of other dosages, the results suggest no diminution of effect down to levels of 0.05 USP U ACTH/100 g but there was no response at 0.005 U/100 g.

When hypophysectomized eels were maintained at 7°C for 12 days in summer, 17-OHCS levels were relatively high (14 μg/100 ml, 2 samples, 6 fish). In this instance, 12.5 USP U ACTH seemed to produce no significant effect over a period of 6 hr and, in fact, the levels appeared to be noticeably depressed after 24 hr (3 μg/100 ml, 2 samples, 6 fish).

The author did not test for significance of the data relating to hypophysectomy or ACTH treatment, and unfortunately it was not possible to confirm statistical significance of much of the above data because there were not sufficient samples analyzed both before and after ACTH administration. Nevertheless, the results suggest a pronounced effect of mammalian ACTH on hypophysectomized eels under specified experimental conditions. It should be noted also that considerable data were presented to establish that the injection of mammalian ACTH in dosages from 0.005 to 12.5 USP U/100 g were reflected in a very significant increase in the weight of the interrenal of this species. It is perhaps surprising that hypophysectomy lowered blood corticoid in the autumn but not in the summer. The most obvious difference between eels at these two times is that the autumn eels were in a more advanced stage of gonad development (gonadosomatic index, 1.77 ± 0.03 as compared with 1.02 ± 0.03) but there was no direct evidence that sexually maturing eels are more sensitive to ACTH. The author suggested that the greater response to ACTH at 16°C as compared to 7°C in the summer animals may be related to the use of mammalian peptide, the responsiveness being greater in the target organ at the higher temperature. It might also be noted that the quantity of ACTH delivered to the adrenal is governed by the concentration of the peptide in the blood and the flow of blood through the gland. During infusion of a constant level of ACTH into hypophysectomized rats, an increase in adrenal blood flow between 0.005 and 0.058 ml/min changed corticosterone output from 1.1 to 6.2 μg/5 min (Porter and Klaiber, 1965). Greater blood flow in the eel at 16°C as compared to 7°C may be a factor in determining the greater response of the animal to injected ACTH at the higher temperature. The beat of the isolated heart of this species is greatly accelerated at 25°C as compared to 2°C (Grodzinski, 1954) and a faster heart rate is reflected in greater cardiac output in fish (Randall 1968, 1970). A degree of structural and species specificity for peptide hormones must be considered (Heller and Pickering, 1961) and anomalous results may sometimes be expected when non mammalian vertebrates are treated with hormones of mammalian origin. Some of the answers to these questions may be found when piscine ACTH is employed in the species from which it was isolated. Extracts of whole fish pituitaries have been shown to stimulate steroidogenesis by fish interrenal tissue but the corticotropic factor has not been isolated for study.

In a brief communication Leloup-Hatey (1967) concluded that actinomycin (concentration not stated) inhibited the ACTH stimulation of pregnenolone synthesis by the European eel *in vivo*. In a later study Leloup-Hatey (1968) used corticosteroid production *in vitro* by interrenal tissue of the eel to measure the effects of hypophysectomy and the injection *in vivo* of mammalian ACTH. Hypophysectomy for 25 days (16°C) resulted in atrophy of the interrenal but did not affect the potential activity of the hydroxylases necessary for the transformation of progesterone to cortisol. However, interrenal tissue from hypophysectomized fish retained only a limited ability to elaborate cortisol from endogenous precursors *in vitro*. Injection of ACTH *in vivo* restored the steroidogenic activity of the interrenal tissue of hypophysectomized eels; the production of cortisol increased tenfold 1 hr after ACTH injection. Preliminary treatment of the hypophysectomized eels with actinomycin D (10 μg/100 g bw), an inhibitor of DNA-dependent RNA synthesis, inhibited the stimulatory effect of ACTH *in vivo*. Thus, in the eel, the response of the interrenal to ACTH stimulation was assumed to be subordinate to the synthesis of RNA. Leloup-Hatey (1968) noted that the inhibition by actinomycin D of ACTH stimulation of steroidogenesis in the eel interrenal was contrary to the effects obtained with rat adrenal *in vitro* (Ferguson and Morita, 1964) but comparable to those obtained with bovine adrenal (Farese, 1966). The author postulated that species differences in response to treatment with actinomycin D might be related to cholesterol content of the adrenal (low in the eel and cattle) and to the stability or half-life of messenger RNA. However, in a review of his own investigations with the guinea pig and of published reports on the effects of actinomycin D on the adrenal cortex, Bransome (1969) observed that results varied with dosage and length of time after administration and frequently represented toxic reactions. He concluded that "interference with a hormonal effect by actinomycin cannot be taken as evidence that the involvement of RNA synthesis is essential to the hormone action; nor can lack of actinomycin effect guarantee that RNA is not involved."

A competitive protein binding assay (CPBA) was used to determine the effect of ACTH and hypophysectomy on plasma cortisol levels of the European eel (Bradshaw and Fontaine-Bertrand, 1968). After hypophysectomy, plasma cortisol decreased from an initial 7 μg/100 ml to zero over a period of 12 days. Plasma cortisol levels returned to normal after injection of porcine ACTH or a carp pituitary extract. The CPBA method was validated by comparing the results obtained for plasma cortisol with those found by a fluorescence procedure which included isolation by thin-layer and paper chromatography and correction for blank values. Unfortunately, 0.015 μC^i cortisol-^{14}C (specific activity 53.8 mC^i/mmole) per milliliter of plasma was added to allow for recoveries and detection of cortisol areas of chromatograms. Thus, cortisol-^{14}C (0.1 μg) added to each sample was higher than endogenous cortisol even in intact animals (0.07 μg/ml). With hypophysectomized fish and low cortisol concentrations, the fluorometric assay used to validate the competitive protein binding assay would be progressively less sensitive. Cortisol concentrations in eel plasma were compared by the two methods over a range of 0–30 μg/100 ml. In the lower ranges, 0–5 μg/100 ml, pertinent to the measurement of cortisol in hypophysectomized fish, the graphic presentation of data does not permit the reader to evaluate the comparison.

Butler *et al.* (1969a) studied the effects of hypophysectomy in the North American eel. Plasmatic cortisol concentration in sham-operated animals averaged 2.3 μg/100 ml ($n = 8$) whereas the concentration dropped to 0.8 μg/100 ml ($n = 8$) within 24 hr of hypophysectomy. The concentration did not decrease further over a 3 week period. Injection of 0.2 IU ACTH daily for 10 days caused a twofold increase in plasmatic cortisol in hypophysectomized eels (4.3 μg/100 ml, $n = 7$).

Similar studies with the Japanese eel gave similar results (Hirano, 1969). The injection of 1 IU ACTH into intact eels resulted in an increase in plasmatic cortisol from 3.8 to 22 μg/100 ml and 10 days after hypophysectomy the concentration was 0.3 μg/100 ml ($p < 0.001$). Transfer of hypophysectomized fish from fresh water to seawater, in contrast to the effect on intact fish, did not affect blood cortisol concentration. Hirano interpreted these data as further evidence that the pituitary–interrenal glands are involved in the adaption of the eel to seawater. Earlier studies had shown that cortisol was involved in the transfer of water in the intestine (Hirano and Utida, 1968) and sodium turnover in the gill (Mayer *et al.*, 1967).

Thus, in *Anguilla* sp. the pituitary–adrenal relationship as evidenced by plasmatic cortisol concentration has been well established. In all cases, except one, the interrenal tissue appears to maintain a low level of activity, i.e., low "basal" levels of cortisol are detectable in the plasma even 3–4 weeks posthypophysectomy. From the data it would seem to be impossible to establish if this residual plasmatic cortisol concentration is real or merely represents the lower limit of sensitivity of the assay methods. To our knowledge, methods sensitive to changes at the submicrogram level have not been used nor has the identity of the fluorogenic compound in plasma of hypophysectomized eel been established as cortisol. However, Leloup-Hatey (1968) found that interrenal tissue of hypophysectomized eels retained its ability, to a limited extent, to elaborate cortisol from endogenous precursors *in vitro*.

b. Ophiocephalus punctatus. Roy (1964) employed the Silber and Porter (1954) procedure to study the effect of ACTH on plasma 17-OHCS levels in *O. punctatus*. Plasma 17-OHCS levels were not affected by the injection of distilled water (18 μg/100 ml, 10 fish). Three hours after the injection of 2 IU of ACTH per fish, plasma 17-OHCS had increased to 54 μg/100 ml (7 fish); essentially the same response was evoked by 1 hr of forced swimming. Plasma 17-OHCS levels (16 μg/100 ml, 8 fish) were maintained for 2 weeks after hypophysectomy, decreased 10–15% in the third week, and finally dropped to 5 μg/100 ml (8 fish) after 4 weeks. During the first and second week after hypophysectomy plasma 17–OHCS levels were elevated by ACTH, but the response was only modest after 3 weeks and there was no increase when ACTH was given 4 weeks after hypophysectomy. The author concluded that true interrenal atrophy occurred in the third and fourth week after hypophysectomy; this was confirmed histologically. The failure of "pitressin" and histamine to elevate plasma 17-OHCS levels after 4 weeks in contrast to their effects 2 weeks posthypophysectomy further confirmed that the interrenal had lost the capacity to be stimulated. The failure of *O. punctatus* to respond to ACTH stimulation 4 weeks after hypophysectomy contrasts with the results obtained with another teleost, the eel.

c. *Salmonids*. Experimental difficulties appear to have frustrated several attempts to determine whether salmonid fishes respond to mammalian ACTH as evidenced by elevation of interrenal steroid concentration in the blood. In the early studies, intact fish were used as experimental animals so that their response to exogenous ACTH could not be distinguished from the response to handling and bleeding which is so evident in the salmonids.

The concentration of 17-OHCS in the blood of immature Pacific king salmon, caught at sea and at the mouth of a river at the beginning of their migration, increased with time in both the control group and ACTH-injected fish (∼ 0.5 IU/kg bw) despite efforts to capture the fish with a minimum of struggle (Hane *et al.*, 1966). King salmon, in an early stage of maturation and trapped "without struggle" at the top of a short fish ladder, had high levels of 17-OHCS (66 μg/100 ml) which increased 2 hr after ACTH treatment (85 μg/100 ml); 17-OHCS levels did not change in untreated fish. The authors concluded that these fish responded to ACTH but statistical treatment of the data was not reported. No response to ACTH could be demonstrated in spawning or postspawned king salmon. Spawning steelhead trout (*Salmo gairdnerii*) showed a marked rise (from 40 to 87 μg/100 ml) in plasma 17-OHCS levels following ACTH injection but there was no mention of a control group, i.e., handled, injected, and bled. Hane *et al.* (1966) noted that although fish with a high initial level of 17-OHCS (∼ 70 μg/100 ml) did respond to ACTH, the response recorded in fish with lower initial values (< 30 μg/100 ml) was approximately five times as great.

Gonadectomized sockeye salmon (*Oncorhynchus nerka*) held in captivity had very low resting cortisol levels (1–2 μg/100 ml) and these were elevated manyfold by the stress of infection and blood sampling after intramuscular injections of high levels of ACTH (8–13.6 IU/kg bw). However, saline-injected controls also responded strongly. The data suggest, but do not prove, a contribution by exogenous ACTH and no claim was made (Fagerlund *et al.*, 1968).

In a more recent study, Fagerlund (1970) examined the relationship between sexual maturity and interrenal response to ACTH in sockeye salmon which had been injected 16 hr previously with sufficient dexamethasone to inhibit endogenous production of ACTH. In contrast to the earlier studies with intact untreated king salmon there was no significant difference in response to ACTH as measured by plasmatic cortisol concentration between immature, maturing, and sexually mature fish. In all cases, a maximal response was recorded 3–5 hr after injection of porcine ACTH (0.5 IU/kg bw). Ten hours after the injection of ACTH, blood cortisol levels remained elevated, especially so in mature and spawned fish indicating that the half-life of ACTH was prolonged or that the catabolism and clearance of cortisol was impaired. Maximal plasmatic cortisol concentrations in the male fish were approximately 60% of those in the female. Hane *et al.* (1966) reported that, with the exception of fish caught at the beginning of their fluvial migration, plasmatic 17-OHCS concentrations were higher in female than in male king salmon (238 samples).

Donaldson and McBride (1967) presented evidence for a pituitary–interrenal relationship in rainbow trout. Plasma cortisol levels were determined by fluorometry following solvent partition between water and carbon tetrachloride (Donaldson *et al.*, 1968). Cortisol levels were reduced significantly from 7.4 to 3.6 μg/100 ml ($p < 0.005$) the day after hypophysectomy by comparison with sham-hypophysectomized fish (8.1 μg/100 ml). In the interval from 2 to 17 days, plasmatic cortisol in the hypophysectomized animals diminished still further to 1.6 μg/100 ml ($p < 0.001$). When the fish were stressed by rapidly lowering the water level to the point where the fish were not totally submerged, the sham-hypophysectomized animals showed a significant increase in cortisol levels while there was a slight but not significant increase in the hypophysectomized animals. The plasma cortisol levels in these fish, held in the laboratory, were very low compared to total 17-OHCS as reported by Hane *et al.* (1966): 8.1 $\pm$ 5.8 versus 40 μg/100 ml. There were probably at least two contributory factors: (a) cortisone as well as cortisol can accumulate in blood of *Salmo* and would not be measured by Donaldson's method; (b) the life histories of the fish were different (i.e., hatchery-reared versus captured adults on their spawning migration from the sea). It would seem that the rainbow trout responded more rapidly to hypophysectomy than did the European eel (Leloup-Hatey, 1964b), but as in the eel, "cortisol" as measured by acid fluorescence was still detectable in the plasma of trout for 2–17 days after hypophysectomy.

Hill and Fromm (1968) could not detect an effect on plasma "cortisol" concentration as a result of administration of exogenous ACTH to intact hatchery-bred rainbow trout. However, "cortisol" levels in the control group of fish, i.e., saline injected, were high (~ 56 μg/100 ml) and apparently unable to further respond to stimulation. Basal "cortisol" levels in trout used in this study were approximately three to five times higher than those found by Donaldson and McBride (1967). The difference may have been due in part to physiological and nutritional differences of the experimental fish but also to the methods used to quantify cortisol. In both investigations cortisol was measured by acid fluorescence after purification by solvent partition. Donaldson and McBride (1967) used carbon tetrachloride and water partition of dichloromethane extractables; Hill and Fromm (1968) used an initial extraction with 2,2,4-trimethylpentane. The use of hydrocarbons to purify fish plasma samples for subsequent fluorometric measurement of cortisol has never been shown to be efficient; either other steroids or nonsteroidal compounds remain to contribute to acid-induced fluorescence and thus to high levels of "cortisol."

d. Elasmobranchs. There have been no reports of the effect of hypophysectomy on corticosteroid concentration in the blood of elasmobranchs. The interrenal–pituitary relationship in Chondrichthyes has received little attention although these fish would appear to be eminently suitable for such studies in that cortical tissues is separate from chromaffin tissue and in some species can be surgically removed; hypophysectomy is also possible. Furthermore, hypophysectomy may involve complete removal of the pituitary or removal of any one of the three lobes, rostral, neurointermediate, or ventral (Dodd *et al.*, 1960; Idler *et al.*, 1970). Dittus (1939, 1941) reported that hypophysectomy of *Torpedo* sp. resulted in atrophy of the interrenal tissue and that the activity of the interrenal was restored by injection of corticotropin. However, there was no cytological effect on interrenal tissue of a dogfish (*Scyliorhinus* sp.) 1 year after hypophysectomy (Dodd, 1961).

3. Effect of ACTH on Interrenals in Vitro

A very limited number of experiments specifically designed to study *in vitro* the effects of ACTH on steroidogenesis in fish has been reported, although mammalian ACTH has been used (presumably in the hope of improving the yield of steroid) in tissue incubations. As outlined earlier (Section III,C,4,a) the heterogeneous nature of teleost interrenal tissue makes it less than ideal for this type of experimentation. However, relatively pure cortical tissue can be obtained from the walls of the anterior cardinal vein of the European eel (Leloup-Hatey, 1968). Interrenal tissue of Chondrichthyes is ideal for *in vitro* experiments but results reported to date have been inconclusive.

a. Teleosts. Nandi and Bern (1965) incubated rainbow trout interrenal tissue in the presence and absence of mammalian ACTH. Ultraviolet photographs of the cortisol area of chromatograms suggested that ACTH was stimulatory, but the authors were correctly reserved in their conclusions.

Concurrently with her studies on the effect of ACTH administration *in vivo*, Leloup-Hatey (1968) measured the effect of ACTH addition on cortisol production by interrenal tissue of the European eel. Mammalian ACTH did not stimulate corticosteroidogenesis in interrenal tissue of intact eels but resulted in a marked increase in the production of cortisol (from 0.12 to 1.1 μg/hr) in interrenal tissue from eels which had been hypophysectomized 25 days previously. Stimulation of interrenal tissue by the addition of ACTH to the excised tissue was comparable to that obtained by administration of ACTH *in vivo*. Leloup-Hatey concluded that the magnitude of the response to ACTH *in vitro* was dependent upon a low initial secretion.

As a result of their discovery that luteinizing hormone (LH) and corticosteroids were ovulating agents in the catfish *Heteropneustes fossilis*, Sundararaj and Goswami (1969) investigated the production of corticosteroids by the interrenal *in vitro* and the effects of mammalian hypophyseal hormones on their production. Cortisol and a lesser amount of 11-deoxycorticosterone were the principal products. Prolactin and follicle-stimulating hormones had no significant effect on endogenous production of cortisol or 11-deoxycorticosterone. Addition of ACTH doubled the production of both cortisol and deoxycorticosterone; LH also stimulated both cortisol and 11-deoxycorticosterone but preferentially the latter. In these experiments, 0.1 IU mammalian ACTH/100 mg tissue was used to evoke a twofold increase in steroid production, but increasing the concentration of ACTH to 1 IU/100 mg tissue did not further enhance the production of cortisol and 11-deoxycorticosterone. It is not clear whether the interrenal tissue used for *in vitro* experiments was excised from intact catfish or from fish previously hypophysectomized (cf. intact and hypophysectomized eel, Leloup-Hatey, 1968). The effect of pituitary hormones on corticosteroidogenesis in the catfish was not the principal goal of these experiments but did substantiate the proposition that mammalian LH acts upon the interrenal to induce the production of corticosteroids which, in turn, promote ovulation and spawning. It would be of interest to attempt to identify the plasmatic corticosteroids in the spawning catfish since 11-deoxycorticosterone has not previously been shown to occur in detectable amounts in fish blood and the products of *in vitro* incubations need not necessarily duplicate the composition of interrenal secretions *in vivo*.

b. Elasmobranchs. The failure to obtain ACTH stimulation of dogfish

(*Squalus acanthias*) and skate (*Raja rhina*) interrenals *in vitro* (Bern *et al.*, 1962) is of doubtful significance because the principal corticoid, 1α-hydroxycorticosterone, was unknown at the time. The interrenal of *R. erinacea* responded *in vitro* to large doses (1 U/100 mg) of mammalian ACTH with an increased output of blue-tatrazolium-positive material and substances which absorbed 240 mμ light (Macchi and Rizzo, 1962). The increase in blue-tetrazolium-positive material calculated as cortisol (0.8–2.1 μg/100 mg hr) was greater than the increase (1.05– 1.8 μg/100 mg hr) found by ultraviolet absorption.

   In our laboratory aliquots of 100 mg interrenal tissue of thorny skate ($n = 10$) were prepared and incubated as described by Macchi and Rizzo (1962) except that the tissue was preincubated for 1 hr and then incubated for 1 hr at 25°C. 1α-Hydroxycorticosterone was purified by paper chromatography and quantified by fluorescence (Idler and Truscott, 1969) after addition of 1α-hydroxycorticosterone-^{3}H to calculate recoveries. The production rate of 1α-hydroxycorticosterone without ACTH was 3.45 ±0.25 μg/100 mg hr, and amounts of porcine ACTH varying from 5 to 500 mU increased the rate by 40% to 4.83 ±0.16 μg/100 mg hr (0.005 > p > 0.001). An acid extract of the acetone powder prepared from skate pituitary equivalent to 0.4–4.0 mg/100 mg resulted in a production rate of 5.45 ±0.51 μg/100 mg hr, which was not significantly different from the response to porcine ACTH. There was no suggestion of a dose-response relationship, and several other attempts to demonstrate an effect of mammalian ACTH or acid extract of skate pituitary *in vitro* have thus far been unsuccessful (Idler and Truscott, 1970). To date, we have found that the *in vitro* response of skate interrenal tissue to ACTH is insignificant or small compared to the response reported for rat adrenal.

H. Sexual Maturation and Reproductive Cycle

1. Teleosts

   Neither qualitative nor quantitative comparisons of plasmatic corticosteroids have been reported for sexually immature and mature teleosts, with the exception of some salmonids. Leloup-Hatey (1964b) found no significant difference in the concentration of total 17-OHCS in the blood of Atlantic salmon captured at the beginning of their upriver migration and on the spawning grounds. Cortisol and cortisone were always the major corticosteroids; in a few cases corticosterone was present as a major component in plasma of salmon at the beginning of their river migration but not in any samples taken from spawning fish. Leloup-Hatey suggested that this qualitative change may have resulted from prolonged exercise and fatigue; a similar phenomenon was demonstrated experimentally in carp (Leloup-

Hatey, 1960). As mentioned earlier (Section IV, B, 1), this apparent inhibition of 17α-hydroxylation by stress is worthy of investigation.

Sufficient quantities of several C_{21} steroids to permit their identification were isolated from plasma of post spawned Pacific salmon, *Oncorhynchus* sp. (Table A. VIII), although not all were necessarily products of interrenal tissue. Cortisol and cortisone were generally the principal C_{21} steroids; in most samples cortisone was the major component in mature, spawning, and spawned fish (Schmidt and Idler, 1962). It is of interest that plasma cortisol and cortisone were at relatively low concentration in fish captured at Siwash Bridge, British Columbia by dipnet and bled immediately, even though these animals were in an advanced state of sexual maturity.

The high levels of 17–OHCS measured in the blood of maturing and spawning Pacific salmon, *Oncorhynchus* sp. (Table A.VIII), coupled with the demonstration of hyperplasia of the interrenal tissue, led to the suggestion that increased production of corticosteroids was associated with sexual maturation and perhaps the postspawning death of these fish (Hane and Robertson, 1959; Robertson and Wexler, 1959). Interpretation of the data reported for salmon captured in their natural environment is difficult since several factors could contribute to the high concentration of 17-OHCS found in these fish, e.g., motor activity of migration, stress of capture and restraint in nets or traps, and in the case of *Oncorhynchus* sp. the moribund condition of postspawned fish. Plasmatic cortisol levels of sockeye salmon caught in quiet pools during their migration and of fish maintained in captivity during sexual maturation were found to be relatively low ($<$ 5 μg/100 ml) indicating that sexual maturation does not necessarily result in a large sustained increase in blood cortisol (Fagerlund, 1967). In sockeye salmon the concentration of total 17-OHCS and cortisol need not be comparable since the ratio of cortisol to cortisone probably is not constant. Idler *et al.* (1963) reported that the greatly diminished slope of the later portions of the clearance curve for radioactivity from the blood of spawning sockeye salmon compared to that of immature salmon indicated that the metabolism of corticosteroids was impaired in the sexually mature fish. Since plasma concentrations are a function of production rates and metabolic clearance rates, Idler *et al.* (1963) proposed that impaired metabolism (clearance) could explain the elevated levels of corticosteroids measured in spawned sockeye salmon and that impaired clearance need not necessarily be accompanied by increased cortisol production rates. In more recent years cortisol production rates, as estimated by the measurement of metabolic clearance rates and plasma concentration, have been reported to be higher in sockeye salmon held to maturity in captivity (not necessarily moribund). These experiments, the subject of several papers, are reviewed in Section VI.

2. *Elasmobranchs*

Interrenal activity as a function of sexual maturity or of the reproductive cycle, as measured by plasmatic corticosteroid concentration, has received little attention although the elasmobranchs include viviparous, ovoviviparous, and oviparous species (Chieffi, 1967; van Tienhoven, 1968). Lupo di Prisco *et al.* (1967) measured the concentration of free plus glucuronic-acid-conjugated cortisol, cortisone, corticosterone, and deoxycorticosterone in the plasma of female *Torpedo marmorata*, an ovoviviparous species. Plasma was collected from fish in four stages of reproductive development, immature, pregestational, gestational, and post- or intergestational. The authors concluded that their results indicated total corticosteroids of the plasma may be lower during gestation in *T. marmorata*; cortisol and cortisone concentrations were higher in immature and pregestational fish although corticosterone was highest in the plasma of fish at the gestation period. These results must be viewed with some skepticism since, as the authors pointed out, analyses were done on pooled blood samples so that the range of individual values is not known and the significance of differences in the four samples cannot be statistically evaluated. Identification and quantification were done by gas–liquid chromatography and ultraviolet absorption of extracts of fractions off thin-layer silica gel, without allowance for recovery through the isolation procedures. Limitations of the methodology are discussed elsewhere (see Section III, B, 2b).

At this time any relationship between the reproductive cycle and interrenal secretion as evidenced by plasmatic concentration of corticosteroids in elasmobranchs remains an open question. Histological changes in interrenal tissue during reproductive cycles have been recorded for both ovoviviparous (*T. marmorata* and *T. ocellata*) and oviparous species (*Scyliorhinus stellaris* and *S. caniculus*) but no corresponding change was found in the intensity of the histochemical reaction for 3β-hydroxysteroid dehydrogenase in the interrenal of these species (Chieffi, 1967).

I. Diurnal Rhythm

In several mammals a diurnal rhythm in the concentration of free corticosteroids in the blood plasma has been demonstrated. Whether such a diurnal variation exists in teleosts is unknown. Unfortunately, the only study reported on this subject (Boehlke *et al.* 1966) does not provide sufficient irrefutable data to accept without reservations its conclusion that in a teleost, the channel catfish *Ictalurus punctatus*, the concentration of total glucocorticoids increases significantly in midafternoon. The individual corticosteroids (cortisol, cortisone, and corticosterone) were identified only in interrenal incubates but not in the plasma. Corticosteroids in the plasma were quantified by methods developed for the clinical assay of glucocorticosteroids in human plasma and were not shown to be applicable to the plasma under study. The concentration of cortisone, reportedly the major corticosteroid, was determined by subtracting the amount of cortisol as measured by fluorescence after carbon tetrachloride partition (Rudd *et al.*, 1963) from total 17-OHCS as measured by the phenylhydrazine reaction (Silber and Porter, 1954). The text fails to provide sufficient information regarding the physical conditions of the experiment; e.g., were precautions taken against stress due to handling and other external stimuli and was there control of duration and intensity of light? Rather elaborate experimental procedures would be required to demonstrate conclusively that a variation in plasmatic corticosteroid concentration in a teleost was solely the result of a diurnal rhythm in corticosteroid production.

J. Stanniectomy

The physiological effects of ablation of the corpuscles of Stannius have been studied in the European eel (see Chapter 8). Leloup-Hatey (1966a, 1970) reported that 1 week after Stanniectomy there was a threefold increase in plasmatic 17-OHCS and a similar increase in the production of corticosteroids from endogenous precursor by interrenal tissue *in vitro*. However, 2, 6 and 9 weeks after surgery the steroid output of the interrenal of the Stanniectomized fish was significantly lower both *in vivo* and *in vitro* than the output before surgery (with the exception of an anomalous result after 6 weeks for cortisol synthesis *in vitro*). There was no significant difference either qualitatively or quantitatively in the transformation of progesterone-^{14}C to its hydroxylated derivatives by interrenal tissue of control and experimental fish. Interrenal weights and plasma calcium levels increased after Stanniectomy; plasma calcium reached its maximal level after 4 weeks. Leloup-Hatey (1970) attributed the inhibition of steriodogenesis, at least in part, to the higher levels of plasma calcium resulting from Stanniectomy. The complete manuscript describing these experiments has not been published as anticipated; it would seem from the summary table (Leloup-Hatey, 1970) that most of the values for corticosteroids were obtained for single animals.

V. Protein Binding of Corticosteroids

A. INTRODUCTION

Plasma corticosteroid levels have been determined in fish under a variety of circumstances (see Section IV). These determinations refer to total solvent-extractable steroids and there are limited data available from which one can calculate the level of steroids bound to plasma proteins of fish (Idler and Freeman, 1968). In mammals it has been suggested that certain plasma proteins bind steroid hormones rendering them biologically inactive; by this criterion, the biological activity of a plasma hormone is not indicated by the total concentration in the plasma but rather is dependent on the concentration of the unbound steroid (for a review see Sandberg *et al.*, 1966). Protein binding is also thought to protect steroids from metabolism and thereby to maintain blood levels by decreasing the metabolic clearance rate (Tait and Burstein, 1964; Bird *et al.*, 1969). Keller *et al.* (1969) proposed a new hypothesis concerning the physiological role of corticosteroid-binding proteins. They postulated that these proteins increase the specificity of the adrenocortical system by determining the distribution of corticosteroid signals. Increases in the levels of the binding proteins were thought to distribute adrenocortical hormonal signals toward organs with protein-permeable vascular beds. Keller *et al.* (1969) fround this hypothesis to have physiochemical consistency by computer simulation of the multiple mass action and transport equations involved.

It would appear then that the relationship between protein binding and activity is not a simple phenomenon. Protein–steroid interaction is not a static system but rather is a dynamic one with free and bound steroids in equilibrium with each other and with conjugated steroids; synthesis, metabolism, and clearance of the hormone must all be considered. If the equilibrium is disturbed in any part of this system, adjustments are made to maintain the equilibrium. When a steroid hormone is bound to protein it is not necessarily out of the picture. The protein binding of a steroid hormone is seen as a storage and buffer system in which the steroid–protein complex serves as a biologically inert reservoir where the hormone is protected from metabolism or excretion; by dissociation the hormone becomes readily available as a physiologically active entity (Hoffman *et al.*, 1969). There is evidence that tissues differ in their abilities to respond to protein-bound steroids (Tait and Burstein, 1964, Keller *et al.*, 1969). Binding of a specific hormone at the tissue level therefore depends on the affinity of the tissue receptors relative to the affinity of the plasma binding proteins. It also depends on the relatively free passage from the plasma to the cell (cell membrane effect), which is determined partly by the size of the molecule. These parameters affect the level of a hormone within the tissue at any given secretion rate, but saturation of the tissue receptors is a further limiting factor. Thus it appears that all steroid-binding proteins, even those with low association constants, have a part to play in regulating the metabolism of steroid hormones in this complex system.

Mammalian corticosteroid-binding globulin (CBG or transcortin) has been isolated and characterized by Slaunwhite *et al.* (1966), Seal and Doe (1966), and Chader and Westphal (1968a,b). It is a protein with a high binding affinity for many steroids and in humans the binding of corticosteroids at normal physiological levels is attributed to transcortin. When plasma corticosteroid levels become abnormally high, or when transcortin sites become saturated, albumin binding occurs; albumin has a weaker binding affinity than transcortin (Daughaday and Kozak, 1958) but possesses an almost unlimited capacity for certain steroids. Albumin type of binding must be determined by a technique that permits slow equilibration, such as dialysis, or that minimizes dissociation, such as rapid filtration through a semipermeable membrane. By contrast, mammalian transcortin can be determined on a Sephadex column without excessive dissociation of the protein–steroid complex. However, even for transcortin the binding values determined by gel filtration are generally minimal since partial dissociation of the complex occurs on the gel during development. To minimize dissociation during gel filtration it is necessary to have a short column, a high flow rate, and a low operating temperature.

B. Protein Binding in Fish

Mammalian transcortin has not been identified in fish, although binding of corticosteroids has been determined using gel filtration methods developed for mammalian transcortin and the results sometimes reported as "transcortin-type" binding to indicate that the protein–steroid complex survived gel filtration intact. The extent of protein binding of corticosteroids determined by gel filtration appears to increase as one moves from the fish to mammals (Seal and Doe, 1965; Steeno and De Moor, 1966). Of 23 fish species studied by Seal and Doe the plasma of 18 bound less than $5\mu g/100$ ml of cortisol or corticosterone. In the light of further investigations we shall discuss below the reason for these consistently low values among several species; the study did demonstrate that there was little "transcortin-type" protein in many fish. Similarly, only $4–7\%$ of the cortisol in the plasma of the female Atlantic salmon *Salmo salar* was bound to protein as determined by gel filtration (Freeman and Idler, 1966). This type of binding was low in four salmonids under a variety of physiological conditions; thus cortisol binding ranged from 2.3 to 5.6% and averaged only 5% of that reported for human plasma at 4°C (Idler and Freeman, 1968). Cortisol binding in the Atlantic cod *Gadus morrhua* was similar in magnitude to that found in salmonids. Cortisol binding, determined by gel filtration, in bowfin (*Amia calva*) and halibut (*Hippoglossus hippoglossus*) plasma was in the range reported for other species of fish (Table II) as was the binding of cortisone by halibut plasma. 1α-Hydroxycorticosterone is a principal corticoid of at least 18 species of elasmobranchs and "transcortin-type" binding of this steroid was low in both female (7%) and male (5%) thorny skate (*Raja radiata*); this

TABLE II

Cortisol Binding by Salmonid Plasma (Equilibrium Dialysis, 4°C)[a]

Species[b]	No. of fish	Sex	Maturity	Cortisol (μg/100 ml)[c]	Cortisol bound (%)[c]
Atlantic salmon	4	F	Immature	10.9	48.8
	3	F	Mature	20.0	34.5
	4	M	Immature	12.0	45.7
	6	M	Mature	15.9	32.9
Brown trout	10	F	Immature		53.7
	20	F	2½ Months postspawned	18.1	52.5
	10	M	Immature		44.0
	20	M	2½ Months post-spawned	13.1	39.7
Chum salmon	10	F	Mature and maturing	17.2	43.2
	10	F	2 Weeks from maturity	15.2	45.6
	10	M	Mature and Maturing	19.5	29.8
	10	M	2 Weeks from maturity	16.0	40.5
Sockeye salmon	3	F	Immature	21.0	55.0
	2	F	Mature	14.8	40.9
	2	M	Immature	15.2	45.6
	1	M	Mature	95.7	33.0
Spring salmon	5	F	Mature	56.4	42.6
	5	M	Mature	64.3	41.1

[a]From Idler and Freeman (1968).

[b]Atlantic salmon, *Salmo salar*; brown trout, *S. trutta*; chum salmon, *Oncorhynchus keta*; sockeye salmon, *O. nerka*; spring salmon, *O. tshawytscha*.

[c]Values determined from a single plasma sample which was a pooled sample when representing more than one fish.

degree of binding was comparable to that of cortisol in the plasma of salmonids (Idler and Freeman, 1968).

The effect of temperature on cortisol binding in Atlantic salmon plasma has been determined with gel filtration (Freeman and Idler, 1966). The total plasma cortisol concentration including added cortisol was 34 μg/100 ml. There was only a slight loss of cortisol binding as the temperature was increased from 2° to 20°C and even at 40°C the plasma of Atlantic salmon bound 40% of that bound at 20°C. Thus, for all practical purposes binding of cortisol, as determined by gel filtration, was determined not to be temperature dependent over the physiological temperature range of the salmon.

The percentage of cortisol bound by plasma proteins of Atlantic salmon (sexually mature females) remains fairly constant over a very wide range of concentrations, resulting in an increasing quantity of free cortisol as the plasma cortisol level is increased (Freeman and Idler, 1966). Thus, it is apparent that the saturation method for determining transcortin binding capacity, as used for human plasma, may give misleading results for Atlantic salmon plasma since the binding capacity would be proportional to the cortisol load used. For this reason we preferred, in our studies, to determine the percent corticosteroid bound at physiological levels or percent bound under a specific load and did not stress binding capacity, which in this case *appears* to be almost unlimited. However, there was a more serious problem unknown to us at this time.

In an evaluation of the above results with fish, three points should be borne in mind: (a) Binding determinations with gel filtration depend for success on a very stable protein–steroid complex; (b) in one study, 200μg cortisol/100 ml of plasma were used to saturate binding sites prior to Sephadex chromatography (Seal and Doe, 1965) but this amount is not sufficient to saturate binding sites in the plasma of the one species of fish for which the binding capacity has been studied, the Atlantic salmon (Freeman and Idler, 1966); and (c) the steroids selected in one study (cortisol and corticosterone) are not the principal plasma corticosteroids of all species investigated (i.e., elasmobranchs). For purposes of this discussion, (a) is by far the most important factor. Therefore our group set out to determine the stability of protein–corticosteroid complexes in fish plasma. The low association constants for three steroids and three species of fish clearly demonstrated that this was the answer to low and monotonously uniform binding as determined by gel filtration. Thus, a plasma protein like that which binds cortisol (2×10^5) in Atlantic salmon dissociates more readily during gel filtration than does transcortin (3×10^7) (Table III), but not as readily as human serum albumin (HSA) (1×10^4). Do the low values found by gel filtration indicate a small quantity of a "transcortinlike" protein or simply incomplete breakdown of a protein–steroid complex with a moderate dissociation constant? There is no direct evidence for the existence of a cortisol-binding protein in fish with an association constant as high as that for transcortin. The binding of cortisone by plasma of Atlantic salmon is most interesting; the association constant is sufficiently high ($K_1 = 3.5 \times 10^6$) that a substantial portion of the protein–cortisone complex survives gel filtration when the column length is just sufficient to permit a separation of the free and bound steroid (~ 20 cm) (Table IV). The data of Seal and Doe (1965), obtained with gel filtration, suggest to the writers that the lungfish *Lepidosiren paradoxa* (51 µg cortisol bound/100 ml plasma), the porcupine fish *Diodon hystrix* (45 µg corticosterone bound/100 ml), and possibly the paddlefish *Polyodon spathula* (13 µg cortisol bound/100 ml) are similarly of great interest; these species may also have a plasma protein with an association constant for corticosteroids higher than those reported in Table III for cortisol. The results for the paddlefish are particularly interesting since the capacity of plasma to bind corticosterone is high while cortisol binding is low (2.4 µg bound/100 ml). Nothing is known of the nature of the steroids of paddlefish but the results with another chondrostean, the sturgeon *Acipenser oxyrhynchus* (Sangalang *et al.*, 1971), suggest that cortisol is probably the principal plasma corticosteroid of paddlefish.

Several, if not all, species of fish require special consideration since the association constant of the high-affinity binding system is intermediate between the weak albumin and strong transcortin types found in man. The association constants, determined in our laboratory by the use of equilibrium dialysis data and a Scatchard type of plot, for the principal corticosteroids in three species of fish are given in Table III (Freeman and Idler, 1971). It is noted that, as in man, salmon and cod have two principal corticosteroid-binding systems. In both species the association constants K_1 (3°C) for cortisol range from 1.7 to 2.6 × 10^5 for both sexes; these values are ~1% of those for man and the rabbit, and only about 10 times the value of K (0.5–1.0 × 10^4) for HSA (Sandberg *et al.*, 1957). In the salmon and cod, however the association constants K_2 (0.8–2.8 × 10^4) of the low-affinity system at 3°C are close to those for HSA at 37°C.

Total binding, determined by equilibrium dialysis, in three species of Pacific salmon (*Oncorhynchus tshawytscha*, *O. keta*, and *O. nerka*) ranged from 30 to 55% at 4°C (Table II) in marked contrast to the small amount of binding measured by gel filtration. Binding was somewhat greater in females (average 45%) than in males of the same species (average 37%). Binding decreased in both sexes of sockeye salmon during the final stage of sexual maturation. In Atlantic salmon and brown trout (*Salmo trutta*) the plasma from immature fish also bound more cortisol than did the plasma from mature fish; for these species plasma from the female bound more cortisol than did male plasma when both sexes were in a comparable state of

TABLE III

Association Constants at 3°C of Corticosteroids Bound to fish Plasma[a]

Species[b]	Sex	Maturity	No. of fish[c]	Steroid	$K_1{}^d$	$K_2 (\times 10^4)^d$
Atlantic salmon	M	Immature	31	Cortisol	1.7×10^5	2.8
	F	Immature	21	Cortisol	2.6×10^5	2.2
	M	Immature	31	Cortisone	2.3×10^6	3.0
	F	Immature	21	Cortisone	4.7×10^6	4.0
Atlantic cod	M	Immature	9	Cortisol	2.1×10^5	0.8
	F	Immature	3	Cortisol	1.7×10^5	1.1
	M	Immature	9	Cortisone	3.1×10^5	0.5
	F	Immature	6	Cortisone	4.7×10^5	0.5
Thorny skate	M	Immature	3	$1\alpha\text{-OH-B}^e$	1.2×10^4	
	F	Immature	4	$1a\text{-OH-B}^e$	0.9×10^4	

[a]From Freeman and Idler (1971).
[b]Atlantic salmon, *Salmo salar*; Atlantic cod, *Gadus morrhua*; thorny skate, *Raja radiata*.
[c]A pooled plasma sample was used.
[d]In liters per mole.
[e]1α-Hydroxycorticosterone.

TABLE IV

Binding of Cortisol and/or Cortisone by the Bowfin *Amia calva*, the Atlantic Salmon *Salmo salar*, and the Halibut *Hippoglossus hippoglossus*[a]

Species	No. of fish	Sex	State of maturity	Steroid	Binding(%)[b] Gel filtration at 4°C[c]	Dialysis at 3°C
Bowfin	4 (pooled)	M	Mature	Cortisol	2.08	33.6
Atlantic salmon	5	M	Mature	Cortisone	30.3 ± 3.9^d	79.7 ± 1.6^d
Halibut	1	F	Immature	Cortisol	5.05	25.2
	1	F	Immature	Cortisone	3.70	38.9

[a]Freeman and Idler (1970).
[b]Binding was determined in serum or plasma at physiological steroid levels.
[c]The column packing was kept to a minimal length necessary to separate bound from free steroid (~ 20 cm).
[d]Standard error.

sexual maturity. At physiological temperatures the extent of total binding (equilibrium dialysis) of cortisol in salmonids is comparable to that found for transcortin in man. Thus, the average binding at 4° C for salmonids (5 species, 135 fish) was 43.8% (Table II), which compares with 35% at 37°C for human transcortin under conditions in which 90% was bound at 2°C (Seal and Doe, 1962).

Plasma cortisol levels are elevated in human pregnancy but symptoms of hypercorticism are not manifested; this is attributed to elevated transcortin levels induced by estrogen. A similar elevation in transcortin binding during pregnancy has been reported in dogs, mice, rabbits, and guinea pigs (Seal and Doe, 1963; Rosenthal *et al.*, 1969), but pregnant or estrogen-treated sheep did not display this phenomenon (Lindner, 1964). Thus, when compared to mammals, it may seem paradoxical that the plasma of immature salmonids consistently bound more cortisol than did mature fish of the same species. However, this failure to increase binding during sexual matura-ation may help to explain the symptoms of Cushing's syndrome sometimes observed in Pacific salmon (Robertson and Wexler, 1960). Salmon cease to feed during the freshwater phase of spawning migration and expend very large quantities of fat and protein (Idler and Bitners, 1960; Robertson *et al.*, 1961a). For example, there was a decrease of 25% in plasma protein of both male and female sockeye salmon during the migration to Stuart Lake, British Columbia (Jonas and MacLeod, 1960). The change in total plasma protein correlates well with the difference in binding observed for immature and mature sockeye (Table II). It therefore seems reasonable to postulate that the decrease of binding protein in mature fish is not primarily due to a decrease in a specific steroid-binding protein but rather to a general protein depletion. Similarly, plasma of both immature and mature female sockeye contained 17% more plasma protein than did males and it is there-fore not necessary to postulate that the greater binding observed in female salmonids is due to a specific elevation of cortisol-binding protein.

Cortisone in the Atlantic salmon and Atlantic cod is also bound by two binding systems (Table III). The association constants K_2 for both species are similar to those for HSA; but the association constants K_1 for cortisone in the salmon are about 10 times those for cortisol in this species, while K_1 for cortisone in cod is of the same order as K_1 for cortisol. Possibly cortisol and cortisone are bound by the same binding sites in the cod since their association constants are similar. At physiological concentra-tions the percent cortisone bound by Atlantic salmon plasma is high (Table IV). This is the highest degree of binding of any corticosteroid in any species of fish found to date in our investigation. The substantial binding of cortisone is of interest in that cortisol is converted to cortisone readily *in vivo* while there is little (Idler *et al.*, 1963) or no (Donaldson and Fagerlund, 1968) conversion of cortisone to cortisol. In mammals it is believed that cortisol is the active hormone and cortisone is active because it is converted to cortisol; if cortisol is the active hormone in salmon, the animal has a double protection against cortisol toxicity. The conversion of weakly bound cortisol to more strongly bound cortisone could explain how the salmon is able to tolerate high plasma levels of 17-OHCS at certain times in its life. A greater association constant of the cortisone–protein complex relative to that for cortisol may explain the accumulation of cortisone in the blood (Schmidt and Idler, 1962) because of lower metabolic clearance rate (Fagerlund and Donaldson, 1970).

Interpretation of data from studies on steroid binding by certain fish proteins has been hampered by lack of knowledge on the principal steroids of many species. For example, reports that some elasmobranchs contain substantial quantities of cortisol and corticosterone have been questioned (Idler and Truscott, 1969). The association constants (0.9×10^4 and 1.2×10^4) for the binding of 1α-hydroxycorticosterone for the female and male thorny skate, respectively, are of the same order of magnitude as those for HSA (Table III). It appears that the skate has only one principal binding system for 1α-hydroxycorticosterone and if a second system exists its capacity is so low that it has not been detected. Total binding (equilibrium dialysis) of 1α-hydroxycorticosterone by plasma of thorny skate is only 18 and 25% in the male and female, respectively (Idler and Freeman, 1968); this value is relatively low by comparison with cortisol binding in salmonids. However, when the frequently high plasma cortisol levels for salmonids (Table II) are compared with the concentration of 1α-hydroxycorticosterone in the plasma of the thorny skate (Idler and Truscott, 1968) the "active" cortisol levels generally exceed those of "active" 1α-hydroxycorticosterone.

From the foregoing it may be concluded that a protein of the mammalian "transcortin type" does not exist as a major corticosteroid-binding protein in fish investigated to date. Much work is still needed in order to elucidate the precise nature of steroid–protein interactions in fish and to evaluate their role in the regulation of metabolism and biological activity of corticosteroids.

VI. Production and Clearance of Corticosteroids

A. Production and Metabolic Clearance Rates

1. Elasmobranchs

The principal corticosteroid produced *in vitro* by the interrenal of all 18 species investigated to date is 1α-hydroxycorticosterone (Table A.II).

The disappearance of 1α-hydroxycorticosterone-^{3}H from plasma of an unanesthetized thorny skate (*Raja radiata*) following a single injection of the radioactive steroid is shown in Fig. 1. The clearance curve is clearly more complex than some reported in mammals (e.g., Little *et al.*, 1966) and four exponentials were fitted by the method of least squares compared with two exponentials frequently reported for humans. The metabolic clearance rate (MCR) was 2.3 liters/kg per 24 hr (five males) when the data were fitted to two slopes and calculations made from the equation for a two-compartment model. Mechanical integration to 12 hr gave an MCR of 2.1 liters/kg per 24 hr. A mean MCR of 2.2 liters/kg per 24 hr (four males, five females) obtained by continuous infusion at 5°–7°C compares with 3.3 liters/kg per 24 hr for cortisol in normal humans (Tait and Burstein, 1964). The production rate *in vivo*, obtained as a product of the MCR and plasma level of 1α-hydroxycorticosterone, was 100 ± 12 μg/kg per 24 hr at 5°–7°C (seven

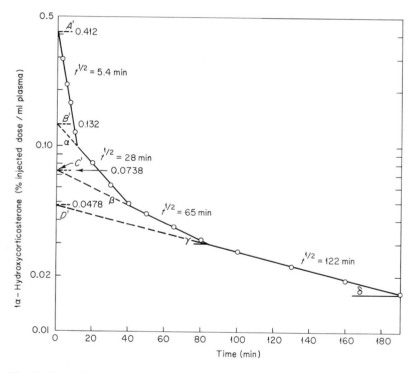

Fig. 1   Rate of disappearance from plasma of 1α-hydroxycorticosterone-7-^{3}H (average 3.4 μCi) injected into five male skates (*Raja radiata*); O, means experimental points; MCR $= 1/[(A/\alpha) + (B/\beta) + (C/\gamma) + (D/\delta)] = 1.01$ liters/kg per 24 hr; production rate $=$ MCR $\times$ plasma steroid level $= 34$ μg/kg per 24 hr.

fish). When interrenal glands were excised from the infused fish the production *in vitro* at 26°C averaged 50% of the production *in vivo* at 5°–7°C. Glands that produced well *in vivo* also produced well *in vitro* ($P < 0.001$) (Idler and Truscott, 1969).

2. Teleosts

Only the Atlantic salmon, cod, and one species of Pacific salmon have been investigated. The freshwater phase of the spawning migration of Pacific salmon is an extremely interesting phenomenon. All five species cease feeding when they begin the migration and die when they have completed it. Some runs are short and others are many hundreds of miles. Migration is accompanied by rapid gonad development and severe depletion of fat and protein (Idler and Bitners, 1958, 1959) and involves sustained as well as frequent vigorous activity. Interpretation of steroid studies on these animals is often difficult because so many things happen at once. One investigator found an essentially steady progression of plasma corticoid levels with increasing maturation, but others have not. Assessment of all data now available does not establish a progressive increase in plasma corticoids during spawning migration. Even if such a progression accompanied sexual maturation it would be difficult to establish experimentally for fish in the natural environment. In fact, low corticoid levels have been observed in salmon well advanced in sexual maturity (Schmidt and Idler, 1962; Fagerlund, 1967).

Interrenal hyperplasia occurs in Pacific king salmon during the river phase of the spawning migration (Robertson and Wexler, 1959), and there is some similarity between changes in the blood biochemistry of these fish and those noted in Cushing's syndrome in man (Robertson *et al.*, 1961a). These authors postulated that hypersecretion of corticoids from the interrenal during the spawning migration would explain the elevated plasma corticoid levels observed in these fish. However, elevated corticoid levels could arise equally well from impaired clearance in the presence of either a decreased or increased secretion. In our opinion it is important to distinguish between high corticoid levels associated with stress or sexual maturation and those associated with a moribund state from whatever cause.

Let us first consider the moribund state. A change in the metabolic clearance curve following infusion of cortisol-^{14}C has been noted for moribund humans and the phenomenon was independent of the cause of death (Sandberg *et al.*, 1956). Moribund humans invariably showed an impaired clearance of cortisol and elevated plasma cortisol levels. There was some increase in plasma 17-OHCS following administration of ACTH. However, the authors concluded that impaired clearance made a major contribution to the elevated plasma corticosteroid levels. For example, when cortisol was injected into moribund patients the average 17-OHCS level rose from 74 to 183 μg/100 ml while that of normal subjects increased from 14 to 77 μg/100 ml. The important point is that after 6 hr plasma 17-OHCS returned to 14 μg/100 ml in normal subjects but 163 μg/100 ml remained in the plasma of moribund patients. Impairment of metabolism in moribund humans presumably involves failure to reduce ring A of the steroid molecule since tetrahydrocortisone was cleared normally. The development of high plasma 17-OHCS levels in humans as a result of stress was variable but was most reproducible in "life-threatening" situations. In Pacific salmon, very large quantities of corticoids can occur in the plasma and exceptionally elevated levels have been observed between the time of spawning and death (Table A. VIII). It has been reported that disease and fungal infections common in postspawned Pacific salmon may produce high plasma cortisol concentrations (Fagerlund, 1967). However, sustained elevated levels of cortisol may contribute to a diseased condition by a diminution of the immunological defence mechanism rather than result from the disease. Intraperitoneal implantation of pellets composed of cortisol and cholesterol in immature rainbow trout produced concentrations of plasma 17-OHCS comparable to those found in mature Pacific salmon (Robertson et al., 1963). During a 5 week period, many of these fish developed severe skin infections and histological examination of tissues showed deteriorative changes typical of spawning salmon. The effects of cortisol implants were dependent upon the amount of cortisol liberated from the pellet into the body and the water temperatures; death occurred more quickly and with lower doses of cortisol when the water temperature was increased from 13° to 17°C. Roth (1967) reported that treatment of the white sucker *Catostomus commersonnii* with cortisol or cortisone permitted the development of fungal infections. Modifications to plasma corticoid levels resulting from various forms of stress and chemical agents are discussed elsewhere (see Section IV).

The clearance curves for radioactive cortisol and cortisone measured as total extractable radioactivity were quite different for spawned sockeye salmon when compared to those for immature fish (Idler et al. 1963). Following an initial rapid clearance of steroid from the peripheral plasma of spawned fish (large distribution volume) the plasma radioactivity fell very slowly for the next several hours. By contrast, the distribution volume of the immature fish was smaller but clearance then continued at a more rapid rate. Atlantic salmon, which frequently survive spawning, showed a fairly rapid and continuous clearance of cortisone-^{14}C for the duration of the experiment (11 hr). Calculation of metabolic clearance rate by the usual two-compartment model is probably not meaningful for moribund fish; the slope of the later portion of the clearance curve is so slight that extrapolation to the X axis is probably not feasible. The pitfalls inherent in the use of such models have been discussed (Gurpide and Mann, 1970). A failure of spawned Pacific salmon to continue to clear radioactivity from the blood is evident also in the data of other investigators (see Fig. 2 in Donaldson and Fagerlund, 1968). However, these authors calculated that anesthetized spawned sockeye salmon had an MCR of 1.1 liters/kg per 24 hr compared with 0.5 liters/kg per 24 hr for maturing fish. The calculations are based on total and extractable radioactivity following injection of cortisol-^{14}C. It should be noted that these fish were matured and spawned in captivity and therefore may not be comparable to salmon which have matured and spawned under their natural conditions. From inspection of the published clearance curves, the point made above with reference to applicability of the two-compartment model may also be pertinent. Hane *et al.* (1966) modified their earlier view that hypersecretion of adrenocortical tissue was the cause of the elevated plasma corticoid level in Pacific salmon at maturity. They noted that extensive liver damage and capillary glomeruloscleroses, which occur in terminal stages of life, could explain the impaired clearance observed by Idler's group. These workers further suggested that increased levels of steroid-binding protein, under the influence of estrogen, might help to explain the elevated blood corticoid levels; however, this seems unlikely since a diminution in protein binding has been reported at this stage in the life cycle (Idler and Freeman, 1968). It would seem worthwhile to explore the possibility that impaired reduction of ring A occurs in spawning Pacific salmon as in moribund humans.

Normal and moribund Atlantic cod gave clearance curves similar to those observed with corresponding Pacific salmon. The early decline in radioactivity in the plasma of moribund fish was greater than for normal fish but the clearance then became very slow for the moribund animals (Idler and Freeman, 1965). A direct measure of the effect of the altered clearance curve in moribund animals on plasma cortisol levels was obtained by holding numerous cod in captivity and taking blood samples at intervals. In cases where animals died during the course of the study elevated plasma cortisol levels were observed in the days prior to death. Unlike the moribund Pacific salmon the cod were sexually immature, which permits the conclusion that impaired hormone metabolism is associated with the agonal state rather than with sexual maturity and spawning. This conclusion is supported by the results with sexually mature Atlantic salmon; an impairment in cortisone clearance was observed for a single Atlantic salmon that died during the course of the experiment (Idler *et al.*, 1963).

Cortisol dynamics including distribution volumes, "half-life," MCR, and production rates as a function of gonad development and gonadal steroids has been studied most intensively in the Pacific sockeye salmon. The distribution volumes of injected cortisol was greater in spawned sockeye salmon of both sexes than in maturing or sexually immature fish (Idler *et al.*, 1963; Donaldson and Fagerlund, 1968). When sockeye salmon were matured in the laboratory there was an increase in distribution volumes, MCR, and cortisol secretion rate. These changes were reversed in fish which were gonadectomized prior to reaching functional maturity (Donaldson and Fagerlund, 1970). Similar results were obtained when cortisone was injected (Fagerlund and Donaldson, 1970), except, as noted below, the MCR for cortisone was low relative to that for cortisol.

In the Pacific sockeye salmon, cortisol-^{14}C was rapidly converted to cortisone-^{14}C but there was little (Idler *et al.*, 1963) or no detectable (Donaldson and Fagerlund, 1968) conversion of cortisone-^{14}C to cortisol-^{14}C. The MCR of total steroid (cortisol + cortisone) is small in comparison to the MCR of cortisol (Fagerlund and Donaldson, 1969). The substantially lower MCR of cortisone relative to cortisol (Fagerlund and Donaldson, 1970) may be explained by the substantially greater association constant which has been reported for the cortisone–protein complex (10^6) as compared to that for cortisol (10^5) in plasma of Atlantic salmon (see Section V). The capacity of the protein is sufficient (30–60 μg/100 ml) to bind more than the total cortisone normally found in plasma (Freeman and Idler, 1971). Androgen or estrogen injection increased the distribution volume of cortisol in gonadectomized male and female salmon, respectively (Donaldson and Fagerlund, 1969; Fagerlund and Donaldson, 1969). The MCR and secretion rates were also increased in estrogen-treated fish with the overall result that plasma cortisol levels decreased. 11-Ketotestosterone is a naturally occurring androgen in salmon where it very effectively promotes the development of secondary characteristics (Idler *et al.*, 1961b; Arai, 1967b). It is the most potent naturally occurring androgen (17 times more potent than testosterone) in bringing about sex reversal in female medaka, *Oryzias latipes* (Hishida and Kawamoto, 1970). Gonadectomized male sockeye salmon treated with 11-ketotestosterone for seven weeks had significantly lower plasma cortisol levels following anesthesia stress than did controls; this was attributed primarily to a greater MCR of cortisol for the androgen-injected fish (Fagerlund and Donaldson, 1969). The MCR of total steroids was low in both groups and the data suggest to us that the conversion of cortisol to cortisone was enhanced by the androgen treatment (see Section V).

Further studies to establish MCR and production rates of corticoids in teleosts are required. Continuous infusion without anesthetic has not been employed but is clearly the method of choice; the products of infusion should be carefully purified. In order to achieve a steady-state system, the experiment should not begin until animals have recovered from surgery. These conditions have not been employed in experiments on teleosts reported to date.

B. CATABOLISM

Information on the catabolic products of corticosteroids in fish is scarce. To the writers' knowledge there have been no intensive studies of the catabolism of C_{21} steroids in organs or tissues of fish. Any summary must be speculative and deduced in some degree from data obtained from studies on other features of steroid metabolism. Perhaps the most pertinent information regarding the possible means of catabolism has been obtained from investigations into the metabolic fate of organic substances and drugs in marine vertebrates (Adamson, 1967; Williams, 1967). Similarities between steroid hydroxylases and drug-metabolizing oxidases in liver tissue of rodents suggest that steroid hormones are the normal substrates for such oxidative microsomal enzyme systems (Kuntzman *et al.*, 1964).

In marine vertebrates, examination of liver tissue with standard test compounds has demonstrated their ability to effect azo and nitro reduction, aromatic hydroxylation, *N*-demethylation, and *O*-dealkylation as well as conjugation reactions to form glucuronosides, sulfates, and glycine derivatives. Although relatively few species have been tested and differences between species were noted, drug-metabolizing enzymes were found in both elasmobranchs and teleosts. Metabolic reactions of particular interest here would include conjugation reactions and oxidation and reduction of the parent steroidal compound (Adamson, 1967).

A corticosteroid (1α-hydroxycorticosterone) as well as an androgen (testosterone), both conjugated with glucuronic acid, have been identified in plasma of the elasmobranch *Raja radiata*. The conjugated steroid was not isolated as such but its identity was presumed on the basis of the identification of the steroid after hydrolysis with β-glucuronidase and inhibition of hydrolysis with glucosaccharo-1,4-lactone (Idler and Truscott, 1966b, 1968). Incubation of 100 ml plasma from mature male *R. radiata* with β-glucuronidase released five compounds which were detectable by absorption of ultraviolet light at 240 mμ and/or reduction of blue tetrazolium. Two of the unknowns again behaved chromatographically as 1α-hydroxycorticosterone and testosterone but the identity of the other three compounds has not been established (Idler and Truscott, 1966c). In the blood of a closely related species, *R. ocellata*, there was no evidence of testosterone glucuronoside, although acid hydrolysis suggested that testosterone may occur as a conjugate with some other substance (e.g., sulfate) (Idler and Truscott, 1966b). Plasma of R. ocellata was not examined for corticosteroid conjugates. No attempt has been made to identify the source of the plasmatic steroid conjugates in these elasmobranchs. In vitro studies with microsomal enzyme fractions of elasmobranch liver tissue and corticosteroid substrates have not been recorded.

In teleosts, information concerning catabolites of corticosteroids is extremely limited although studies with androgenic and estrogenic compounds indicate that at least some products of liver metabolism are similar in representative species of vertebrates. In the liver of the trout Salmo iridens, metabolites of C_{19} steroids established the presence of 5α- and 5β-reductases and 3α-, 3β-, and 17β-hydroxysteroid oxidoreductases (Lisboa and Breuer, 1966). A C_{18} hydroxylase, estradiol-17β hydroxylase, demonstrable in liver of a frog, appeared to be absent in the trout (Ozon and Breuer, 1963), although 16α-, 16β, and 17β-hydroxysteroid dehydrogenase were present in the supernatant fractions of three lower vertebrates (Breuer et al., 1963). Similar studies with C_{21} corticosteroids as substrates have not been recorded. Arai et al. (1969) identified 5α- and 5β-pregnanedione, 3α- and 3β-hydroxy-5α-pregnan-20-one, and 3α- and 3β-hydroxy-5β-pregnan-20-one metabolites in vitro of kidney tissue of rainbow trout.

In postspawned and thus moribund sockeye salmon (Oncorhynchus nerka), Idler et al. (1962) isolated 20β-dihydrocortisone from the plasma; in the same plasma, 20β-dihydrocortisol was not detected. 20β-Dihydro-17α-hydroxyprogesterone was identified in plasma of spawned sockeye salmon (Idler et al., 1960a); it also occurred at other stages of development as well as in plasma of Atlantic salmon (Schmidt and Idler, 1962). It is not known if these two steroids are secretions of endocrine tissue or metabolites resulting from reduction of the parent compounds elsewhere in the animal (e.g., liver). 20β-Dihydrocortisone has the same activity as cortisone in the eosinophil test (Carvajal et al., 1959) and other 20β-dihydrocorticosteroids are biologically active.

Although corticosteroid conjugates have not been reported in plasma of teleosts, testosterone conjugated with glucuronic acid was identified in the plasma and testes of O. nerka (Grajcer and Idler, 1963). Furthermore, uridine diphosphate glucuronic acid (UDPGA) was identified in liver tissue of the spring salmon O. tshawytscha (Tsuyuki et al., 1958) and the trout Salmo fario (Dutton and Montgomery, 1958). In S. fario glucuronyl transfer from UDPGA was demonstrable at 22°C in the liver slices but the enzyme was thermolabile at 37°C. Conjugation of glucuronic acid with aminobenzoic acids was reported for the goosefish Lophius americanus and the flounder *Pseudopleuronectes americanus* (Huang and Collins, 1962). Sulfation of steroids in mammalian liver occurs via adenosine 3'-phosphate-5'–phosphosulfate (De Meio *et al.*, 1958). To the writers' knowledge, this compound has not yet been reported in fish but a related substance, succinoadenosine 5'-phosphosulfate (peptide), has been isolated from the acid-soluble nucleotides of salmon (*O. tshawytscha*) liver (Tsuyuki and Idler, 1957).

C. EXCRETION

Patterns of excretion of inorganic ions and end products of nitrogen metabolism in fish have received considerable attention (Hoar and Randall, 1969) but little work has been reported on the excretion of corticosteroid metabolites. There are three possible routes of excretion in aquatic vertebrates, namely the gills, kidney and intestine, and, perhaps in some cases, the skin. Lipid-soluble substances, such as the corticosteroids, were at one time considered to present no excretory problem to fish since such compounds could be dialyzed into the external medium through the gills. The excretion of drugs and related organic compounds has been examined particularly in an elasmobranch, the spiny dogfish *Squalus acanthias*. Dixon *et al.* (1967) found that for this species plasma half-times did not indicate rapid diffusion of lipid-soluble substances; 4-aminoantipyrine and sulfanilamide, both lipid soluble, not ionized at plasma pH, and only slightly bound to plasma proteins, gave plasma half-times of 4 and 6 hr, respectively. Further studies, also with dogfish, indicated that only extremely lipid soluble substances (e.g., tricaine methanesulfonate) were excreted by the gills and polar ionizable compounds were excreted by renal tubules (Maren *et al.*, 1968). These authors concluded that in dogfish the rate of excretion across the gill is a function of lipid solubility and, unless tubular secretion occurs, kidney excretion is relatively slow since the glomerular filtration rate is low. Since there is now considerable evidence that many naturally occurring corticosteroids are bound by protein to an appreciable extent both in elasmobranchs and teleosts, excretion through the gill membranes would be expected to be limited. However, the role of the gills in the excretion of corticosteroids and their metabolites does not appear to have been studied experimentally.

Urinary metabolites have contributed greatly to the understanding of steroid metabolism in mammals but to the writers' knowledge there have been no studies on the excretion of steroid catabolites in cyclostomes or elasmobranchs. It has been noted above that 1 α-hydroxycorticosterone and testosterone conjugated with glucuronic acid have been identified in the peripheral plasma of the skate *Raja radiata* but there is no evidence that conjugation is a preliminary step to facilitate their excretion from the animal. In teleosts, as in the mammalian vertebrates, there may be differences in excretory routes among the species, but evidence to date suggests that, in freshwater species at least, the biliary and fecal route of steroid excretion is the major one and steroid excretion in the urine is relatively minor. McKim (1966) examined urine collected from rainbow trout for corticosteroids and their metabolites and tentatively identified cortisol and cortisone in the free steroid fraction, and tetrahydrocortisone, principally as a "sulfate," in the conjugated fraction. Although total 17-OHCS in urine was initially higher after the trout were adapted to confinement in the experimental apparatus, the daily excretion rate averaged only 1.3 μg/24 hr per fish. The experimental fish ranged in weight from 230 to 280 g; thus, the steroid excretion would equal approximately 5 μg/kg per 24 hr. There are no published values for secretion rates in trout which would allow an estimate of the percentage of excretion of 17-OHCS by the kidney. In a "resting" mature sockeye salmon, the secretion rate of cortisol as measured by metabolic clearance rates and plasma concentration was 67 μg/kg per day (Donaldson and Fagerlund, 1968). Although a comparison is not strictly valid, the difference in production and excretion rates suggests that excretion of 17-OHCS in urine represents only a fraction of the total daily excretion.

After radioactive cortisol was injected into the dorsal aorta of a rainbow trout, tissues and body fluids were examined for the distribution of radioactivity. In 1.5 hr the concentration of radioactivity in the bile was twice as high, on a wet weight basis, as in the liver and three to six times higher than in any other organ or tissue (Freeman and Idler, 1969). In the freshwater white sucker the gut was considered to be the main excretory pathway for steroids (Roth, 1967); two incompletely identified metabolites of cortisone were found in the urine.

ACKNOWLEDGMENTS

Thanks are due to Academic Press for their permission to reproduce a table from the paper, "Binding of testosterone, 1α-hydroxycorticosterone and cortisol by plasma proteins of fish," by D. R. Idler and H. C. Freeman, *General and Comparative Endocrinology* 11, 366–372 (1968), and a figure from the paper, "Production of 1α-hydroxycorticosterone *in vivo* and *in vitro* by elasmobranchs," by D. R. Idler and B. Truscott, *General and Comparative Endocrinology*, Supplement 2, p. 328, January 1969. We appreciate too the permission received from J. B. Lippincott Co. and from E. D. Bransome, Jr. to quote from his article, "Actinomycin D *in vivo*: Paradoxical and non-specific effects on adrenal cortex," *Endocrinology*, 85, 1114, (1969). We acknowledge permission from the editor of *Steroids*, Dr. Albert Segaloff, to use data from three tables published in the article, "Binding affinities of blood proteins for sex hormones and corticosteroids in fish," by H. C. Freeman and D. R. Idler, *Steroids* 17(2), 233–249 (1971).

REFERENCES

Adamson, R. H. (1967). *Fed. Proc. Fed. Amer. Soc. Exp. Biol.* **26**, 1047.
Arai, R. (1967a). *Annot. Zool. Jap.* **40**, 136.
Arai, R. (1967b). *Annot. Zool. Jap.* **40**, 1.
Arai, R., and Tamaoki, B. (1967). *J. Endocrinol.* **39**, 453.
Arai, R., Tajima, H., and Tamaoki, B. (1969). *Gen. Comp. Endocrinol.* **12**, 99.
Axelrod, L. R., Mathijssen, C., Goldzieher, J. W., and Pulliam, J. E. (1965). *Acta Endocrinol. (Copenhagen)* **49**, Suppl. 99, 1–77.
Bara, G. (1968). *Gen. Comp. Endocrinol.* **10**, 126.
Bell, G. R. (1964). *Bull. Fish. Res. Bd. Can.* No. 148, 1–4.
Berliner, D. L., Cazes, D. M., and Nabors, C. J. (1962). *J. Biol. Chem.* **237**, 2478.
Bern, H. A. (1967). *Science* **158**, 455.
Bern, H. A., deRoos, C. C., and Biglieri, E. G. (1962). *Gen. Comp. Endocrinol.* **2**, 490.
Bird, C. E., Green, R. N., and Clark, A. F. (1969). *J. Clin. Endocrinol. Metab.* **29**, 123.
Black, E. C. (1957a). *J. Fish. Res. Bd. Can.* **14**, 117.
Black, E. C. (1957b). *J. Fish. Res. Bd. Can.* **14**, 807.
Boehlke, K. W., Church, R. L., Tiemeier, O. W., and Eleftheriou, B. E. (1966). *Gen. Comp. Endocrinol.* **7**, 18.
Bondy, P. K., and Upton, G. V. (1957). *Proc. Soc. Exp. Biol. Med.* **94**, 585.
Bondy, P K., Upton, G. V., and Pickford, G. E. (1957). *Nature (London)* **179**, 1354.
Botte, V., Buonanno, C., and Chieffi, G. (1964). *Boll. Zool.* **31**, 461.
Botticelli, C. R., and Hisaw, F. L., Jr. (1964). *Amer. Zool.* **4**, 119.
Boyd, G. S., and Simpson, E. R. (1968). *In* "Functions of the Adrenal Cortex" (K. W. McKerns, ed.), Vol. 1, pp. 49–76. Appleton, New York.
Bradshaw, S. D., and Fontaine-Bertrand, E. (1968). *C.R. Acad. Sci. Ser. D* **267**, 894.
Bransome, E. D., Jr. (1969). *Endocrinology* **85**, 1114.
Breuer, H., Ozon, R., and Mittermayer, C. M. (1963). *Hoppe-Seyler's Z. Physiol. Chem.* **333**, 272.
Brodie, A. H., Shimizu, N., Tait, S. A. S., and Tait, J. F. (1967). *J. Clin. Endocrinol. Metab.* **27**, 997.
Bush, I. E., and Ferguson, K. A. (1953). *J. Endocrinol.* **10**, 1.
Bush, I. E., and Sandberg, A. A. (1953). *J. Biol. Chem.* **205**, 783.
Butler, D. G. (1965). *Comp. Biochem. Physiol.* **16**, 583.
Butler, D. G., Donaldson, E. M., and Clarke, W. C. (1969a). *Gen. Comp. Endocrinol.* **12**, 173.
Butler, D. G., Clarke, W. C., Donaldson, E. M., and Langford, R. W. (1969b). *Gen. Comp. Endocrinol.* **12**, 503.
Carballeira, A., Mehdi, A. Z., and Venning, E. H. (1965). *Proc. Soc. Exp. Biol. Med.* **119**, 751.
Carvajal, F., Vitale, O. F., Gentles, M. J., Herzog, H. L., and Hershberg, E. B. (1959). *J. Org. Chem.* **24**, 695.
Chader, G. J., and Westphål, U. (1968a). *J. Biol. Chem.* **243**, 928.
Chader, G. J., and Westphal, U. (1968b). *Biochemistry* **7**, 4272.
Chavin, W. (1956). *J. Exp. Zool.* **133**, 1.
Chavin, W. (1967). Personal communication.
Chester Jones, I. (1969). Private communication.
Chester Jones, I., and Phillips, J. G. (1960). *Symp. Zool. Soc. (London)* **1**, 17.
Chester Jones, I., Phillips, J. G., and Holmes, W. N. (1959). *In* "Comparative Endocrinology" (A. Gorbman, ed.), pp. 582–612. Wiley, New York.
Chester Jones, I., Phillips, J. G., and Bellamy, D. (1962). *Gen. Comp. Endocrinol. Suppl.* **1**, 36.

Chester Jones, I., Henderson, I. W., and Mosley, W. (1964). *J. Endocrinol.* **30**, 155.
Chester Jones, I., Chan, D. K. O., Henderson, I. W., Mosley, W., Sandor, T., Vinson, G. P., and Whitehouse, B. (1965). *J. Endocrinol.* **33**, 319.
Chieffi, G. (1967). *In* "Sharks, Skates and Rays" (P. W. Gilbert, R. F. Mathewson, and D. P. Rall, eds.), pp. 553–580. Johns Hopkins Press, Baltimore, Maryland.
Chieffi, G., and Botte, V. (1963). *Nature (London)* **200**, 793.
Chuiko, V. A. (1968a). *J. Evol. Biochem. Physiol.* **4**, 384.
Chuiko, V. A. (1968b). *J. Evol. Biochem. Physiol.* **4**, 411.
Coghlan, J. P., and Blair-West, J. R. (1967). *In* "Hormones in Blood" (C. H. Gray and A. L. Bacharach, eds.), Vol. 2, pp. 391–488. Academic Press, New York.
Coghlan, J. P., and Scoggins, B. A. (1967). *J. Clin. Endocrinol. Metab.* **27**, 1470.
Daughaday, W. H., and Kozak, I. (1958). *J. Clin. Invest.* **37**, 511.
De Meio, R. H., Lawycka, C., Wizerkaniuk, M., and Salciunas, O. (1958). *Biochem. J.* **68**, 1.
deRoos, R., and deRoos, C. (1967). *Gen. Comp. Endocrinol.* **9**, 267.
Dittus, P. (1939). *Biol. Zentralbl.* **59**, 627.
Dittus, P. (1941). *Z. Wiss. Zool. Abt. A* **154**, 40.
Dixon, R. L., Adamson, R. H., and Rall, D. P. (1967). *In* "Sharks, Skates and Rays" (P. W. Gilbert, R. F. Mathewson, and D. P. Rall, eds.), pp. 547–552. Johns Hopkins Press, Baltimore, Maryland.
Dodd. J. M. (1961). *Abstr. Pacific Sci. Congr., 10th*, 167.
Dodd, J. M., Evennett, P. J., and Goddard, C. K. (1960). *Symp. Zool. Soc. (London)* **1**, 77.
Donaldson, E. M., and Fagerlund, U. H. M. (1968). *Gen. Comp. Endocrinol.* **11**, 552.
Donaldson, E. M., and Fagerlund, U. H. M. (1969). *J. Fish. Res. Bd. Can.* **26**, 1789.
Donaldson, E. M., and Fagerlund, U. H. M. (1970). *J. Fish. Res. Bd. Can.* **27**, 2287.
Donaldson, E. M., and McBride, J. R. (1967). *Gen. Comp. Endocrinol.* **9**, 93.
Donaldson, E. M., Fagerlund, U. H. M., and Schmidt, P. J. (1968). *J. Fish. Res. Bd. Can.* **25**, 71.
Dorfman, R. I., and Ungar, F. (1965). "Metabolism of Steroid Hormones." Academic Press, New York.
Dutton, G. J., and Montgomery, J. P. (1958). *Biochem. J.* **70**, 17P.
Eik-Nes, K. B. (1957). *J. Clin. Endocrinol. Metab.* **17**, 502.
Eik-Nes, K. B. (1968). *In* "Methods in Hormone Research. Chemical Determinations" (R. I. Dorfman, ed.), 2nd ed., Vol. 1, pp. 271–322. Academic Press, New York.
Eik-Nes, K. B., Nelson, D. H., and Samuels, L. T. (1953). *J. Clin. Endocrinol. Metab.* **13**, 1280.
Fagerlund, U. H. M. (1967). *Gen. Comp. Endocrinol.* **8**, 197.
Fagerlund, U. H. M. (1970). *J. Fish. Res. Bd. Can.* **27**, 1169.
Fagerlund, U. H. M., and Donaldson, E. M. (1969). *Gen. Comp. Endocrinol.* **12**, 438.
Fagerlund, U. H. M., and Donaldson, E. M. (1970). *J. Fish. Res. Bd. Can.* **27**, 2323.
Fagerlund, U. H. M., and McBride, J. R. (1969). *Gen. Comp. Endocrinol.* **12**, 651.
Fagerlund, U. H. M. McBride, J. R., and Donaldson, E. M. (1968). *J. Fish. Res. Bd. Can.* **25**, 1465.
Farese, R. V. (1966). *Endocrinology* **78**, 929.
Ferguson, J. J., Jr., and Morita, Y. (1964). *Biochim. Biophys. Acta* **87**, 348.
Fontaine, M. (1936). *C. R. Acad. Sci.* **202**, 1312.
Fontaine, M., and Hatey, J. (1954). *C.R. Acad. Sci.* **239**, 319.
Fontaine, M., and Leloup-Hatey, J. (1959). *J. Physiol. (Paris)* **51**, 468.
Fontaine, M., Bertrand, E., Lopez, E., and Callamand, O. (1964). *C.R. Acad. Sci.* **259**, 2907.
Ford, P. (1959). *In* "Comparative Endocrinology" (A. Gorbman, ed.), pp. 728–734. Wiley, New York.
Freeman, H. C., and Idler, D. R. (1966). *Gen. Comp. Endocrinol.* **7**, 37.

Freeman, H. C., and Idler, D. R. (1969). Unpublished results.

Freeman, H. C., and Idler, D. R. (1970). Unpublished results.

Freeman, H. C., and Idler, D. R. (1971). *Steroids* **17**, 233.

Garrett, F. D. (1942). *J. Morphol.* **70**, 41.

Germain, P., and Gagnon, A. (1968). *Comp. Biochem. Physiol.* **26**, 371.

Grajcer, D., and Idler, D. R. (1963). *Can. J. Biochem. Physiol.* **41**, 23.

Grant, J. K., ed. (1967). *In* "The Gas–Liquid Chromatography of Steroids." Memoirs of the Society for Endocrinology, No. 16, pp. 265–282. Cambridge Univ. Press. London and New York.

Grimm, Y., and Kendall, J. W. (1968). *Neuroendocrinology* **3**, 55.

Grodzinski, Z. (1954). *Bull. Acad. Polon. Sci. Cl. 2*, **2**, 19.

Grollman, A., Firor, W. M., and Grollman, E. (1934). *Amer. J. Physiol.* **108**, 237.

Guillemin, R., Dear, W. E., Nichols, B., Jr., and Lipscomb, H. S. (1959). *Proc. Soc. Exp. Biol. Med.* **101**, 107.

Gurpide, E., and Mann, J. (1970). *J. Clin. Endocrinol. Metab.* **30**, 707.

Hane, S., and Robertson, O. H. (1959). *Proc. Nat. Acad. Sci. U.S.* **45**, 886.

Hane, S., Robertson, O. H., Wexler, B. C., and Krupp, M. A. (1966). *Endocrinology* **78**, 791.

Hanke, W., Bergerhoff, K., and Chan, D. K. O. (1967). *Gen. Comp. Endocrinol.* **9**, 64.

Hartman, F. A., Lewis, L. A., Brownell, K. A., Angerer, C. A., and Sheldon, F. F. (1944). *Physiol. Zool.* **17**, 228.

Hatey, J. (1954). *Arch. Int. Physiol.* **62**, 313.

Heller, H., and Pickering, B. T. (1961). *J. Physiol. (London)* **155**, 98.

Heyl. H. L. (1970). *Gen. Comp. Endocrinol.* **14**, 43.

Hill, C. W., and Fromm, P. O. (1968). *Gen. Comp. Endocrinol.* **11**, 69.

Hirano, T. (1969). *Endocrinol. Jap.* **16**, 557.

Hirano, T., and Utida, S. (1968). *Gen. Comp. Endocrinol.* **11**, 373.

Hishida, T., and Kawamoto, N. (1970). *J. Exp. Zool.* **173**, 279.

Hoar, W. S., and Randall, D. J., eds. (1969). "Fish Physiology," Vol. 1. Academic Press, New York.

Hochachka, P. W., and Somero, G. N. (1968). *Comp. Biochem. Physiol.* **27**, 659.

Hoffman, W., Forbes, T. R., and Westphal, U. (1969). *Endocrinology* **85**, 778.

Huang, K. C., and Collins, S. F. (1962). *J. Cell. Comp. Physiol.* **60**, 49.

Idler, D. R. (1969). *In* "Fish in Research" (O. W. Neuhaus and J. E. Halver, eds.), pp. 121–133. Academic Press, New York.

Idler, D. R. (1971). *Excerpta Med. Found. Int. Congr. Ser.* **219**, 14.

Idler, D. R., and Bitners, I. (1958). *Can. J. Biochem. Physiol.* **36**, 793.

Idler, D. R., and Bitners, I. (1959). *J. Fish. Res. Bd. Can.* **16**, 235.

Idler, D. R., and Bitners, I. (1960). *J. Fish. Res. Bd. Can.* **17**, 113.

Idler, D. R., and Freeman, H. C. (1965). *Can. J. Biochem.* **43**, 620.

Idler, D. R., and Freeman, H. C. (1966). *J. Fish. Res. Bd. Can.* **23**, 1249.

Idler, D. R., and Freeman, H. C. (1968). *Gen. Comp. Endocrinol.* **11**, 366.

Idler, D. R., and O'Halloran, M. J. (1970). *J. Endocrinol.* **48**, 621.

Idler, D. R., and Sangalang, G. B. (1970). *J. Endocrinol.* **48**, 627.

Idler, D. R., and Sangalang, G. B. (1971). Unpublished results.

Idler, D. R., and Szeplaki, B. J. (1968), *J. Fish. Res. Bd. Can.* **25**, 2549.

Idler, D. R., and Truscott, B. (1966a). *J. Fish. Res. Bd. Can.* **23**, 615.

Idler, D. R., and Truscott, B. (1966b). *Gen. Comp. Endocrinol.* **7**, 375.

Idler, D. R., and Truscott, B. (1966c). Unpublished results.

Idler, D. R., and Truscott, B. (1967a). *Steroids* **9**, 457.

Idler, D. R., and Truscott, B. (1967b). *Excerpta Med. Found Int. Congr. Ser.* **132**, 1041.

Idler, D. R., and Truscott, B. (1967c). Unpublished results.

Idler, D. R., and Truscott, B. (1968). *J. Endocrinol.* **42**, 165.

Idler, D. R., and Truscott, B. (1969). *Gen. Comp. Endocrinol. Suppl.* **2**, 325.

Idler, D. R., and Truscott, B. (1970). Unpublished results.

Idler, D. R., Ronald, A. P., and Schmidt, P. J. (1959a). *J. Amer. Chem. Soc.* **81**, 1260.

Idler, D. R., Ronald, A. P., and Schmidt, P. J. (1959b). *Can. J. Biochem. Physiol.* **37**, 1227.

Idler, D. R., Fagerlund, U. H. M., and Ronald, A. P. (1960a). *Biochem. Biophys. Res. Commun.* **2**, 133.

Idler, D. R., Schmidt, P. J., and Ronald, A. P. (1960b). *Can. J. Biochem. Physiol.* **38**, 1053.

Idler, D. R., McBride, J. R., Jonas, R. E. E., and Tomlinson, N. (1961a). *Can. J. Biochem. Physiol.* **39**, 1575.

Idler, D. R., Bitners, I. I., and Schmidt, P. J. (1961b). *Can. J. Biochem. Physiol.* **39**, 1737.

Idler, D. R., Schmidt, P. J., and Ronald, A. P. (1962). *Can. J. Biochem. Physiol.* **40**, 549.

Idler, D. R., Truscott, B., Freeman, H. C., Chang, V., Schmidt, P. J., and Ronald, A. P. (1963). *Can. J. Biochem. Physiol.* **41**, 875.

Idler, D. R., Freeman, H. C., and Truscott, B. (1964). *Can. J. Biochem.* **42**, 211.

Idler, D. R., Truscott, B., and Stewart, H. C. (1969). *Excerpta Med. Found. Int. Congr. Ser.* **184**, 724.

Idler, D. R., Truscott, B., and O'Halloran, M. J. (1970). *J. Fish. Res. Bd. Can.* **27**, 2339.

Idler, D. R., Sangalang, G. B., and Weisbart, M. (1971). *Excerpta Med. Found. Int. Congr. ser.* **219**, 983.

Idler, D. R., Sangalang, G. B., and Truscott, B. (1972). *Gen. Comp. Endocrinol. Suppl.* 3, (in press).

Ito, Y., Takabatake, E., and Ui, H. (1952). *J. Pharm. Soc. Jap.* **72**, 1029.

Janssens, P. A. (1965). *Excerpta Med. Found. Int. Congr. Ser.* **83**, 95.

Janssens, P. A., Vinson, G. P., Chester Jones, I., and Mosley, W. (1965). *J. Endocrinol.* **32**, 373.

Jonas, R. E. E., and MacLeod, R. A. (1960), *J. Fish. Res. Bd. Can.* **17**, 125.

Keller, N., Richardson, U. I., and Yates, F. E. (1969). *Endocrinology* **84**, 49.

Kliman, B., and Peterson. R. E. (1960). *J. Biol. Chem.* **235**, 1639.

Koch, H. J. A. (1968). *In* "Perspectives in Endocrinology: Hormones in the Lives of Lower Vertebrates" (E. J. W. Barrington and C. B. Jørgensen, eds.), pp. 305–349. Academic Press, New York.

Krishnamurthy, V. G. (1968). *Gen. Comp. Endocrinol.* **11**, 92.

Kuntzman, R., Jacobson, M., Schneidman, K., and Conney, A. H. (1964). *J. Pharmacol. Exp. Ther.* **146**, 280.

Leloup-Hatey, J. (1958). *C.R. Acad. Sci.* **246**, 1088.

Leloup-Hatey, J. (1960). *J. Physiol. (Paris)* **52**, 145.

Leloup-Hatey, J. (1961). *J. Physiol. (Paris)* **53**, 405.

Leloup-Hatey, J. (1964a). *Arch. Sci. Physiol.* **18**, 293.

Leloup-Hatey, J. (1964b). *Ann. Inst. Océanogr. (Monaco)* **42**, 221.

Leloup-Hatey, J. (1966a). *Excerpta Med. Found. Int. Congr. Ser.* **111**, 367.

Leloup-Hatey, J. (1966b). *Comp. Biochem. Physiol.* **19**, 63.

Leloup-Hatey, J. (1967). *Gen. Comp. Endocrinol.* 9, 514.

Leloup-Hatey, J. (1968). *Comp. Biochem. Physiol.* **26**, 997.

Leloup-Hatey, J. (1969). Personal communication.

Leloup-Hatey, J. (1970). *Comp. Biochem. Physiol.* **32**, 353.

Lindner, H. R. (1964). *J. Endocrinol.* **28**, 301.

Lisboa, B. P., and Breuer, H. (1966). *Gen. Comp. Endocrinol.* **6**, 414.

Little, B., Tait, J. F., Tait, S. A. S., and Erlenmeyer, F. (1966). *J. Clin. Invest.* **45**, 901.

Lockwood, A. P. M. (1961). *Comp. Biochem. Physiol.* **2**, 241.

Lopez, E. (1969). *Gen. Comp. Endocrinol.* **12**, 339.

Lucis, R. (1966). "Comparative Studies of Adrenal Steroid Biosynthesis in Various Species." Thesis, McGill University, Montreal, Canada.

Lupo di Prisco, C., Vellano, C., and Chieffi, G. (1967). *Gen. Comp. Endocrinol.* **8**, 325.

Macchi, I. A., and Rizzo, F. (1962). *Proc. Soc. Exp. Biol. Med.* **110**, 433.

McFarland, W. N., and Norris, K. S. (1958). *Calif. Fish Game* **44**, 291.

McKim, J. M. (1966). "Stress Hormone Metabolites and their Fluctuations in the Urine of Rainbow Trout." Thesis, University of Michigan, Ann Arbor.

Maetz, J. (1968). *In* "Perspectives in Endocrinology: Hormones in the Lives of Lower Vertebrates" (E. J. W. Barrington and C. B. Jørgensen, eds.), pp. 47–162. Academic Press, New York.

Mahesh, V. B., and Ulrich, F. (1959). *Nature (London)* **184**, 1147.

Maren, T. H., Embry, R., and Broder, L. E. (1968). *Comp. Biochem. Physiol.* **26**, 853.

Mayer, N., Maetz, J., Chan, D. K. O., Forster, M., and Chester Jones, I. (1967). *Nature (London)* **214**, 1118.

Nandi, J. (1962). *Univ. Calif. Publ. Zool.* **65**, 129.

Nandi, J., and Bern, H. A. (1960). *Endocrinology* **66**, 295.

Nandi, J., and Bern, H. A. (1965). *Gen. Comp. Endocrinol.* **5**, 1.

Nelson, D. H., and Samuels, L. T. (1952). *J. Clin. Endocrinol. Metab.* **12**, 519.

Nishimura, H., Oguri, M., Ogawa, M., Sokabe, H., and Imai, M. (1970). *Amer. J. Physiol.* **218**, 911.

Nomura, T. (1962a). *J. Jap. Chem.* **16**, 345.

Nomura, T. (1962b). *J. Jap. Chem.* **16**, 406.

Ogawa, M. (1963). *Sci. Rep. Saitama Univ. Ser. B* **4**, 181.

Olivereau, M. (1962). *Gen. Comp. Endocrinol.* **2**, 565.

Olivereau, M. (1964). *Amer. Zool.* **4**, 170.

Ozon, R., and Breuer, H. (1963). *Hoppe-Seyler's Z. Physiol. Chem.* **333**, 282.

Pasqualini, J. R., Lafoscade, G., and Jayle, M. F. (1964). *Steroids* **4**, 739.

Phillips, J. G. (1959). *J. Endocrinol.* **18**, xxxvii.

Phillips, J. G., and Chester Jones, I. (1957). *J. Endocrinol.* **16**, iii.

Phillips, J. G., and Mulrow, P. J. (1959a). *Nature (London)* **184**, 558.

Phillips, J. G., and Mulrow, P. J. (1959b). *Proc. Soc. Exp. Biol. Med.* **101**, 262.

Phillips, J. G., Holmes, W. N., and Bondy, P. K. (1959). *Endocrinology* **65**, 811.

Phillips, J. G., Chester Jones, I., Bellamy, D., Greep, R. O., Day, L. R., and Holmes, W. N. (1962). *Endocrinology* **71**, 329.

Pickford, G. E. (1957). *In* "The Physiology of the Pituitary Gland of Fishes" (G. E. Pickford and J. W. Atz, eds.), pp. 485–487. New York Zoological Society, New York.

Pickford, G. E., and Atz, J. W., eds. (1957). "The Physiology of the Pituitary Gland of Fishes." New York Zoological Society, New York.

Porter, J. C., and Klaiber, M. S. (1965). *Amer. J. Physiol.* **209**, 811.

Porter, C. C., and Silber, R. H. (1950). *J. Biol. Chem.* **185**, 201.

Purrott, R. J., and Sage, M. (1969). *Pfluegers Arch.* **309**, 107.

Randall, D. J. (1968). *Amer. Zool.* **8**, 179.

Randall, D. J. (1970). *In* "Fish Physiology" (W. S. Hoar and D. J. Randall, eds.), Vol. 4, pp. 133–172. Academic Press, New York.

Rasquin, P. (1956). *Biol. Bull.* **111**, 399.

Rinfret, A. P., and Hane, S. (1955). *Proc. Soc. Exp. Biol. Med.* **90**, 508.

Robertson, O. H., and Wexler, B. C. (1959). *Endocrinology* **65**, 225.

Robertson, O. H., and Wexler, B. C. (1960). *Endocrinology* **66**, 222.

Robertson, O. H., Krupp, M. A., Favour, C. B., Hane, S., and Thomas, S. F. (1961a). *Endocrinology* **68**, 733.

Robertson, O. H., Krupp, M. A., Thomas, S. F., Favour, C. B., Hane, S., and Wexler, B. C. (1961b). *Gen. Comp. Endocrinol.* **1**, 473.

Robertson, O. H., Hane, S., Wexler, B. C., and Rinfret, A. P. (1963). *Gen. Comp. Endocrinol.* **3**, 422.

Rosenfeld, G., and Bascom, W. D. (1956). *J. Biol. Chem.* **222**, 565.

Rosenthal, H. E., Slaunwhite, W. R., and Sandberg, A. A. (1969). *Endocrinology* **85**, 825.

Roth, R. R. (1967). "Some Aspects of Steroid Metabolism and Excretion in *Catostomus commersonii.*" Thesis, University of Alberta, Edmonton, Canada.

Roy, B. B. (1964). *Calcutta Med. J.* **61**, 223.

Rudd, B. T., Sampson, P., and Brooke, B. N. (1963). *J. Endocrinol.* **27**, 317.

Sage, M., and Purrott, R. J. (1969). *Z. Vergl. Physiol.* **65**, 85.

Sandberg, A. A., Eik-Nes, K., Migeon, C. J., and Samuels, L. T. (1956). *J. Clin. Endocrinol. Metab.* **16**, 1001.

Sandberg, A. A., Slaunwhite, W. R., and Antoniades, H. N. (1957). *Recent Progr. Horm. Res.* **13**, 209.

Sandberg, A. A., Rosenthal, H. E., Schneider, S. L., and Slaunwhite, W. R. (1966). *In* "Steroid Dynamics" (G. Pincus, T. Nakao, and J. F. Tait, eds.), pp. 1–61. Academic Press, New York.

Sandor, T., Vinson, G. P., Chester Jones, I., Henderson, I. W., and Whitehouse, B. J. (1966). *J. Endocrinol.* **34**, 105.

Sandor, T., Lanthier, A., Henderson, I. W., and Chester Jones, I. (1967a). *Endocrinology* **81**, 904.

Sandor, T., Henderson, I. W., Chester Jones, I., and Lanthier, A. (1967b). *Gen. Comp. Endocrinol.* **9**, 490.

Sandor, T., Chan, S. W. C., Phillips, J. G., Ensor, D., Henderson, I. W., and Chester Jones, I. (1970). *Can. J. Biochem.* **48**, 553.

Sangalang, G. B., Weisbart, M. L., and Idler, D. R. (1971). *J. Endocrinol.* **50**, 413–421.

Sayers, G., and Sayers, M. A. (1948). *Recent Progr. Horm. Res.* **2**, 81.

Schmidt, P. J., and Idler, D. R. (1962). *Gen. Comp. Endocrinol.* **2**, 204.

Seal, U. S., and Doe, R. P. (1962). *Cancer Chemother. Rep.* No. 16, 329.

Seal, U. S., and Doe, R. P. (1963). *Endocrinology* **73**, 371.

Seal, U.S., and Doe, R. P. (1965). *Steroids* **5**, 827.

Seal, U.S., and Doe, R. P. (1966). In "Steroid Dynamics" (G. Pincus, T. Nakao and J. F. Tait, eds.), pp. 63–88. Academic Press, New York.

Seiler, K., Seiler, R., and Sterba, G. (1970). *Acta Biol. Med. Ger.* **24**, 553.

Shiffman, R. H. (1959). *Progr. Fish. Cult.* **20**, 151.

Shimizu, K., Shimao, S., and Tanaka, M. (1965). *Steroids* **5**, Suppl. 1, 85.

Silber, R. H., and Porter, C. C. (1954). *J. Biol. Chem.* **210**, 923.

Simpson, T. H., and Wright, R. S. (1970). *J. Endocrinol.* **46**, 261.

Simpson, T. H., Wright, R. S., and Gottfried, H. (1963a). *J. Endocrinol.* **26**, 489.

Simpson, T. H., Wright, R. S., and Hunt, S. V. (1963b). *J. Endocrinol.* **27**, 131.

Simpson, T. H., Wright, R. S., and Renfrew, J. (1964a). *J. Endocrinol.* **31**, 11.

Simpson, T. H., Wright, R. S., and Hunt, S. V. (1964b). *J. Endocrinol.* **31**, 29.

Simpson, T. H., Wright, R. S., and Hunt, S. V. (1969). *Gen. Comp. Endocrinol.* **13**, 532.

Slaunwhite, W. R., Schneider, S., Wissler, F. C., and Sandberg, A. A. (1966). *Biochemistry* **5**, 3527.

Smith, H. W. (1931). *Amer. J. Physiol.* **98**, 279.

Sokabe, H. (1968). *J. Jap. Med. Ass.* **59**, 502.

Somero, G. N., and Hochachka, P. W. (1969). *Nature (London)* **223**, 194.

Steeno, O., and De Moor, P. (1966). *Bull. Soc. Roy. Zool. D'Anvers* No. 38, 1–24.

Stenlake, J. B., Davidson, A. G., Williams, W. D., and Downie, W. W. (1970). *J. Endocrinol.* **46**, 209.

Sundararaj, B. I., and Goswami, S. V. (1969). *Gen. Comp. Endocrinol. Suppl.* **2**, 374.

Tait, J. F., and Burstein, S. (1964). *In* "The Hormones" (G. Pincus, K. V. Thimann, and E. B. Astwood, eds), Vol. 5, pp. 441–557. Academic Press, New York.

Thorson, T. B. (1967). *In* "Sharks, Skates and Rays" (P. W. Gilbert, R. F. Mathewson, and and D. P. Rall, eds.), pp. 265–270. Johns Hopkins Press, Baltimore, Maryland.

Truscott, B., and Idler, D. R. (1968a). *J. Endocrinol.* **40**, 515.

Truscott, B., and Idler, D. R. (1968b). *J. Fish. Res. Bd. Can.* **25**, 431.

Truscott, B., and Idler, D. R. (1969). *Gen. Comp. Endocrinol.* **13**, 535.

Truscott, B., and Idler, D. R. (1970) Unpublished results.

Tsang, C. P. W., and Stachenko, J. (1970). *Can. J. Biochem.* **48**, 740.

Tsuyuki, H., and Idler, D. R. (1957). *J. Amer. Chem. Soc.* **79**, 1771.

Tsuyuki, H., Chang, V. M., and Idler, D. R. (1958). *Can. J. Biochem. Physiol.* **36**, 465.

Urist, M. R., and Van de Putte, K. (1967). *In* "Sharks, Skates and Rays" (P. W. Gilbert, R. F. Mathewson, and D. P. Rall, eds.), pp. 271–285. Johns Hopkins Press, Baltimore, Maryland.

van Tienhoven, A. (1968). "Reproductive Physiology of Vertebrates." Saunders, Philadelphia, Pennsylvania.

Venning, E. H., Kazmin, V. E., and Bell, J. C. (1946). *Endocrinology* **38**, 79.

Vinson, G. P., and Whitehouse, B. J. (1969). *Acta Endocrinol. (Copenhagen)* **61**, 695.

Wallace, E. Z., Silverberg, H. O., and Carter, A. C. (1957). *Proc. Soc. Exp. Biol. Med.* **95**, 805.

Wedemeyer, G. (1969). *Comp. Biochem. Physiol.* **29**, 1247.

Weisbart, M., and Idler, D. R. (1970). *J. Endocrinol.* **46**, 29.

Whitehouse, B. J., and Vinson, G. P. (1968). *Steroids* **11**, 245.

Williams, R. T. (1967). *Fed. Proc. Fed. Amer. Soc. Exp. Biol.* **26**, 1029.

Woodhead, A. D. (1960). *J. Endocrinol.* **21**, 295.

Appendix

TABLES A. I–A. XI

TABLE A. I

Corticosteroids in Cyclostomes (Class Agnatha)

STEROIDS IDENTIFIED *IN VITRO* AND IN BODY FLUIDS

Species	Steroid	Source of steroid[a]	Quantity (μg/100 ml)	Major criteria[b]	Rating[b] Identity	Rating[b] Quantity	Reference
MYXINOIDEA							
Myxine glutinosa L. (Atlantic hagfish)	Cortisol Corticosterone	Serum	10.6	PC, CT, UV, Ip–nmc	Su	Te, T	Phillips *et al.* (1962)
	Cortisol		27.2 <0.06	PC, CT, UV, Ip–nmc TLC, Der(r), DIDA	Su Te[c]	Te, T Pr, T	Weisbart and Idler (1970)
After injection of ACTH *in vivo*	Cortisol	Plasma	0.022	TLC, Der(r), DIDA	Te[c]	Pr, T[d]	Weisbart and Idler (1970)
	Corticosterone		0.013	TLC, Der(r), CryC ³H/¹⁴C, DIDA	Te[c]	Pr, T[d]	
After serial injections of ACTH or saline *in vivo*	Cortisol	Serum		TLC, Der(r), Ip–mrc, CryC³H/¹⁴C, DIDA	Pr[e]	Po, T	Idler *et al.* (1971)

Species	Steroid	Condition	Value	Methods			Reference
	Cortisone	(1) + ACTH	0.09				
		(2a) + saline	0.07				
		(2b) + ACTH	0.12		Pr[e]	Po, T	
	Corticosterone	(1) + ACTH	1.38				
		(2a) + saline	0.03				
		(2b) + ACTH	0.99		Pr[e]	Po, T	
	11-Deoxycortisol	(1) + ACTH	0.37				
		(2a) + saline	0.02				
		(2b) + ACTH	0.02		Pr[e]	Po, T	
		(1) ACTH	0.34				
		(2a) + saline	0				
		(2b) ACTH	0.27				
Polistotrema stoutii (Pacific hagfish)	Cortisol	Plasma	9.6	PC, CT, AlkFl	Su	Te, S	Phillips (1959)
	Corticosterone		14.0		Su	Te, S	
PETROMYZONTIA *Petromyzon marinus* L. (lamprey)							
Anadromous and landlocked	17α-Hydroxy-progesterone-^{14}C	Posterior cardinal vein incubate + progesterone-^{14}C		TLC, PC, Ox, Ip–nmrc, Ip–mrc, CryC ^{3}H/^{14}C	Pr	NA	Weisbart and Idler (1970)
Anadromous	17-OHCS	Plasma	♂ 2.2 ♀23	AC, PSCr	SNI	Te, S	Leloup-Hatey (1964b)
Landlocked	Cortisol	Plasma	♂47 ♀28	PC, CT, AlkFl	Su	Te, S	Phillips (1959)
	Corticosterone		♂ 4.4 ♀ 5.3		Su	Te, S	
Landlocked	Cortisol	Plasma	0.005	TLC, Der(r), Ip–mrc, CryC ^{3}H/^{14}C, DIDA	Pr	Pr, T	Weisbart and Idler (1970)
	Cortisone		0.002	TLC, Der(r), DIDA	Su[f]	Te, T[d]	
	Corticosterone		0.002	TLC, Der(r), DIDA	Su[f]	Te, T[d]	

[a] Numbers in parentheses refer to separate experiments (see text for details).

[b] For an explanation of abbreviations and rating system, see Chapter 2, Tables I–IV.

[c] Identity rated as tentative only, since both isopolarity and isomorphism not fully established.

[d] Quantitative values represent maximal concentration.

[e] Presumptive identification of each steroid depends upon samples in which isopolarity and isomorphism were demonstrated and ratios were significantly higher than theoretical values.

[f] Assay extended to limit of its sensitivity.

TABLE A.II

Corticosteroids in Elasmobranchs (Class Chondrichthyes)

STEROIDS IDENTIFIED *IN VITRO*

Species	Steroid	Source of steroid[a]	Yield (μg/100 mg tissue or % transformation)[b]	Major criteria[c]	Rating[c] Identity	Rating[c] Quantity	Reference
SELACHII							
Carcharhinus falciformis (sickle shark)	1α-Hydroxycorticosterone-14C	(F) Interrenal incubate + corticosterone-14C	7%	TLC, PC, Ip–nmrc, Der, C³H/¹⁴C SD	Pr	NA	Truscott and Idler (1968a)
Carcharhinus longimanus (white-tip shark)	1α-Hydroxycorticosterone-14C	(F) Interrenal incubate + corticosterone-14C	54%	TLC, PC, Ip–nmrc, Der, C³H/¹⁴C SD	Pr	NA	Truscott and Idler (1970)
Carcharhinus obscurus (dusky shark)	1α-Hydroxycorticosterone	(F) Interrenal incubate	4/hr	TLC, PC, UV, CT, Ip–nmc, Der(r), Ip–mrc, C³H/¹⁴C SD	Pr	Te, P	Truscott and Idler (1968a)
	Corticosterone		Trace	TLC, UV, CT	Ex	NA	
	1α-Hydroxycorticosterone-14C		66%	TLC, PC, Ip–nmrc, Der, C³H/¹⁴C SD	Pr	NA	
Galeus melastomus	Progesterone-14C	(F) Interrenal homogenate + pregnenolone-14C	2.7%[d]	TLC, PC, Ip–nmrc, EnzRe, Der, Ip–mrc, Ip–SD	Pr	NA	Simpson and Wright (1970)
	11-Deoxycorticosterone-14C		1.2%	TLC, PC, Ip–nmrc, Der, EnzRe, Ox, Ip–mrc, Ip–SD	Pr	NA	
	Corticosterone-14C		0.2%		Pr	NA	
Isurus oxyrinchus (mako shark)	1α-Hydroxycorticosterone	(F) Interrenal incubate	11/hr	TLC, PC, UV, CT, Ip–nmc, Der(r), Ip–mrc, C³H/¹⁴C SD	Pr	Te, P	Truscott and Idler (1968a)
	Corticosterone	(F) Interrenal incubate + corticosterone	Trace	TLC, UV, CT	Ex	NA	
	1α-Hydroxycorticosterone			TLC, PC, UV, CT, Der(r), Ip–mrc, C³H/¹⁴C SD	Pr	NA	

Species	Product	Substrate	Yield	Methods			Reference
Prionace glauca (blue shark)	1α-Hydroxycorticosterone	(F) Interrenal incubate	2/hr	TLC, PC, UV, CT, Ip-nmc, Der(r), Ip-mrc, $C^3H/^{14}C$ SD	Pr	Te, P	Truscott and Idler (1968a)
	Corticosterone	(F) Interrenal incubate	2/hr	TLC, PC, UV, CT, Der(r), CryCSA	Pr	Te, P	
	11-Deoxycorticosterone		0.2/hr		Pr		
	1α-Hydroxycorticosterone-^{14}C	(F) Interrenal incubate + corticosterone-^{14}C	43%	TLC, PC, Ip-nmrc, $C^3H/^{14}C$ SD, Der	Pr	Te, P	
Scyliorhinus caniculus	Progesterone-^{14}C	(F) Interrenal homogenate + pregnenolone-^{14}C	48%[d]	TLC, PC, Ip-nmrc, EnzRe, Der, Ip-mrc, Ip-SD	Pr	NA	Simpson and Wright, (1970)
	11-Deoxycorticosterone-^{14}C		19%	TLC, PC, Ip-nmrc, Der, EnzRe, Ox, Ip-mrc, Ip-SD	Pr	NA	
	Corticosterone-^{14}C	Interrenal homogenate + progesterone-^{14}C	0.3%[d]		Pr	NA	
	Corticosterone-^{14}C		36%[d]		Pr	NA	
	11-Deoxycorticosterone-^{14}C		32%	TLC, PC, Der, Ox, Ip-mrc, Ip-SD	Pr	NA	
	1α-Hydroxycorticosterone-^{14}C		6%	TLC, PC, UV, CT, CSAD	Pr	NA	
Scyliorhinus stellaris	1α-Hydroxycorticosterone	Interrenal incubate + corticosterone	68%		Te	NA	Truscott and Idler (1968a)
Sphyrna lewini (scalloped hammerhead shark)	1α-Hydroxycorticosterone	(F) Interrenal incubate	1/hr	TLC, PC, UV, CT, Ip-nmrc, Der(r), Ip-mrc, $C^3H/^{14}C$ SD	Pr	Te, P	Truscott and Idler (1968a)
	1α-Hydroxycorticosterone-^{14}C	(F) Interrenal incubate + corticosterone-^{14}C	27%	TLC, PC, Ip-nmrc, Der, $C^3H/^{14}C$ SD	Pr	NA	
Sphyrna zygaena (smooth hammerhead shark)	11-Dehydrocorticosterone-^{14}C	(F) Interrenal + corticosterone-^{14}C	27%	TLC, PC, Ip-nmrc, CryCSA	Pr	NA	Truscott and Idler (1970)
	1α-Hydroxycorticosterone-^{14}C		55%	TLC, PC, Ip-nmrc, Der, $C^3H/^{14}C$SD	Pr	NA	

TABLE A.II (cont.)

Species	Steroid	Source of steroid[a]	Yield (μg/100 mg tissue or % transformation)[b]	Major criteria[c]	Rating[c] Identity	Rating[c] Quantity	Reference
Squalus acanthias (spiny dogfish)	Corticosterone	Interrenal extract	0.3[e]	PC, UV, Der, AlkFl, ACr, DIDA	Pr	Pr, p[f]	Bern et al. (1962)
	Aldosterone	Interrenal incubate	0.06/hr[e]	DIDA	Pr	Pr, p[f]	
		Interrenal extract	0.01[e]	DIDA	Te	Te, p[f]	
		Interrenal incubate	0.03/hr[e]	PC, AlkFl	Te	Te, p[f]	
	11-Dehydrocorticosterone	Interrenal incubate		PC, AlkFl	Ex		
	11-Deoxycorticosterone-14C	Semen incubate + progesterone-14C or + pregnenolone-14C	60%[d]	PC, Ip-nmrc, Der, EnzRe, Ip-mrc, Ip-SD	Pr	NA	Simpson et al. (1964a)
	11-Deoxycorticosterone-14C	Testis incubate + progesterone-14C	38%	PC, Ip-nmrc, Der, EnzRe, Ip-SD	Pr	NA	Simpson et al. (1964b)
	11-Deoxycortisol-14C		1.8%	PC, Ip-nmrc, Ox, EnzRe, Ip-SD	Te	NA	
	17α,20β,21-Trihydroxypregn-4-en-3-one-14C		1.3%	PC, Ip-nmrc, Der, Enz, Ox, Ip-SD	Te	NA	
	20β,21-Dihydroxypregn-4-en-3-one-14C		1.1%		Te	NA	
	1α-Hydroxycorticosterone	Interrenal incubate	4/hr	TLC, PC, UV, CT, Ip-nmc, Der(r), Ip-mrc, C3H/14C SD	Pr	Te, P	Truscott and Idler (1968a)
	Corticosterone	Interrenal incubate + corticosterone-14C	Trace	TLC, UV, CT	Ex	NA	
	1α-Hydroxycorticosterone-14C		53%	TLC, PC, Ip-nmrc, Der, C3H/14C SD	Pr	NA	
	Progesterone-14C	(F) Interrenal homogenate[g] + (a) Pregnenolone-14C + (b) Progesterone-14C	(a) 1.5%	TLC, PC, Ip-nmrc, EnzRe, Der, Ip-mrc, Ip-SD	Pr	NA	Simpson and Wright (1970)

216

Species / Compound	Incubation	Yield	Methods			Reference
11-Deoxycorticosterone-¹⁴C	(F) Interrenal incubate + corticosterone-¹⁴C	(a) 27% (b) 42%	TLC, PC, Ip-nmrc, Der, EnzRe, Ox, Ip-SD	Pr	NA	Truscott and Idler (1968a)
Corticosterone-¹⁴C	(F) Interrenal incubate + corticosterone-¹⁴C	(a) 36% (b) 25%		Pr	NA	Truscott and Idler (1970)
BATOIDEA						
Dasyatis violacea (stingray)						
1α-Hydroxycorticosterone-¹⁴C	Interrenal incubate + corticosterone-¹⁴C	73%	TLC, PC, Ip-nmrc, Der, C³H/¹⁴C SD	Pr	NA	Truscott and Idler (1968a)
Potamotrygon circularis (freshwater stingray)						
1α-Hydroxycorticosterone-¹⁴C	Interrenal incubate[g]	1%	TLC, PC, Ip-nmrc, Der, C³H/¹⁴C SD, CryC³H/¹⁴C D	Pr	NA	Macchi and Rizzo (1962)
Raja clavata (thornback ray)						
1α-Hydroxycorticosterone	Interrenal incubate		TLC, PC, UV, CT, Der(r), Ip-mrc, C³H/¹⁴C SD	Pr	NA	Truscott and Idler (1968a)
Raja erinacea (little skate)						
α-Ketolic	Interrenal incubate + corticosterone-¹⁴C	♂5.1/hr[e] ♀4.2/hr	CT	SNI	Te, T	
Δ⁴-3-Keto		♂8.6/hr[e] ♀7.0/hr	UV	SNI	Te, T	Truscott and Idler (1968a)
1α-Hydroxycorticosterone	Interrenal incubate	9/hr	TLC, PC, UV, CT, Ip-nmc, Der(r), Ip-mrc, C³H/¹⁴C SD	Pr	Te, P	Truscott and Idler (1968a)
1α-Hydroxycorticosterone-¹⁴C	Interrenal incubate + corticosterone	82%	TLC, PC, Ip-nmrc, Der C³H/¹⁴C SD	Pr	NA	Idler and Truscott (1966a, 1967a)
Raja laevis (barndoor skate)						
1α-Hydroxycorticosterone	Interrenal[h] incubate (3.6 g) + corticosterone (4.6 mg)	6/hr	TLC, PC, UV, CT, Ip-nmc, Der(r), Ip-mrc, C³H/¹⁴C SD	Pr	Te, P	Idler and Truscott (1966a, 1967a)
	Interrenal incubate			Pr	NA	
Raja ocellata and *R. radiata*						
1α-Hydroxycorticosterone	Interrenal incubate	2.3 mg	TLC, PC, UV, CT, AcFl, Ox, Der, ACr–Der, IR, IR–Der, NMR, NMR–Der, mp, mp–Der	Po	NA	Idler and Truscott (1967a)
Raja ocellata						
1α-Hydroxycorticosterone		6.4/hr	TLC, PC, UV, CT, Ip-nmc, AcFl	Te	Te, P	

217

TABLE A.II (cont.)

STEROIDS IDENTIFIED *IN VITRO*

Species	Steroid	Source of steroid[a]	Yield (μg/100 mg tissue or % transformation)[b]	Major criteria[c]	Rating[c] Identity	Rating[c] Quantity	Reference
Raja radiata	1α-Hydroxycorticosterone	Interrenal incubate	4.4/hr	TLC, PC, UV, CT, Ip-nmc, AcFl	Te	Te, P	Idler and Truscott (1967a)
	1α-Hydroxycorticosterone		57 μg/kg fish /24 hr[e]	TLC, PC, UV, Ip-nmc, CT, AcFl	Te	Pr, T	Idler and Truscott (1969)
	1α-Hydroxycorticosterone-[3]H	Interrenal incubate + progesterone-[3]H		TLC, PC, Ip-nmrc, Der, Ip–SD, Cry CSAD	Pr	NA	Truscott and Idler (1968a)
Raja rhina	Cortisol	Interrenal incubate	0.01/hr[e]	DIDA	Te	Te, p[f]	Bern *et al.* (1962)
	Corticosterone		0.14/hr[e]	DIDA	Te	Te, p[f]	
	Aldosterone		0.005/hr[e]	DIDA	Te	Te, p[f]	
Raja senta (smooth skate)	1α-Hydroxycorticosterone-[14]C	Interrenal incubate + corticosterone-[14]C	57%	TLC, PC, Ip-nmrc, Der, C[3]H/^{14}C SD	Pr	NA	Truscott and Idler (1970)
Torpedo nobiliana (Atlantic electric ray)	1α-Hydroxycorticosterone-[14]C	(F) Interrenal incubate + corticosterone-[14]C	39%	TLC, PC, Ip-nmrc, Der, C[3]H/^{14}C SD	Pr	NA	Truscott and Idler (1970)

[a] The letter F indicates tissue was stored in frozen state prior to incubation.
[b] In this and subsequent tables in which mixed data are presented, the numerical values always refer to micrograms per 100 mg tissue (or per 100 ml) unless otherwise indicated (e.g., as percent).
[c] For an explanation of abbreviations and rating system, see Chapter 2, Tables I–IV.
[d] Yield expressed as percent total recovered radioactivity.
[e] Average value calculated from published data.
[f] Quantity represents maximal values; insufficient data to asses adequacy of assay.
[g] Partial summary; data from one experiment only recorded here.
[h] Preparative biosynthesis of 1α-hydrocorticosterone for chemical description.

TABLE A.III

Corticosteroids in Elasmobranchs (Class Chondrichthyes)

STEROIDS IDENTIFIED IN BODY FLUIDS

Species	Steroid	Source of steroid	Quantity (μg/100 ml)[a]	Major criteria[b]	Rating[b] Identity	Rating[b] Quantity	Reference
SELACHII							
Carcharhinus leucas (bull shark)	Cortisol	Plasma	♂ 0.9 ♀ 2.9	PC, CT, AlkFl	Su	Te, S	Phillips (1959)
	Corticosterone		♂ 1.8 ♀ 1.7		Su	Te, S	
Carcharhinus maculipinnis (black-tipped shark)	Cortisol	Plasma	♂ 2.9	PC, CT, AlkFl	Su	Te, S	Phillips (1959)
	Corticosterone		♂ 0.8		Su	Te, S	
Carcharhinus milberti (brown shark)	Cortisol	Plasma	♀ 2.6	PC, CT, AlkFl	Su	Te, S	Phillips (1959)
	Corticosterone		♀ 5.9		Su	Te, S	
Carcharhinus obscurus (dusky shark)	Cortisol	Plasma	♀ 3.3	PC, CT, AlkFl	Su	Te, S	Phillips (1959)
	Corticosterone		♀ 2.7		Su	Te, S	
Galeocerdo cuvieri (tiger shark)	Cortisol	Plasma	♀ 1.6	PC, CT, AlkFl	Su	Te, S	Phillips (1959)
	Corticosterone		♀ 5.2		Su	Te, S	
Scyliorhinus caniculus (dogfish)	Cortisol	Cardiac blood	2	PC, CT, UV, AlkFl	Su	Te, S	Phillips and Chester Jones (1957), Chester Jones and Phillips (1960)
Scyliorhinus stellaris (cat shark)	17-OHCS[c]	Plasma	46.6 0	AC, PSCr	SNI	Te, S	Leloup-Hatey (1964b)
Squalus acanthias (spiny dogfish)	11-OHCS[d]	Plasma	25 ± 2 (9)	SPa, AcFl	SNI	Te, P	Chuiko (1968a)
	11-Deoxycorticosterone	Semen	500 μg/100 g	PC, CT, UV, Ip–nmc, Der, Re, Ip–mc, IR	Po	Pr, T	Simpson *et al.* (1963a)
	Aldosterone			PC, CT, UV	Ex		
BATOIDEA							
Dasyatis americana (stingray)	Cortisol	Plasma	♀ 4.3	PC, CT, AlkFl	Su	Te, S	Phillips (1959)
	Corticosterone		♀ 4.0		Su	Te, S	
Dasyatis pastinaca (stingray)	11-OHCS[d]	Plasma	12 ± 2 (11)	SPa, AcFl	SNI	Te, P	Chuiko (1968a)

TABLE A.III (cont.)

Species	Steroid	Source of steroid	Quantity (μg/100 ml)[a]	Major criteria[b]	Rating[b] Identity	Rating[b] Quantity	Reference
Myliobatus freminvillii (eagle ray)	Cortisol	Cardinal sinus plasma	6.8	PC, CT, AlkFl	Su	Te, S	Chester Jones et al. (1959)
Raja clavata (thornback ray)	Corticosterone	Cardiac plasma	20.4	PC, CT, UV, AlkFl	Su	Te, S	Phillips and Chester Jones (1957), Chester Jones and Phillips (1960)
	Corticosterone		8				
	11-OHCS[d]	Plasma	6 ± 1 (9)	SPa, AcFl	SNI	Te, P	Chuiko (1968a)
	1α-Hydroxy-corticosterone	Plasma	1.5 (3)	TLC, PC, Ip-nmc, SPa, AcFl	Te	Pr, S	Idler and Truscott (1969)
Raja eglanteria (clearnose skate)	Cortisol	Plasma	♀ 5.3	PC, CT, AlkFl	Su	Te, S	Phillips (1959)
Raja erinacea (little skate)	1α-Hydroxy-corticosterone	Plasma	♂ 0.9	TLC, PC, Ip-nmc, SPa, AcFl	Te	Pr, S	Idler and Truscott (1969)
Raja laevis (barndoor skate)	1α-Hydroxy-corticosterone	Plasma	0.9	TLC, PC, Ip-nmc, SPa, AcFl	Te	Pr, S	Idler and Truscott (1969)
Raja ocellata (winter skate)	1α-Hydroxy-corticosterone	Plasma	0.4	TLC, PC, Ip-nmc, SPa, AcFl	Te	Pr, S	Idler and Truscott (1969)
Raja radiata (thorny skate)	1α-Hydroxy-corticosterone	Plasma	0.5–2.0	TLC, PC, CT, UV, Ip-nmc, Der, Ip-SD, AcFl	Te	Te, S	Idler and Truscott (1966a, 1967b)
	Cortisol	Plasma	0.1	TLC, PC, DIDA	Te, ID[e]	Te, S	Idler and Truscott (1966a)
	Corticosterone	Plasma	0.1		Te, ID[e]	Te, S	
	1α-Hydroxy-corticosterone	Plasma	1.6	TLC, PC, CT, UV, Ip-nmc, Der, AcFl, Ip-SD ACr-Der	Pr	Pr, P	Idler and Truscott (1967a)
	1α-Hydroxy-corticosterone	Plasma	2.1 ± 0.5 (9)	TLC, PC, UV, Ip-nmc, SPa, AcFl	Te	Te, P	Idler and Truscott (1968)
		Cranial fluid	0.8 ± 0.3 (4)		Te	Te, P	
		Perivisceral fluid	23 ± 4.4 (12)	TLC, PC, CT, UV, AcFl, Der(r), $C^3H/^{14}C$ SD	Pr	Pr, P	

Condition	Steroid	Sample	Value	Methods			Reference
	1α-Hydroxy-corticosterone glucuronoside[f]	Pericardial fluid	17 ±5.6 (7)	TLC, PC, UV, Ip-nmc, SPa, AcFl	Te	Te, P	Idler and Truscott (1968)
		Plasma	2	TLC, PC, Ip-nmc, AcFl	Su	Te, S	
		Cranial fluid	2		Su	Te, S	
		Perivisceral fluid	1		Su	Te, S	
		Pericardial fluid	4		Te	Pr, P	
Anesthetized	1α-Hydroxy-corticosterone	Plasma	1.6 ±0.5 (9)	TLC, PC, UV, Ip-nmc, SPa, AcFl	Te	Pr, P	Idler and Truscott (1969)
	1α-Hydroxy-corticosterone glucuronoside[f]		2.2 ±0.3 (4)		Su	Te, S	
Spinal cord severed	1α-Hydroxy-corticosterone glucuronoside[f]	Plasma	4.3 ±0.6 (7)	TLC, PC, UV, Ip-nmc, SPa, AcFl	Te	Pr, P	
After MCR measurements *in vivo* by (a) and (b)	1α-Hydroxy-corticosterone	Plasma		TLC, PC, UV, Ip-nmc, SPa, AcFl	Te	Pr, T	
		(a) Continuous infusion	4.7 ±0.5 (7)				
		(b) Single injection	3.2 ±0.2 (5)				
Torpedo marmorata (at 4 stages of sexual maturity)	Cortisol	Plasma[g]	37–56[g]	AC, TLC, UV, GLC	Su, ID[h]	Te, T	Lupo di Prisco *et al.* (1967)
	Cortisone		5–18		Su, ID[h]	Te, T	
	Corticosterone		1–58		Su, ID[h]	Te, T	
	11-Deoxycorti-costerone		0.2–6		Su, ID[h]	Te, T	

[a]Numbers in parentheses record the number of samples analyzed.
[b]For an explanation of abbreviations and rating system, see Chapter 2, Tables I–IV.
[c]Calculated as cortisol equivalents.
[d]Calculated as corticosterone equivalents.
[e]Quantity represents maximal values; insufficient data to assess adequacy of assay.
[f]Steroid quantified after hydrolysis with β-glucuronidase.
[g]Total steroid (free and conjugated) quantified after hydrolysis with β-glucuronidase; range of four values reported in original publication.
[h]Data from GLC reported for authentic steroids only.

221

TABLE A. IV

Corticosteroids in Holocephalans (Class Chondrichthyes)

STEROIDS IDENTIFIED *IN VITRO*

Species	Steroid	Source of steroid	Yield (μg/100 mg tissue or % transformation)	Major criteria[a]	Rating[a] Identity	Rating[a] Quantity	Reference
Hydrolagus colliei (Pacific ratfish)	Cortisol	Interrenal extract	0.23	PC, UV, CT, DIDA, ACr	Pr	Pr, P[b]	Bern *et al.* (1962)
		Interrenal incubate	0.24/hr[c]		Pr	Pr, P[b]	
	Aldosterone	Interrenal extract	0.01	DIDA	Te	Te, P[b]	
		Interrenal incubate	0.01/hr[c]		Te	Te, P[b]	
	Cortisol	Interrenal incubate	0.6/hr	TLC, PC, Ip-nmc, UV, CT, AcFl	Te	Te, P	Idler *et al.* (1969)
	Corticosterone		0.01/hr	TLC, PC, Ip-nmc	Su	Te, P	
	Cortisone			TLC, PC, UV	Ex	Te, P	
	Cortisol-14C	Interrenal incubate + corticosterone-14C	32%	TLC, PC, Ip-nmrc, UV, CT, CryC, 3H/14C	Pr	NA	
	Cortisol-14C	Interrenal incubate + progesterone-14C	37%	TLC, PC, Ip-nmrc, UV, CT, CryC, 3H/14C	Pr	NA	
	11-Deoxy-cortisol-14C		28%		Pr	NA	
	Corticosterone-14C		0.1%		Pr	NA	
	17α-Hydroxyprogesterone-14C		5.2%		Pr	NA	

[a] For an explanation of abbreviations and rating system, see Chapter 2, Tables I–IV.

[b] Quantities represent maximal values; insufficient data to assess applicability of assay to these samples.

[c] Average of two or more analyses.

TABLE A.V

Corticosteroids in Chondrosteans (Class Osteichthyes)

STEROIDS IDENTIFIED *IN VITRO* AND IN BODY FLUIDS

Species	Steroid	Source of steroid	Quantity (μg/100 ml or % Transformation)		Major criteria[a]	Rating[a]		Reference
						Identity	Quantity	
Acipenser oxyrhynchus Mitchill (American Atlantic sturgeon)	Cortisol-^{3}H, ^{14}C	Interrenal incubate (4 hr) + pregnenolone-^{3}H and progesterone-^{14}C	[^{3}H]	54.3%	TLC, PC, Der, Ip–nmrc, CryC ^{3}H/^{14}C, Ip–mrc, CryC ^{3}H/^{14}C D	Pr	NA	Idler and Sangalang (1970)
			[^{14}C]	55.1%				
	Cortisone-^{3}H, ^{14}C		[^{3}H]	2.75%	TLC, PC, Der, Ip–nmrc, CryC ^{3}H/^{14}C, Ip–mrc, Cry C ^{3}H/^{14}C D	Pr	NA	
			[^{14}C]	2.75%				
	Corticosterone-^{3}H, ^{14}C		[^{3}H]	0.45%		Pr	NA	
			[^{14}C]	1.02%				
	11-Deoxycortisol-^{3}H, ^{14}C		[^{3}H]	0.08%	TLC, PC, Der, Ip–nmrc, Ip–mrc, Cry ^{3}H/^{14}C D	Pr	NA	
			[^{14}C]	0.06%				
	17α-Hydroxyprogesterone-^{3}H, ^{14}C		[^{3}H]	0.023%	TLC, PC, Ip–nmrc, Cry ^{3}H/^{14}C	Pr	NA	
			[^{14}C]	0.015%				
	Progesterone-^{3}H [^{3}H]		[^{3}H]	0.016%	TLC, PC, EnzRe, Ip–nmrc, Ip–mrc, Cry ^{3}H/^{14}C D	Pr	NA	
	17α-Hydroxypregnenolone-^{3}H				TLC, PC, Der, Ip–nmrc, Ip–mrc	Te		
	Cortisol-^{3}H	Interrenal incubate (4 hr) + cholesterol-^{3}H		0.061%	TLC, PC, Der, Ip–nmrc, Ip–mrc, Cry ^{3}H/^{14}C D	Pr	NA	

TABLE A.V (cont.)

Steroids Identified *in Vitro*

Species	Steroid	Source of steroid	Quantity (μg/100 ml or % Transformation)	Major criteria[a]	Rating[a] Identity	Quantity	Reference
	Cortisone-³H		0.004%	TLC, PC, Ip–nmrc, Cry ³H/¹⁴C	Pr	NA	
	Corticosterone-³H		0.001%	TLC, PC, Ip–nmrc, Cry ³H/¹⁴C	Pr	NA	
	11-Deoxycortisol-³H		0.047%	TLC, PC, Der, Ip–nmrc, Ip–mrc, Cry ³H/¹⁴C D	Pr	NA	
	17α-Hydroxyprogesterone-³H		0.023%	TLC, PC, Ip–nmrc, Cry ³H/¹⁴C	Pr	NA	
	Progesterone-³H		0.091%	TLC, PC, EnzRe, Ip–nmrc, Ip–mrc, Cry ³H/¹⁴C D	Pr	NA	
	Pregnenolone-³H		0.43%	TLC, PC, Ip–nmrc, Cry ³H/¹⁴C	Pr	NA	
	17α-Hydroxypregnenolone-³H			TLC, PC, Der, Ip–nmrc, Ip–mrc	Te	NA	
	Cortisol	Plasma	0.18	TLC, PC, Der(r), Ip–mrc, Cry C ³H/¹⁴C, DIDA	Pr	Po, P	Idler et al. (1971), Sangalang et al. (1971)
	Cortisone		0.02		Pr	Po, P	
	Corticosterone		0.007		Pr	Po, P	
	11-Deoxycortisol		0.007	TLC, PC, Der(r), Ip–mrc, DIDA	Te	Te, P[b]	
	11-Deoxycorticosterone		0.008		Te	Te, P[b]	

[a] For an explanation of abbreviations and rating system, see Chapter 2, Tables I–IV.
[b] Quantitative values represent maximal concentration.

224

TABLE A. VI

Corticosteroids in Holosteans (Class Osteichthyes)

STEROIDS IDENTIFIED IN BODY FLUIDS

Species	Steroid	Source of steroid	Quantity (μg/100 ml)	Major criteria[a]	Rating[a]			Reference
					Identity	Quantity		
Amia calva (bowfin)	17-OHCS	Plasma	13	PSCr	SNI	Te, S		Seal and Doe (1963)
	Cortisol	Plasma	0.76	TLC, Der(r), Ip–mrc, CryC^{3}H/^{14}C, DIDA	Pr	Po, P		Idler *et al.* (1971)
	Corticosterone		0.11	TLC, Der(r), CryC ^{3}H/^{14}C, DIDA	Su[b]	Pr, P		

[a] For an explanation of abbreviations and rating system, see Chapter 2, Tables I–IV.
[b] Yield of purified acetylated derivative too low to claim identification (authors).

225

TABLE A.VII

Corticosteroids in Teleosts (Class Osteichthyes)

STEROIDS IDENTIFIED *IN VITRO*

Species	Steroid	Source of steroid[a]	Yield (µg/100 mg tissue or % transformation)	Major criteria[b]	Rating[b] Identity	Rating[b] Quantity	Reference
Anguilla anguilla (European eel) Silver freshwater	Cortisol	CV Extracts	5.9	PC, UV, Ip–nmc, PSCr	Te	Pr, P	Leloup-Hatey (1961, 1964b, 1969)
Freshwater	Cortisone		0.22		Te	Pr, P	Butler (1965)
	Cortisol-^{14}C	HK + CV Incubate (4 hr) + progesterone-^{14}C	1.7%[c]	PC, Ip–nmrc, Der, Ip–mrc	Te	NA	
	Cortisone-^{14}C		0.4%		Te	NA	
	Corticosterone-^{14}C		0.1%		Ex	NA	
	11-Deoxycorticosterone-^{14}C		13.3%		Su	NA	
Silver freshwater	Cortisol-^{14}C	CV Incubate (3 hr) + progesterone-^{14}C	20–40%	PC, TLC, UV, CT, Ip–nmrc, Ox, Der, C^{3}H/^{14}C SD	Pr	NA	Leloup-Hatey (1966b)
	Cortisone-^{14}C		5–10%	PC, Ip–nmrc, CT, Der, Ip–mrc	Te	NA	
	Corticosterone-^{14}C		2–6%	PC, TLC, UV, CT, Ip–nmrc, Ox, Der, C^{3}H/^{14}C SD	Te–Pr	NA	
	11β-Hydroxyprogesterone-^{14}C		1–5%	PC	Ex	NA	
	Cortisol	CV Incubate	2.9[d]	ID	SPIsp	ID	Leloup-Hatey (1966a, 1970)[e]
Post-Stanniectomy		1 week	10.3				
		2 weeks	0.8				
		6 weeks	0.9				

226

	Substrate	Incubation	% Conversion	Methods			Reference
yellow and silver fresh- and salt-water adapted	Cortisol-14C	HK + CV Incubate (3–4 hr) + progesterone-14C	1.6–7.1%	PC, Ip-nmrc, Der, Ip-mrc, Cry CSAD	Pr	NA	Sandor et al. (1966)
yellow freshwater	Cortisone-14C Corticosterone-14C		0.7–1.7%	PC	Pr Ex	NA NA NA	
	Cortisol-14C, 3H	HK + CV Incubate (3–4 hr) + progesterone-14C and pregnenolone-3H	[3H] 4.8% [14C] 4.5%	PC, Ip-nmrc, Der, Ip-mrc, CryC 3H/14C, Cry CSAD	Pr	NA	
	Cortisone-14C,3H		[3H] 1.1% [14C] 1.2%	PC, Ip-nmrc, Der, Ip-mrc, CryC 3H/14C, Cry CSAD	Pr	NA	
	17α-Hydroxyprogesterone-14C, -3H			PC, Ip-nmrc, CryCSA, Ox, Cry CSAD	Pr	NA	
	17α-Hydroxypregnenolone-14C, -3H			PC, Der, Ox, Ip-mrc	Te	NA	
	Cortisol-14C,-3H	HK + CV Incubate (3–4 hr) + progesterone-14C and corticosterone-3H		PC, Ip-nmrc, Der, CryC 3H/14C D	Te–Pr	NA	
	Cortisol-3H	HK + CV Homogenate (3 hr) + cholesterol-3H	0.5–1%	PC, Ip-mrc, Der, Cry 3H/14C D	Pr	NA	Sandor et al. (1967a)
	Pregnenolone-3H		0.25–1%	PC, EnzRe, Der, C 3H/14C SD	Te	NA	
	Cortisol-14C,3H	HK + CV Homogenate (3 hr) + progesterone-14C and pregnenolone-3H	[3H] 17% [14C] 28%	TLC, PC, Der, Ox, CryC 3H/14C, CryC 3H/14C D	Pr	NA	
	11-Deoxycortisol-14C, 3H		[3H] 16% [14C] 26%	TLC, Der, EnzRe, Ox, CryC 3H/14C, CryC 3H/14C D	Pr	NA	

TABLE A.VII (cont.)

Species	Steroid	Source of steroid[a]	Yield (μg/100 mg tissue or % transformation)	Major criteria[b]	Rating[b] Identity	Rating[b] Quantity	Reference
	Cortisol-^{14}C,^{3}H	HK + CV Homogenate (3 hr) + 17α-OH-progesterone-^{14}C and progesterone-^{3}H	[^{14}C] 5%	PC, TLC, Der, CryC^{3}H/^{14}C D	Pr	NA	
	11-Deoxycortisol-^{14}C,-^{3}H		[^{14}C] 46%	PC, TLC, EnzRe, Ox, C^{3}H/^{14}C SD	Pr	NA	
Silver freshwater intact	Cortisol + cortisol-^{14}C	CV Incubate (3 hr) + progesterone-^{14}C	3.3^{d} (3.4%)	PC, Ip-nmrc, PSCr	SPIsp	Pr, P	Leloup-Hatey (1968)
	Cortisone + cortisone-^{14}C		(0.3%)		SPIsp	Te, P	
	Cortisol + cortisol-^{14}C		0.12 (3.7%)		SPIsp	Pr, P	
	Cortisone + cortisone-^{14}C		0.52 (0.3%)		SPIsp	Te, P	
25 Days posthypophysectomy	Cortisol + cortisol-^{14}C	As before + ACTH in vitro	1.1 (5.3%)	PC, Ip-nmrc, PSCr	SPIsp	Pr, P	
	Cortisone + cortisone-^{14}C		0.01 (0.5%)		SPIsp	Te, P	
	Cortisol + cortisol-^{14}C	+ ACTH in vivo	1.5 (5.8%)		SPIsp	Te, P	
	Cortisone + cortisone-^{14}C		0 (0.3%)		SPIsp		
Freshwater (FW) and seawater (SW) adapted	18-Hydroxycorticosterone-^{14}C	HK + CV "Mitochondrial" fraction (2 hr) + corticosterone-^{14}C	FW 0.13% SW 0.09%	PC, TLC, Ip-nmrc, Ox, Ip-mrc, C^{3}H/^{14}C SD	Pr	NA	Sandor et al. (1970)
Anoplopoma fimbria (sablefish)	Cortisol	HK Incubate (2 hr)		PC, CT	Su		Nandi and Bern (1960)

Species	Compound	Method	Yield	Identification		NA	Reference
Bodianus bilunu-latus (a'awa)	Cortisol	HK Incubate (3.5 hr)	Low	TLC, CT	Ex	NA	Nandi and Bern (1965)
	11-Deoxycortisol		Low		Ex	NA	
	Corticosterone		Low		Ex	NA	
Carassius auratus (Japanese goldfish), held in 33% seawater	Cortisone	HK Incubate (3 hr)		PC, CT	Ex	NA	Ogawa (1963)[e]
Catla catla	Cortisol	HK Incubate (1.5–3 hr)		PC, CT, UV, Der, AcFl, PSCr	Su–Te		Roy (1964)[e]
	Corticosterone			PC, CT, UV, Der, AcFl	Su		
Cirrhina mrigala	Aldosterone	HK Incubate (1.5–3 hr)		PC, CT, UV	Ex		Roy (1964)[e]
	Cortisol			PC, CT, UV, Der, AcFl, PSCr	Su–Te		
	Corticosterone			PC, CT, UV, Der, AcFl	Su		
Clupea harengus (Atlantic herring)	Aldosterone	HK + CV Incubate (5 hr) + corticosterone-³H		PC, CT, UV	Ex	NA	Truscott and Idler (1968b)
	Aldosterone-³H			TLC, PC, Ip–nmrc, CryC³H/¹⁴C	Pr		
Colisa lalia	18-Hydroxycorticosterone-³H	HK Extract		TLC, PC, IP–nmrc, Der, Ox, Ip–mrc	Te	NA	Krishnamurthy (1968)[e]
	Cortisone			PC, UV, CT, ACr	Su–Te		
	Corticosterone				Su		
Conger conger (marine eel)	Cortisol-¹⁴C	HK + CV Incubate (3 hr) + progesterone-¹⁴C	0.96%[c]	PC, Ip–nmrc, Der, Ip–mrc	Te	NA	Butler (1965)
	Corticosterone-¹⁴C		0.44%	PC, Ip–nmrc, Der, Ip–mrc	Su	NA	
Fundulus hetero-clitus (killfish)	Cortisol-³H	HK Incubate (3 hr) + progesterone-³H		PC, Ip–nmrc, Der, Ip–mrc	Te	NA	Phillips and Mulrow (1959b)
	Cortisone-³H			PC	Ex	NA	
	Aldosterone-³H			PC, Ip–nmrc, Der, Ip–mrc	Su	NA	

TABLE A.VII (cont.)

Species	Steroid	Source of steroid[a]	Yield (μg/100 mg tissue or % transformation)	Major criteria[b]	Rating[b] Identity	Rating[b] Quantity	Reference
Gadus morrhua (cod)	18-Hydroxycorticosterone-³H	HK Homogenate (4 hr) + corticosterone-³H	0.04%	TLC, PC, Ip–nmrc, Ox, Ip–mrc, C³H/¹⁴C SD	Pr	NA	Sandor *et al.* (1970)
	Cortisol-³H			PC, Ip–nmrc	ID		
Heteropneustes fossilis (catfish)	Cortisol	HK Incubate (3 hr) + LH	0.35/hr 0.95/hr.	TLC, UV, CT, Ip–nmc, AcFl, Der, ACr	Te	Pr, P	Sundararaj and Goswami (1969)[e]
	11-Deoxycorticosterone	HK Incubate (3hr) + LH	0.25/hr 0.68/hr		Su–Te	Pr, P	
Ictalurus punctatus (channel catfish)	Cortisone	HK Incubate (3.5 hr)		TLC, CT, UV, ACr	Su		Boehlke *et al.* (1966)[e]
	Cortisol				Su		
	Corticosterone				Su		
Labeo rohita	Cortisol	HK Incubate (1.5–3hr)		PC, CT, UV, Der, AcFl, PSCr	Su–Te		Roy (1964)[e]
	Corticosterone			PC, CT, UV, Der, AcFl	Su		
	Aldosterone			PC, CT, UV, AlkFl	Ex		
Melanogrammus aeglefinus (haddock)	18-Hydroxycorticosterone-³H	HK homogenate (4 hr) + corticosterone-³H	0.012%	TLC, PC, Ip–nmrc, Ox, Ip–mrc, C³H/¹⁴C SD	Pr	NA	Sandor *et al.* (1970)
	Cortisol-³H			PC, Ip–nmrc	ID		
Mugil cephalus (mullet)	Cortisol	HK Incubate (3.5 hr)		PC, CT	Su		Nandi and Bern (1960)
	Cortisone				Su		
Ophiocephalus punctatus (2 weeks post-hypophysectomy)	Cortisol	(a) HK + CV Incubate (1.5–3 hr)	(a) 0.8/hr	PC, CT, UV, Der, AcFl, PSCr	Su–Te	Te, P	Roy (1964)[e]
		(b) + ACTH *in vivo*	(b) 1.5/hr				
	Corticosterone		(a) 0.2/hr (b) 0.4/hr	PC, CT, UV, Der, AcFl	Su	Te, P	

Salmo gairdnerii (rainbow trout)	HK Incubate (3.5 hr)		Major				Nandi and Bern (1965)
		Cortisol		TLC, PC, UV, CT, Ip–nmc, ACr, PSCr	Te		
		Cortisone		TLC, PC, UV, CT, Ip–nmc, ACr	Te		
		Corticosterone		TLC, PC, UV, CT, Ip–nmc, ACr	Su–Te		
	HK Homogenate (0.5 hr) + progesterone-^{14}C	Cortisol-^{14}C	31.9%[c]	TLC, Ip–nmrc, Der, Ox, Ip–mrc, CrySA	Pr	NA	Arai (1967a)
		11-Deoxycortisol-^{14}C	14.0%	TLC, Ip–nmrc, Der, Ox, Ip–mrc, CrySA	Pr	NA	
		Corticosterone-^{14}C	1.2%	TLC, Ip–nmrc, Der, Ox, Ip–mrc, CrySA	Te	NA	
		11-Deoxycorticosterone-^{14}C	14.1%	TLC, Ip–nmrc, Der, Ox, Ip–mrc, CrySA	Pr	NA	
	Body kidney homogenate + progesterone-^{14}C	Pregnanedione-^{14}C	42.7%	TLC, Ip–nmrc, Der, CrySA	Pr	NA	
	HK Homogenate (0.5 hr) + 11-deoxycorticosterone-^{14}C	18-Hydroxy-11-deoxycorticosterone-^{14}C	2.2%	TLC, Ip–nmrc, CrySA	Pr	NA	Arai and Tamaoki (1967)
	HK Homogenate (2.5 hr) + pregnenolone-^{14}C	Cortisol-^{14}C	2.5%[c]	TLC, Ip–nmrc, Der, Ox, Ip–mrc, CrySA	Pr	NA	Arai et al. (1969)
		17α-Hydroxy-pregnenolone-^{14}C	65.3%	TLC, Der, Ox, CrySA	Te–Pr	NA	
	HK Homogenate (2.5 hr) + 17α-hydroxyprogesterone-^{14}C	11-Deoxycortisol-^{14}C	45.8%	TLC, Ip–nmrc, Der, Ox, Ip–mrc, CrySA	Pr	NA	

TABLE A. VII (cont.)

Species	Steroid	Source of steroid[a]	Yield (μg/100 mg tissue or % transformation)	Major criteria[b]	Rating[b] Identity	Rating[b] Quantity	Reference
	Corticosterone-14C	HK Homogenate (2.5 hr) + 11-deoxycorticosterone-14C	16.8%	TLC, Ip-nmrc, Der, Ox, Ip-mrc, CryCSA	Pr	NA	
	18-Hydroxy-11-deoxycorticosterone		2.0%	TLC, Ip-nmrc, Der, Ox, Ip-mrc, CryCSA	Pr	NA	
	3β-Hydroxy-5α-pregnan-20-one-14C	Body kidney homogenate (2.5 hr) + pro-gesterone-14C	6.8%	TLC, Der, Ox, CryCSA	Pr	NA	
	3α-Hydroxy-5β-pregnan-20-one-14C		1.4%	TLC, Der, Ox, CryCSA	Pr	NA	
	3β-Hydroxy-5β-pregnan-20-one-14C		2.4%	TLC, Der, Ox, CryCSA	Pr	NA	
	3α-Hydroxy-5α-pregnan-20-one-14C		5.1%	TLC, Der, Ox, CryC ^{3}H/^{14}C	Pr	NA	
Salmo salar (Altantic salmon) Smolts	Cortisol	HK Extracts	415 μg/100 g^f	PC, CT, UV, Ip-nmc, PSCr	Te	Pr, T	Fontaine and Leloup-Hatey (1959), Leloup-Hatey (1964b)
	Cortisone		79	PC, CT, Ip-nmc, AcFl	Te	Pr, T	
	Corticosterone		8.1		Su	Te, T	
Adults, upriver migrants	Cortisol	HK Extracts	♂167 ♀111	PC, CT, UV, Ip-nmc, PSCr	Te	Pr, T	Leloup-Hatey (1964b)
	Cortisone		♂2.1 ♀26	PC, CT, Ip-nmc, AcFl	Te	Pr, T	
	Corticosterone		♂4.5 ♀1.7		Su	Te, T	
Spawning	Cortisol		♂137 ♀46	PC, CT, UV, Ip-nmc, PSCr	Te	Pr, T	

	Cortisone		♂6.6 ♀1.8	PC, CT, Ip–nmc, AcFl	Te	Pr, T	
	Corticosterone		♂2.2 ♀6.0		Su	Te, T	
Postspawned, recovered	Cortisol		♀38	PC, CT, UV, Ip–nmc, PSCr	Te	Pr, T	
	Cortisone		♀–	PC, CT, Ip–nmc, AcFl		Pr, T	
	Corticosterone		♀2.7		Su	Te, T	
Tilapia mossambica (cichlid)	Cortisol	HK Incubate (3.5 hr)	Major	TLC, CT, UV, Ip–nmc, ACr	Te	Te, T	Nandi and Bern (1960, 1965)
	Cortisone		Major	PC, TLC, CT, Ip–nmc	Su	Te, T	
	11-Deoxycortisol		Minor	TLC, CT, Ip–nmc	Su	Te, T	
	11-Dehydrocorticosterone		Minor	TLC, CT, Ip–nmc	Su	Te, T	

[a] Head kidney (HK) and cardinal vein (CV) tissue containing interrenal cells.

[b] For an explanation of abbreviations and rating system, see Chapter 2, Tables I–IV.

[c] Yield expressed as percent total recovered radioactivity.

[d] Production of radioinert steroid expressed as micrograms per hour per kilogram of fish.

[e] Partial summary; identification of steroids not the primary subject of original publication.

[f] Steroid concentration in HK extracts of Salmo salar as micrograms per 100 g tissue rather than micrograms per 100 mg tissue.

233

TABLE A. VIII

Corticosteroids in Teleosts (Class Osteichthyes)

STEROIDS IDENTIFIED IN BODY FLUIDS

Species[a]	Steroid	Source of steroid	Quantity (μg/100 ml)[b]	Major criteria[c]	Rating[c] Identity	Rating[c] Quantity	Reference
Alosa alosa (shad)							
Migrating into fresh water	17-OHCS[d]	Plasma	♂34.5 ± 14.7 (2) ♀12.5 ± 6.3(3)	AC, PSCr	SNI	Te, P	Leloup-Hatey (1964b)
Anguilla anguilla (European eel)							
Silver freshwater (GSI = 1.78)	Cortisol	Plasma	21.6	PC, Ip-nmc, PSCr	Te	Te, P	Leloup-Hatey (1961, 1964b, 1969)
Spring-summer Yellow freshwater (GSI = 0.63)	Cortisone Cortisol Cortisone	Plasma	1.6 10.7 1.9	PC, Ip-nmc, PSCr	Te Te	Te, P Te, P	
Autumn (GSI = 1.77)	Corticosterone 17-OHCS[d]	Plasma	1.3 4.6 ± 0.7 (62)	PC, Ip-nmc, AcFl AC, PSCr	Su SNI	Te, P Pr, T	Leloup-Hatey, (1961, 1964b, 1969)
28 days posthypophysectomy (16°C)		Hypox control + 12.5 U ACTH (1 hr)[e]	0.4–0.8 (2) 4.7		SNI	Pr, T	
Summer (GSI = 1.02)	17-OHCS[d]	Plasma	9.1 ± 1.9 (19)	AC, PSCr	SNI	Pr, T	
12 days posthypophysectomy (16°C)		Hypox control + 12.5 U ACTH (1 hr)[e]	9.8 (2) 25.7 (2)				
(7°C)		Hypox control + 12.5 U ACTH	11.8–16.5(2) 5.9–9.7 (2)	AC, PSCr	SNI	Pr, T	
Silver freshwater	17-OHCS[d]	Plasma	♀2.7 ±1.1 (15)	AC, PSCr	SNI	Pr, T	Leloup-Hatey

Group	Steroid	Condition	Value	Method			Reference
Freshwater	17-OHCS[d]	Plasma	♀5.3 ± 0.5 (103)	AC, PSCr	SNI	Pr, T	Leloup-Hatey, (1964b)
	17-OHCS[d]	Plasma 1 week	3.1	PSCr	SNI	ID	Leloup-Hatey (1966a, 1970)
		6 weeks	9.1 8.0				
		9 weeks	1.5				
			1.4				
Post-Stanni-ectomy Freshwater	Cortisol	Plasma	♀7.1 ± 0.8	TLC, PC, Der, AcFl	Te	Te, T	Bradshaw and Fontaine-Bert-rand (1968)
Posthypo-physectomy (20°C)	Cortisol	Plasma 1 day	♀4.5 ± 1.0	CPBA	SNI	Te, T	
		12 days	♀0		SNI	Te, T	
		Hypox control	♂0 (20)		SNI	Te, T	
		+ 50 mU ACTH (0.5 hr)	♂7.6 ± 2.5 (25)	CPBA	SNI	Te, T	
		+ 200 μg carp pituitary (0.5 hr)	♂5.2 ± 1.5 (4)				
Anguilla japonica (Japanese eel) Seawater (SW) adapted	Cortisol	Plasma Intact control	4.4 ± 0.8 (5)	SPa, AcFl	SNI	Pr, T	Hirano (1969)
		Into Fw (2 hr)	6.0 ± 2.9 (5)				
Freshwater (FW) adapted (20°C)		Intact control + 1 U ACTH (2 hr)	3.8 ± 0.9 (5)	SPa, AcFl	SNI	Pr, T	
			21.9 ± 1.8 (5)				
		Into SW (2 hr)	7.8 ± 1.0 (5)				
10 days post-hypophysectomy		Hypox control	0.28 ± 0.17 (5)	SPa, AcFl	SNI	Pr, T	
		Into SW (2 hr)	0.19 ± 0.19 (5)				
Anguilla rostrata (North American eel)	Cortisol	Plasma Intact control + Saline	2.0 ± 0.3 (8)	SPa, AcFl	SNI	Pr, T	Butler *et al.* (1969a)
Silver freshwater		+ Saline	2.1 ± 0.3 (10)		SNI	Pr, T	
		+ 0.6 mg dexa-methasone[e]	1.1 ± 0.1 (9)		SNI	Pr, T	

TABLE A.VIII (cont.)

Species[a]	Steroid	Source of steroid	Quantity (μg/100 ml)[b]	Major criteria[c]	Rating[c]		Reference
					Identity	Quantity	
6 days post-hypophysectomy	Cortisol	Hypox control +10 × 0.2 U/day ACTH[e]	0.8 ± 0.1 (8) 4.3 ± 0.5 (7)	SPa, AcFl	SNI SNI	Pr, T Pr, T	Butler et al. (1969b)[f]
Silver freshwater, 21 days post-surgery	Cortisol	Plasma intact control Sham-op control Interrenalectomy	3.29 ± 0.14 (10) 2.43 ± 0.88 (7) 0.58 ± 0.24 (8)	SPa, AcFl	SNI SNI	Pr, T Pr,T Pr, T	
Yellow freshwater, 21 days post-surgery	Cortisol	intact control Sham-op control Interrenalectomy	3.93 ±0.56 (7) 3.02 ±0.33 (10) 1.05 ±0.11 (11)	SPa, AcFl	SNI SNI SNI	Pr,T Pr,T Pr,T	
Anoplopoma fimbria sablefish	17-OHCS[d]	Plasma	♂22.9	SPa, PSCr	SNI	Pr, P	Schmidt and Idler (1962)
Catostomus catostomus (long-nosed sucker)	Cortisol Corticosterone	Plasma	♂29.8 ♀18 ♂11.4 ♀3.8	PC, CT, AlkFl	Su Su	Te, S Te, S	Phillips (1959)
Catostomus comersoni (short-nosed sucker)	Cortisol Corticosterone	Plasma	♂44 ♀20 ♂7.7 ♀18.5	PC, CT, AlkFl	Su Su	Te, S Te, S	Phillips (1959)
Clupea harengus (Atlantic herring)	Aldosterone	Plasma	0.008 0.065	TLC, PC, Der(r), Ip-mrc, Ip-SD, CryC ^{3}H/^{14}C D	Pr	Po, S	Truscott and Idler (1969)
Conger conger	17-OHCS[d]	Plasma	♀14.4 ± 4.7 (6)	AC, PSCr	SNI	Pr, P	Leloup-Hatey (1964b)
Cyprinus carpio (carp)	Cortisol	Plasma	♂24.4 ♀43.8	PC, UV, CT, Ip-nmc, AlkFl	Su—Te	Te, P	Bondy et al. (1957)

236

Species / Condition	Steroid	Material	Concentration	Method			Reference
	17-OHCS[d] Cortisol Corticosterone	Plasma	1.8 ± 0.5 (11) 7.2–12 (3) 0 (3)	AC, PSCr PC, UV, CT, PSCr	SNI Te	Pr, T Pr, T	Leloup-Hatey (1958, 1960, 1964a)[f]
After 30 min forced exercise	17-OHCS[d] Cortisol Corticosterone	Plasma	27.5 ± 3.3 (4) 12–36 (3) 0–26 (3)	AC, PSCr PC, UV, CT, PSCr PC, UV, CT, AcFl	SNI Te Su	Pr, T Pr, T Te, T	Leloup-Hatey (1964b)
Diplodus annularis (gilthead)	17-OHCS[d]	Cardiac plasma	♂6.5 ± 2.1 (36) ♀4.8 ± 2.4 (22)	AC, PSCr	SNI	Pr, P	Leloup-Hatey (1964b)
	11-OHCS[g]	Plasma	65 ± 5 (6)	SPa, AcFl	SNI	Pr, P	Chuiko (1968a)
Fundulus heteroclitus (killfish)	Cortisol	Plasma	♂5.2 ♀8.2	PC, Ip-nmc, AlkFl	Su–Te	Te, S	Chester Jones et al. (1959)
Gadus morrhua (Atlantic cod)	Cortisol	Cardiac blood	1.0	PC, UV, CT	Su	Te, S	Phillips and Chester Jones (1957), Chester Jones and Phillips (1960)
In Captivity	Cortisol	Plasma controls moribund	♂9.1 (4) ♀24.5 (1) ♂25–83 (4) 12 ± 2 (6)	PC, Ip-nmc, AcFl	Su–Te	Te, P	Idler and Freeman (1965)[f]
Gobius catrachocephalus (toad goby)	11-OHCS[g]	Plasma	<38	SPa, AcFl	SNI	Pr, P	Chuiko (1968a)
Gobius melanostomus (round goby)	11-OHCS[g]	Plasma	1–12 (25)	SPa, AcFl	SNI	Te, P	Chuiko (1968a)
Ictalurus punctatus (channel catfish)	Cortisol Cortisone Corticosterone	Plasma	35–86 (25) 18–36 (25) 21.5	SPa, AcFl SPa, PSCr SPa, AcFl	Su, SNI Ex, SNI Su, SNI	Te, P Te, P Te, P	Boehlke et al. (1966)[f]
Menticirrhus americanus (southern kingfish)	Cortisol	Plasma		PC, AlkFl	Su	Te, S	Chester Jones et al. (1959)

TABLE A.VIII (cont.)

Species[a]	Steroid	Source of steroid	Quantity (μg/100 ml)[b]	Major criteria[c]	Rating[c] Identity	Rating[c] Quantity	Reference
Mugil cephalus (mullet)	11-OHCS[g]	Plasma	68 ± 2 (7)	SPa, AcFl	SNI	Pr, P	Chuiko (1968a)
Oncorhyncus gorbuscha (pink salmon), marine, immature	17-OHCS[d]	Plasma	♀ 31.5	SPa, PSCr	SNI	Pr, P	Schmidt and Idler (1962)
Oncorhyncus kisutch (coho salmon) marine, immature	17-OHCS[d]	Plasma	♂ 0–22 (4) ♀ 0–31 (5)	SPa, PSCr	SNI	Pr, P	Schmidt and Idler (1962)
Freshwater, immature	Cortisol	Serum		SPa, AcFl	Su, SNI	Pr, P	Wedemeyer (1969)[f]
		Controls	13 ± 1 (6)				
		Rapid anesthesia	12 ± 2 (6)				
		"Stressed", cold shock (15 min)	47 ± 3 (6)				
		Exercise (1–2 hr)	~90				
Oncorhyncus nerka (sockeye salmon)	Cortisol	Plasma	♂11♀26	PC, CT, UV, Ip–nmc, ACr, PSCr, Ox, Ip–mc, Der, IR	Po	Pr, P	Idler *et al* (1959a,b)
Migrating, prespawning	Cortisone		♂41♀22		Po	Pr, P	
	17α-Hydroxyprogesterone		♂5.2	PC, UV, Ip–nmc, ACr, Re, Ox, Ip–mc	Pr		Idler *et al.* (1959b)
Spawning, postspawned	Cortisol	Plasma	♂6.1	PC, UV, CT, Ip–nmc, AlkFl	Te	Pr, T	Phillips *et al.* (1959)
	Cortisone		♂7.3		Te	Te, T	
	Corticosterone				Su[h]	Te, T	
	Aldosterone		♂0.12		Su	Te, T	

238

Condition	Tissue	Steroid		Value	Method			Reference
Postspawned	Plasma	17α, 20β-Dihydroxyprogesterone		♀ 5.5	PC, UV, CT, Ip–nmc, ACr, Ox, Ip–mc, IR	Po	Pr, P	Idler et al. (1960a)
	Plasma	17-OHCS[d]						Idler et al. (1960b)
		Cortisol		♂32♀86	SPa, PSCr	SNI	Pr, P	
		Cortisol		♂15.6♀36.3	PC, UV, Ip–nmc, AcFl	SPIsp	Pr, P	
		Cortisone		♂13.6♀53.7	PC, UV, Ip–nmc, PSCr	SPIsp	Pr, P	
		11-Deoxycortisol		♂0.6	PC, UV	Ex	Te, P	
		Corticosterone		♂0.27♀0.24	PC, UV, CT, Ip–nmc, AcFl	Te	Pr, P	
	Plasma	20β-Dihydrocorti-sone		♀2.1	PC, UV, CT, Ip–nmc, Der, Ox, Re, ACr, Ip–mc	Pr	Pr, P	Idler et al. (1962)
Migrating	Plasma	17-OHCS[d]			SPa, PSCr	SNI	Pr, P	Schmidt and Idler (1962)
(a) Immature			(a)	79.4 ± 12.8 (13)				
(b) Maturing			(b)	7.8–9.4 (2)				
(c) Mature			(c)	41–105(2)				
(d) Post-spawned			(d)	20–102(4)				
		Cortisol	(a)	16–33(2)	PC, UV, Ip–nmc	SPIsp	Pr, P	
			(b)	3.0–13 (4)	PSCr, AcFl	SPIsp	Pr, P	
			(c)	8.9–32 (4)				
			(d)	9.5–39 (4)				
		Cortisone	(a)	19–26(2)	PC, UV, Ip–nmc, PSCr	SPIsp	Pr, P	
			(b)	4.5–14(4)				
			(c)	20–40(4)				
			(d)	11–46(4)				
		17α-Hydroxypro-gesterone	(a)	2.5–2.6 (2)	PC, UV, Ip–nmc	SPIsp	Te, P	
			(b)	<1 (3)				
			(c)	0.6–20 (4)				
			(d)	<1–14 (4)				
		20β-Dihydro-17α-hydroxypro-gesterone	(a)	1.8–3.1 (2)	PC, UV, Ip–nmc, AcFl	SPIsp	Te, P	
			(b)	<1 (4)				
			(c)	<1–24 (4)				
			(d)	3.3–13.4 (4)				
In captivity, Freshwater immature→mature	Plasma Resting	Cortisol		♂2.1 ± 1.3 (20) ♀2.5 ± 1.7 (20)	SPa, AcFl	SPIsp	Pr, T	Fagerlund (1967)

239

TABLE A.VIII (cont.)

Species[a]	Steroid	Source of steroid	Quantity ($\mu g/100$ ml)[b]	Major criteria[c]	Rating[c] Identity	Rating[c] Quantity	Reference
Wild, freshwater migrating	Cortisol	Active (3 hr)	♂24.0 (3) ♀38.3 ± 13.9 (7)	SPa, AcFl	SPIsp	Pr, T	Fagerlund et al. (1968)[f]
		Moribund	6.8–198 (18)				
		Postspawned	<5 (14)				
		Resting (from pools)	1.7 ± 1.2 (7)				
		Active (from rapids)	♂14.0 ± 1.8 (5) ♀10.0–15.0 (3)				
		Spawning and postspawned	♂5.1–35.6 (6) ♀5.1–98.8 (7)				
♀,6 months postgonadectomy	Cortisol	Plasma	0.7–10.8 (9)	SPa, AcFl	SPIsp	Pr, T	
(a) Resting and		(a) + Oil (controls)	18.2				
(b) Stressed		(b)	42.3				
		(a) +10 × 1.67 mg/day Metopirone[e]	15.5				
		(b)	18.2				
		(a) + Saline (controls)	31.6				
		(b)	83.1				
		(a) +3 × 1.4 U ACTH[e]	83.0				
In captivity, Freshwater, resting	Cortisol	Plasma Maturing	2.9 (4)	SPa, AcFl	SPIsp	Pr, T	Donaldson and Fagerlund (1968)[f]
		Mature	1.3 (2)			Pr, T	
5 months post-gonadectomy		Postspawned	8.5 (6)			Pr, T	
			4.1 (2)			Pr, T	
♀,6 months postgonadectomy	Cortisol	Plasma		SPa, AcFl	SPIsp	Pr, T	Donaldson and Fagerlund (1969)[f]

240

(a) Resting and[i] (b) Stressed	Cortisol	+ Oil (controls) + 16 × 2.5 mg estradiol (8 weeks) Plasma	(a) 1.3 ± 0.4 (5) (b) 36.4 ± 15.2 (5) (a) 7.0 ± 2.9 (5) (b) 14.9 ± 2.7 (5)	SPa, AcFl	SPIsp	Pr, T	Fagerlund and Donaldson (1969)[f]
♂,3 months postgonadectomy (a) Resting and[i] (b) Stressed	Cortisol	+ Oil (controls) + 14 × 2.5 mg 11-ketotestosterone (7 weeks) Plasma	(a) 1.4 ± 1.4 (4) (b) 25.6 ± 4.8 (4) (a) 1.2 ± 0.3 (3) (b) 7.3 ± 2.5 (3)	SPa, AcFl	SPIsp	Pr, T	Fagerlund and McBride (1969)[f]
In captivity, maturing (a) Resting and[i] (b) Stressed 24 hr post-injection	Cortisol	Untreated controls + 0.1 mg dexamethasone[e]	(a) ♂1.6 ± 1.3 (8) ♀2.0 ± 0.9 (9) (b) ♂12.5 ± 4.0 (8) ♀31.2 ± 11.2 (9) (a) ♂1.5 ± 0.4 (6) ♀1.6 ± 0.5 (6) (b) ♂2.1 ± 0.7 (6) ♀3.7 ± 2.2 (6)	SPa, AcFl	SPIsp	Pr, T	Fagerlund (1970)[f]
In captivity, maturing 16 hr post-dexamethasone injection	Cortisol	Plasma Controls + 0.05 U ACTH[e]	♂1.2–3.4 (11) ♀2.0–3.6 (12) ♂23.0–32.2 (11) ♀42.1–55.6 (12)	SPa, AcFl	SPIsp	Pr, T	Fagerlund (1970)[f]
Oncorhynchus tshawytscha (king salmon) Marine	Cortisol Cortisone 17-OHCS[d]	Plasma Bled at capture Confined for 3–48 hr	Major Minor 11.8 (12) ~45 (10)	PC, UV, CT Ip–nmc, ACr PSCr	Te Te SNI	NA NA Pr, T	Hane and Robertson (1959), Hane et al. (1966)[e] Hane and Robertson (1959), Hane et al. (1966)[f]

TABLE A.VIII (cont.)

Species[a]	Steroid	Source of steroid	Quantity (μg/100 ml)[b]	Major criteria[c]	Rating[c] Identity	Rating[c] Quantity	Reference
Freshwater, migrating, maturing		Plasma	♂49.0 ±21 (7) ♀53.4 ±13 (7)	PSCr	SNI	Pr, T	
Spawning and postspawned		Plasma	♂32.4 ± 13 (24) ♀77.4 ± 28 (26)		SNI	Pr, T	
Spring run, migrating 2–3 months in river	17-OHCS[a]	Plasma	51.5 (14)	PSCr	SNI	Pr, T	Robertson *et al.* (1961a)[f]
Spawning 5–6 months in river			105 (14) ♂108♀100	PSCr	SNI	Pr, T	
Fall run, migrating 1–2 months in river		Plasma	41.4 (7)	PSCr	SNI	Pr, T	
Spawning 2–3 months in river			54.9 (36) ♂31♀79	PSCr	SNI	Pr, T	
Active, on spawning grounds	Cortisol	Plasma	♂ 24–296 (4) ♀ 35–317 (6)	SP4, AcFl	SNI	Pr, T	Fagerlund, 1967
Ophiocephalus punctatus	17-OHCS[d]	Plasma					Roy (1964)[f]
Intact controls			18.0 (10)	PSCr	SNI	Pr, P	
After exercise (1 hr)			53.6 (8)	PSCr	SNI	Pr, P	
+ 2 U ACTH			49.6 (7)				
+ Water controls			15.7 (8)	PSCr	SNI	Pr, P	
2 weeks post-hypophysec-tomy + 2 U ACTH			40.4 (8)				
+ Water controls			13.9 (8)	PSCr	SNI	Pr, P	
3 weeks post-hypophysec-tomy + 2 U ACTH			18.3 (8)				

242

Species	Steroid	Sample	Value	Method			Reference
4 weeks post-hypophysectomy		+ Water controls + 2 U ACTH	5.0 (8) 4.1 (8)	PSCr	SNI	Pr, P	
Ophiodon elongatus (lingcod)	17-OHCS[d]	Plasma	♂5.1	SPa, PSCr	SNI	Pr, P	Schmidt and Idler (1962)
Pogonias cromis (Channel bass)	Cortisol	Plasma	2.0	PC, AlkFl	Su	Te, S	Chester Jones et al. (1959)
Pseudopleuronectes americanus (flounder)	Cortisol	Plasma	16	PC, UV, CT, AlkFl	Su	Te, P	Bondy et al. (1957)
Salmo fario (river trout)	17-OHCS[d]	Plasma	♂12.5 ± 2.3 (5)	AC, PSCr	SNI	Pr, P	Leloup-Hatey (1964b)
Salmo gairdnerii migrating steelhead trout	Cortisol Cortisone	Plasma	Major Minor	PC, UV, CT, Ip-nmc, ACr	Te Te	NA NA	Hane and Robertson (1959), Robertson et al (1961b)[f]
Spawning	17-OHCS[d]	Plasma	♂28.1 (16) ♀41.2 (24)	PSCr	SNI	Pr, T	
Wild, non-migratory rainbow trout Immature	17-OHCS[d]	Plasma	♂10.6 (13) ♀13.7 (10)	PSCr	SNI	Pr, T	
Spawning			♂26.9 (7) ♀58.4 (8)	PSCr	SNI	Pr, T	
Salmo gairdnerii (rainbow trout)	17-OHCS[d]	Plasma controls Exercise (<24 hr) Prolonged exercise	4.7 ± 1.1 (14) 6.7 ± 2.3 16.2 ± 3.7	AC, PSCr	SNI	Pr, T	Leloup-Hatey (1964a)[f]
	17-OHCS[d]	Controls Prolonged exercise	3.9 ± 1.1 (3) 5.1 ± 2.3 (4)	AC, PSCr	SNI	Pr, T	
	17-OHCS[d]	Plasma	♂3.5 ± 1.4 (24) ♀6.9 ± 1.2 (26)	AC, PSCr	SNI	Pr, T	Leloup-Hatey (1964b)
	Total 17-OHCS[j]	Urine	21.5 (4)	SPa, PSCr, PC, UV, CT, Ip-nmc	SNI	Pr, T	McKim (1966)[f]

TABLE A.VIII (cont.)

Species[a]	Steroid	Source of steroid	Quantity (μg/100 ml)[b]	Major criteria[c]	Rating[c] Identity	Rating[c] Quantity	Reference
	Cortisol	Urine	Major	PC, CT, Ip–nmc	Su		
	Cortisone	Urine			Su		
	Tetrahydrocortisone (conjugate)[j]	Urine			Su		
	Cortisol	Plasma	7.4 (8)	SPa, AcFl	SNI	Pr, T	Donaldson and McBride (1967)[f]
2–17 days Post-Sham-hypophysectomy (a) Resting and[i] (b) stressed. 0.5 hr	Cortisol	Plasma	(a) 8.1 ± 5.8 (37) (b) 13.4 ± 5.7 (12)	SPa, AcFl	SNI	Pr, T	
2–17 days post hypophysectomy	Cortisol	Plasma	(a) 1.6 ± 1.8 (19) (b) 2.5 ± 3.2 (4)	SPa, AcFl	SNI	Pr, T	
Salmo gairdnerii	Cortisol	Plasma + Oil (controls) + 3 × 10 mg/day[e] metopirone	4.0 ± 1.5 (4) 3.0 ± 1.2 (4) 1.8 ± 0.8 (6)	SPa, AcFl SPa, AcFl	SNI SNI	Pr, T Pr, T	Fagerlund *et al.* (1968)[f]
	Cortisol	Plasma Controls Exercise (4 hr)	35.2–66.2 (72) 54.4 ± 3.5 (5) 64.2 ± 4.3 (5)	SPa, AcFl SPa, AcFl	SNI SNI	Te, T Te, T	Hill and Fromm (1968)[f]
Salmo salar (Atlantic salmon) Parr Smolt Adult migrating spawning	17-OHCS[d]	Plasma	12.7 (1) 99.4 (5) ♂31.4 (8)♀34.7 (14) ♂21.2 (8)♀25.7 (15)	AC, PSCr AC, PSCr AC, PSCr	SNI SNI SNI	Pr, P Pr, P Pr, P	Fontaine and Hatey (1954)
Spawning	Glucocorticoid	Plasma	116[k]	Liver glycogen mouse bioassay	NA	NA	Hatey (1954)
Postspawned	17-OHCS[d]	Plasma	♂23.0	SPa, PSCr	SNI	Pr, P	Schmidt and Idler (1962)

244

Stage	Steroid	Sample	Concentration	Methods			Reference
	Cortisol		♂16.49±4	PC, UV, Ip-nmc, PSCr, AcFl	Te	Pr, P	
	Cortisone		♂5.29±7.2	PC, UV, Ip-nmc, PSCr	Te	Pr, P	
	17a-Hydroxyprogesterone		♂ .29±1	PC, UV, Ip-nmc	Su	Te, P	
	17a,20β-Dihydroxyprogesterone		♂12.59±.6	PC, UV, Ip-nmc, AcFl	Su	Pr, P	
Winter parr, ♂ precocious, mature	17-OHCS[d] Glucocorticoid	Plasma	♂31.8 ±30.4 / ♀30?	SPa, PSCr / Liver glycogen mouse bioassay	SNI / NA	Pr, T / NA	Idler et al. (1964)
	Cortisol		?13.2	PC, CT, UV, Ip-nmc, PSCr, Ox, 1p-mc	Pr	Pr, T	
	Cortisone		?15.8	PC, CT, UV, Ip-nmc, PSCr, Ox, 1p-mc	Pr	Pr, T	
Parr–smolt ♂	17-OHCS[d]	Plasma	12.7	AC, PSCr	SNI	Pr, T	Leloup-Hatey (1964b)[f]
Smolt			22.4-36.3 (2)		SNI	Pr, T	
Winter parr, ♂			96.5 ±17.8 (16)		SNI	Pr, T	
	Cortisol	Plasma	♂136[m]	PC, UV, CT, Ip-nmc, PSCr	Te	Pr, T	
Parr–smolt	Cortisol		217[m]	PC, UV, CT, Ip-nmc, PSCr	Te	Pr, T	
	Cortisone		115	PC, UV, CT, Ip-nmc, AcFl	Te	Pr, T	
	Corticosterone		3.2		Su	Te, T	
Smolt, migrating to sea	Cortisol		134[m]	PC, UV, CT, Ip-nmc, PSCr	Te	Pr, T	
	Cortisone		22		Te	Te, T	
	Corticosterone		2.3	PC, UV, CT, Ip-nmc, AcFl	Su	Te, T	
Adults (a) Migrating into fresh water	17-OHCS[d]	Plasma	(a) ♂29.0 ± 3.16 (13) ♀26.7 ± 4.15 (24)	AC, PSCr	SNI	Pr, T	Leloup-Hatey (1964b)[f]

245

TABLE A.VIII (cont.)

Species[a]	Steroid	Source of steroid	Quantity (μg/100 ml)[b]	Major criteria[c]	Rating[c] Identity	Rating[c] Quantity	Reference
(b) Spawning			(b) ♂31.5 ± 6.54 (18) ♀29.5 ± 2.04 (24)	AC, PSCr	SNI	Pr, T	
(c) Post-spawned, recovered	Glucocorticoid	Plasma	(c) ♂11.3(2) ♀23.5 ± 15.5 (13)	AC, PSCr	SNI	Pr, T	
			(a) ♂67 ♀184 (b) ♂98 ♀122 (c) ♀129	Liver glycogen mouse bioassay	NA	NA	
	Cortisol	Plasma	(a) ♂110 ♀77.5 (b) ♂44.3 ♀143 (c) ♀107	PC, UV, CT, Ip–nmc, PSCr	Te	Pr, P	
	Cortisone	Plasma	(a) ♂18.9 ♀16.5 (b) ♂21.8 (c) ♀22.7	PC, UV, CT, Ip–nmc, PSCr	Te	Pr, P	
	Corticosterone	Plasma	(a) ♂0 ♀0.7 (b) 0.3 0 (c) ♂3.2	PC, Ip–nmc, AcFl	Su	Te, P	
	Cortisol	Plasma	(a) ♂0–23 (5) ♀0–19 (9) ♂21–68 (4) (b) ♀47–143 (2) ♂0–14 (2) (c) ♀7–23 (4)	PC, UV, CT, Ip–nmc, PSCr	Te	Pr, T	
	Corticosterone	Plasma	(a) ♂1.7–22 (5) ♀0–71 (9) (b) ♂0–0.1 (c) ♂0 ♀0	PC, UV, CT, Ip–nmc, AcFl	Su / NA	Te, T	
Sciaena umbra (black drum)	11-OHCS[g]	Plasma	16 ± 2 (7)	SPa, AcFl	SNI	Pr, P	Chuiko (1968a)
Scorpena porcus (sea perch)	11-OHCS[g]	Plasma	14 ± 2 (38)	SPa, AcFl	SNI	Pr, P	Chuiko (1968a)

246

11-OHCS[g]	Plasma		SPa, AcFl	SNI	Pr, T	Chuiko (1968b)[f]
	Upon capture	18 ± 2 (6)		SNI	Pr, T	
	3 hr after capture	45 ± 3 (7)		SNI	Pr, T	
	1 week in captivity	16 ± 2 (6)			Pr, T	
	+ Pituitary extract	55 ± 3 (7)		SNI	Pr, T	
Spicara smaris (pickerel) 11-OHCS[g]	Plasma	66 ± 3 (11)	SPa, AcFl	SNI	Pr, P	Chuiko (1968a)
Trachurus mediterraneus ponticus (horse mackerel) 11-OHCS[g]	Plasma	50 ± 3 (13)	SPa, AcFl	SNI	Pr, P	Chuiko (1968a)
Uranoscopus scaber (sea cow) 11-OHCS[g]	Plasma	20 ± 2 (11)	SPa, AcFl	SNI	Pr, P	Chuiko (1968a)

[a]The value GSI = gonadosomatic index.
[b]Numbers in parentheses record the number of samples analyzed (individual samples may represent several fish); hypox, hypophysectomized; +, injected.
[c]For an explanation of abbreviations and rating system, see Chapter 2, Tables I–IV.
[d]Calculated as cortisol equivalents.
[e]Dose of injected compound expressed per 100 g body weight.
[f]Partial summary of data recorded in original publication.
[g]Total corticosteroid measured by acid fluorescence, e.g., corticosterone and cortisol but not cortisone; quantity calculated as cortisol equivalents.
[h]Identified as 11-ketotestosterone by Idler *et al.* (1960b).
[i]Plasmatic steroid measured at beginning of experiment (resting) and after experimental procedures, e.g., injections and blood sampling (stressed).
[j]Steroids extracted after hydrolysis with helix enzyme (sulfatase + β-glucuronidase).
[k]Bioassay and chemical assay for 17-OHCS not applied to the same plasma sample.
[l]Bioassay and chemical assay for 17-OHCS applied to same plasma sample.
[m]Author reported that high levels of cortisol and cortisone found in these samples, relative to total 17-OHCS found in other samples, were real and not attributable to methods used.

TABLE A.IX

Corticosteroids in Corpuscles of Stannius of Teleosts (Class Osteichthyes)

STEROIDS IDENTIFIED *IN VITRO*

Species	Steroid	Source of steroid[a]	Quantity μg/100 mg or % transformation	Major Criteria[b]	Rating[b] Identity	Rating[b] Quantity	Reference
Anguilla anguilla (European eel)	None	CS Incubate + progesterone-14C and pregnenolone-3H (37°C, 3 hr)	0	PC, Der, No radioactivity isopolar with 17α,21,11β- or 18-hydroxy derivatives	NA		Chester Jones *et al.* (1965)
Carassius auratus (held in 33% seawater)	11-Deoxycorticosterone	CS Incubate (~20°C, 3 hr)		PC, CT	Ex		Ogawa (1963)
Cottus lalia	Cortisol	CS Extract		PC, UV, CT, Ip–nmc, ACr	Te		Krishnamurthy (1968)
	11-Deoxycortisol			PC, UV, CT, ACr	Su		
Gadus morrhua (Atlantic cod)	Progesterone-14C	CS Incubate + pregnenolone-14C (~23°C, 3.5 hr)	~ 1%[c]	TLC, PC, Ip–nmrc, EnzRe, Der; Ip–mrc, Cry CSAD	Pr	NA	Idler and Freeman (1966)
	11-Deoxycorticosterone-14C	CS Incubate + progesterone-14C (~23°C, 3.5 hr)	0.03%	TLC, PC, Ip–nmrc, Der, EnzRe, Ip–mrc	Te	NA	
Pseudopleuronectes americanus (winter flounder)	None	CS Incubate + progesterone-3H (37°C, 3 hr)		PC, No radioactivity isopolar with 17α,21,11β- or 18-hydroxy derivatives	NA		Phillips and Mulrow (1959a)

Salmo gairdnerii (rainbow trout)	5α- and 5β-Pregnanedione-^{14}C	CS Homogenate + progesterone-^{14}C (37°C, 0.5 hr)		TLC, Ip–nmrc, Ox, Der, Ip–mrc, CSAD, no radioactivity isopolar with 17α,21,11β- or 18-hydroxy derivatives	Pr	NA	Arai et al. (1969)
	None	CS Homogenate + 11-deoxy-corticosterone-^{14}C (37°C, 0.5 hr)	0	TLC; no radioactivity isopolar with 11β- or 18-hydroxy derivatives	NA		
Salmo salar (Atlantic salmon) Migrating into freshwater	Cortisol	CS Extract	♂0.44 ♀0.19	PC, CT, PSCr	Su	Te, P	Fontaine and Leloup-Hatey (1959)
Spawning	Corticosterone		♂0 ♀0.02	PC, AcFl	Su	Te, P	
	Cortisol		♂0.04 ♀0.04	PC, CT, PSCr	Su	Te, P	
	Corticosterone		♂0 ♀0				

[a] Corpuscles of Stannius, CS.
[b] For an explanation of abbreviations and rating system, see Chapter 2, Tables I–IV.
[c] Yield expressed as percent total recovered radioactivity.

TABLE A.X

Corticosteroids in Dipnoi (Class Osteichthyes)

STEROIDS IDENTIFIED IN VITRO AND IN BODY FLUIDS

Species	Steroid	Source of steroid	Quantity (μg/100 ml or % transformation)	Major criteria[a]	Rating[a] Identity	Rating[a] Quantity	Reference
Lepidosiren paradoxa Fitzinger (South American lungfish)	Cortisol	Plasma	0.60	TLC, Der(r), Ip-mrc, CryC^{3}H/^{14}C, DIDA	Pr	Po, T	Idler *et al.* (1972)
	Corticosterone		0.16		Pr	Po, T	
	11-Deoxycortisol		0.03		Pr	Po, T	
	Aldosterone		0.58		Pr	Po, T	
Protopterus annectens (African lungfish) Aestivating	Corticosterone-^{14}C	Interrenal incubate + progesterone-^{14}C	0.05%	PC, Der, Ip-mrc, C^{3}H/^{14}C SD	Te	NA	Janssens *et al.* (1965)
Free-living aquatic	17-OHCS	Plasma	12.0	AC, PSCr	SNI	Te, P	Leloup-Hatey (1964b)
	Cortisol	Plasma	15	PC, Ip-nmc, CT, UV, AlkFl	Su	Te, S	Phillips and Chester Jones (1957)

[a]For an explanation of abbreviations and rating system, see Chapter 2, Tables I–IV.

TABLE A.XI

Corticosteroids Identified in Body Fluids of Fish: A Summary[a]

Species	Source	Steroid	Reference
Cyclostomes			
Myxine glutinosa	Serum	Cortisol, cortisone	Weisbart and Idler (1970); Idler *et al.* (1971)
(+ ACTH *in vivo*)	Serum	Cortisol, cortisone, corticosterone, 11-deoxycortisol	Idler *et al.* (1971)
Petromyzon marinus	Plasma	Cortisol	Weisbart and Idler, 1970
Elasmobranchs			
Raja clavata	Plasma	1α-Hydroxycorticosterone	Idler and Truscott (1969)
Raja erinacea	Plasma	1α-Hydroxycorticosterone	Idler and Truscott (1969)
Raja laevis	Plasma	1α-Hydroxycorticosterone	Idler and Truscott (1969)
Raja ocellata	Plasma	1α-Hydroxycorticosterone	Idler and Truscott (1969)
Raja radiata	Plasma	1α-Hydroxycorticosterone	Idler and Truscott (1966a, 1967a, 1968, 1969)
	Perivisceral fluid	1α-Hydroxycorticosterone	Idler and Truscott (1968)
	Pericardial fluid	1α-Hydroxycorticosterone	Idler and Truscott (1968)
	Cranial fluid	1α-Hydroxycorticosterone	Idler and Truscott (1968)
Squalus acanthias	Semen	11-Deoxycorticosterone	Simpson *et al.* (1963a)
Chondrosteans			
Acipenser oxyrhynchus	Plasma	Cortisol, cortisone, corticosterone	Idler *et al.* (1971), Sangalang *et al.* (1971)
Holosteans			
Amia calva	Plasma	Cortisol	Idler *et al.* (1971)
Teleosts			
Anguilla anguilla	Plasma	Cortisol	Leloup-Hatey (1961, 1964b), Bradshaw and Fontaine-Bertrand (1968)
		Cortisone	Leloup-Hatey (1961, 1964b)
		Aldosterone	Truscott and Idler (1969)
Clupea harengus	Plasma	Cortisol	Bondy *et al.* (1957), Leloup-Hatey (1958, 1960, 1964a)
Cyprinus carpio	Plasma		
Fundulus heteroclitus	Plasma	Cortisol	Chester Jones *et al.* (1959)

251

TABLE A.XI (cont.)

Corticosteroids Identified in Body Fluids of Fish: A Summary[a]

Species	Source	Steroid	Reference
Gadus morrhua	Plasma	Cortisol	Idler and Freeman (1965)
Oncorhynchus nerka	Plasma	Cortisol	Idler et al. (1959a,b), Phillips et al. (1959)
		Cortisone	Idler et al. (1959a,b), Phillips et al. (1959)
		Corticosterone	Idler et al. (1960b)
		17α-Hydroxyprogesterone	Idler et al. (1959b)
		17α,20β-Dihydroxyprogesterone	Idler et al. (1960a)
		20β-Dihydrocortisone	Idler et al. (1962)
Oncorhynchus tshawytscha	Plasma	Cortisol, cortisone	Hane and Robertson (1959); Hane et al. (1966)
Salmo gairdnerii	Plasma	Cortisol, cortisone	Hane and Robertson (1959)
Salmo salar	Plasma	Cortisol, cortisone	Schmidt and Idler (1962), Leloup-Hatey (1964b), Idler et al. (1964)
Dipnoans			
Lepidosiren paradoxa	Plasma	Cortisol, corticosterone, aldosterone, 11-deoxycortisol	Idler et al. (1972)

[a]This table refers only to publications concerned with isolation and identification of corticosteroids and includes only those in which the identification was rated as tentative, presumptive, or positive.

252

Chapter 5

CORTICOSTEROIDS IN AMPHIBIA, REPTILIA, AND AVES

THOMAS SANDOR

I. Introduction

The main objective of this chapter is to review the available evidence in connection with the chemical identity of corticosteroid hormones in Amphibia, Reptilia, and Aves and, at the same time, to make an assessment of the possible biosynthetic pathways by which these steroid hormones are produced in the adrenal glands of these animals. While this review is far from being complete, it is hoped that it will enable the reader to form a tentative picture of the corticosteroid secretion pattern in the three vertebrate classes to be discussed.

Once the vertebrates obtained a dominant position in water, their eventual invasion of the dry land became inevitable. Romer (1967) pointed out that a water dweller, who by means of air breathing could stay alive during prolonged periods of droughts, possessed a surviving potential superior to that of the obligatory water-dwelling form. This positive surviving potential became even more accentuated by the adaptation of limbs to dry-land locomotion.

The transition from water to dry land required profound physiological changes to ensure the survival of both the individual and the species. The protoamphibian, which undoubtedly evolved from a bony fish ancestor, had to modify its electrolyte and fluid metabolisms, learn to cope with the sharp fluctuation of environmental temperature, and, finally, adopt means of propagation, involving neither the incubation of fertilized ova in water, nor the fishlike, gill-breathing larval form. Thus, it is not surprising that while amphibians made the first big step, they still could not completely sever their ties with the watery environment. The finalization of the total physiological transition to life in a gaseous *milieu extérieur* became the lot of the reptilians and their winged descendants, the birds. The emergence of the amniotic egg together with homoiothermic regulation in birds assured the dominance of vertebrates in the gaseous zoosphere of the earth and made possible the evolution of mammals as the dominant animal class.

II. The Nature of Corticosteroids in Amphibia, Reptilia, and Aves

In the following section, a large part of the published evidence will be presented on the isolation and chemical identification of corticosteroids from lower-vertebrate sources. Tables I–V give a partial list of these data, analyzed according to the principles discussed in Chapter 2. Steroids isolated *in vivo* are grouped separately from those isolated following *in vitro* experiments. In addition, these tables contain data from experiments in which the biosynthesis of an already known steroidal substance has been investigated. The evidence presented will be discussed and evaluated from two points of view: first, in relation to the chemical nature of corticosteroids secreted by lower-vertebrate adrenal glands and, second, in connection with the possible biosynthetic sequence by which these substances are produced by the adrenal cortical cells.

It has been customary in the literature to refer to the adrenals of certain nonmammalian vertebrates as *interrenals*. However, it is believed that these interrenals are homologous biochemically with the mammalian adrenal gland in spite of their gross anatomical appearance. Gorbman and Bern (1966) have suggested the use of the designation *interrenal* to denote the portion of nonmammalian vertebrate adrenals corresponding functionally to the mammalian *adrenal cortex*. However, if we consistently differentiate between the adrenal and interrenal, the term *corticosteroid* becomes a misnomer since it refers to substances elaborated by the adrenal cortex and in lower vertebrates the cortical and chromaffin cells are not organized separately. Thus, in this review, the noun *adrenal* and the adjective *adrenal* or *adrenal cortical* will be used for the sake of simplicity, without prejudice to the real anatomical or histological conformation of the secreting cells or organs thus denoted.

A detailed description of the control of adrenal cortical function is outside the scope of this chapter. However, some data on the stimulatory or inhibitory effect of hypophyseal, renal, or synthetic substances on the secretion pattern of adrenocortical steroid hormones have been included. These data were in many instances an integral part of the proof that a given steroidal substance was indeed a genuine secretory product of adrenal cells. In this context, it seems to be in order to briefly review the present concept of the pituitary control of adrenocortical steroid secretion.

It is generally accepted that the hypothalamus, hypophysis, and organs that produce steroid hormones form a functional unit for the regulation of secretion of these hormones. This also seems to be true for the adrenal gland. Schriefers (1967) envisages this system as an automatic control loop consisting of an error-sensing device (hypothalamus), servomotor (hypophysis), and final control element (steroid-hormone-producing gland). Regulation of steroid hormone secretion is mediated by polypeptides elaborated by the hypophysis. In the case of adrenal tissue, the pituitary regulating polypeptide is adrenocorticotropin or ACTH.

Mammalian ACTH is a polypeptide consisting of 39 amino acids. The sequence of amino acids for porcine, bovine, and human ACTH differs only in a short part of the chain, at positions 23–33 (Schwyzer and Sieber, 1963; Li, 1963; Lee *et al.*, 1961). Interestingly, the whole chain of 39 amino acids is not necessary for biological action. Although loss of one amino acid from the N-terminal of the chain results in complete loss of biological activity, loss of amino acids from 20 to 39 has little or no effect on the ability of ACTH to stimulate adrenal steroidogenesis (Sayers, 1967). There is no report to the present author's knowledge on any chemical study of nonmammalian ACTH. Nevertheless, as will be seen, lower-vertebrate pituitary tissue has ACTH-like activity and mammalian ACTH does have, with certain exceptions, a tropic effect, both *in vivo* and *in vitro* on the steroidogenic activity of nonmammalian adrenocortical tissue.

While it is by no means certain that native ACTH has the same mechanism of action on lower-vertebrate adrenals as has mammalian ACTH, it seems to be in order to give a short review of the current concept of ACTH action on adrenal steroidogenesis. All these theories have been developed from experiments on laboratory mammals.

It has been known for some time that ACTH administration, either *in vivo* or *in vitro*, increases the rate of transformation of cholesterol to corticosteroids. Haynes and Berthel (1957) and Haynes (1958) suggested that the physiological effect of ACTH upon adrenal cells is mediated through a rise in concentration of cyclic 3′,5′-AMP. Subsequently, Haynes *et al.* (1959) demonstrated the direct stimulatory effect of the nucleotide on steroidogenesis in the rat adrenal by *in vitro* methodology. The theory was formulated that ACTH, through a rise in cyclic 3′,5′-AMP concentration, elicits increased phosphorylase activity and increased glucose 6-phosphate production, and this in turn results in the increased formation of NADPH (Karaboyas and Koritz, 1965; Satoh *et al.*, 1966). Recently, several developments have put a different light on the mechanism of action of the corticosteroid-stimulating effect of ACTH.

Stimulation of the adrenal with ACTH has been shown to result in an increased growth of adrenal cells and a concomitant increase in adrenal protein synthesis (Farese and Reddy, 1963). Addition of puromycin could effectively inhibit the effect of ACTH *in vitro* (Ferguson, 1962). Thus, some indirect indications have been obtained that the action of ACTH on adrenal steroidogenesis might involve the synthesis of specific protein(s). This thesis was further developed by Farese (1967) and Farese and Schnure (1967). He has shown that the increased cholesterol side chain cleavage in rat adrenals which is apparently induced by ACTH or cyclic 3′,5′-AMP seems, in fact, to be an inductive process not attributable directly to either ACTH or cyclic AMP. He postulated the presence of a labile protein factor, "steroidogenin," present in the 60,000 g supernatant of ACTH-stimulated adrenals. In addition, he demonstrated the presence of a "steroidohibin" in nonstimulated adrenals which also exhibited proteinlike chemical behavior and inhibited cholesterol side chain cleavage. He advanced the theory that ACTH might act through the induced synthesis of "steroidogenin," which would make possible the stimulatory action of ACTH by the reversal of the inhibition exerted by "steroidohibin." However, this interpretation of ACTH action needs further experimental proof.

A. AMPHIBIA

The group of Chester Jones was the first to demonstrate the presence of corticosteroids in the blood of amphibians, reptiles, and birds (Phillips and

Chester Jones, 1957; Chester Jones et al., 1959). These preliminary studies did not clarify entirely the chemical nature of these steroid hormones but strongly suggested that the peripheral or adrenal venous blood of a number of nonmammalian vertebrates, including amphibians, contains steroidal substances of the pregn-4-ene-3-one type, with an α-ketol group in the side chain. These findings were in accord with the earlier observations of Macchi (1955, 1956) that bullfrog (Rana catesbeiana) adrenal preparations elaborated substances that reduced blue tetrazolium. The amount of these substances increased significantly following the addition of mammalian ACTH to the reaction mixture. The chemical nature of these "reducing" substances was investigated in more detail by Carstensen and associates (1959, 1961). They could tentatively identify corticosterone and aldosterone as the major steroid hormones produced in vitro by bullfrog adrenal preparations from endogenous precursors. In addition, Carstensen et al. (1961) noted that the secretion of the presumed corticosterone and aldosterone was significantly increased following the addition of mammalian ACTH or crude frog pituitary extract to the incubation medium.

Prompted by the known mammalian adrenal biosynthetic pattern, Ulick and Solomon (1960) incubated Rana catesbeiana adrenal minces with progesterone-4-^{14}C and confirmed the ability of bullfrog adrenals to synthesize aldosterone. In addition to aldosterone, progesterone-^{14}C was metabolized to another substance, subsequently identified by Ulick and Kusch (1960) as 18-hydroxycorticosterone-^{14}C. The authors also indicated the presence of corticosterone and 11-deoxycorticosterone, both biosynthetic metabolites of progesterone. Formal proof that in vitro, R. catesbeiana adrenals synthesize corticosterone was furnished by Nicolis and Ulick (1965). Mehdi and Carballeira (1971a,b) have shown that in addition to corticosterone, 18-hydroxycorticosterone, and aldosterone, bullfrog adrenal preparations biosynthesized 11-deoxycorticosterone and 11β-hydroxyprogesterone from exogenous precursors in vitro.

The isolation of 18-hydroxycorticosterone from bullfrog adrenal incubates marked the first instance that this steroid was obtained from natural sources. Its presence could be demonstrated subsequently in a variety of experiments using progesterone as substrate and mammalian adrenal preparations as enzyme donors (rat: Péron, 1962; beef zona glomerulosa slices and human adrenal slices: Sandor and Lanthier, 1963a). The substance was chemically synthesized by Schmidlin and Wettstein (1961) and was shown to exist mainly in the 20→18 cyclic hemiketal form (Fig. 1). 18-Hydroxycorticosterone is apparently an important member of the adrenal cortical secretion pattern of most vertebrate classes. Until recently, it was thought that bony fish adrenal tissue was incapable of 18-oxygenating exogenous steroidal substrates (Sandor et al., 1966b, 1967). However, it has been demonstrated

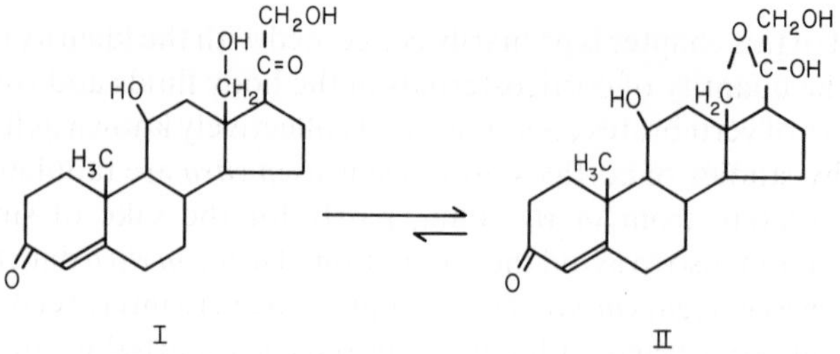

Fig. 1. I, 18-Hydroxycorticosterone; II, 18-hydroxycorticosterone 20——⟶18 cyclic hemiketal. 18-Hydroxy-11-deoxycorticosterone and 18-hydroxy-11-dehydrocorticosterone also form 20——⟶18 cyclic hemiketals when in solution.

that under certain conditions, head kidney tissue of some teleost species transforms corticosterone to 18-hydroxycorticosterone and aldosterone *in vitro* (Truscott and Idler, 1968). We shall discuss later in more detail its possible role in the biosynthesis of aldosterone.

The secretion *in vivo* of corticosterone and aldosterone by bullfrog adrenals was validated when Johnston *et al*. (1967) established the presence of these two hormones in the peripheral plasma and postcaval vein plasma of *Rana catesbeiana*.

Corticosterone and aldosterone were demonstrated in the adrenal secretion of other amphibians. Crabbé (1961, 1963) has shown that fortified adrenal gland homogenates of the toad *Bufo marinus* transformed exogenous progesterone-¹⁴C to steroids tentatively identified as corticosterone, 11-deoxycorticosterone, and aldosterone. In addition, he measured corticosterone and aldosterone in the peripheral blood of these animals by a double-isotope derivative assay (Crabbé, 1961). Adrenal gland incubates from the leopard frog *Rana pipiens* yielded substances from endogenous precursors possibly identical with aldosterone, corticosterone, and 18-hydroxycorticosterone (Kraulis and Birmingham 1964). The adrenals of the same species transformed a mixture of pregnenolone-³H and progesterone-¹⁴C to ³H- and ¹⁴C-labeled progesterone, 11-deoxycorticosterone, corticosterone, aldosterone, and 18-hydroxycorticosterone (Lamoureux, 1966). Similar steroid metabolic patterns have been established under *in vitro* conditions for the frog *Rana rugulosa* (Chan *et al*., 1969) and the South African toad *Xenopus laevis* (Chan and Edwards, 1970).

The question whether amphibian adrenals are capable of 17-hydroxylation of steroids has not been decisively answered. Chester Jones *et al*. (1959) reported the presence of cortisol in the blood of the giant salamander *Amphiuma tridactyla* and Crabbé (1963) adduced preliminary evidence that *Bufo marinus* adrenal gland homogenates produce cortisol from exogenous progesterone. This claim could not be fully substantiated. The reported conversion of progesterone to cortisol was extremely small and there were no follow-up studies to develop this highly interesting but still preliminary observation. It has to be mentioned that Johnston *et al.* (1967) could not find any cortisol in either the peripheral or postcaval plasma of *Rana catesbeiana*.

Under *in vitro* conditions, without the addition of exogenous precursors, bullfrog and leopard frog adrenals synthesized more aldosterone than corticosterone (Nicolis and Ulick 1965; Kraulis and Birmingham, 1964). The ratio of aldosterone to corticosterone was 5.8 in the bullfrog. *In vitro*, amphibian adrenals have a very high capacity to biosynthesize aldosterone. Psychoyos and co-workers (1966) reported that the maximal aldosterone-producing capacity of bullfrog adrenal mitochondria was 2.1 μg/mitochondria equivalent to 50 mg adrenal tissue/10 min. While these data represent conversion rates from exogenous corticosterone rather than secretion rates from endogenous precursors, the substrate was present at saturation level and thus this figure gives a good quantitative indication of the abilities of these adrenals.

The extent to which quantitative data obtained in incubation experiments can be extrapolated to *in vivo* conditions is highly speculative. We have no data on the secretory rate of corticosterone in the intact amphibian and the secretion rate of aldosterone was determined only in the bullfrog (Ulick and Feinholtz, 1968). This was found to be 19 μg/kg body weight per day in bullfrogs kept in tap water. Values obtained for the amount of circulating aldosterone and corticosterone in intact animals have shown that both in the toad *Bufo marinus* (Crabbé, 1961) and in the bullfrog (Johnston *et al.*, 1967) the ratios obtained by *in vitro* experiments are reversed *in vivo*. In the latter animal, the aldosterone–corticosterone ratio was 0.14 in the peripheral plasma and 0.17 in the postcaval vein plasma. To what extent these figures can be extrapolated to actual production rates is open to question. No similar data exist for either secretion rate or blood level of 18-hydroxycorticosterone or 11-deoxycorticosterone.

The regulation of corticosteroid secretion in members of the amphibian class has not been fully worked out. The secretion of both aldosterone and corticosterone was stimulated *in vitro* and *in vivo* in the bullfrog, the leopard frog, and the South African toad by the addition of mammalian ACTH or frog pituitary extracts (Carstensen *et al.*, 1961; Kraulis and Birmingham, 1964; Nicolis and Ulick, 1965; Macchi and Phillips, 1966; Johnston *et al.*, 1967; Chan and Edwards, 1970). In the bullfrog, a corticoid-pituitary negative-feedback mechanism was demonstrated by Piper and deRoos (1966) and, in the same animal, Johnston *et al.* (1967) reported that both circulating aldosterone and corticosterone increase following the intravenous infusion of a frog kidney extract considered to contain frog renin. Details of the experimental data on amphibian corticosteroids are shown in Tables I (*in vivo* experiments) and II (*in vitro* experiments).

Quite recently, some new evidence was obtained on the adrenocortical steroid secretion of a urodele, the giant Chinese salamander, *Megalobatrichus davidianus*. In collaboration with Dr. S. T. H. Chan and Professor B. Lofts of the Department of Zoology, University of Hong Kong, this reviewer incubated an NADPH fortified whole homogenate of the adrenal tissue of this salamander in the presence of tritiated pregnenolone and progesterone-¹⁴C. Though at present time (Christmas 1971) the experiment is not yet fully worked up, it is apparent, that the major transformation products of both precursors are corticosterone, 11-deoxycorticosterone, 18-hydroxycorticosterone, and aldosterone.

While most of the available published reports on the chemical nature of corticosteroids isolated from amphibians have been reviewed here, it has to be pointed out that of the total number of living amphibian species, only about 0.2% have been investigated. The reasoning that the most common and, to us, most familiar forms are representative of the whole class is obviously fallacious. With the exception of the giant salamander, all the species investigated were Anura, and there are very few data on Urodela and Apoda. Similarly, corticosteroids of the larval, gill-bearing forms of Anura were not investigated beyond the exploratory stages (Dale 1962; Rapola 1963). This lack of knowledge can partly be explained by anatomical peculiarities present in some amphibian forms. A projected investigation of *in vitro* corticosteroidogenesis by the larvae of *Ambystoma tigrinum* (axalotl), started by this reviewer and the University of Sheffield group (Prof. I. Chester Jones, Dr. I. W. Henderson, Mr. W. Mosley), never materialized due to the failure of localizing, beyond a few scattered clumps, any significant concentration of adrenal tissue in the experimental animal. Thus, at present it can be accepted that in amphibians, as represented by a few Anura, the major circulating corticosteroid is corticosterone, followed in quantitative importance by aldosterone. The isolated adrenal gland of frogs and toads elaborates aldosterone, 18-hydroxycorticosterone, and corticosterone, their relative amounts being in the above order. In incubation experiments, important amounts of 11-deoxycorticosterone were also demonstrated, but we have no information on the quantities of this steroid and 18-hydroxycorticosterone that are secreted in the intact animal or are present in the circulating blood. The possible biosynthetic routes of adrenal corticosteroid formation will be discussed later.

TABLE I

Corticosteroids in Amphibia *in Vivo*

Species	Steroid	Source of steroid	Quantity (μg/100 ml plasma)[a]	Major criteria[a]	Rating[a] Identity	Rating[a] Quantity	Reference
Amphiuma tridactyla (giant salamander)	Corticosterone	Adrenal venous blood	♂41.1 ♀22.1	PC, Ip–nmc, CT, UV, Fl	Su	Te, P	Chester Jones *et al.* (1959)
	Cortisol		♂11.5 ♀11.3	PC, Ip–nmc, CT, UV, Fl	Su	Te, P	
Xenopus laevis (South African toad)	Cortisol	Mixture of adrenal and renal blood	7.0	PC, Ip–nmc, CT, UV, Fl	Su	Te, P	Phillips and Chester Jones (1957)
	17-Ketogenic steroids	Excreta from tadpoles	Stage 52–53, — Stage 55–56, 0.58[b] Stage 58, 1.39[b] Stage 58–59, 1.57[b] Stage 62–63, 0.93[b] Adult (2 weeks), 1.40[b] Adult (4 months), 0.88[b]	SNI, CT[c]	NA	Te, P	Rapola (1963)
Rana pipiens (leopard frog)	Cortisol (Porter–Silber material)[d]	Excreta from tadpoles	Stages 23–30, 0.45–0.79 mg/1000 larval hr	PC, CT, UV	Ex	Te, P	Dale (1962)
Rana catesbeiana (bullfrog)	Aldosterone	Secretory rate of aldosterone following administration of aldosterone-[3H]	Animals kept in tap water (TW), 16.3 ± 4.8[e] Animals kept in saline(S), 4.5 ± 1.0[e] TW + Angiotensin[f], 19.0 ± 3.5[e] S + Angiotensin, 4.3 ± 0.5[e] TW + ACTH,[g] 50.2 ± 11.2[e]	DIDA	Pr	Po, T	Ulick and Feinholtz (1968)

TABLE I (cont.)

Species	Steroid	Source of steroid	Quantity (μg/100 ml plasma)[a]	Major criteria[a]	Rating[a] Identity	Rating[a] Quantity	Reference
	Corticosterone	Peripheral plasma	5.05 ± 0.79	DIDA	Pr	Po, T	Johnston et al. (1967)
		Postcaval(PC) vein plasma	8.84 ± 1.13	DIDA	Pr	Po, T	
		PC after saline infusion	14.1 ± 6.5				
		PC after infusion of ACTH[h]	18.0 ± 0.6				
		PC after infusion of frog renin	7.2 ± 1.4				
	Corticosterone	Hypophysectomy, PC	1.3 ± 0.4				Johnston et al. (1967)
		PC, hypophysectomy, after infusion of frog renin	1.7 ± 0.5				
	Aldosterone	Peripheral plasma[i]	0.73 ± 0.18	DIDA	Pr	Po, T	
		Postcaval(PC) vein plasma[i]	1.50 ± 0.29				
		PC after saline infusion	Control, 0.29 ± 0.10 Exp, 0.21 ± 0.09				
		PC after infusion of ACTH	Control, 0.20 ± 0.07 Exp, 1.80 ± 0.47				
		PC after infusion of frog renin	Control, 0.22 ± 0.08 Exp, 0.53 ± 0.17				
		PC after hypophysectomy	0.15 ± 0.08				

		PC after hypophysectomy + frog renin					
			Control, 0.15 ±0.08				
			Exp, 0.25 ±0.04				
Bufo marinus (toad)	Corticosterone	Peripheral plasma Animals kept in distilled water (DW)	2.64	Pr	DIDA	Po, T	Crabbé (1961)
		Animals kept in saline	3.42				
	Aldosterone	Peripheral plasma		Pr	DIDA	Po, T	
		DW	1.17				
		Saline	0.68				

[a]For an explanation of abbreviations and rating system, see Chapter 2, Tables I–IV.
[b]17-Ketogenic steroids (Norymberski, 1952), micrograms per gram of body weight.
[c]Norymberski (1952).
[d]Porter and Silber (1950).
[e]Secretory rate expressed in micrograms per kilogram body weight per day.
[f]Daily dosage q12h: 10 μg/kg angiotensin.
[g]1IU
[h]0.17 IU ACTH/min.
[i]Values obtained from bled, pithed frogs.

TABLE II

Corticosteroids in Amphibia in Vitro

Species	Steroid[a]	Source of steroid[a]	Quantity (μg/100 mg tissue or % transformation)[b]	Major criteria[c]	Rating[c] Identity	Rating[c] Quantity	Reference
Rana catesbeiana (bullfrog)	Corticosteroids	Adrenal mince + ACTH (10.0 IU)[d]	1.23 ± 0.11/hr 2.37 ± 0.46/hr	Blue-tetrazolium-reducing lipids[e]	SNI	Te, S	Macchi (1955)
	Corticosteroids	Adrenal mince + ACTH (10.0 IU)[d]	1.50 ± 0.53/hr 2.90 ± 0.89/hr	Blue-tetrazolium-reducing lipids	SNI	Te, S	Macchi (1956)
	Corticosterone	Adrenal mince + ACTH (1.09 IU)	NA	SPa, PC, Ip-nmc, UV, CT, ACr, Fl	Te	NA	Carstensen et al. (1961)
	Aldosterone	Adrenal mince + ACTH (1.09 IU)	NA	SPa, PC, Ip-nmc, UV, CT, ACr, Ba	Te	NA	
	Corticosterone	Adrenal mince + ACTH (porcine, 1.09 IU) + ACTH (bovine, 1.09 IU) + FAP[g]	0.07/2 hr 0.40/2 hr 1.24–1.02/2 hr	PC, SPa, Ip-nmc, UV, CT, ACr, Fl	Te	Pr, T	Carstensen et al. (1961)
	Aldosterone	Adrenal mince + ACTH (porcine, 1.09 IU) + ACTH (bovine, 1.09 IU) + FAP[h]	Not detectable 0.29–0.69/2 hr 1.09/2 hr 3.53–4.49/2 hr 0.69–3.34/2 hr	SPa, PC, Ip-nmc, UV, CT, ACr	Te	Pr, T	

Compound	Incubation system	Yield	Methods			Reference
Aldosterone-^{14}C	Adrenal mince + progesterone-^{14}C (aldosterone-^{3}H added as carrier)	4.4%	PC, Der, 1p-nmc-Der, C ^{3}H)/^{14}C D	Pr	NA	Ullick and Solomon (1960)
18-Hydroxycorticosterone-^{14}C	Adrenal mince + progesterone-^{14}C (reduced aldosterone etiollactone-^{3}H added as carrier)	3.0%	PC, AC, Ox, Re, C ^{3}H)/^{14}C D, IR–Der	Po	NA	Ullick and Kusch (1960)
Corticosterone	Adrenal slices + ACTH (1.0 IU) (corticosterone-^{3}H added as carrier)	1.2–4.2/4 hr 12.8/4 hr	PC, Der, 1p-nmc-Der, CSA-D	Pr	Pr, T	Nicolis and Ulick (1965)
Aldosterone	Adrenal slices + ACTH (1.0 IU) (aldosterone-^{3}H added as carrier)	11.3–17.8/4 hr 55.2/4 hr	PC, Der, Ox, AC, 1p-nmc-Der, CSA-SD	Pr	Pr, T	
18-Hydroxycorticosterone	Adrenal slices + ACTH (1.0 IU)	3.8–9.3/4 hr 25.1/4 hr				
Aldosterone-^{3}H	Adrenal slices + corticosterone-^{3}H	8.9–26.0%	PC, Der, Ox, AC, 1p-nmc-Der, CSA-SD	Pr	NA	Nicolis and Ulick (1965)
	Adrenal homogenate + corticosterone-^{3}H	6.7%		Pr	NA	
18-Hydroxycorticosterone-^{3}H	Adrenal slices + corticosterone-^{3}H	4.0–10.0%	PC, Der(Ox), 1p-nmc-Der, CSA-D	Pr	NA	
	Adrenal homogenate + corticosterone-^{3}H	12.0%		Pr	NA	

TABLE II (cont.)

Species	Steroid[a]	Source of steroid[a]	Quantity (μg/100 mg tissue or % transformation)[b]	Major criteria[c]	Rating[c] Identity	Rating[c] Quantity	Reference
	Aldosterone-³H	Adrenal slices + 18-hydroxycorticosterone-³H	0.16–0.92%	PC, Der(Ox), Ip–nmrc–Der, CSASD	Pr	NA	Nicolis and Ulick (1965)
		Adrenal homogenate + 18-hydrocorticosterone-³H	0.31%		Pr	NA	
	Aldosterone-³H	Adrenal slices + progesterone-³H	18.3%		Pr	Na	
		Adrenal slices + 18-hydroxyprogesterone-³H	0.21%		Pr	NA	
		Adrenal slices + 11-deoxycorticosterone-³H	14.0–19.6%		Pr	NA	
		Adrenal slices + 18-hydroxy-11-deoxycorticosterone-³H	0.7–1.3%		Pr	NA	
Rana pipiens (leopard frog)	Corticosterone	Quartered adrenals + ACTH (1.3 IU)	2.1/4 hr[h]	PC, CT, UV, Ip–nmc	Su	Te, P	Kraulis and Birmingham (1964)
		Quartered adrenals + corticosterone (85 μg)	68.1 ± 0.5/4 hr[i] 62.0 ± 0.7/4 hr[j]		Su	Te, P	
		Quartered adrenals + corticosterone	89.0/8 hr[i] 95.0/8 hr[j]		Su	Te, P	

	Quartered adrenals + progesterone (100 μg)	7.4/8 hr[i] 6.0/8 hr[j]		Su	Te, P
	Quartered adrenals + 11-deoxycorticosterone (108 μg)	10.0 ± 2.0/8 hr[i] 10.6 ± 2.8/8 hr[j]		Su	Te, P
Corticosterone	Quartered adrenals + 11β-hydroxyprogesterone (98 μg)	18.6 ± 0.3/8 hr[i]		Su	Te, P
Aldosterone	Quartered adrenals + ACTH (1.3 IU)	4.5/8 hr[i] 2.5/8 hr[j]	PC, CT, UV, Ip–nmc	Su	Te, P
	Quartered adrenals + corticosterone (104 μg)	6.3/8 hr[i] 3.1/8 hr[j]		Su	Te, P
	Quartered adrenals + progesterone (100 μg)	5.3/8 hr[i] 2.8/8 hr[j]		Su	Te, P
	Quartered adrenals + 11-deoxycorticosterone (108 μg)	4.6 ± 0.9/8 hr[i] 3.3 ± 0.0/8 hr[j]		Su	Te, P

TABLE II (cont.)

Species	Steroid[a]	Source of steroid[a]	Quantity (μg/100 mg tissue or % transformation)[b]	Major criteria[c]	Rating[c] Identity	Rating[c] Quantity	Reference
		Quartered adrenals · 11β-hydroxyprogesterone (98 μg)	4.0 ± 1.0/8 hr[i]; 2.5 ± 0.6/8 hr[j]		Su	Te, P	Lamoureux (1966)
	Corticosterone-^{3}H, ^{14}C	Adrenal slices + pregnenolone-^{3}H + progesterone-^{14}C	^{3}H, 8.3%; ^{14}C, 8.4%	PC, TLC, Der, Ip-nmrc-Der, CryC ^{3}H/^{14}C D	Pr	NA	
	Aldosterone-^{3}H, ^{14}C		^{3}H, 0.5%; ^{14}C, 0.9%	PC, TLC, Ip-nmrc-Der, C ^{3}H/^{14}C D	Pr	NA	
	18-Hydroxycorticosterone-^{3}H, ^{14}C		^{3}H, 2.0%; ^{14}C, 3.0%	PC, TLC, Der(Ox), Ip-nmrc-Der, C ^{3}H/^{14}C SD	Te[k]	NA	
	11-Deoxycorticosterone-^{3}H, ^{14}C		^{3}H, 3.3%; ^{14}C, 3.0%	PC, TLC, Der, Ip-nmrc-Der, CryC ^{3}H/^{14}C D	Pr	NA	
	Progesterone-^{3}H		^{3}H, 11.7%	PC, TLC, Ip-nmrc, CryC ^{3}H/^{14}C-nmrc	Te	NA	
Bufo marinus (toad)	Corticosterone-^{14}C	Adrenal homogenate + progesterone-^{14}C	Animals kept in dist. water, 0.56% in saline, 0.69%	PC, Der, Ip-nmrc-Der	Su	NA	Crabbé (1961)
	Aldosterone-^{14}C		Animals kept in dist. water, 0.24% in saline, 0.31%	PC, Der, Ip-nmrc-Der	Su	NA	
	Corticosterone-^{14}C	Adrenal homogenate + pro-	NA	PC, Der, Ip-nmrc-Der, CSAD	Pr	NA	Crabbé (1963)

268

Aldosterone-^{14}C		NA	PC, Der, Ip–nmrc–Der	Te	NA	
11-Deoxycorticosterone-^{14}C		NA	PC, Der, Ip–nmrc–Der, SCAD	Pr	NA	
Cortisol-^{14}C	Adrenal homogenate + progesterone-^{14}C	NA	PC, Der, Ip–nmrc–Der	Su[l]	NA	
Rana catesbeiana (bullfrog) Aldosterone-^{3}H	Adrenal mitochondria + corticosterone-^{3}H	4.2/10 min	PC, Der(Ox), Ip–nmrc–Der	Te	Pr, T	Psychoyos *et al.* (1966)
18-Hydroxycorticosterone-^{3}H		2.2/10 min	PC, Ip–nmrc	Su	Te, P	Chan *et al.* (1969)
Rana rugulosa (frog) ^{3}H-labeled progesterone, ^{14}C- and ^{3}H-labeled 11-deoxycorticosterone, corticosterone, 18-OH B, and aldosterone	Adrenal mince + pregnenolone-16-^{3}H + progesterone-4-^{14}C; progesterone-4-^{14}C + DOC-1,2-^{3}H; DOC-1,2-^{3}H + corticosterone-4-^{14}C	Kinetic study[m]				
Xenopus laevis (South African toad) 11-Deoxycorticosterone-^{3}H,^{14}C	Adrenal homogenate + pregnenolone-16-^{3}H + progesterone-4-^{14}C; DOC-1,2-^{3}H + corticosterone-4-^{14}C	NA	PC, Der, Ip–nmrc–Der, Cry CSAD	Pr	NA	Chan and Edwards (1970)
Corticosterone-^{3}H,^{14}C		NA	PC, Der, Ip–nmrc–Der, Cry CSAD	Pr	NA	
18-Hydroxycorticosterone-^{3}H,^{14}C		NA	PC	ID	NA	

269

TABLE II (cont.)

Species	Steroid[a]	Source of steroid[a]	Quantity (μg/100 mg tissue or % transformation)[b]	Major criteria[c]	Rating[c] Identity	Rating[c] Quantity	Reference
	Aldosterone-³H, ¹⁴C		NA	PC, Der, Ip–nmrc–Der, Cry CSAD	Pr	NA	Chan and Edwards (1970)
	Progesterone-³H		NA		ID	NA	
	¹⁴C-Labeled 11-deoxycorticosterone, corticosterone, 18-OH B, and aldosterone	Adrenal homogenate + progesterone-4-¹⁴C	Kinetic study	See previous experiments			
	³H-Labeled progesterone, 11-deoxycorticosterone, corticosterone, 18-OH B, and aldosterone; no ¹⁴C steroids detected	Adrenal homogenate + cholesterol-4-¹⁴C + pregnenolone-16-³H from animals: ACTH injected, 2 IU/animal/8 hr for 8 days;	Kinetic study[n]	See previous experiments	Pr	Pr, P	
		Adenohypophysectomized for 9 days;			Pr	Pr, P	
		Adenohypophysectomy + ACTH, 2 IU/animal/8 hr for 8 days 24 hr after operation;			Pr	Pr, P	
		Control group: distilled water injected, 0.1 ml/animal/8 hr			Pr	Pr, P	

270

Species	Substrate	Incubation conditions	Yield	Methods			Reference
Rana catesbeiana (bullfrog)	Progesterone-14C	Adrenal homogenate + cholesterol-4-14C + NADPH + fumarate + 3H marker	1.0%	PC, Ip-nmrc-Der, CryC ^{3}H/^{14}C	Pr	Po, T	Mehdi and Carballeira (1971b)
	11-Deoxycorticosterone-14C		0.2%	PC, Ip-nmrc-Der, CryC ^{3}H/^{14}C	Pr	Po, T	
	Corticosterone-14C		0.2%	PC, Ip-nmrc-Der, CryC ^{3}H/^{14}C	Pr	Po, T	
	18-Hydroxycorticosterone-14C		0.3%	PC, Ip-nmrc-Der (Ox)	Te	Pr, T	
	Aldosterone-14C		0.3%	PC, Ip-nmrc-Der, CryC ^{3}H/^{14}C	Pr	Po, T	
	Corticosterone-14C	Adrenal mitochondria + cholesterol-4-14C + NADPH + fumarate	0.3%	PC, Ip-nmrc-Der, CryC ^{3}H/^{14}C	Pr	Po, T	Mehdi and Carballeira (1971b)
	18-Hydroxycorticosterone-14C		0.3%	PC, Ip-nmrc-Der (Ox)	Te	Pr, T	
	Aldosterone-14C		0.3%	PC, Ip-nmrc-Der, CryC ^{3}H/^{14}C	Pr	Po, T	
	Progesterone-14C	Adrenal slices + pregnenolone-4-14C + 3H markers; 3 hr incubation	5.8%	PC, Ip-nmrc-Der (Re), CryC ^{3}H/^{14}C	Pr	Po, T	Mehdi and Carballeira (1971a)
	11-Deoxycorticosterone-14C		4.4%	PC, Ip-nmrc-Der, CryC ^{3}H/^{14}C	Pr	Po, T	
	Corticosterone-14C		14.1%	PC, Ip-nmrc-Der, CryC ^{3}H/^{14}C	Pr	Po, T	

TABLE II (cont.)

Species	Steroid[a]	Source of steroid[a]	Quantity (μg/100 mg tissue or % transformation)[b]	Major criteria[c]	Rating[c] Identity	Rating[c] Quantity	Reference
	18-Hydroxycorticosterone-14C		3.5%	PC, Ip–nmrc–Der(Ox)	Te	Pr, T	
	Aldosterone-14C		11.9%	PC, Ip–nmrc–Der, CryC 3H/14C	Pr	Po, T	
	Progesterone-14C	Adrenal homogenate + pregnenolone-4-14C (113 μg/100 mg tissue) + NADPH + fumarate; 3 hr incubation	3.8	PC, Ip–nmrc–Der(Re), CryC 3H/14C	Pr	Po, T	Mehdi and Carballeira (1971a)
	11β-Hydroxyprogesterone-14C		3.2	PC, Ip–nmrc–Der(Ox), Cry CSAD	Pr	Pr, T	
	11-Deoxycorticosterone-14C		11.8	PC, Ip–nmrc–Der, CryC 3H/14C	Pr	Po, T	
	Corticosterone-14C		3.1	PC, Ip–nmrc–Der, CryC 3H/14C	Pr	Po, T	
	18-Hydroxycorticosterone-14C		1.0	PC, Ip–nmrc–Der(Ox)	Te	Pr, T	
	Aldosterone-14C		2.3	PC, Ip–nmrc–Der, CryC 3H/14C	Pr	Po, T	
	Progesterone-14C	Adrenal mitochondria + pregnenolone-4-14C (113 μg/100 mg tissue) + NADPH + fumarate; 3 hr	4.0	Criteria and ratings as above			Mehdi and Carballeira (1971a)

11β-Hydroxyprogesterone-^{14}C		1.0			
11-Deoxycorticosterone-^{14}C		3.3			
Corticosterone-^{14}C		0.6			
18-Hydroxycorticosterone-^{14}C		0.3			
Aldosterone-^{14}C		0.3			
11β-Hydroxyprogesterone-^{14}C	Adrenal slices + progesterone-4-^{14}C + ^{3}H markers; 3 hr incubation	0.8%	PC, Ip–nmrc– Der(Ox), CryC ^{3}H/^{14}C	Pr	Po, T	Mehdi and Carbal- leira (1971a)
11-Deoxycorticos- terone-^{14}C		3.9	PC, Ip–nmrc– Der, CryC^{3}H/^{14}C	Pr	Po, T	
11-Dehydrocorti- costerone-^{14}C		1.9%	PC, Ip–nmrc–Der, CryC^{3}H/^{14}C	Pr	Po, T	
Corticosterone-^{14}C		18.6	PC, Ip–nmrc–Der, CryC^{3}H/^{14}C	Pr	Po, T	
18-Hydroxycorti- costerone-^{14}C		4.8%	PC, Ip–nmrc– Der(Ox)	Te	Pr, T	
Aldosterone-^{14}C		12.9%	PC, Ip–nmrc–Der, CryC^{3}H/^{14}C	Pr	Po, T	
11β-Hydroxypro- gesterone-^{14}C	Adrenal homoge- nate + progeste- rone-4-^{14}C (113 μg/100 mg tissue) + NADPH + fumarate; 3 hr incubation	4.5	Criteria and ratings as above			Mehdi and Carbal- leira (1971a)
11-Deoxycorticos- terone-^{14}C		12.0				
Corticosterone-^{14}C		11.2				
18-Hydroxycorti- costerone-^{14}C		2.2				
Aldosterone-^{14}C		2.1				
11β-Hydroxypro- gesterone-^{14}C	Adrenal mitochon- dria + proges-	5.6	Criteria and ratings as above			Mehdi and Carbal- leira (1971a)

TABLE II (cont.)

Species	Steroid[a]	Source of steroid[a]	Quantity (μg/100 mg tissue or % transformation)[b]	Major criteria[c]	Rating[c] Identity	Rating[c] Quantity	Reference
		terone-4-[14]C (113 μg/100 mg tissue) + NADPH + fumarate; 3 hr incubation					
	11-Deoxycorti-costerone-[14]C		1.5				
	Corticosterone-[14]C		1.9				
	18-Hydroxycorti-costerone-[14]C		0.3				
	Aldosterone-[14]C		0.2				

[a] Abbreviations: 18-OH B, 18-hydroxycorticosterone; DOC, deoxycorticosterone.

[b] In this and subsequent tables in which mixed data are presented, the numerical values always refer to micrograms per 100 mg tissue, unless otherwise indicated (e.g., as percent).

[c] For an explanation of abbreviations and rating system, see Chapter 2, Tables I–IV.

[d] In this and subsequent tables, the amount of ACTH indicated is always per 100 mg tissue incubated.

[e] Mader and Buck (1952).

[f] Meyer and Lindberg (1955).

[g] FAP, frog anterior pituitaries.

[h] Mean value of amount measured by ultraviolet spectrophotometry and by blue tetrazolium reaction.

[i] Value obtained by ultraviolet spectrophotometry.

[j] Value obtained by blue tetrazolium reaction.

[k] Rating changed from Pr to Te as no authentic carrier was available.

[l] Rating changed from Te to Su due to the small amount biosynthesized.

[m] For major criteria and rating, see Table V, data of Whitehouse and Vinson (1967).

[n] No numerical values reported: quantitative results shown in graph form. Claim for increased corticosterone and aldosterone formation after ACTH and decreased formation following adenohypophysectomy.

274

B. Reptilia

While the first vertebrates venturing onto dry land were the protoamphibians, reptiles occupy a unique position in the evolution of water-dwelling animals to terrestrial tetrapods and are considered today as the direct ancestors of the homoiothermic vertebrates, the birds and mammals. Romer (1967) casts doubt on the direct evolutionary relationship between anuran amphibians and reptiles. According to his thesis, anuran amphibians are of separate and more recent ancestry than reptiles. As most of our knowledge on amphibian secretion of adrenal cortical steroids came from anuran species, reptilian steroid biochemistry might better represent the primitive vertebrate pattern.

Our knowledge of the nature of corticosteroids secreted by reptiles is very limited. Corticosteroids isolated from intact animals have been identified only tentatively whereas chemically valid evidence has originated from *in vitro* incubation of reptilian adrenals with or without added exogenous precursors. Eight species have been investigated, including four species of turtles, two species of snakes, and one species each of lizard and alligator.

Phillips and Chester Jones (1957) analyzed the adrenal effluent blood of the grass snake *Natrix natrix* and Chester Jones *et al.* (1959) reported on the corticosteroid content of the blood of a turtle (*Lepidochelys kempi*). In the grass snake, cortisol and corticosterone and in the turtle cortisol were tentatively identified. With the availability of better analytical tools, the adrenal cortical secretion of the snake *Natrix natrix* was reinvestigated by several workers. Phillips and associates (1962) incubated grass snake adrenal slices in the presence of tritiated progesterone and tentatively identified corticosterone and aldosterone. The authors reported some sex difference in the biosynthesis of these hormones, the adrenals of the female snake being more active. This animal was further investigated by Macchi and Phillips (1966) and Macchi (1967). Their data confirmed the previous reports on the transformation of exogenous progesterone to aldosterone and corticosterone. The corticosteroids produced *in vitro* by adrenal slices of another species of snake, the cobra *Naja naja*, were studied by Gottfried *et al.* (1967). In these experiments no precursors were added to the medium prior to incubation. The surviving adrenals of the cobra produced corticosterone, aldosterone, and 18-hydroxycorticosterone. The isolation of 18-hydroxycorticosterone from the cobra adrenal incubate was not unexpected. Phillips *et al.* (1962) reported the presence of relatively large amounts of a corticosteroid (presumably of the 4-ene–3-one type) biosynthesized from progesterone by snake adrenals. This steroid, on the basis of available published evidence was equated with 18-hydroxycorticosterone by Sandor and Lanthier (1963b). Convincing identification of corticosterone, aldosterone, and especially 18-hydroxycorticosterone endogenously produced from a reptile source gave additional weight to the adrenal secretory pattern previously described. In addition to the three corticosteroids mentioned above, the work of Gottfried and co-workers suggested the presence of cortisone in the *Naja* incubates. Incubation of adrenal minces of this same species of snake with radioactive pregnenolone and progesterone resulted in the isolation of radioactive 11-deoxycorticosterone, corticosterone, 18-hydroxycorticosterone, and aldosterone (Huang *et al.*, 1969).

Turtles are easily obtainable experimental animals of the reptilian class; thus several species of turtles were investigated. Sandor and co-workers (1963a, 1964) reported on the *in vitro* metabolism of progesterone-^{14}C by adrenal slices of the slider turtle *Pseudemys scripta elegans* and on the simultaneous biotransformation of pregnenolone plus progesterone, both radioactively labeled, by adrenal slices of the painted turtle *Chrysemys picta picta*. The adrenal tissue of both species of turtles transformed the exogenous substrates to radioactive corticosterone, aldosterone, 18-hydroxycorticosterone, and 11-deoxycorticosterone. The biosynthetic capabilities of the *Chrysemys* adrenals were further investigated in a thorough study by Mehdi (1969). He was able to demonstrate the incorporation of exogenous cholesterol into corticosteroids by turtle adrenal preparations *in vitro* and added 11β-hydroxyprogesterone to the list of steroid metabolites biosynthesized by the adrenal gland of these animals. Other studies with quartered adrenals of *Pseudemys* and another species of turtle (*Emys orbicularis*) suggested that aldosterone and corticosterone are produced by these glands even in the absence of an added substrate (Macchi and Phillips, 1966).

In addition to snakes and turtles, the adrenal cortical secretion pattern of one species of lizard and one species of alligator was investigated. Phillips *et al.* (1962) incubated adrenal slices from the green lizard *Lacerta viridis* with tritiated progesterone and noted the formation of labeled aldosterone, corticosterone, and a 4-ene–3-keto substance which might have been 18-hydroxycorticosterone. Gist and deRoos (1966) worked with adrenals of the alligator *Alligator mississipiensis*. Sliced adrenal glands of these animals were incubated either in the absence of exogenous substrates or following the addition of non radioactive progesterone. In both series of experiments, the formation of aldosterone and corticosterone was noted. While 18-hydroxycorticosterone was not identified, the authors mentioned two presumably 4-ene–3-ketosteroids, present in all experiments and exhibiting paper chromatographic mobilities not inconsistent with a pregn-4-ene–polyhydroxyl structure.

While the anuran adrenal incubated *in vitro* in the absence of exogenous precursors produces aldosterone, 18-hydroxycorticosterone, and corticosterone in roughly 6:3:1 ratio (Nicolis and Ulick, 1965), quite different ratios have been found for reptilian adrenals. Corticosterone was found to be on the whole the quantitatively most important steroid produced both in the presence or absence of added pregnenolone and/or progesterone. 18-Hydroxycorticosterone was synthesized in quantities approximating or even surpassing in some instances that of corticosterone. However, in every experiment reported, the amount of aldosterone isolated was always much lower than any of the above two steroid hormones. Unfortunately, no detailed studies were done on either the blood level or secretion rates of corticosteroids in reptiles. Phillips and Chester Jones (1957) found in the postcaval blood of the grass snake 156 μg of corticosterone, 8.5 μg of cortisol, and 2μg of cortisone per 100 ml whole blood. However, the identity and quantity of these substances were never reinvestigated by subsequently introduced modern methods and thus they have only a suggestive value. The same is true for the analysis of adrenal effluent blood from the turtle *Lepidochelis kempi* (Chester Jones *et al.*, 1959).

There is no doubt that in the reptilian species investigated, 17-deoxycorticosteroids predominate. Nevertheless, there are indications that the adrenals of this class of animals are not totally devoid of 17α-hydroxylase activity. Gottfried *et al.* (1967) tentatively identified cortisone in adrenal incubates from the cobra and trace amounts of a substance behaving chromatographically as cortisol. In addition cortisol has been reported to be present among the metabolites produced from progesterone by *Pseudemys* adrenal slices (Sandor *et al.*, 1964). The 17α-hydroxylation capability of reptile adrenals clearly needs careful reinvestigation.

While corticosterone, 18-hydroxycorticosterone, and aldosterone are the main recognizable steroid hormonal products of the reptilian adrenals assayed, most workers have reported on the presence of presumably steroidal substances which could not be immediately equated with known corticosteroid structures. Three such substances were found in the grass snake and, while one of them might be indeed identical with 18-hydroxycorticosterone, the identities of the other two are still unknown (Macchi and Phillips, 1966).

Histological evidence adduced by Wright and Chester Jones (1957) has shown the probable involvement of reptilian anterior pituitary in the regulation of adrenal cortical secretion. Until recently, however, experiments designed to demonstrate increased corticosteroidogenesis *in vitro* following the addition of stimulatory additives did not meet with success, in spite of the fact that under similar experimental conditions and using the same additives, positive responses were elicited from amphibian, avian, and mammalian adrenal gland preparations. Mammalian ACTH did not increase the steroid production *in vitro* of grass snake and green lizard adrenals (Phillips *et al.*, 1962; Macchi and Phillips, 1966). It was similarly without effect when added to turtle (Macchi and Phillips 1966) or alligator (Gist and deRoos, 1966) adrenal gland preparations. Snake pituitary HCl extracts or snake whole anterior pituitary tissue failed to stimulate steroidogenesis *in vitro* of *Natrix natrix* adrenal gland preparations (Macchi, 1967), although Gist and deRoos (1966) could demonstrate ACTH-like activity in alligator adenohypophyseal extracts by their effect on chicken adrenal tissue *in vitro*. The first positive report on the action of ACTH on reptilian adreno-cortical function *in vitro* came from Huang *et al* (1969). By using the time course analysis technique, these authors reported an increased formation of corticosterone from an equimolar mixture of exogenous pregnenolone plus progesterone by cobra (*Naja naja*) adrenal tissue minces *in vitro* following the addition of mammalian ACTH. They attributed the failure of earlier studies to detect ACTH effect *in vitro* to the fact that ACTH not only increased corticosterone formation but also resulted in more rapid turnover of this metabolite. Thus by using single time incubation techniques, the ACTH-induced changes were not detectable. While these studies have not yet been confirmed, they do raise interesting possibilities. According to present scientific concensus, ACTH is believed to stimulate enzyme activity from precursors which precede pregnenolone or progesterone in the bio-synthetic sequence. It remains to be seen whether the stimulatory action of ACTH upon C_{21} steroid hydroxylating enzyme systems is a particularity of the cobra or reptilian adrenal tissue in general or whether such actions would be detectable with adrenal gland preparations of other nonmammalian vertebrates as well.

We have recently obtained information on the adrenocortical secretion of an additional lizard species. Incubation of NADPH fortified adrenal whole homogenates of the South American lizard, the tiju (*Tupinambis* sp.) with exogenous, labeled cholesterol, pregnenolone, and progesterone resulted in the formation of radioactive corticosterone, 11-deoxycortico-sterone, 18-hydroxycorticosterone and aldosterone. (Mehdi and Sandor (1971), unpublished observations).

From the preceding discussion it is clear that we are far from having a good understanding of the qualitative and quantitative functioning of the reptilian adrenal gland. Secretory products *in vitro* seem to be identical to those found in Anura. On the other hand, we have no knowledge about the composition or quantity of plasma corticosteroids nor can we hazard a guess about the secretory rates of corticosterone, aldosterone, and 18-hydroxy-corticosterone in the intact animal. In addition, far too few species have undergone close investigation. Data on the experiments discussed in this section are shown in Table III.

TABLE III

Corticosteroids in Reptilia

Species	Steroid[a]	Source of steroid	Quantity (μg/100 ml plasma or μg/100 mg tissue or % transformation)	Major criteria[b]	Rating[b] Identity	Rating[b] Quantity	Reference
Natrix natrix (grass snake)	Corticosterone	Adrenal venous blood after ACTH	156	PC, Ip–nmc, UV, CT Fl	Su	Te, P	Phillips and Chester Jones (1957)
	Cortisol Cortisone		8.5 2	PC, Ip–nmc, UV, CT, Fl	Su	Te, P	
	Corticosterone-³H	Adrenal slices + progesterone-³H + ACTH + Amphenon	♂13.9% ♀16.2% ♀17.8% ♀ + ♂6.0%	PC, Der, Ip–nmrc– Der, CT, UV	Te	NA	Phillips *et al.* (1962)
	Aldosterone-³H	Adrenal slices + progesterone-³H + ACTH + Amphenon	♂1.9% ♀4.6% ♀1.8% ♂ + ♀0.6%	PC, Der, Ip–nmrc– Der, CT, UV	Te	NA	
	Corticosterone-¹⁴C	Adrenal mince + progesterone-¹⁴C	Incubation medium, 10.20 ± 1.25% Adrenal tissue, 1.95 ± 1.23%	PC, Der, Ip–nmrc– Der, CT, UV	Te	Pr, T	Macchi and Phillips (1966)
	Aldosterone-¹⁴C	Adrenal mince + progesterone-¹⁴C	Incubation medium, 4.22 ± 0.70% Adrenal tissue, 0.97 ± 0.33%	PC, Der, Ip–nmrc– Der, CT, UV	Te	Pr, T	
	Corticosterone-¹⁴C	Adrenal mince + progesterone-¹⁴C + ACTH (1.0 IU) + Bell $p_1 + p_2$ ACTH	8.15%; 3.57/2 hr 12.65%; 7.52/2 hr 6.12%; 2.12/2 hr	PC, Der, Ip–nmrc– Der, CT, UV	Te	Pr, T	Macchi and Phillips (1966)

TABLE III (cont.)

Species	Steroid[a]	Source of steroid	Quantity (μg/100 ml plasma or μg/100 mg tissue or % transformation)	Major criteria[b]	Rating[b] Identity	Rating[b] Quantity	Reference
	Aldosterone-[14]C	+ Bell $\nu_1 + \nu_2$ ACTH	10.72%; 4.69/2 hr				
		+ APE[a]	6.82%; 3.88/2 hr				
		+ APT[a]	12.94%; 6.54/2 hr	PC, Der, Ip-nmrc-Der, CT, UV	Te	Pr, T	
		Adrenal mince + Proges-terone-[14]C + ACTH (1.0.IU)	4.61%; 4.36/2 hr				
		+ Bell $\nu_1 + \nu_2$ ACTH	5.98%; 4.68/2 hr				
		+ Bell $\nu_1 + \nu_2$ ACTH	4.56%; 2.07/2 hr				
		+ APE[a]	4.24%; 2.11/2 hr				
		+ APT[a]	3.66%; 2.01/2 hr				
			3.13%; 2.84/2 hr				
Naja naja (cobra)	Corticosterone	Adrenal slices	0.87	TLC, Der, Ip-nmc-SD, Re	Pr	Te, P	Gottfried *et al.* (1967)
	Aldosterone		0.17	TLC, Der(Ox), GLC, Ip-nmc-Der	Te	Pr, T	
	18-Hydroxycorti-costerone		0.98	TLC, Der(Ox), GLC, Ip-nmc-Der, IR-Der	Pr	Pr, T	
	Cortisone		0.12	TLC, Der, GLC, Ip-nmc-Der	Te-Su	Pr, T	
Lacerta viridis (green lizard)	Corticosterone-[3]H	Adrenal slices + progesterone-[3]H	16.9%	PC, Der, Ip-nmrc-Der, CT, UV	Te	NA	Phillips *et al.* (1962)
	Aldosterone-[3]H		2.9%	PC, Der, Ip-nmrc-Der, CT, UV	Te	NA	

280

Species	Precursor	Preparation	Yield	Methods			Reference
Pseudemys scripta (slider turtle)	Corticosterone-^{14}C	Adrenal slices + progesterone-^{14}C	14.7%; 0.41[c]	PC, Der, Ox, Ip–nmrc–Der, CSASD	Pr	Pr, P	Sandor et al. (1964)
	Aldosterone-^{14}C		2.2%; 0.27	PC, Der(Ox), Ip–nmrc–Der, CSA–nmrc–Der, UV	Pr	Te, P	
	18-Hydroxycorticosterone-^{14}C		6.1%; 0.37	PC, Der (Ox), Ip–nmrc–Der, UV	Te	Te, P	
	11-Deoxycorticosterone-^{14}C		1.2%; d	PC, Ip–nmrc, CSA–nmrc, Der, Cry CSAD	Pr	NA	
Chrysemys picta (painted turtle)	Cortisol-^{14}C	Adrenal slices + pregnenolone-^{3}H + progesterone-^{14}C	Trace: d	PC, Ip–nmrc	Su	NA	Sandor et al. (1964)
	Corticosterone-^{3}H, ^{14}C		^{3}H, 8.8%; ^{14}C, 19.7%; 1.29[c]	PC, Ip–nmrc, CSA–nmrc, CryCSA–nmrc–CSAD	Pr	Pr, P	
	Aldosterone-^{3}H,		^{14}C^{3}H, 2.4% 1.63	PC, Ip–nmrc, CSA–nmrc–CSAD	Pr nmrc, Cry	Pr, P	
	18-Hydroxycorticosterone-^{3}H,		^{3}H, 5.5%; ^{14}C, 14.2% 1.96	PC, Der(Ox), Ip–nmrc–SD, CSAD	Pr	Pr, P	
	11-Deoxycorticosterone-^{3}H, ^{14}C		^{3}H, 0.5% ^{14}C, 1.2%	PC, Ip–nmrc, CSA–nmrc, Der, Cry CSAD	Pr	NA	
	Progesterone-^{3}H		^{3}H, 1.3%	PC, IP–nmrc, Cry CSA–nmrc	Te	NA	
Emys orbicularis (turtle)	Corticosterone-^{14}C	Quartered adrenals + progesterone-^{14}C + ACTH	16.22%; 3.10/2 hr[c]	PC, Ip–nmc, Der, Ip-Der, CT, UV, Fl	Te	Pr, T	Macchi and Phillips (1966), Macchi (1967)
	Aldosterone-^{14}C	+ ACTH	16.12%; 3.08/2 hr 1.49%; 0.10/2 hr 5.26%; 0.84/2 hr	PC, Der, Ip–nmrc–Der, CT, UV, Fl	Te	Pr, T	

TABLE III (cont.)

Species	Steroid[a]	Source of steroid	Quantity (μg/100 ml plasma or μg/100 mg tissue or % transformation)	Major criteria[b]	Rating[b] Identity	Rating[b] Quantity	Reference
Alligator mississippiensis (alligator)	Corticosterone	Adrenal slices + ACTH (1.0 IU) + progesterone (50 ug/100 mg tissue)	1.1 ± 0.3 1.2 ± 0.6 11.8 ± 2.4	PC, Der, Ox, Ip–nmc–SD, CT, UV, ACr	Pr	Pr, T	Gist and deRoos (1966)
		+ ACTH + progesterone	6.5 ± 1.8				
	Aldosterone	Adrenal slices + ACTH (1.0 IU) + Progesterone (50 ug/100 mg tissue)	1.2 ± 0.1 0.9 ± 0.5 2.5 ± 0.2	PC, Ip–nmc, CT, ACr, UV	Te	Te, T	
		+ ACTH + progesterone	1.1 ± 0.3				
Naja naja (cobra)	³H-Labelled progesterone, ¹⁴C and ³H-labeled 11-deoxycortico-sterone, cortico-sterone, 18-hydroxycorti-costerone and aldosterone	Adrenal slices + ACTH (1.0 IU) + Progesterone 4-¹⁴C	Kinetic Study[c]				Huang et al. (1969)
Chrysemys picta picta (painted turtle)	Progesterone-¹⁴C	Adrenal homogenate + cholesterol-4-¹⁴C + NADPH + fumarate; ³H markers added; 3 hr	0.6%	PC, Ip–nmrc–Der(Re), Cry C³H/¹⁴C	Pr	Po, T	Mehdi (1969)

282

Substrate	Conditions	Yield	Methods			Reference
11-Deoxycorticosterone-^{14}C	incubation	0.2%	Pc, Ip-nmrc–Der, CryC ^{3}H/^{14}C	Pr	Po, T	
Corticosterone-^{14}C		0.2%	Pc, Ip-nmrc–Der, CryC	Pr	Po, T	
18-Hydroxycorticosterone-^{14}C		0.5%	PC, Ip-nmrc–Der(Ox) ^{3}H/^{14}C	Te	Pr, T	
Aldosterone-^{14}C		0.2%	Pc, Ip-nmrc–Der, CryC ^{3}H/^{14}C	Pr	Po, T	
Pregnenolone-^{14}C	Adrenal mitochondria + cholesterol-4-^{14}C + NADPH + fumarate; 3 hr incubation; ^{3}H markers added	1.0%	PC, Ip-nmrc–Der, CryC ^{3}H/^{14}C	Pr	Po, T	Mehdi (1969)
Progesterone-^{14}C		0.8%	PC, Ip-nmrc–Der (Re), CryC ^{3}H/^{14}C	Pr	Po, T	
18-Hydroxycorticosterone-^{14}C		0.2%	PC, Ip-nmrc–Der(Ox)	Te	Pr, T	
Aldosterone-^{14}C		0.1%	PC, Ip-nmrc–Der, CryC ^{3}H/^{14}C	Pr	Po, T	
Progesterone-^{14}C	Adrenal homogenate + pregnenolone-4-^{14}C (113 μg/100 mg tissue) + NADPH + fumarate; 3 hr incubation; ^{3}H markers added	19.6	PC, Ip-nmrc–Der, CryC ^{3}H/^{14}C	Pr	Po, T	Mehdi (1969)

TABLE III (cont.)

Species	Steroid[a]	Source of steroid	Quantity (μg/100 ml plasma or μg/100 mg tissue or % transformation)	Major criteria[b]	Rating[b] Identity	Quantity	Reference
	11β-Hydroxy-progesterone-^{14}C		2.0	PC, Ip–nmrc–Der (Ox), CSAD	Pr	Pr, T	
	11-Deoxycorti-costerone-^{14}C		30.1	PC, Ip–nmrc–Der, CryC ^{3}H/^{14}C	Pr	Po, T	
	Corticosterone-^{14}C		16.9	PC, Ip–nmrc–Der, CryC ^{3}H/^{14}C	Pr	Po, T	
	18-Hydroxycor-ticosterone-^{14}C		1.1	PC, Ip–nmrc–Der(Ox)	Te	Pr, T	
	Aldosterone-^{14}C		0.5	PC, Ip–nmrc–Der, CryC ^{3}H/^{14}C	Pr	Po, T	
	Progesterone-^{14}C	Adrenal mitochondria + pregnenolone-4-^{14}C (113 μg/100 mg tissue) + NADPH + fumarate; ^{3}H markers added; 3 hr incubation	4.5	PC, Ip–nmrc–Der(Re), Cry C ^{3}H/^{14}C	Pr	Po, T	Mehdi (1969)
	11β-Hydroxy-progesterone-^{14}C		0.7	PC, Ip–nmrc–Der(Ox), CSAD	Pr	Pr, T	
	11-Deoxycorti-costerone-^{14}C		1.2	PC, Ip–nmrc–Der, CryC ^{3}H/^{14}C	Pr	Po, T	

11β-Hydroxy-progesterone-^{14}C	Adrenal homogenate + progesterone-4-^{14}C (113 μg/100 mg tissue) + NADPH + fumarate; 3 hr incubation; ^{3}H	8.5	Criteria and rating as above	Mehdi (1969)
11-Deoxycorticosterone-^{14}C		24.1		
Corticosterone-^{14}C		14.8		
18-Hydroxycorticosterone-^{14}C		1.7		
Aldosterone-^{14}C		0.4		
11β-Hydroxy-progesterone-^{14}C	Adrenal mitochondria + progesterone-^{14}C (113 μg/100 mg tissue) + NADPH + fumarate; ^{3}H markers added; 3hr incubation	3.9	Criteria and rating as above	Mehdi (1969)
11-Deoxycorticosterone-^{14}C		1.4		
Corticosterone-^{14}C		0.7		

[a] Abbreviations: APE, anterior pituitary HCl extract; APT, anterior pituitary tissue.
[b] For an explanation of abbreviations and rating system, see Chapter 2, Tables I–IV.
[c] Endogeneous steroid production.
[d] Could not be measured.
[e] For criteria and rating, see Table V, data of Whitehouse and Vinson (1967).

C. Aves

Phillips and Chester Jones (1957) reported that in the caponized cockerel, corticosterone might be the major plasmatic corticosteroid. Subsequently, Newcomer (1959a) quantified the total free and conjugated (liberated following enzymic hydrolysis with β-glucuronidase and hot HCl hydrolysis) corticosteroids in the peripheral plasma and the adrenal gland of the chicken *Gallus domesticus*. The steroid level was assayed by the isonicotinic acid hydrazide (INH) method of Weichselbaum and Margraf (1957), believed to be specific for 4-ene–3-one steroids. Newcomer noted that following chronic ACTH treatment, the corticosteroid content of the adrenal glands decreased, while the plasma levels increased. Administration of o,p'-DDD (2-o-chlorophenyl-2-p-chlorophenyl-1,1-dichloroethane) elicited a decrease in the amount of the circulating INH-positive material. From these studies he concluded that the INH material, probably corticosterone, was of adrenal origin, in spite of the fact that hypophysectomy hardly decreased its plasma level (Newcomer, 1959b). Further studies by Urist and Deutch (1960) in the chicken demonstrated that plasma dichloromethane extracts contained material showing corticosteronelike fluorescent reaction in 80% sulfuric acid (Silber *et al.*, 1958). The circulating levels of this fluorigen, presumably identical with Newcomer's INH-positive substance and labeled as corticosterone by the authors, exhibited an increase following chronic treatment of the chicken with mammalian ACTH. Using a similar fluorimetric method, Nagra and associates (1960) measured this fluorigen in the peripheral plasma and adrenal venous effluent of gallinaceous birds and found significantly higher levels in the blood originating directly from the adrenal gland. The first attempts to establish the identity of the circulating fluorigen, undoubtedly of adrenal origin, came from Brown (1961), who isolated relatively large amounts from the peripheral plasma of the turkey *Meleagris gallopavo* and suggested that the steroid might indeed be identical with corticosterone. This contention was supported by the *in vitro* studies of de Roos (1960, 1961a, 1963). Incubation of adrenal minces of the chicken, the western gull *Larus occidentalis*, the white king pigeon *Columbia livia*, and the white Pekin duck *Anas platyrhynchos* has shown that the adrenal glands of all these avian species biosynthesize corticosterone. In addition, again in all four species, the *in vitro* biosynthesis of aldosterone could be tentatively advanced. The *in vitro* biosynthesis of corticosteroids by avian adrenals was further investigated by Sandor and Lanthier (1963b), Sandor *et al.* (1963b), and Lamoureux *et al.* (1964). Incubation of adrenal gland slices of the domestic duck, the chicken, and the goose *Anser anser* with a mixture of tritiated pregnenolone and ^{14}C-labeled progesterone resulted in the formation of ^{3}H- and ^{14}C-labeled corticosterone, aldosterone, and 18-hydroxycorticosterone. In addition, small amounts of 11-deoxycorticosterone, 11β-hydroxyprogesterone, and 11-dehydrocorticosterone were formed. These results were in agreement with those previously obtained by deRoos and added 18-hydrocorticosterone to the list of major avian corticosteroids.

The findings of Sandor *et al.* (1963b) on the chemical nature of the adrenal cortical steroids of the duck were confirmed by Donaldson *et al.* (1965). They demonstrated the *in vitro* formation of corticosterone, aldosterone, and 18-hydroxycorticosterone by duck adrenal slices in the absence of exogenous substrates and established corticosterone as the immediate precursor of 18-hydroxycorticosterone and possible aldosterone. By the use of a double-isotope derivative assay they identified corticosterone as the major plasmatic corticosteroid of the duck.

The steroid biochemistry of the domestic duck adrenal gland continued to be a subject of interest to several research groups. Duck adrenals are very efficient producers of 18-hydroxycorticosterone and aldosterone and thus furnished excellent test material for the study of depth of 18-oxygenated hormones. In addition, the duck, basically a water or even marine bird, has a functional nasal gland for the extrarenal excretion of sodium chloride. It has been suggested that this organ is dependent on the adrenal gland (Holmes *et al.*, 1961; Phillips *et al.*, 1961; Macchi *et al.*, 1967), and, in consequence, the precise definition of the steroid biosynthetic events taking place in the duck adrenal gland assumed added importance.

Duck, chicken, and goose adrenal slices produce *in vitro* relatively large amounts of corticosterone, 18-hydroxycorticosterone, and aldosterone from exogenous progesterone and pregnenolone (Sandor *et al.*, 1963b; Lamoureux *et al.*, 1964). It is believed, however, that especially the high conversion rates of substrates into 18-hydroxycorticosterone is an artificial phenomenon and is probably due to the accumulation of intermediaries. Thus, it could be shown that duck adrenal preparations have a very high 18-hydroxylating capability; although in the intact animal, with its very high circulatory rate, most of the corticosterone formed is washed out from the gland, under *in vitro* conditions this corticosterone is available for 18-oxygenation to form 18-hydroxycorticosterone and aldosterone. The circulating corticosterone level was found to be in the neighborhood of 6 μg/100 ml peripheral plasma in the duck (Donaldson and Holmes, 1965) and in the chicken (Frankel *et al.*, 1967a). Donaldson and Holmes (1965) estimated the secretory rate of corticosterone in the intact duck at 2.4 μg/kg body weight per minute. Peripheral plasma aldosterone levels in intact 8-week-old male domestic ducks were found to be around 0.014 μg/100 ml plasma when measured by the double-isotope derivative assay of Nowaczynski *et al.* (1967). (This determination was performed through the kind cooperation of Dr. W. J. Nowaczynski, Montreal). By this assay, the aldosterone level of human peripheral blood is between 0.002 and 0.016 μg/100 ml. Taylor *et al.* (1970) measured the level of corticosterone and aldosterone in the adrenal vein blood of the chicken. They found 6.5 μg corticosterone and 0.21 μg aldosterone per 100 ml plasma. Infusion of mammalian ACTH significantly increased the corticosterone secreted by the adrenal, while aldosterone values remained unchanged. These same authors demonstrated the presence of a renal pressor system in the chicken, although no steroidogenic action of this system was demonstrable. No reports exist on the plasma level or secretory rates of 18-hydroxycorticosterone in any avian species. We shall need *in vivo* secretion rate data before it can be decided whether the dichotomy between the *in vitro* production rates of steroids and their plasma level does indeed reflect genuine quantitative differences due to the differences in the experimental procedures or peripheral metabolism.

It seems appropriate at this point to discuss briefly some points on the regulation of adrenal cortical secretion in birds. In the hypophysectomized mammal, the adrenal gland atrophies and loses its capability for corticosteroid synthesis. This can be restored by the administration of exogenous ACTH. In birds, hypophysectomy is not followed by the complete cessation of steroid hormone synthesis (Nagra *et al.*, 1960; Brown, 1961; Nagra *et al.*, 1963; Resko *et al.*, 1964; Frankel *et al.*, 1967b). The work of Frankel and associates (1967b) has shown that following hypophysectomy, about 37% of the preoperative steroid-biosynthesis ability remains. In a subsequent study, Frankel and associates (1967c) concluded that adrenal function in the hypophysectomized chicken is probably supported by an extrahypophyseal adrenocorticotropin, the identity of which has not been established (Frankel *et al.*, 1967d). The possible identity of an extrahypophyseal ACTH was reinvestigated by Salem *et al.* (1970a,b). They presented evidence that chicken hypothalami contain an ACTH-like material as assayed by the adrenal ascorbic acid depletion test. They advanced the hypothesis that this hypothalamic factor might be identical with α-melanocyte-stimulating hormone.

Details of the experimental data on avian corticosteroids are listed in Tables IV (*in vivo* experiments) and V (*in vitro* experiments).

It can be concluded from our survey that corticosterone and aldosterone are the main corticosteroid components of the adrenal secretion of amphibians, reptiles and birds. 18-Hydroxycorticosterone is also present in quantities approximating or even surpassing those of the two other hormones. However, it is not known whether 18-hydroxycorticosterone is a steroid with a distinct physiological role or whether it is the intermediary in the transformation of corticosterone to aldosterone. In addition, 18-hydroxycorticosterone has not been isolated from the plasma of any of the lower vertebrates.

The pioneering studies of Stachenko and Giroud (1959, 1962) have estab-

TABLE IV

Corticosteroids in Aves *in Vivo*

Species	Steroid	Source of steroid	Quantity (μg/100 ml plasma)	Major criteria[a]	Rating[a]		Reference
					Identity	Quantity	
Gallus domesticus (chicken)	Corticosterone	Adrenal venous (AV) effluent blood +ACTH	312.0	PC, Ip-nmc, UV, CT	Su	Te, P	Phillips and Chester Jones (1957)
	Aldosterone	AV Effluent +ACTH	65.5	PC, Ip-nmrc, UV, CT	Su	Te, P	
	Cortisol	AV Effluent +ACTH	3.0	PC, Ip-nmc, UV, CT	Su	Te, P	
	Cortisone	AV Effluent +ACTH	2.5	PC, Ip-nmc, CT, UV	Su	Te, P	
	Corticosteroids	Adrenal gland extract	Total, 43.6[b]; Free, 27.0; Gluc, 10.9[d]; SO_4, 6.5[e]	SNI, IN[b]H reaction[c]	NA	Te, P; Te, P	Newcomer (1959a)
			Total, 12.2; Gluc, 5.8[d]; SO_4, 5.8[e]	SNI, INH reaction[c]	NA	Te, P	
	Corticosterone	Peripheral plasma	♂ 6.5 ±2; ♀ 8.0 ±3	SNI, Fl reaction[f]		Te, P	Urist and Deutch (1960)
		Peripheral plasma–ACTH	♂12.0 ±5; ♀15.0 ±4			Te, P	
	Corticosterone	Peripheral plasma	7.3 ±0.3	SNI Fl reaction[f]		Te, P	Nagra *et al.* (1960)
		AV Effluent	44.3 ±5.5			Te, P	
		AV Effluent after ACTH	143.7			Te, P	
	Corticosterone	Left adrenal vein plasma	NA	AC, PC, TLC, Ip-nmc, UV	Su	NA	Nagra *et al.* (1963)

TABLE IV (cont.)

Species	Steroid	Source of steroid	Quantity (μg/100 ml plasma)	Major criteria[a]	Rating[a] Identity	Rating[a] Quantity	Reference
		AV Effluent	Intact, 15.1 Bleeding, 67.8 Intact + ACTH, 105.8 Hypox[h], 8.9	SNI Fl reaction[g]	NA	Te, T	Resko et al. (1964)
	Corticosterone	Adrenal venous plasma	NA	PC, TLC, Ip-nmc, CT	Su	NA	
		AV Plasma	Intact, 24.4 + ACTH, 43.4 + CPE[j], 73.5 Hypox[h], 15.7	Fl reaction[i]	NA	Te, T	
	Corticosterone	AV Plasma	Intact, 7.3 ±0.5 Hypox[h], 2.7 ±0.6 + Metopirone, 0.2 + ACTH, 52.0 ±5.6 Stress, 18.3 ±3.6	SPa, PC, Ip-nmc, Fl[k] Verified by DIDA	Pr	Po, T	Frankel et al. (1967b)
	Corticosterone	Adrenal venous blood	Surgical stress, 6.58 ±1.47	DIDA	Pr	Po, T	Taylor et al. (1970)
			ACTH infusion (0.09 IU/min for 30 min), 15.16 ±3.51	DIDA	Pr	Po, T	
			Hypophysectomy, 1.06 ±0.20	DIDA	Pr	Po, T	
			Hypophysectomy + chicken kidney extract, 0.78 ±0.12	DIDA	Pr	Po, T	
			Sodium depletion, 3.40 ±1.60	DIDA	Pr	Po, T	

290

Compound	Species	Sample	Concentration	Method			Reference
Aldosterone		Surgical stress, 0.21 + 0.06		DIDA	Pr	Po, T	
		ACTH infusion (0.09 IU/min for 30 min), 0.11 ±0.02		DIDA	Pr	Po, T	
		Hypophysectomy, 0.06 ±0.01		DIDA	Pr	Po, T	
		Hypophysectomy + chicken kidney extract, 0.08 ±0.02		DIDA	Pr	Po, T	
		Sodium depletion, 0.17 ±0.06		DIDA	Pr	Po, T	
	Meleagris gallo-pavo (turkey)	Corticosterone	Peripheral plasma	NA	AC, PC, Ip-nmc, CT, ACr Fl reaction[f]	Te	NA	Nagra et al. (1960)
		Corticosterone	Peripheral plasma	Normal, 12.5 + ACTH, 28.7	Fl reaction[f]	NA	Te, P	
	Catheturus sp. (broad-breasted bronz turkey)	Corticosterone	Peripheral plasma AV plasma	7.4 ±0.4 42.4 ± 5.3	SNI Fl reaction[f]			Brown (1961)[,f]
	Phasianus colchicus (ring-necked pheasant)	Corticosterone	Peripheral plasma AV effluent	Intact, 8.6 ±0.8 Castrated, 7.8 ±0.7 Intact, 34.8 ±4.7 Castrated, 33.1 ±7.2	SNI Fl reaction[f]			Nagra et al. (1960)
		Corticosterone	Left adrenal vein plasma AV plasma	NA Intact, 23.2 Stressed, 106.6	AC, PC, TLC, Ip-nmc, UV Fl reaction[g]	Su	NA	Nagra et al. (1963)

TABLE IV (cont.)

Species	Steroid	Source of steroid	Quantity (μg/100 ml plasma)	Major criteria[a]	Rating[a] Identity	Rating[a] Quantity	Reference
Anas platyrhynchos (domestic duck)	Corticosterone	Peripheral plasma	5.1 ± 0.49	DIDA	Pr	Po, T	Donaldson and Holmes (1965)
	Corticosterone		Secretion rate, $2.43 \pm 0.13\ \mu g/kg/min$	DIDA	Pr	Po, T	
	Aldosterone	Peripheral plasma	0.014	DIDA	Pr		Sandor (1970)[l]

[a]For an explanation of abbreviations and rating system, see Chapter 2, Tables I–IV.
[b]Micrograms per 100 mg adrenal tissue.
[c]Weichselbaum and Margraf (1957).
[d]Substances liberated by enzymic hydrolysis with β-glucuronidase.
[e]Substances liberated by hot acid (10% HCl) hydrolysis.
[f]Silber et al. (1958).
[g]Nagra et al. (1963).
[h]Hypophysectomized.
[i]Zenker and Bernstein (1958).
[j]Crude chicken pituitary acid extract.
[k]Frankel et al. (1967a).
[l]Measurement performed by the DIDA method of Nowaczynski et al. (1967) through the kind cooperation of Dr. W. Nowaczynski, Montreal.

292

TABLE V

Corticosteroids in Aves *in Vitro*

Species	Steroid[a]	Source of steroid	Quantity (μg/100 mg tissue or % transformation)	Major criteria[b]	Rating[b] Identity	Rating[b] Quantity	Reference
Gallus domesticus (chicken)	Corticosterone	Adrenal mince	NA	PC, Der, Ip–nmc–Der, CT, ACr, Fl, UV	Te	NA	deRoos (1960)
	Aldosterone		NA	PC, Ip–nmc, CT, UV	Su	NA	
	Cortisol		NA	PC, Ip–nmc, CT, UV	Su	NA	
	Corticosterone	Adrenal mince + ACTH (0.5 IU) + ACTH (1.0 IU)	0.9. ±0.26 / 9.0 / 13.0 ±1.11	PC, Der, Ip–nmc–Der, Ox, CT, ACr, UV	Pr	Pr, T	deRoos (1961a)
	Aldosterone	Adrenal mince + ACTH (0.5 IU) + ACTH (1.0 IU)	0.3 / 0.3 / 0.6 ±0.28	PC, Ip–nmc, ACr, CT, UV, DIDA	Pr	Pr, T	
	Corticosterone	Adrenal mince + Angiotensin II[c] + ACTH (1.0 IU) + Angiotensin II[d] + ACTH (1.0 IU)	0.23 ±0.08 / 0.00 – 0.18 / 6.64 ±0.66 / 4.90	PC, Der, Ip–nmc–Der, Ox, CT, ACr, UV	Pr	Pr, T	deRoos and deRoos (1963)
	Aldosterone	Adrenal mince + Angiotensin II[c] + ACTH (1.0 IU) + Angiotensin II[d] + ACTH (1.0 IU)	0.33 ±0.11 / 0.00–0.18 / 1.39 ±0.19 / 0.73	PC, Ip–nmc, ACr, CT, UV	Te	Pr, T	

TABLE V (cont.)

Species	Steroid[a]	Source of steroid	Quantity (μg/100 mg tissue or % transformation)	Major criteria[b]	Rating[b] Identity	Rating[b] Quantity	Reference
Corticosterone	Corticosterone	Adrenal mince + ACTH (1.0 IU) + CAP[e]	0.2 ± 0.07 6.6 ± 0.66 5.4 ± 0.47	PC, Der, Ip–nmc–Der, Ox, CT, ACr, UV	Pr	Pr, T	deRoos and deRoos (1964)
	Aldosterone	Adrenal mince + ACTH (1.0 IU) + CAP[e]	0.4 ± 0.09 1.4 ± 0.19 1.5 ± 0.10	PC, Ip–nmc, ACr, CT, UV			
	Corticosterone-^{3}H, [14]C	Adrenal slices + pregnenolone-7-[3]H + progesterone-4-[14]C	[3]H, 10.9% [14]C, 18.1%	PC, Der, Ip–nmrc–Der, CSAD	Pr	NA	Sandor et al. (1963b)
	Aldosterone-^{3}H, [14]C		[3]H, 0.9% [14]C, 1.5%	PC, Der, Ip–nmrc–Der, CSAD	Pr	NA	
	18-Hydroxycorticosterone-^{3}H, [14]C		[3]H, 3.5% [14]C, 5.9%	PC, Der(Ox), Ip–nmrc–Der, C ^{3}H/^{14}C SD	Te–Pr	NA	
	11-Deoxycorticosterone-^{3}H, [14]C		[3]H, 0.3% [14]C, 0.6%	PC, Der, Ip–nmrc–Der, Cry CSAD	Pr	NA	
	11β-Hydroxyprogesterone-^{3}H, [14]C		Traces	PC, Ox, Ip–nmrc–Der	Su	NA	
	Progesterone-[3]H		[3]H, 1.2%	PC, Ip–nmrc, Cry CSA–nmrc	Te	NA	
	Corticosterone	Adrenal slices + progesterone-4-[14]C Tissue from intact animals	13.4/2 hr, 5.1%	PC, TLC, Ip–nmrc, Fl, UV	Te	Po, T	Frankel et al. (1967b)

294

Organism	Product	Incubation conditions	Yield	Identification			Reference
	Corticosterone-³H	Tissue from hypox[f] animals / Adrenal slices + progesterone-4-¹⁴C + Dexamethasone (5 μg/flask)	9.1/2 hr, 4.0% / 4.7/2 hr, 7.1% / 6.2/2 hr, 11.6%	PC, Der, Ip–nmrc–Der, Cry CSA–nmrc–Der	Pr	NA	Hall and Koritz (1966)
Anas platyrhynchos (domestic duck)	Corticosterone	Quartered adrenals + cholesterol-7-³H + ATCH (0.08 IU) / Adrenal mince + ACTH (1.0 IU)	0.001% / 0.8 ± 1.1 / 12.2 ± 2.75	PC, Der, Ip–nmc–Der, Ox, CT, ACr, UV	Pr	Pr, T	deRoos (1961a)
	Aldosterone	Adrenal mince + ACTH (1.0 IU)	0.008% / 1.0–2.2 / 1.8 ± 0.38	PC, Ip–nmc, UV, ACr, DIDA	Pr	Pr, T	
	Corticosterone-¹⁴C	Adrenal slices + progesterone-4-¹⁴C	11.4%	PC, Der, Ip–nmrc–Der, Ox, CSASD	Pr	NA	Sandor and Lanthier (1963b)
	Aldosterone-¹⁴C		6.8%	PC, Der, Ip–nmrc–Der, CSAD	Te	NA	
	18-Hydroxycorticosterone-¹⁴C		15.5%	PC, Der(Ox), Ip–nmrc–Der, CSASD	Pr	NA	
	11-Deoxycorticosterone-¹⁴C		0.38%	PC, Der, Ip–nmrc–Der, Cry CSAD	Pr	NA	
	Cortisol-¹⁴C		0.05%	PC, Der(Ox), Ip–nmrc–Der CSAD	Su-Te	NA	
	Corticosterone-³H, ¹⁴C	Adrenal slices + pregnenolone-7-³H + progesterone-4-¹⁴C	³H, 5.0% / ¹⁴C, 10.3%	PC, Der, Ip–nmrc–Der, CSAD	Pr	NA	Sandor et al. (1963b)
	Aldosterone-³H, ¹⁴C		³H, 3.4% / ¹⁴C, 6.2%	PC, Der, Ip–nmrc–Der, C³H/¹⁴C D	Pr	NA	

TABLE V (cont.)

Species	Steroid[a]	Source of steroid	Quantity (μg/100 mg tissue or % transformation)	Major criteria[b]	Rating[b] Identity	Rating[b] Quantity	Reference
	18-Hydroxycorticosterone-³H, ¹⁴C		³H, 6.8% ¹⁴C, 13.8%	PC, Ox, Ip–nmrc–Der,C ³H/¹⁴C SD	Pr–Te	NA	Donaldson et al. (1965)
	11-Deoxycorticosterone-³H, ¹⁴C		³H, 0.1% ¹⁴C, 0.4%	PC, Der, Ip–nmrc, Ip–Der, Cry CSAD	Pr	NA	
	11β-Hydroxyprogesterone-³H, ¹⁴C		³H, 0.08% ¹⁴C, 0.1%	PC, Der(Ox), Ip–nmrc–Der	Su	NA	
	Progesterone-³H		0.1%	PC, Ip–nmrc, Cry CSA–nmrc	Te	NA	
	Corticosterone	Adrenal slices + ACTH (1.0 IU)	0.14 ± 0.03 23.66 ± 1.80	PC, Der(r), Ip–nmrc–Der(r), Ox, CT, ACr, UV, DIDA	Pr	Po, T	
	Aldosterone	Adrenal slices + ACTH (1.0 IU)	1.00 ± 0.16 6.20 ± 0.43	As above	Pr	Po, T	
	18-Hydroxycorticosterone	Adrenal slices + ACTH (1.0 IU)	At limit of detection, 16.30	SNI PC, Der(r), Ip–nmrc, Ip–Der(r), CT, UV, ACr	NA Pr	NA Po, T	
	Aldosterone-¹⁴C	Adrenal slices + corticosterone-4-¹⁴C	Time–concentration study	PC, Der(r), C ³H/¹⁴C D	Pr	NA	
	Cholesterol-¹⁴C	Adrenal slices + Na acetate-1-¹⁴C + ACTH (0.9 IU)	0.008%	AC, TLC, Ip–nmrc–Ip–Der, CT, Cry CSAD, IR	Po	NA	Sandor et al. (1965)
	Corticosterone-¹⁴C		0.25%	PC, TLC, Der, Ip–nmrc–Der, UV, CT, Cry CSAD	Pr	NA	

Compound	Substrate/conditions	Yield	%	Analytical methods	Tissue	Te, P	Reference
Aldosterone-^{14}C			0.17%	PC, Der, Ip–nmrc–Der(Ox), CT, UV, CSAD	Pr	NA	
18-Hydroxycorticosterone-^{14}C			0.12%	PC, Der(Ox), Ip–nmrc–Der, UV, CSASD	Pr	NA	
Corticosterone-^{14}C	Adrenal whole homogenate + cholesterol-4-^{14}C		0.75%	AC, PC, TLC, Der, Ip–nmrc–Der, Cry CSAD	Pr	NA	Sandor et al. (1965)
Corticosterone	Adrenal mince + ACTH (1.0 IU) + ACTH (Bell $\gamma_1 + \gamma_2$, 1.0 IU) + AAHE[h] (equivalent to 550 mU ACTH) + Cyclic 3',5'-AMP(50 mM)	0.45/2 hr[g]; 4.25/2 hr; 5.92/2 hr; 2.42/2 hr; 2.08–5.92/2 hr		PC, Der, Ip–nmc–Der, CT, UV	Te	Te, P	Macchi (1967)
Aldosterone	Adrenal mince + ACTH (1.0 IU) + ACTH (Bell $\gamma_1 + \gamma_2$, 1.0 IU) + AAHE[h] (equivalent to 550 mU ACTH) + Cyclic 3',5'-AMP(50 mM)	0.96/2 hr[g]; 3.05/2 hr; 2.78/2 hr; 3.22/2 hr; 1.51/2 hr		PC, Der, Ip–nmc–Der, CT, UV	Te	Te, P	
Corticosterone + aldosterone	Adrenal mince + Progesterone-4-^{14}C + ACTH (1.0 IU) + ACTH (Bell, 1.0 IU)	10.98/2 hr; 19.94/2 hr; 16.61/2 hr	21.33%; 25.16%; 23.77%	PC, Der, Ip–nmc–Der, CT, UV	Te	Te, P	Macchi (1967)

TABLE V (cont.)

Species	Steroid[a]	Source of steroid	Quantity (μg/100 mg tissue or % transformation)	Major criteria[b]	Rating[b]		Reference
					Identity	Quantity	
	[3]H,[14]C-Labeled corticosterone, aldosterone, 18-OH B and DOC	Adrenal slices + progesterone-4-[14]C + 11-deoxy-corticosterone 1,2-[3]H	Kinetic study[i]				Sandor et al. (1966a)
	[3]H,[14]C-Labeled corticosterone, aldosterone, and 18-OH B	Adrenal slices + 11-deoxycorti-costerone-1,2-[3]H + corticosterone-4-[14]C	Kinetic study[i]				Sandor et al. (1966a)
	^{14}C-Labeled aldosterone and 18-OH B	Adrenal slices + corticosterone-4-[14]C	Kinetic study[i]				Sandor (1969a)
		Adrenal slices + pregnenolone-7-[3]H + progesterone-4-[14]C	Kinetic study[j]				Sandor (1969a)
		Adrenal whole homogenate + NADPH-generating system + pregnenolone-7-[3]H + progesterone-4-[14]C	Kinetic study[j]				Sandor (1969a)

Aldosterone-^{14}C	Adrenal mitochondria (6000 g) + NADPH-generating system + corticosterone-4-^{14}C	2.4/10 min	PC, TLC, Der Ip–nmrc–Der	Te	Pr, T	Sandor and Lanthier (1966), Sandor et al. (1972b)
18-Hydroxycorticosterone-^{14}C	Adrenal mitochondria (6000 g) + NADPH-generating system + progesterone-4-^{14}C	10.4/10 min	PC, TLC, Der, Ip–nmrc–Der	Te	Pr, T	Sandor and Lanthier (1966), Sandor et al. (1972b)
	Adrenal mince + pregnenolone-16-^{3}H + progesterone-4-^{14}C; progesterone-4-^{14}C + DOC-1,2-^{3}H; DOC-1,2-^{3}H + corticosterone-4-^{14}C	Kinetic study[k]				Whitehouse and Vinson (1967)
		Kinetic study[l]				
Anser anser (goose)						
Corticosterone-^{3}H, ^{14}C	Adrenal slices + pregnenolone-7-^{3}H + progesterone-one-4-^{14}C	^{3}H, 5.1%; ^{14}C, 9.1%	PC, Der, Ip–nmrc–Der, Cry CSAD	Pr	NA	Lamoureux et al. (1964), Lamoureux (1966)
Aldosterone-^{3}H, ^{14}C		^{3}H, 2.7%; ^{14}C, 5.4%	PC, TLC, Der, Ip–nmrc–Der, C ^{3}H/^{14}C D	Pr	NA	
18-Hydroxycorticosterone-^{3}H, ^{14}C		^{3}H, 5.1%; ^{14}C, 9.9%	PC, Ip–nmrc, CSA–nmrc	Te	NA	
11-Deoxycorticosterone-^{3}H, ^{14}C		^{3}H, 0.13%; ^{14}C, 0.14%	PC, TLC, Ip–nmrc, C ^{3}H/^{14}C–nmrc	Te	NA	

TABLE V (cont.)

Species	Steroid[a]	Source of steroid	Quantity (μg/100 mg tissue or % transformation)		Major criteria[b]	Rating[b]		Reference
						Identity	Quantity	
	11-Dehydrocorticosterone-³H, ¹⁴C		³H,	0.1%	PC, Der, Ip–nmrc–Der, Cry CSAD	Pr	NA	
			¹⁴C,	0.4%				
	11β-Hydroxyprogesterone-³H, ¹⁴C		³H,	Trace	PC, Der(Ox), Ip–nmrc–Der	Su	NA	
			¹⁴C,	Trace				
	Cholesterol-¹⁴C	Adrenal slices + 1.45 IU ACTH + Na acetate-1-¹⁴C	0.003%		AC, TLC, Ip–nmrc, IR	Pr	NA	Sandor et al. (1965)
	Corticosterone-¹⁴C		0.53%		PC, TLC, Ip–nmrc, CSA–nmrc	Te	NA	
	Aldosterone-¹⁴C		0.49%		PC, Ip–nmrc, CSA–nmrc	Te	NA	
	18-Hydroxycorticosterone-¹⁴C		0.37%		PC, Ip–nmrc, CSA–nmrc	Te	NA	
Columbia livia (white king pigeon)	Corticosterone	Adrenal mince + ACTH (1.0 IU)	1.1 ±0.41 7.6 ±1.00		PC, Der, Ip–nmc–Der, Ox, CT, ACr, UV	Pr	Pr, T	deRoos (1961a)
	Aldosterone	Adrenal mince + ACTH (1.0 IU)	0.4 ±1.30 1.1 ±0.56		PC, Ip–nmc, UV, CT, ACr	Te	Te, T	
Larus occidentalis (western gull)	Corticosterone	Adrenal mince + ACTH (1.0 IU)	4.4 ±0.52 9.7 ±0.88		PC, Der, Ip–nmc–Der, Ox, CT, ACr, UV	Pr	Pr, T	deRoos (1961a)
	Aldosterone	Adrenal mince + ACTH (1.0 IU)	0.2 ±0.06 0.4 ±0.05		PC, Ip–nmc, CT, ACr, UV	Te	Te, T	
	11-Dehydrocorticosterone	Adrenal mince + ACTH (1.0 IU)	0.3 ±0.07 0.7 ±0.09		PC, Der, Ip–nmc–Der, UV, CT	Te	Te, T	

Species	Compound	System	Value	Methods			Reference
Pipilo fuscus (brown towhee)	Corticosterone	Adrenal slices + ACTH (2.0 IU)	NA 24.0	PC, Ip-nmc, ACr, UV	Te	Te, P	deRoos (1961b)
	Aldosterone	Adrenal slices + ACTH (2.0 IU)	NA 3.4	PC, Ip-nmc, ACr, UV	Te	Te, P	
Anas platyrhynchos (domestic duck)	11β-Hydroxyprogesterone-14C	Adrenal slices + pregnenolone-4-14C (50 µg/100 mg tissue)	1.08/60 min	PC, Ip-nmrc–Der(Re, Ox), CSAD	Pr	Te, P	Sandor (1969b)
	11β-Hydroxyprogesterone-14C	Adrenal slices + progesterone-4-14C (50 µg/100 mg tissue)	0.49/60 min	As above	Pr	Te, P	Sandor (1969b)
	11β-Hydroxyprogesterone-14C	Adrenal mitochondria (1.6 mg protein equivalent) + progesterone-4-14C (20 µg)	4.42/60 min	As above	Pr	Te, P	Sandor and Lanthier (1970)
	Corticosterone-14C; 18-Hydroxycorticosterone-14C; aldosterone-14C	Adrenal slices + 11β-hydroxyprogesterone-4-14C	Kinetic study[m]				Sandor and Lanthier (1970)
	11-Deoxycorticosterone-14C	Adrenal microsomes (105,000 g sediment) + progesterone-14C	3.85 µg/mg protein/min; enzymic study[m]				Leblanc *et al.* (1970) Leblanc (1970)
	19-Hydroxy-11-deoxycorticosterone-14C	Adrenal mitochondria + 11-deoxycorticosterone-4-14C; 3H marker added	1.0%	PC, TLC, Ip-nmrc, Der, C 3H/14C D	Pr	NA	Mehdi and Sandor (1971)

301

TABLE V (cont.)

Species	Steroid[a]	Source of steroid	Quantity (μg/100 mg tissue or % transformation)	Major criteria[b]	Rating[b]		Reference
					Identity	Quantity	
	11β-Hydroxyand-rost-4-ene-3,17-dione-[14]C	Adrenal mito-chondria + tes-tosterone-4-^{14}C; ^{3}H markers added	3.0%	PC, Ip-nmrc–Der(Ox), CryC ^{3}H/[14]C D	Pr	Po, T	Mehdi and Sandor (1971)
	11β,17β-Dihyd-roxyandrost-4-en-3-one-[14]C		60.0%	PC, Ip-nmrc–Der(Ox), CryC ^{3}H/[14]C D	Pr	Po, T	
	17β, 18-Dihyd-roxyandrost-4-en-3-one-[14]C		2.0%	PC, TLC, Ip-nmrc	Su	NA	
	11β-Hydroxyand-rost-4-ene-3,17-dione-[14]C	Adrenal mito-chondria + androst-4-ene-3,17-dione-4-[14]C	38.0%	PC, Ip-nmrc–Der(Ox), CryC ^{3}H/[14]C D	Pr	Po, T	Mehdi and Sandor (1971)
	19-Hydroxyand-rost-4-ene-3,17-dione-[14]C		1.0%	PC, TLC, Ip-nmrc, CryCSA	Te	NA	
	Testosterone-[14]C		32.0	PC, Ip-nmrc–Der, CryC ^{3}H/[14]C D	Pr	Po, T	
Gallus domesticus (chicken)	11-Deoxycorti-costerone-[14]C	Adrenal homo-genate of 14-day-old chicken embryo adrenal explants in-cubated with sodium acetate-1-^{14}C for 24 hr	ID	TLC, Ip-nmrc–SD	Su	NA	Bonhommet and Weniger (1967)

| Corticosterone-^{14}C | ID | TLC, Ip–nmrc–SD | Su | NA |
| Aldosterone-^{14}C | ID | TLC, Ip–nmrc–SD | Su | NA |

[a] Abbreviations: 18-OH B, 18-hydroxycorticosterone; DOC, deoxycorticosterone.

[b] For an explanation of abbreviations and rating system, see Chapter 2, Tables I–IV.

[c] 50 μg angiotensin II per 100 mg tissue.

[d] 25 μg angiotensin II per 100 mg tissue.

[e] Chicken adenohypophysis extract.

[f] Hypophysectomized.

[g] Mean of values obtained by ultraviolet spectrophotometry and colorimetric reaction with blue tetrazolium.

[h] Avian adenohypophyseal HCl extract.

[i] For criteria and rating see under Sandor et al. (1963b).

[j] For substances isolated, criteria, and rating see under Sandor et al. (1963b).

[k] Same compounds isolated as in Sandor et al. (1963b), labeled with ^{3}H, ^{14}C; for criteria and rating see under Sandor et al. (1963b) and Sandor and Lanthier (1963b).

[l] Same compounds isolated as in Sandor et al. (1966a). Sample identification of progesterone-^{3}H (Te). 11-deoxycorticosterone-^{14}C (Pr), corticosterone-^{3}H, ^{14}C. (Pr), 18-hydroxycorticosterone-^{14}C,^{3}H (Te), and aldosterone-^{3}H, ^{14}C. Kinetic data obtained on nonmodified radioactive compounds following paper partition chromatography in two systems. Identity rating: Su: Quantity rating: Te, S.

[m] For criteria and rating see under Sandor et al. (1963b) and Sandor and Lanthier (1963b).

303

lished that in rat and beef adrenals, the zona glomerulosa is the only source of aldosterone, while all the 17-hydroxylating activity is localized in the two inner zones. The main steroids produced by the zona glomerulosa of beef adrenals are corticosterone, aldosterone, and 18-hydroxycorticosterone. This pattern is qualitatively extremely similar to the steroid-secretion pattern of amphibian, reptilian, and bird adrenals. However, histologically, adrenal cells from nonmammalian vertebrates resemble the cells of the zona fasciculata of mammals (Gorbman and Bern, 1966). The functional zonation of the mammalian adrenal is not as complete as it was previously thought to be. Mitochondria and homogenates of the two inner zones of beef adrenals were shown to form 18-hydroxycorticosterone from corticosterone, although no aldosterone synthesis was detected (Marusic and Mulrow, 1967). In addition, the adrenals in the order Rodentia do not produce 17-hydroxycorticosteroids although histological zones common to mammalian adrenals are present (Dorfman and Ungar, 1965). In consequence, the adrenals of nonmammalian vertebrates cannot be represented as incomplete mammalian adrenals. The capacity of most mammalian adrenals to hydroxylate steroids at the C-17 position does not represent a higher evolutionary step, as this capacity is shared with the teleost fish. (Chapter 4). It is believed that evolutionary ranking of the adrenal secretory pattern of vertebrates is not justified at the present state of our knowledge.

III. The Biosynthesis of Corticosteroids in the Amphibian, Reptilian, and Avian Adrenal Gland

We have seen in the previous sections that the adrenals of all three vertebrate classes investigated secrete corticosterone, aldosterone, and 18-hydroxycorticosterone as the major steroid hormones. While none of these substances was positively identified according to the criteria of classical organic chemistry (a possible exception might be 18-hydroxycorticosterone-^{14}C, which has been isolated from *Rana catesbeiana* incubates by Ulick and Kusch, 1960), enough presumptive evidence has been accumulated to accept the identity of these steroids as genuine. Thus, there is justification to take a closer look at the biochemical processes which are responsible for the biosynthesis of these steroids in the various adrenal glands. The nature of adrenal hormone secretion in amphibian, reptilian, and avian adrenal glands seems to be, on the whole, identical and there is a close relation with the biochemical profile of the mammalian zona glomerulosa. Ideally, the biosynthesis of corticosteroids should be discussed separately for each vertebrate class. However, we do not have enough data for such a detailed review.

Our review of the available information on the biosynthetic routes operating in lower-vertebrate adrenals will hardly be more than the description and evaluation of experiments performed on a single species of any class. In addition, all the major corticosteroids isolated from amphibian, reptilian, or avian adrenals have been previously described as occurring in mammalian adrenals. Thus, while reviewing their biosynthesis in lower vertebrates, it is necessary to discuss the results obtained in experiments using mammalian adrenals. This should not mean that a given corticosteroid is biosynthesized in all adrenal cells by identical processes. This cannot be determined until the adrenal steroid secretion of a statistically significant number of non-mammalian species has been investigated.

The review of the biosynthesis of corticosteroids will be essentially limited to the investigation of the sequence by which a given precursor is transformed to presumed end products, although in later sections the possible mechanism of these transformations will be discussed. Thus, we shall attempt to establish precursor–product relationships even though it is fully realized that the experimental methods are full of uncertainties and hedged in by restrictive qualifications. It will take some time until sufficient data have accumulated to give more authoritative opinions. It is hoped that all the qualifying statements and contradictory interpretations will have a stimulatory rather than discouraging effect on the reader.

A. The Mechanism of Steroid Hydroxylation

In the last few years, some important advances have been made regarding our understanding of steroid hydroxylation reactions. Since most reactions in the vertebrate adrenocortical cells in connection with steroid hormone synthesis involve the introduction of primary, secondary, or tertiary alcohol groups, it was felt that a brief review of the modern biochemical aspects of steroid hormone biosynthesis might be in order. Most of these studies have been performed with mammalian adrenal gland preparations although some of the results obtained have been applied to or even expanded by using lower-vertebrate adrenal tissue.

Studies with mammalian cell-free preparations have shown that there is no common intracellular site of location of steroid-metabolizing enzymes. The cholesterol side chain cleavage system was found in the mitochondria (Halkerston *et al.*, 1961) as were the 11β-hydroxylase (Sweat, 1951) and 18-oxygenase systems. These latter systems will be discussed in some detail in Section III,D. On the other hand, the enzyme systems responsible for 17α-hydroxylation and 21-hydroxylation were found to be associated with the microsomes (endoplasmic reticulum) (Ryan and Engel, 1957). Thus, according to the present concept, the steroid molecule is transported back and forth between mitochondria and microsomes, although apparently the mechanism of mitochondrial and microsomal hydroxylation is not dissimilar.

Studies undertaken in this reviewer's laboratory demonstrated a very similar intracellular distribution of steroid hydroxylating enzyme systems in the adrenal cells of nonmammalian vertebrates. A comparative study of the microsomal C-21 hydroxylase (EC 1.14.1.8) in the bullfrog *Rana catesbeiana*, the snake *Natrix sp.* and the duck *Anas platyrhynchos* yielded data showing that microsomal 21-hydroxylation is accomplished by very similar mechanisms in the above mentioned three species of nonmammalian vertebrates and differed very little from those established in the adrenocortical microsomes of mammals (Leblanc, 1970; Sandor *et al.* 1972a).

About 15 years ago, Tomkins and co-workers (1957) indicated that adrenal steroid hydroxylating systems were multicomponent. A better understanding of the nature of these systems was achieved following the studies of Estabrook *et al.* (1963) of adrenocortical microsomal 21-hydroxylation of 17α-hydroxyprogesterone. They have established that this hydroxylation reaction is catalyzed by a mixed-function oxidase and uses NADPH as cofactor. In addition, they have shown that a hemoprotein, denoted as cytochrome P-450, is the oxygen-activating enzyme. The stoichiometry for 21-hydroxylation of steroids was represented as follows:

$$17\alpha\text{-Hydroxyprogesterone} + H^+ + O_2 + NADPH \longrightarrow$$
$$17\alpha,21\text{-dihydroxypregn-4-ene-3,20-dione} + H_2O + NADP$$

Cytochrome P-450 was isolated from bovine liver microsomes (Omura and Sato, 1964). adrenocortical microsomes (Estabrook *et al.*, 1963), and adrenocortical mitochondria (Harding *et al.*, 1964). In rat adrenal mitochondria, P-450 was found in concentrations from two to seven times that of any of the other cytochromes of the respiratory chain (Harding and Nelson, 1966). Subsequently, the presence of the pigment was demonstrated in bullfrog (*Rana catesbeiana*) and human adrenal mitochondria (Greengard *et al.*, 1967; Wilson *et al.*, 1968). Cytochrome P-450 is a hemoprotein and in its reduced (Fe^{2+}) form readily combines with carbon monoxide. The P-450–Fe^{2+}–CO complex is inactive and exhibits a characteristic light absorption band with a unique maximum at 450 mμ. The CO complex undergoes photochemical dissociation by irradiation with monochromatic light of 450 mμ wavelength (Estabrook *et al.*, 1963; Cooper *et al.*, 1965).

Further studies have shown that P-450 is the terminal oxygenase of an electron-transport system consisting of a NADP-linked flavoprotein dehydrogenase (Fp) and a nonheme iron protein similar to spinach ferredoxin. The latter substance was isolated from pig adrenal mitochondria and termed adrenodoxin by Suzuki and Kimura (1965). Omura *et al.* (1966) isolated the NADP-linked flavoprotein, adrenodoxin, and cytochrome P-450 from beef adrenal mitochondria. They succeeded in fragmenting and reconstituting the system and established that it is obligatory for adrenal 11β-hydroxylation. They proposed the following scheme:

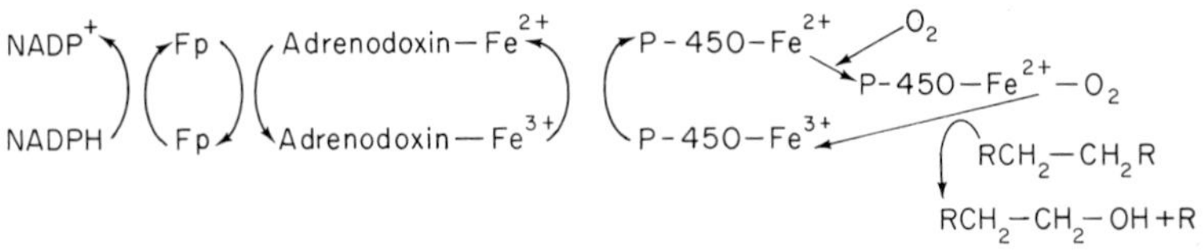

$$
\begin{array}{c}
\text{NADP}^+ \searrow \quad \nearrow \text{Fp} \searrow \quad \nearrow \text{Adrenodoxin} - \text{Fe}^{2+} \nwarrow \quad \nearrow \text{P-450}-\text{Fe}^{2+} \nwarrow \quad \nearrow \text{O}_2 \\
\text{NADPH} \nearrow \quad \searrow \text{Fp} \nearrow \quad \searrow \text{Adrenodoxin} - \text{Fe}^{3+} \nearrow \quad \searrow \text{P-450}-\text{Fe}^{3+}
\end{array}
$$

P-450$-$Fe^{2+} $-$O$_2$

RCH$_2$$-CH_2$R

RCH$_2$$-CH_2$$-$OH $+$R

Metopirone [2-methyl-1,2-bis(3-pyridil)-1-propanone], a known inhibitor of adrenal 11β-hydroxylation, apparently combines with P-450, thereby blocking the interaction of the pigment with the steroid substrate (Wilson *et al.*, 1968).

Thus, P-450$-$Fe^{2+} reacts with molecular oxygen and one atom of oxygen is utilized to reoxidize the pigment, while the other is introduced as a hydroxyl group into the steroid substrate. This electron-transport system is probably paralleled by the "classical" electron-transport chain involving NADH, NADH-reductase, coenzyme Q, cytochrome b and cytochrome c, and a system. The two chains could be linked through a NADH—NADPH transhydrogenase. The P-450 system would allow the entry of Krebs cycle dehydrogenases into the latter.

In addition to the 21- and 11β-hydroxylase systems, the P-450 mechanism is probably involved in the oxidative cleavage of cholesterol [mitochondrial 20α- and 22-hydroxylase (Simpson and Boyd, 1966)] and 18-oxygenation of corticosterone. Details of the last reaction are in Section III,D.

One of the particularities of the mitochondrial and microsomal cytochrome P-450 systems is that addition of various substances to mitochondrial and microsomal suspensions induces so-called difference spectra (spectra of a suspension without the additive read against a suspension containing the additive). Steroids such as 17α-hydroxyprogesterone, 11-deoxycorticosterone, and corticosterone induce difference spectra. In general, two types of steroid-induced difference spectra have been found. The so-called "type I" is characterized by a maximum between 380 and 390 mμ and a trough at 420 mμ, while "type II" is more or less the mirror image of type I and exhibits a trough around 380–390 mμ and a maximum at 420 mμ. Detailed descriptions of these difference spectra are given by Mitani and Horie (1969). Presently, much very relevant work is being done on the mechanism of steroid hydroxylation and it is probably one of the most active fields in steroid biochemistry. For detailed and up-to-date reviews, see Sih and Whitlock (1968) Sih (1969) and Simpson *et al.* (1969).

B. The Incorporation of Acetate and Cholesterol into Corticosteroids

In vivo and *in vitro* studies with mammalian adrenal cortices have established cholesterol as a precursor of corticosteroids. In addition, it has been shown that the mammalian adrenal gland has the capability of synthesizing cholesterol and corticosteroids from two-carbon fragments (Grant, 1962; Dorfman and Ungar, 1965). According to the present concept of mammalian adrenal steroid biochemistry, the initial steps in the synthesis of corticosteroids consist in the building up of the cyclopentanoperhydrophenanthrene skeleton from two-carbon fragments, yielding cholesterol as the key intermediary (Conforth, 1959). Cholesterol in turn undergoes hydroxylation at C-20 and C-22 and under the influence of a side-chain-splitting enzyme yields pregnenolone (Hechter and Pincus, 1954). Pregnenolone serves as precursor for both 17-oxygenated and 17-deoxycorticosteroids in mammals (Grant, 1962). In the previous sections of this chapter we have seen that pregnenolone can be regarded as a universal precursor of corticosteroids in these nonmammalian vertebrates as well. Thus, any discussion of biosynthetic mechanism has to start with the initial steps mentioned above.

The transformation of sodium acetate to adrenal cholesterol and corticosteroids was studied in the American bullfrog by Mehdi and Carballeira (1971b) and in the painted turtle by Mehdi (1969). In spite of the utilization of a variety of experimental conditions, adrenal gland preparations of neither species formed cholesterol and/or corticosteroids from exogenous sodium acetate *in vitro*. On the other hand, using very similar experimental conditions, Sandor *et al.* (1965) were able to demonstrate the transformation of exogenous sodium acetate-1-^{14}C to ^{14}C-labeled adrenal cholesterol and ^{14}C-labeled corticosterone, 18-hydroxycorticosterone, and aldosterone by adrenal slices of the domestic duck and goose. The presence of ACTH was required to obtain significant transformation. The specific activity of the isolated adrenal cholesterol was significantly lower than that of the corticosterone-^{14}C isolated from the same experiment (ratio of specific activities of corticosterone-^{14}C–cholesterol-^{14}C: duck, 31.3; goose, 16.9). Results indicating such an apparent nonparticipation of adrenal cholesterol in steroid synthesis have also been obtained in experiments utilizing mammalian adrenal preparations (Grant, 1962). Several hypotheses were brought forward to explain this phenomenon in mammals (Samuels, 1960; Hechter and Pincus, 1954; Saba and Hechter, 1955). However, none of these hypotheses, including the one postulating the existence of an extracholesterol biosynthetic pathway, has been fully substantiated. It would appear that at least in mammals, the question of whether cholesterol is an obligatory precursor of corticosteroids *in vivo* has been settled partly by feeding experiments in the guinea pig and the dog (Werbin and Chaikoff, 1961; Krum *et al.*, 1964). Thus, the specific activity differences encountered could be explained either by kinetic phenomena (Zilversmit *et al.*, 1943) or by the double pool theory (Saba and Hechter, 1955) or again by a biosynthetic route which under *in vitro* conditions bypasses cholesterol (Heard *et al.*, 1956). Experimental evidence at hand is insufficient to allow a choice of these alternatives.

The capacity of bird adrenals to metabolize acetate to corticosteroids apparently appears very early in life. Bonhommet and Weniger (1967) presented suggestive evidence that adrenals of 14-day-old chick embryos were capable of transforming sodium acetate-1-^{14}C into ^{14}C-labeled corticosterone, 11-deoxycorticosterone, and aldosterone.

The inability of anuran and reptilian adrenals to build up the steroid skeleton from two-carbon fragments might suggest a class-correlated biochemical evolution in the enzyme profile of the adrenal tissue. Such a hypothesis is also supported by the inability of teleost adrenal tissue to incorporate exogenous sodium acetate into cholesterol *in vitro* (Sandor *et al.*, 1966b).

Once cholesterol is available, however, adrenals of amphibians, reptiles, and birds are capable of side chain scission and subsequent hydroxylation. Mehdi and Carballeira (1971b) reported the transformation of cholesterol-^{14}C into radioactive corticosteroids by adrenal homogenates and adrenal mitochondria of the bullfrog, and Mehdi (1969) described similar transformations using adrenal homogenates and adrenal mitochondria of the painted turtle *Chrysemys picta picta* as the sources of enzymes. On the other hand, Chan and Edwards (1970) were unable to obtain the transformation cholesterol ⟶ corticosteroids with adrenal homogenates of the South African toad *Xenopus laevis*. However, their negative results might have been due to a failure to supply exogenous NADPH, which seems to be essential for cholesterol side chain cleavage (see Section III,D). Sandor *et al.* (1965) reported the transformation of radioactive cholesterol to corticosterone by domestic duck adrenal homogenates. The incorporation of cholesterol-^{3}H of high specific activity into quartered chicken adrenals was reported by Hall and Koritz (1966) using Tween 80 as a solubilizing agent. Sandor and associates (1965) reported difficulties in obtaining the biotransformation of cholesterol-4-^{14}C with duck adrenal slices despite the use of several physiological spreading agents (beef serum albumin, egg albumin, homologous duck plasma, sodium taurocholate, etc.), and similar difficulties were encountered by Mehdi and Carballeira (1971b) when bullfrog adrenal gland sections were used, even when Tween 80 was added. The use of this detergent allowed Hall and Koritz to demonstrate the stimulating effect *in vitro* of mammalian ACTH in the utilization of exogenous cholesterol. However, it is not quite clear why the penetration of cholesterol into the isolated adrenal gland should take place only in the presence of a synthetic nonphysiological spreading agent. It has to be mentioned that duck adrenal slices failed to incorporate cholesteryl-4-^{14}C oleate or cholesteryl-4-^{14}C linoleate.

Thus, at present we can conclude that the biosynthetic sequence acetate $\longrightarrow$ cholesterol does not exist in the one species of each of the amphibians and reptiles investigated, but in the three species of bird, namely the domestic duck, the goose, and the chicken, the formation of cholesterol from two-carbon fragments can be accepted as proven. On the other hand, adrenal gland preparations of the frog, turtle, duck, and chicken were capable of cholesterol side chain cleavage *in vitro*. These data seem to support the hypothesis that in vertebrates, plasma cholesterol is the only or the chief substrate of adrenal corticosteroid hormone synthesis (Werbin and Chaikoff, 1961).

C. The Biosynthetic Pathway Pregnenolone $\longrightarrow$ Corticosteroids

Mammalian adrenal steroid biochemistry has established that the transformation of cholesterol to corticosteroids involves pregnenolone as an obligatory intermediary. This steroid can be regarded as the common precursor of both 17-deoxy- and 17-hydroxycorticosteroids. There is general agreement that the biosynthesis of corticosterone from pregnenolone involves the transformation of pregnenolone to progesterone by the action of the Δ^5-3β-hydroxysteroid dehydrogenase-isomerase. The sequence of hydroxylation is normally accepted as occurring at C-21 and C-11, in that order, giving rise to the pathway pregnenolone $\longrightarrow$ progesterone $\longrightarrow$ 11-deoxycorticosterone $\longrightarrow$ corticosterone (Grant, 1962). Corticosterone in turn was shown to be the precursor of aldosterone and 18-hydroxycorticosterone in the mammalian adrenal (Mulrow and Cohn, 1959; Stachenko and Giroud, 1962, 1964; Sandor and Lanthier, 1963a; Davis *et al.*, 1966). In mammalian steroid biochemistry it is customary to deal separately with the biosynthesis of corticosterone and aldosterone. This rather illogical distinction stems no doubt from the observation that in mammalian adrenals, aldosterone is specifically elaborated by the *zona glomerulosa* (Ayres *et al.*, 1956; Stachenko and Giroud, 1959), while corticosterone is synthesized by the outer and the two inner zones. Such functional zonation has not yet been detected in the adrenals of any of the nonmammalian vertebrates. Thus in discussing the biosynthesis of corticosteroids in these animal classes, the entire pathway from pregnenolone to aldosterone has to be considered.

Data presented in Sections III,B and C clearly show that the above-described corticosteroid biosynthetic pathway found in mammalian adrenals is present in the adrenals of amphibians, reptiles, and birds and constitutes the main sequence of transformation of pregnenolone to aldo-sterone. However, in the last few years evidence has accumulated that this pathway is not necessarily the only one by which pregnenolone is transformed to corticosteroids. The presence of alternate biosynthetic routes has been suggested both in mammalian and lower-vertebrate adrenals.

In the generally accepted scheme of steroid biosynthesis, pregnenolone has to be transformed to progesterone before it can enter the chain of sequen-tial hydroxylation. Studies on the formation of cortisol in vitro by mamma-lian adrenals have shown that this is not always true. Cortisol is synthesized from pregnenolone via 17α-hydroxypregnenolone or 21-hydroxypre-gnenolone by adrenal glands of several mammalian species (Weliky and Engel, 1962; Mulrow et al., 1962; Pasqualini et al., 1964; Klein and Giroud, 1967; Cameron et al., 1968a) and by adrenal tissue preparations of a teleost fish, the European eel (Sandor et al., 1966b; Sandor et al., 1967). This so called Δ^5 pathway is quantitatively more important in the biosynthesis of cortisol than the one proceeding through progesterone. Indications have been obtained that a similar mechanism exists in the adrenal gland of birds, al-though these glands do not synthesize appreciable amounts of cortisol. Sandor and associates (1963b) noted that incubation of a mixture of tritiated pregnenolone and ^{14}C-labeled progesterone with duck adrenal slices yielded only small amounts of progesterone-^3H. This observation was later confirmed by experiments in which the time course of the incorporation in vitro of pregnenolone into progesterone was studied again using duck adrenal slices (Sandor et al., 1966a; Sandor, 1969a,b). While no hydroxylated pregn-5-en-3β-ol intermediary was isolated, circumstantial evidence suggested that the transformation of pregnenolone to aldosterone proceeds in part through the sequential hydroxylation of pregn-5-en-3β-ol intermediaries. The existence of more than one biosynthetic sequence in the adrenal gland of the duck was disputed by Whitehouse and Vinson (1967). They reported data obtained by the incubation of duck adrenal minces with tritium- and ^{14}C-labeled precursor–product pairs in an experimental setup very similar to that of Sandor et al., (1966a). While the results obtained by the two groups were not dissimilar, Whitehouse and Vinson interpreted the temporal variations of the isotope content of the metabolites as indicative of a pregnenolone $\longrightarrow$ progesterone $\longrightarrow$ 11-deoxycorticosterone sequence. More recently, Vinson and Whitehouse (1969a) reported studies in which duck adrenal minces were incubated with an equimolar mixture of tritiated pregnenolone and ^{14}C-

labeled progesterone. The course of the reaction was followed for 6hr and samples withdrawn from the incubation mixture were analyzed for the presence of radioactive steroid transformation products. At the same time, the mass of these metabolites was also measured by a gas–liquid chromatographic technique (Vinson and Whitehouse, 1969b). They drew the conclusion that exogenous precursors did not form a homogeneous pool with endogenous substrates originating from the tissue. On the other hand, they underlined their previous contention (Whitehouse and Vinson, 1967) that progesterone and especially 11-deoxycorticosterone were important intermediaries in corticosterone biosynthesis both from added substrates and from endogenous precursors. While the large-scale transformation of pregnenolone to progesterone by duck adrenal gland preparations could not be confirmed (Sandor, 1969a,b), the intermediary role of 11-deoxycorticosterone was investigated in more detail.

Hydroxylations of progesterone play a leading role in the biosynthesis of corticosteroids and the study of the sequence of these hydroxylations has some biochemical interest. It was originally suggested that hydroxylation at the 11β position could not be followed by hydroxylation at another position. However, evidence to the contrary has been forthcoming from experiments using both mammalian and lower-vertebrate adrenal gland preparations. Brownie *et al.* (1954) demonstrated the formation of 11β-hydroxyprogesterone by mammalian adrenal mitochondrial preparations and suggested its possible intermediary role. Giroud *et al.* (1958) and Stachenko and Giroud (1959, 1964) found that 11β-hydroxyprogesterone was freely transformed to corticosterone and aldosterone. They concluded that in the zona glomerulosa of beef adrenals the sequence of hydroxylation may proceed in the order $11 \longrightarrow 21$ as efficiently as, if not more efficiently than, in the reverse order. Subsequently, Kraulis and Birmingham (1964) presented preliminary evidence for the transformation of 11β-hydroxyprogesterone to corticosterone and aldosterone by adrenal preparations of the leopard frog *Rana pipiens*. Sandor and associates (1963b) isolated and tentatively identified [3]H- and ^{14}C-labeled 11β-hydroxyprogesterone following the incubation of a mixture of pregnenolone-^{3}H and progesterone-^{14}C with duck adrenal slices. The isotope composition of the presumed 11β-hydroxyprogesterone-^{3}H,[14]C was not inconsistent with the $11\beta \longrightarrow 21$ hydroxylation sequence. Further studies along these lines showed that under condition of substrate saturation, pregnenolone-^{14}C was transformed in good yield to corticosterone, and the presence of significant amounts of 11β-hydroxyprogesterone could also be demonstrated (Sandor, 1969b) when duck adrenal slices were used as the metabolizing tissue. Further proof that in the duck adrenal 11β-hydroxyprogesterone can serve as an efficient precursor of corticosterone, 18-hydroxycorticosterone, and aldosterone was furnished by Sandor and Lanthier

(1970). From these experiments it was concluded that in the duck adrenal, both the C-11, C-21 and C-21, C-11 hydroxylation sequences are equally important under *in vitro* conditions. Similar conclusions were arrived at by Tsang and Stachenko (1969) working with rat adrenal preparations.

It was mentioned earlier in this section that corticosterone has been regarded as the immediate precursor of aldosterone in the mammalian adrenal. The transformation of exogenous progesterone, 11β-hydroxyprogesterone, and 11-deoxycorticosterone to aldosterone could be visualized through the transformation of these substrates to corticosterone, which in turn would be metabolized to aldosterone. The position of corticosterone as the immediate precursor of aldosterone was challenged, however, following the discovery of 18-oxygenated steroids of adrenal origin. One of these compounds was 18-hydroxy-11-deoxycorticosterone, secreted in large amounts by the adrenal gland of the rat (Birmingham and Ward, 1961; Péron, 1961); the other, 18-hydroxycorticosterone, was first isolated by Ulick and Kusch (1960) from *in vitro* incubation systems using adrenal slices of the bullfrog and progesterone as exogenous substrate. 18-Hydroxycorticosterone was subsequently identified as a product of the adrenal glands of the rat (Péron, 1962), the ox (Ulick and Kusch-Vetter, 1962; Sandor and Lanthier, 1963a), the duck (Sandor and Lanthier, 1963b) and the turtle (Sandor *et al.*, 1964). The biosynthesis of 18-hydroxycorticosterone by human adrenal glands has been demonstrated both *in vitro* (Sandor and Lanthier, 1963a) and *in vivo* (Ulick and Kusch-Vetter, 1965). These latter studies have shown that the production of 18-hydroxycorticosterone is on the average two to three times greater than aldosterone and the production rate of both substances changes in a parallel manner under physiological stimuli. Thus, according to our present knowledge, all adrenal glands which synthesize aldosterone also produce 18-hydroxycorticosterone. This is not true for 18-hydroxy-11-deoxycorticosterone. This steroid is secreted only by the adrenals of some mammalian species and teleost fish (Chapter 4).

18-Hydroxycorticosterone seems to be produced by the zona glomerulosa of mammalian adrenals, although contrary evidence has been presented by Marusic and Mulrow (1967).

All these findings strongly suggest that 18-hydroxycorticosterone is the immediate precursor of aldosterone in all vertebrate aldosterone-producing species and the adrenal biosynthetic sequence corticosterone $\longrightarrow$ 18-hydroxycorticosterone $\longrightarrow$ aldosterone should be the main route for aldosterone biosynthesis. However, direct incubation of avian or amphibian adrenal gland preparations with exogenous corticosterone did not yield any aldosterone (Nicolis and Ulick, 1965; Lamoureux, 1966; Psychoyos *et al.*, 1966; Sandor, 1969b). On the other hand, mammalian adrenals when reacted in the presence of exogenous 18-hydroxycorticosterone, yielded small but identifiable amounts of aldosterone (Sandor and Lanthier, 1963a; Pasqualini, 1964; Kahnt and Neher, 1965; Raman *et al.* 1966; Fazekas and Sandor, 1969). There seem to be indications that mammalian and nonmammalian adrenals differ in their ability to accept 18-hydroxycorticosterone as aldosterone substrate, and also in their ability to form aldosterone through 11-dehydrocorticosterone and 11-dehydro-18-hydroxycorticosterone (Fazekas and Sandor, 1969; Sharma, 1970). It has to be emphasized, however, that even when mammalian adrenal preparations are used, the yield of aldosterone from 18-hydroxycorticosterone is much smaller than the yield from corticosterone or other 18-deoxysteroids of the biosynthetic chain. The question of aldosterone biosynthesis will be discussed in more detail in Section III,D.

While their biochemical or physiological significance is still not well understood, some reactions recently shown to be performed by duck adrenal mitochondria should be mentioned. These reactions are 19-hydroxylation of 11-deoxycorticosterone and androstenedione, the presumed 18-hydroxylation of testosterone, the 11β-hydroxylation of testosterone and androstenedione, and the reversible interconversion of testosterone and androstenedione. The biosynthesis of both testosterone and androstenedione is thought to require 17α-hydroxylating enzyme systems. These systems are absent in avian adrenals; thus the acceptence of duck adrenal mitochondria of these C_{19} substances as substrates for hydroxylation and oxidoreductase reactions might be regarded as an artificial but interesting biochemical event (Mehdi and Sandor, 1971).

While in all three vertebrate classes reviewed the biosynthesis of corticosteroids seems to be accomplished by mechanisms more or less identical, in experiments using reptilian adrenal gland preparations an apparent dissociation has been noticed between the secretion of steroids from endogenous precursors and the metabolism of added substrates. All authors have mentioned this lack of correlation (Phillips *et al.*, 1962; Sandor *et al.*, 1964; Macchi and Phillips, 1966). Following the incubation of turtle adrenal slices with progesterone-^{14}C, Sandor and associates (1964) found that the specific activity of the resultant corticosterone was four times higher than aldo-

---

Fig. 2. Schematic representation of the biosynthesis of corticosteroids by the adrenals of amphibians, reptiles, and birds. Validated pathways are shown by heavy arrows, possible or hypothetical ones by broken arrows. Key to compounds: I, acetyl-CoA; II, cholesterol; III, pregnenolone; IV, progesterone; V, 11-deoxycorticosterone; VI, corticosterone; VII, aldosterone; VIII, 18-hydroxycorticosterone 20——→ 18 cyclic hemiketal; IX, 11-hydroxyprogesterone; X, 11-dehydrocorticosterone; XI, cortisol; XII, 19-hydroxy-11-deoxycorticosterone. A detailed rating of the validity of these reactions, together with relevant references, are shown in Table VI.

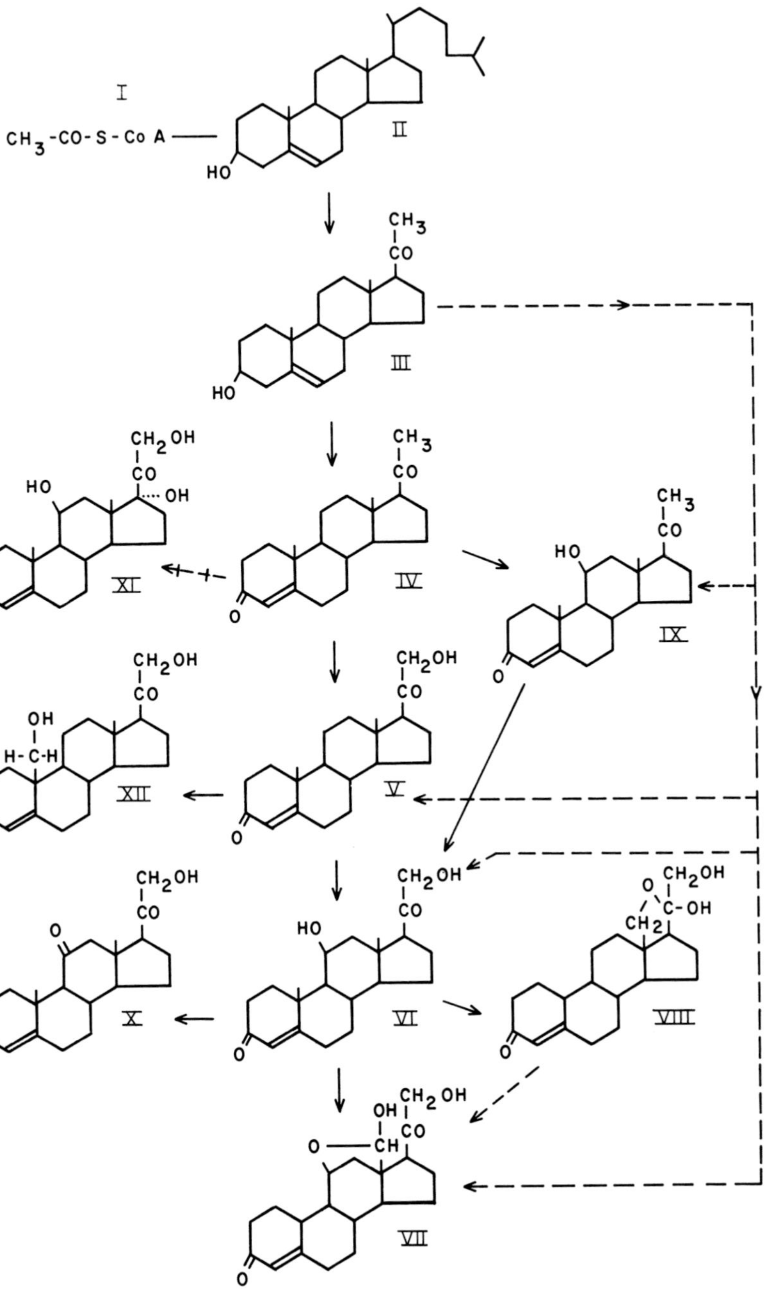
I
CH3-CO-S-CoA
II
HO
CH3
CO
III
HO
CH2OH
CO
HO
OH
XI
O
CH3
CO
IV
O
CH3
CO
HO
IX
O
CH2OH
CO
OH
H-C-H
XII
O
CH2OH
CO
V
O
CH2OH
CO
O
X
O
CH2OH
CO
HO
VI
O
O
CH2OH
C-OH
CH2
VIII
O
CH2OH
OH
CO
O
CH
VII
O

sterone and twice that of the biosynthetic 18-hydroxycorticosterone. A straightforward explanation of this phenomenon is rather difficult. Several possibilities have been envisaged: leaching-out of preformed metabolites from the adrenal tissue during incubation, the existence of biosynthetic pathways bypassing progesterone, etc. However, the most plausible explanation of these unequal specific activities can be derived from the principles laid down by Zilversmit *et al.* (1943) on the temporal behavior of specific activities of precursor–product pairs. In none of the reptile experiments quoted were the changes in specific activities measured at different time intervals during the incubations. Thus more work is necessary to find an explanation for this apparent divergence between the metabolism of endogenous and exogenous substrates.

On the basis of our present knowledge, Fig. 2 and Table VI show a composite picture of the known biosynthetic reactions that occur in the adrenal glands of amphibians, reptiles, and birds. The biotransformations have been given a rating in Table VI. This rating simply serves to distinguish well-established reactions from doubtful or hypothetical ones.

The general conclusion one can draw from Fig. 2 could be summarized as follows. None of the biotransformations, either established on the basis of irrefutable chemical data or postulated on the basis of circumstantial evidence, is unique for any one of the vertebrate classes here reviewed. In addition, all these reactions have their parallels in mammalian adrenals. It has to be emphasized that all we know today about lower-vertebrate adrenal steroid hormone biosynthesis has been obtained by the *in vitro* methodology, using exogenous substrates. Thus all we can say at present is that a given steroidal substrate incubated with surviving adrenals of an amphibian, reptile, or bird, will be metabolized along the lines indicated in Fig. 2. Whether this picture represents the biosynthesis of the native steroid hormones as well is still very much an open question.

D. The Biosynthesis of Aldosterone by Adrenal Mitochondria

In the previous sections we described the biosynthesis of steroids by adrenal slices, minces, and homogenates and occasionally we referred to experiments performed with adrenal mitochondria. In nonmammalian vertebrates, study of the steroid-metabolizing enzymes in the intracellular fractions of adrenal cells is still in its infancy. However, an understanding of the intimate mechanism of the biosynthetic process can be achieved only through the study and characterization of the different enzyme systems involved. The transformation of corticosterone to aldosterone and 18-hydroxycorticosterone is one of the few systems which has been studied in some

TABLE VI

Biosynthesis of Corticosteroids by the Adrenals of Amphibians, Birds, and Reptiles *in Vitro*

Transformation[a]	Class	Species	Rating[b]	Reference
I→II	Aves	*Anas platyrhynchos*	Po	Sandor *et al.* (1965)
	Aves	*Anser anser*	Po	Sandor *et al.* (1965)
I→VI,VII,VIII	Aves	*Anas platyrhynchos*	Po	Sandor *et al.* (1965)
	Aves	*Anser anser*	Po	Sandor *et al.* (1965)
II→VI	Aves	*Anas platyrhynchos*	Po	Sandor *et al.* (1965)
	Aves	*Gallus domesticus*	Po	Hall and Koritz (1966)
III→IV,V,VI,VII,VIII	Amphibia	*Rana pipiens*	Po	Lamoureux (1966)
	Reptilia	*Chrysemys picta*	Po	Sandor *et al.* (1964)
	Aves	*Anas platyrhynchos*	Po	Sandor *et al.* (1963b)
	Aves	*Gallus domesticus*	Po	Sandor *et al.* (1963b)
	Aves	*Anser anser*	Po	Lamoureux *et al.* (1964)
III→V	Aves	*Anas platyrhynchos*	CE	Sandor *et al.* (1963b), Sandor (1969a)
III→VI	Aves	*Anas platyrhynchos*	CE	Sandor *et al.* (1963b), Sandor (1969a)
III→VII	Aves	*Anas platyrhynchos*	CE	Sandor *et al.* (1963b), Sandor (1969a)
IV→V,VI,VII,VIII	Amphibia	*Rana catesbeiana*	Po	Nicolis and Ulick (1965), Ulick and Solomon (1960), Ulick and Kusch (1960)
	Amphibia	*Rana pipiens*	Po	Lamoureux *et al.* (1964)
	Reptilia	*Pseudemys scripta*	Po	Sandor *et al.* (1964)
	Reptilia	*Chrysemys picta*	Po	Sandor *et al.* (1964)
	Aves	*Anas platyrhynchos*	Po	Sandor and Lanthier (1963b)
	Aves	*Gallus domesticus*	Po	Sandor *et al.* (1963b)
	Aves	*Anser anser*	Po	Lamoureux *et al.* (1964)
IV→VI,VII	Amphibia	*Bufo marinus*	Pr	Crabbé (1963)
	Reptilia	*Natrix natrix*	Pr	Phillips *et al.* (1962), Macchi and Phillips (1966)
	Reptilia	*Lacerta viridis*	Pr	Phillips *et al.* (1962)
	Reptilia	*Emys orbicularis*	Pr	Macchi and Phillips (1966)
	Reptilia	*Alligator mississipiensis*	Pr	Gist and de Roos (1966)
IV→IX	Aves	*Anas platyrhynchos*	Po	Sandor *et al.* (1963b)
	Aves	*Gallus domesticus*	Po	Sandor *et al.* (1963b)
IV→XI	Aves	*Anas platyrhynchos*	Pr–CE	Sandor and Lanthier (1963b)

TABLE VI (cont.)

Transformation[a]	Class	Species	Rating[b]	Reference
V→VI	Amphibia	*Rana catesbeiana*	Po	Nicolis and Ulick (1965)
	Amphibia	*Rana pipiens*	Pr	Kraulis and Birmingham (1964)
	Aves	*Anas platyrhynchos*	Po	Sandor (1969a,b)
VI→VII,VIII	Amphibia	*Rana catesbeiana*	Po	Nicolis and Ulick (1965), Psychoyos *et al.* (1966)
	Amphibia	*Rana pipiens*	Pr	Kraulis and Birmingham (1964)
	Aves	*Anas platyrhynchos*	Po	Sandor (1969a,b), Sandor *et al.* (1972b)
VIII→VII	Amphibia	*Rana catesbiana*	CE	Ulick and Solomon (1960)
IX→VI,VII,VIII	Aves	*Amas platyrhynchos*	Po	Sandor and Lanthier (1970)
IX→VI(IV→IX→VI)	Amphibia	*Rana pipiens*	Pr	Kraulis and Birmingham (1964)
	Aves	*Anas platyrhynchos*	Pr—CE	Sandor (1969b), Sandor and Lanthier (1970)
V→XII	Aves	*Anas platyrhynchos*	Pr	Mehdi and Sandor (1971)

[a]For a key to compounds (roman numerals), see legend to Fig. 2.
[b]The genuineness of a biotransformation was rated as follows: Po, positively established; Pr, probably occurring; CE, postulated on the basis of circumstantial evidence.

318

detail in nonmammalian classes by cell-free systems and as this transformation is still not completely understood, the relevant experiments will be described at some length.

In Section III,A, we briefly reviewed the present concept of steroid hydroxylation. It was mentioned that mammalian mitochondrial 11β-hydroxylation and microsomal 21-hydroxylation have been extensively investigated. These studies served as models for the subsequent attempts to resolve the problem of aldosterone synthesis. This reaction has the distinction that most of our recent knowledge of it has been gained from experiments using lower-vertebrate rather than mammalian adrenals.

In 1966, several publications appeared showing that 18-oxygenation of corticosterone was mainly effected by adrenal mitochondria. Raman et al. (1966) worked with mammalian adrenals, the group at Geigy corporation with bullfrog adrenals (Psychoyos et al., 1966), and Sandor and Lanthier (1966) with the adrenals of the domestic duck. The intracellular distribution of the 18-oxygenating systems in these classes is shown in Table VII. The presence of mitochondrial 18-oxygenase has also been demonstrated in the adrenals of the painted turtle (Mehdi, 1969). Both 18-hydroxycorticosterone and aldosterone were produced from corticosterone by these mitochondrial preparations. While at first approximation these 18-oxygenating systems seemed to have similar characteristics, more detailed investigations revealed important differences. All three required NADPH to furnish reducing equi-

TABLE VII

The Formation of Aldosterone and 18-Hydroxycorticosterone from Exogenous Corticosterone by Intracellular Fractions of Adrenal Gland Homogenates of Different Species of Vertebrates.

| | Steroid formation (% of that formed by homogenate) | | | | | |
| | Aldosterone | | | 18-OH-Corticosterone | | |
Adrenal preparation	Sheep[a]	Duck[b]	Frog[c]	Sheep[a]	Duck[b]	Frog[c]
Homogenate	100	100	100	100	100	100
Low-speed sediment (700–750g)		27	3		18	10
Mitochondrial fraction (6000–10,500 g sediment)	100	78	54	100	50	108
Microsomal fraction (105,000g sediment)	Trace	Trace	1	Trace	2	5
Soluble fraction (105,000g supernatant)	Trace	0	0	Trace	0	0

[a] Raman et al. (1966).
[b] Sandor and Lanthier (1966).
[c] Psychoyos et al. (1966).

valents (Sandor, 1969b, Sandor *et al.*, 1972b). In sheep mitochondria, Ca^{2+} was required, while Mg^{2+} and Ca^{2+} were necessary to maintain the reaction in bullfrog adrenals (Psychoyos *et al.*, 1966; Sharma *et al.*, 1967). In duck mitochondria, Ca^{2+} was more important than Mg^{2+}, although for optimal reaction Ca^{2+}, Mg^{2+}, Na^+, and K^+ were necessary (Sandor *et al.*, 1972b). Mitochondria of mammalian and nonmammalian origin showed important differences in substrate specificity. Sheep (Raman *et al.*, 1966) and rabbit (Fazekas and Sandor, 1969) transformed corticosterone to 11-dehydro-18-hydroxycorticosterone similarly to rhesus monkey adrenal homogenates (Sharma, 1970), but this reaction could not be shown to take place with either frog or duck preparations. Rabbit adrenal mitchondria transformed 11-dehydrocorticosterone to 11,18-hydroxycorticosterone and 11-dehydro-aldosterone (Fazekas and Sandor, 1969), a reaction also noted to take place with monkey adrenal homogenates (Sharma 1970). The above-described reaction sequence resulted ultimately in aldosterone and 18-hydroxycorticosterone formation through the reduction of the 11-oxo group to the β-oriented secondary alcohol. These reactions did not take place in either duck or frog adrenals (deNicola *et al.*, 1968; Sharma, 1970). In the sheep, mitochondria transformed exogenous corticosterone to seven times more 18-hydroxycorticosterone than aldosterone. In the duck, maximal formation of 18-oxygenated metabolites was 10.4 μg of 18-hydroxycorticosterone and 2.2 μg of aldosterone/10 min per mitochondria equivalent to 100 mg adrenal tissue (Sandor *et al.*, 1972b), while the corresponding figures for bullfrog preparations were 2.2 μg 18-hydroxycorticosterone and 4.2 μg aldosterone.

It was mentioned earlier that mammalian adrenals did form small but measurable amounts of aldosterone from exogenous 18-hydroxycorticosterone, while such a reaction could not be substantiated with adrenal preparations of lower vertebrates.

Kinetic studies with bullfrog and duck adrenal mitochondria gave K_m values for corticosterone in the range of $6 \times 10^{-6}M$ for both 18-hydroxycorticosterone and aldosterone for both species (Greengard *et al.*, 1968; Sandor *et al.*, 1972b).

The participation of cytochrome P-450 in mitochondrial 18-oxygenation was studied with bullfrog mitochondria by Greengard and associates (1967) and in domestic duck adrenal mitochondria by Sandor and associates (1972b). In both species, the spectrophotometric presence of the hemoprotein could be shown and in quantities quite similar (0.5 nmole/mg mitochondrial protein in the frog and 0.6 nmole/mg mitochondrial protein in the duck). These concentrations differed somewhat from those obtained for mammalian mitochondria (1.3–1.6 nmoles/mg protein in bovine mitochondria (Harding and Nelson, 1966). By measuring the CO inhibition of 18-

oxygenation and subsequently the photochemical action spectrum of the light reversal of the CO-inhibited reaction in the bullfrog, Greengard and his group came to the conclusion that cytochrome P-450 is necessary for aldosterone formation from corticosterone. Thus, a hydroxylation step is involved, implying the intermediary role of 18-hydroxycorticosterone. A mechanism was proposed which would involve the following steps. Once corticosterone were hydroxylated at C-18, an enzyme–18-hydroxycorticosterone complex would be formed. This complex could undergo either dissociation to enzyme plus 18-hydroxycorticosterone or the steroid could be dehydrogenated to aldosterone. The poor ability of exogenous 18-hydroxycorticosterone to yield aldosterone would be due to the fact that the equilibrium constant of the reaction between the enzyme and 18-hydroxycorticosterone would be in favor of dissociation.

With the duck adrenal, addition of corticosterone to mitochondrial suspensions gave so-called type II difference spectra, characterized by a trough between 380 and 390 mμ and a peak at 420 mμ. Similar steroid-induced difference spectra were given by 11-deoxycorticosterone, contrary to mammalian adrenal mitochondria in which this steroid induced type I difference spectra (see Section III, A and Williamson and O'Donnell, 1969). 18-Oxygenation of corticosterone was inhibited competitively by metopirone, and spectrophotometrically the spectrum given by metopirone was indistinguishable from that yielded by corticosterone. Titration of duck mitochondrial P-450 with corticosterone and metopirone revealed that the cytochrome became saturated with both substances at identical concentrations (21.8 μmoles/mg mitochondrial protein). In addition to metopirone, aminopterin, the known folic acid antagonist, inhibited 18-oxygenation in a noncompetitive manner. The reaction was equally inhibited by CO and by mercurials.

Raman *et al.* (1966) noted that the presence of exogenous 18-hydroxycorticosterone inhibited aldosterone formation from corticosterone. These experiments were repeated with duck adrenal mitochondria and radioactively labeled corticosterone. Addition of exogenous 18-hydroxycorticosterone did not result in a dilution effect in the production of aldosterone, but both biosynthetic 18-hydroxycorticosterone and aldosterone were inhibited and this inhibition was proportional to the concentration of the added 18-hydroxycorticosterone. However, throughout this experiment, the ratio 18-hydroxycorticosterone–aldosterone remained constant. From this the conclusion was drawn that the transformation corticosterone ⟶ 18-hydroxycorticosterone ⟶ aldosterone was not a kinetically sequential reaction and in the above experiments exogenous 18-hydroxycorticosterone simply acted as an inhibitor.

Investigation of the kinetics of the 18-oxygenation of exogenous corticosterone by domestic duck adrenal slices and adrenal mitochondria clearly showed that the limiting factor in aldosterone biosynthesis was the availability of corticosterone and not that of 18-hydroxycosticosterone. Further analysis of these curves suggested that in terms of kinetics at least, the transformation of corticosterone to 18-hydroxycorticosterone and aldosterone could be interpreted as a parallel first-order reaction rather than a series first-order reaction (Sandor *et al.*, 1972b).

The biosynthesis of aldosterone will not be explained in detail until the 18-oxygenating enzyme complex can be solubilized. Unfortunately, until now, attempts in these directions were not successful. However, there seems to be little doubt that aldosterone biosynthesis is probably one of those reactions in which the biosynthetic pathways might be different in different animal classes while yielding the same end product.

IV. Summary

By the time the reader has arrived at this section, he has no doubt realized the scarcity of available information on corticosteroids in amphibians, reptiles, and birds. Steroid biochemistry of the nonmammalian vertebrates is now in the same state of development as mammalian steroid biochemistry was about twenty years ago. However, it is quite certain that in the next few years there will be a spectacular expansion of knowledge in this field. First, the results obtained in mammals can be used to advantage in this discipline and, second, we now possess refined research tools which were not available a few years ago.

On the basis of the data obtained up to now, it is probably safe to say that, basically, corticosteroidogenesis in amphibians, reptiles, and birds is not drastically different from that of mammals. There have been no corticosteroids discovered which are unique to any of these vertebrate classes, nor is there evidence for any biosynthetic mechanism which would have no parallel in the mammalian adrenal. Obviously, these statements have only temporary value. It has been pointed out on several occasions that all we know about lower-vertebrate corticosteroids comes from the study of only a few species. It is quite conceivable that as more and more representatives of these vertebrate classes undergo careful study, our whole picture of nonmammalian steroid biochemistry will have to be reevaluated. As far as the biosynthesis of steroids is concerned, there is a lack of valid chemical studies. Almost all of our knowledge about the genesis of corticosteroids in nonmammalian adrenals has been obtained by *in vitro* methods coupled with the use of radioactive substrates. This means that as long as we cannot present results obtained by perfusion studies, feeding experiments, etc., our conclusions remain highly tentative.

Physiologically, there is a very wide gap between an anuran frog, still shackled to his ancestral watery environment, and a warm-blooded bird or mammal. Nevertheless, purely from the point of view of adrenal steroid hormone synthesis, this difference is not all apparent. The adrenal cell, so it seems, attained its evolutionary peak long before other structures attained theirs. Steroid hormone production has a very high survival value and the regulatory effect of these hormones allows the animal to adapt to all possible environments the earth can offer. It has been widely believed that the capability of synthesizing and utilizing steroid hormones is an exclusive feature of vertebrates. This we do not know, and slowly some evidence is emerging that cells containing enzyme systems which can use steroidal substrates are much more ancient than the development of an inner rigid supporting structures (Lehoux and Sandor, 1970). Thus, it is questionable whether from the point of view of the adrenal cell we should distinguish between "lower" and "higher" vertebrates. However, before we can give any authoritative answers, much more extensive work is needed.

ACKNOWLEDGMENTS

Personal research works described or quoted in this chapter were supported by grants from the Medical Research Council of Canada, the National Institute of Arthritis and Metabolic Diseases, U.S.P.H.S., and the CIBA Company, Montreal. The author is holder of a Medical Research Associateship of the Medical Research Council of Canada. In addition to the institutional grants, the author wishes to express his gratitude for the following personal awards: Nuffield Foundation Canadian Travel Grant, Schering Traveling Fellowship, a Science Research Council Senior Visiting Fellowship (U.K.), and an Endocrine Society Traveling Fellowship.

REFERENCES

Ayres, P. J., Gould, R. P., Simpson, S. A., and Tait, J. F. (1956). *Biochem. J.* **63**, 19P.
Birmingham, M. K., and Ward, P. J. (1961). *J. Biol. Chem.* **236**, 1661.
Bonhommet, M., and Weniger, J. P. (1967). *C.R. Soc. Biol.* **161**, 2052.
Brown, K. I. (1961). *Proc. Soc. Exp. Biol. Med.* **107**, 538.
Brownie, A. C., Grant, J. K., and Davidson, D. W. (1954). *Biochem. J.* **58**, 218.
Cameron, E. H. D., Beynon, M. A., and Griffiths, K. (1968a). *J. Endocrinol.* **41**, 319.
Cameron, E. H. D., Beynon, M. A., and Griffiths, K. (1968b). *J. Endocrinol* **41**, 327.
Carstensen, H., Burgers, A. C. J., and Li, C. H. (1959). *J. Amer. Chem. Soc.* **81**, 4109.
Carstensen, H., Burgers, A. C. J., and Li, C. H. (1961). *Gen. Comp. Endocrinol.* **1**, 37.
Chan, S. T. H., and Edwards, B. R. (1970). *J. Endocrinol.* **47**, 183.
Chan, S. W. C., Vinson, G. P., and Phillips, J. G. (1969). *Gen. Comp. Endocrinol.* **12**, 644.
Chester Jones, I., Phillips, J. G., and Holmes, W. N. (1959). *In* "Comparative Endocrinology" (A. Gorbman, ed.), pp. 582–612. Wiley, New York.

Conforth, J. W. (1959). *J. Lipid Res.* **1**, 3.
Cooper, D. Y., Levin, S., Narasimhulu Shakunthala, Rosenthal, O., and Estabrook, R. W. (1965). *Science* **147**, 400.
Crabbé, J. (1961). *Endocrinology* **69**, 673.
Crabbé, J. (1963). "The Sodium Retaining Action of Aldosterone." Presses Académiques Européennes, Brussels.
Dale, E. (1962). *Gen. Comp. Endocrinol.* **2**, 171.
Davis, W. W., Burwell, L. R., Kelley, G., Casper, A. G. T., and Bartter, F. C. (1966). *Biochem. Biophys. Res. Commun.* **22**, 218.
de Nicola, A. F., Kraulis, I., and Birmingham, M. K. (1968), *Steroids* **11**, 165.
deRoos, R. (1960). *Endocrinology* **67**, 719.
deRoos, R. (1961a). *Gen. Comp. Endocrinol.* **1**, 494.
deRoos, R. (1961b). *Amer. Zool.* **1**, 193.
deRoos, R. (1963). *Proc. XIII Int. Ornithol. Congr.* **2**, 1041.
deRoos, R., and deRoos, C. C. (1963). *Science* **141**, 1284.
deRoos, R., and deRoos, C. C. (1964). *Gen. Comp. Endocrinol.* **4**, 602.
Donaldson, E. M., and Holmes, W. N. (1965). *J. Endocrinol.* **32**, 329.
Donaldson, E. M., Holmes, W. N., and Stachenko, J. (1965). *Gen. Comp. Endocrinol.* **5**, 542.
Dorfman, R. I., and Ungar, F. (1965). "Metabolism of Steroid Hormones." Academic Press, New York.
Estabrook, R. W., Cooper, D. Y., and Rosenthal, O. (1963). *Biochem. Z.* **338**, 741.
Farese, R. V. (1967). *Fed. Proc. Fed. Amer. Soc. Exp. Biol.* **26**, 423.
Farese, R. V., and Reddy, W. J. (1963). *Biochim. Biophys. Acta* **76**, 148.
Farese, R. V., and Schnure, J. J. (1967). *Endocrinology* **80**, 872.
Fazekas, A. G., and Sandor, T. (1969). *Steroids* **14**, 161.
Fazekas, A. G., and Webb, J. L. (1966). *Eur. J. Steroids* **1**, 389.
Ferguson, J. J., Jr. (1962). *Biochim. Biophys. Acta* **57**, 616.
Frankel, A. I., Cook, B., Graber, J. W., and Nalbandov, A. V. (1967a). *Endocrinology* **80**, 181.
Frankel, A. I., Graber, J. W., and Nalbandov, A. V. (1967b). *Endocrinology* **80**, 1013.
Frankel, A. I., Graber, J. W., and Nalbandov, A. V. (1967c). *Gen. Comp. Endocrinol.* **8**, 387.
Frankel, A. I., Graber, J. W., Cook, B., and Nalbandov, A. V. (1967d). *Steroids* **10**, 699.
Giroud, C. J. P., Stachenko, J., and Piletta, P. (1958). *In* "An International Symposium on Aldosterone" (A. F. Muller and C. M. O'Connor, eds.), pp. 56–72. Little, Brown, Boston, Massachusetts.
Gist, D. H., and deRoos, R. (1966). *Gen. Comp. Endocrinol.* **7**, 304.
Gorbman, A., and Bern, H. A. (1966). "A Textbook of Comparative Endocrinology." Wiley, New York.
Gottfried, H., Huang, D. P., Lofts, B., Phillips, J. G., and Tam, W. H. (1967). *Gen. Comp. Endocrinol.* **8**, 18.
Grant, J. K. (1962). *Brit. Med. Bull.* **18**, 99.
Greengard, P., Psychoyos, S., Tallan, H. H., Cooper, D. Y., Rosenthal, O., and Estabrook, R. W. (1967). *Arch. Biochem. Biophys.* **121**, 298.
Greengard, P., Tallan, H. H., and Psychoyos, S. (1968). *In* "Functions of the Adrenal Cortex" (K. W. Mckerns, ed.), Vol. 1, p. 233. Appleton, New York.
Halkerston, I. D. K., Eichhorn, J., and Hechter, O. (1961). *J. Biol. Chem.* **236**, 374.
Hall, P. F., and Koritz, S. B. (1966). *Endocrinology* **79**, 652.
Harding, B. W., and Nelson, D. H. (1966). *J. Biol. Chem.* **241**, 2212.
Harding, B. W., Wong, S. H., and Nelson, D. H. (1964). *Biochim. Biophys. Acta* **92**, 415.

Haynes, R. C. (1958). *J. Biol. Chem.* **233**, 1220.

Haynes, R. C., and Berthel, L. (1957). *J. Biol. Chem.* **225**, 115.

Haynes, R. C., Koritz, S. B., and Péron, F. G. (1959). *J. Biol. Chem.* **234**, 1421.

Heard, R. D. H., Bligh, E. G., Cann, M. C., Jellineck, P. H., O'Donnell, V. J., Rao, B. G., and Webb, J. L. (1956). *Recent Progr. Horm. Res.* **12**, 45.

Hechter, O., and Pincus, G. (1954). *Physiol. Rev.* **34**, 459.

Holmes, W. N., Phillips, J. G., and Butler, D. G. (1961). *Endocrinology* **69**, 483.

Huang, D. P., Vinson, G. P., and Phillips, J. G. (1969). *Gen. Comp. Endocrinol.* **12**, 637.

Johnston, C. I., Davis, J. O., Wright, F. S., and Howards, S. S. (1967). *Amer. J. Physiol.* **213**, 393.

Kahnt, F. W., and Neher, R. (1965). *Helv. Chim. Acta* **48**, 1457.

Karaboyas, G. C., and Koritz, S. B. (1965). *Biochemistry* **4**, 462.

Klein, G. P., and Giroud, C. J. P. (1967). *Steroids* **9**, 113.

Kraulis, I., and Birmingham, M. K. (1964). *Acta Endocrinol.* (*Copenhagen*) **47**, 76.

Krum, A. A., Morris, M. D., and Bennett, L. L. (1964). *Endocrinology* **74**, 543.

Lamoureux, J. (1966). "La Biosynthèse des Stéroides Surréaliens chez les Vertebrés Inférieurs aux Mammiféres." Doctoral thesis, Université de Montréal, Canada.

Lamoureux, J., Sandor, T., and Lanthier, A. (1964). *Proc, Int. Congr. Biochem., 6th.* **32**, VII–90.

Leblanc, H. (1970). "Etude de la Fonction Surrénalienne chez les Oiseaux." M.Sc. thesis, Université de Montréal, Canada.

Leblanc, H., Lehoux, J. G. Lanthier, A., and Sandor, T. (1970). *Proc. Can. Fed. Biol. Soc.* **13**, 525.

Lee, T. H., Lerner, A. B., and Buettner-Janusch, V. (1961). *J. Biol. Chem.* **236**, 2970.

Lehoux, J. G., and Sandor, T. (1970). *Steroids* **16**, 141.

Li, C. H. (1963). *Sci. Amer.* **209**, 46.

Macchi, I. A. (1955). *Biol. Bull.* **3**, 373.

Macchi, I. A. (1956). *J. Clin. Endocrinol.* **16**, 942.

Macchi, I. A. (1967). *Excerpta Med. Found. Int. Congr. Ser.* **132**, 1094.

Macchi, I. A., and Phillips, J. G. (1966). *Gen. Comp. Endocrinol.* **6**, 170.

Macchi, I. A., Phillips, J. G., and Brown, P. (1967). *J. Endocrinol.* **38**, 319.

Mader, W. J., and Buck, J. J. (1952). *Anal. Chem.* **24**, 666.

Marusic, E. T., and Mulrow, P. J. (1967). *Endocrinology* **80**, 214.

Mehdi, A. Z. (1969). "*In vitro* Corticosteroid Biosynthesis by Frog and Turtle Interrenals." Doctoral thesis, Department of Investigative Medicine, McGill University, Montreal, Canada.

Mehdi, A. Z., and Carballeira, A. (1971a). *Gen. Comp. Endocrinol.* **17**, 1.

Mehdi, A. Z., and Carballeira, A. (1971b). *Gen. Comp. Endocrinol.* **17**, 14.

Mehdi, A. Z., and Sandor, T. (1971). *Steroids* **17**, 143.

Meyer, A. S., and Lindberg, M. C. (1955). *Anal. Chem.* **27**, 813.

Mitani, F., and Horie, S. (1969). *J. Biochem.* (*Tokyo*) **65**, 269.

Mulrow, P. J., and Cohn, G. L. (1959). *Proc. Soc. Exp. Biol. Med.* **101**, 731.

Mulrow, P. J., and Cohn, G. L., and Kuljian, A. (1962). *J. Clin. Invest.* **41**, 1584.

Nagra, C. L., Baum, G. J., and Meyer, R. K. (1960). *Proc. Soc. Exp. Biol. Med.* **105**, 68.

Nagra, C. L., Birnie, J. G., Baum, G. J., and Meyer, R. K. (1963). *Gen. Comp. Endocrinol.* **3**, 274.

Newcomer, W. S. (1959a). *Amer. J. Physiol.* **196**, 276.

Newcomer, W. S. (1959b). *Endocrinology* **65**, 133.

Nicolis, G. L., and Ulick, S. (1965). *Endocrinology*, **76**, 514.

Norymberski, J. K. (1952). *Nature* (*London*) **170**, 1074.

Nowaczynski, W., Silah, J., and Genest, J. (1967). *Can. J. Biochem.* **45**, 1919.

Omura, T., and Sato, R. (1964). *J. Biol. Chem.* **239**, 2370.

Omura, T., Sanders, E., Estabrook, R. W., Cooper, D.Y., and Rosenthal, O. (1966). *Arch. Biochem. Biophys.* **117**, 660.

Pasqualini, J. R. (1964). *Nature (London)* **201**, 501.

Pasqualini, J. R., Lafoscade, G., and Jayle, M. F. (1964). *Steroids* **4**, 739.

Péron, F. G. (1961). *Endocrinology* **69**, 39.

Péron, F. G. (1962). *Endocrinology* **70**, 386.

Phillips, J. G., and Chester Jones, I. (1957). *J. Endocrinol.* **16**, iii.

Phillips, J. G., Holmes, W. N., and Butler, D. G. (1961). *Endocrinology* **69**, 958.

Phillips, J. G., Chester Jones, I., and Bellamy, D. (1962). *J. Endocrinol.* **25**, 233.

Piper, G. D., and deRoos, R. (1966). *Gen. Comp. Endocrinol.* **8**, 135.

Porter, C. C., and Silber, R. H. (1950). *J. Biol. Chem.* **185**, 201.

Psychoyos, S., Tallan, H. H., and Greengard, P. (1966). *J. Biol. Chem.* **241**, 2949.

Raman, P. B., Sharma, D. C., and Dorfman, R. I. (1966). *Biochemistry* **5**, 1795.

Rapola, J. (1963). *Gen. Comp. Endocrinol.* **3**, 412.

Resko, J. A., Norton, H. W., and Nalbandov, A. V. (1964). *Endocrinology* **75**, 192.

Romer, A. S. (1967). *Science* **158**, 1629.

Ryan, K. J., and Engel, L. L. (1957). *J. Biol. Chem.* **225**, 103.

Saba, N., and Hechter, O. (1955). *Fed. Proc. Fed. Amer. Soc. Exp. Biol.* **14**, 775.

Salem, M. H., Norton, H. W., and Nalbandov, A. V. (1970a). *Gen. Comp. Endocrinol.* **14**, 270.

Salem, M. H., Norton, H. W., and Nalbandov, A. V. (1970b). *Gen. Comp. Endocrinol.* **14**, 281.

Samuels, L. T. (1960). *In* "Metabolic Pathways" (D. M. Greenberg, ed.), pp. 431–480. Academic Press, New York.

Sandor, T. (1969a). *Gen. Comp. Endocrinol. Suppl.* **2**, 284.

Sandor, T. (1969b). *Excerpta Med. Found. Int. Congr. Ser.* **184**, 730.

Sandor, T. (1970). Unpublished data.

Sandor, T., and Lanthier, A. (1963a). *Acta Endocrinol. (Copenhagen)* **42**, 355.

Sandor, T., and Lanthier, A. (1963b). *Biochem. Biophys. Acta* **74**, 756.

Sandor, T., and Lanthier, A. (1966). "Abstract Book," IUPAC 4th International Symposium on the Chemistry of Natural Products, Stockholm, 3–15.

Sandor, T., and Lanthier, A. (1970). *Endocrinology* **86**, 552.

Sandor, T., Lanthier, A., and Lamoureux, J. (1963a). *Fed. Proc. Fed. Amer. Soc. Exp. Biol.* **22**, 65.

Sandor, T., Lamoureux, J., and Lanthier, A. (1963b). *Endocrinology* **73**, 629.

Sandor, T., Lamoureux, J., and Lanthier, A. (1964). *Steroids* **4**, 213.

Sandor, T., Lamoureux, J., and Lanthier, A. (1965). *Steroids* **6**, 143.

Sandor, T., Vinson, G. P., Whitehouse, B., Lamoureux, J., and Lanthier, A. (1966a). *Excerpta Med. Found. Int. Congr. Ser.* **111**, 213.

Sandor, T., Vinson, G. P., Chester Jones, I., Henderson, I. W., and Whitehouse, B. (1966b). *J. Endocrinol.* **34**, 105.

Sandor, T., Lanthier, A., Henderson, I. W., and Chester Jones, I. (1967). *Endocrinology* **81**, 904.

Sandor, T., Lehoux, J. G., and Mehdi, A. Z. (1972a). *Gen. Comp. Endocrinol. Suppl.* **3**, In press.

Sandor, T., Fazekas, A., Lehoux, J. G., Leblanc, H., and Lanthier, A. (1972b). *J. Steroid Biochem.* **3**. In press.

Satoh, P., Constantopoulos, G., and Tehen, T. T. (1966). *Biochemistry* **5**, 1646.

Sayers, G. (1967). *In* "Hormones in Blood" (C. H. Gray and A. L. Bacharach, eds.), Vol. 1, pp. 170–192. Academic Press, New York.

Schmidlin, J., and Wettstein, A. (1961). *Helv. Chim. Acta* **44**, 1596.

Schriefers, H. (1967). *Vitam. Horm. (New York)* **25**, 271.

Schwyzer, R., and Sieber, P. (1963). *Nature (London)* **199**, 172.

Sharma, D. C. (1970). *Acta Endocrinol. (Copenhagen)* **62**, 299.

Sharma, D. C., Nerenberg, C. A., and Dorfman, R. I. (1967). *Biochemistry* **6**, 3472.

Sih, C. J. (1969). *Science* **163**, 1297.

Sih, C. J., and Whitlock, H. W., Jr. (1968). *Annu. Rev. Biochem.* **37**, 661.

Silber, R. H., Busch, R. D., and Oslapas, R. (1958). *Clin. Chem.* **4**, 278.

Simpson, E. R., and Boyd, G. S. (1966). *Biochem. Biophys. Res. Commun.* **24**, 10.

Simpson, E. R., Cooper, D. Y., and Estabrook, R. W. (1969). *Recent Progr. Horm. Res.* **25**, 523.

Stachenko, J., and Giroud, C. J. P. (1959). *Endocrinology* **64**, 730.

Stachenko, J., and Giroud, C. J. P. (1962). *In* "The Human Adrenal Cortex" (A. R. Currie, T. Symington, and J. K. Grant, eds.), pp. 30–43. Livingstone, Edinburgh.

Stachenko, J., and Giroud, C. J. P. (1964). *Can. J. Biochem.* **42**, 1777.

Suzuki, K., and Kimura, T. (1965). *Biochem. Biophys. Res. Commun.* **19**, 340.

Sweat, M. L. (1951). *J. Amer. Chem. Soc.* **77**, 5185.

Taylor, A. A., Davis, J. O., Breitenbach, R. P., and Hartroft, P. M. (1970). *Gen. Comp. Endocrinol.* **14**, 321.

Tomkins, G. M., Michael, P. J., and Curran, J. F. (1957). *Biochim. Biophys. Acta* **92**, 415.

Truscott, B., and Idler, D. R. (1968). *J. Fish. Res. Bd. Can.* **25**, 431.

Tsang, C. P. W., and Stachenko, J. (1969). *Can. J. Biochem.* **47**, 1109.

Ulick, S., and Feinholtz, E. (1968). *J. Clin. Invest.* **47**, 2523.

Ulick, S., and Kusch, K. (1960). *J. Amer. Chem. Soc.* **82**, 6421.

Ulick, S., and Kusch-Vetter, K. (1962). *Excerpta Med. Found. Int. Congr. Ser.* **51**, 213.

Ulick, S., and Kusch-Vetter, K. (1965). *J. Clin. Endocrinol. Metab.* **25**, 1015.

Ulick, S., and Solomon, S. (1960). *J. Amer. Chem. Soc.* **82**, 249.

Urist, M. R., and Deutch, N. M. (1960). *Proc. Soc. Exp. Biol. Med.* **104**, 35.

Vinson, G. P., and Whitehouse, B. J. (1969a). *Acta Endocrinol. (Copenhagen)* **61**, 695.

Vinson, G. P., and Whitehouse, B. J. (1969b). *Acta Endocrinol. (Copenhagen)* **61**, 709.

Weichselbaum, T. E., and Margraf, H. W. (1957). *J. Clin. Endocrinol. Metab.* **17**, 959.

Weliky, I., and Engel, L. L. (1962). *J. Biol. Chem.* **237**, 2089.

Werbin, H., and Chaikoff, I. L. (1961). *Arch. Biochem. Biophys.* **93**, 476.

Whitehouse, B., and Vinson, G. P. (1967). *Gen. Comp. Endocrinol.* **9**, 161.

Williamson, D. G., and O'Donnell, V. J. (1969). *Biochemistry* **8**, 1306.

Wilson, L. D., Oldham, S. B., and Harding, B. W. (1968). *J. Clin. Endocrinol. Metab.* **28**, 1143.

Wright, C., and Chester Jones, I. (1957). *J. Endocrinol.* **15**, 83.

Zenker, N., and Bernstein, D. S. (1958). *J. Biol. Chem.* **231**, 695.

Zilversmit, D. B., Entenman, C., and Fischler, M. C. (1943). *J. Gen. Physiol.* **26**, 325.

Chapter 6

ANDROGENS IN FISHES, AMPHIBIANS, REPTILES, AND BIRDS

R. OZON

I. Introduction

The anatomical location as well as the histological structure of the testes differ little throughout the vertebrate phylum. They are paired glands situated within the abdominal cavity, except in sexually mature mammals where they occupy an extraabdominal pouch, the scrotum (see Chapter 3). The testes of vertebrates have a double function of secretion: (a) exocrine (spermatozoa) and (b) endocrine (androgenic hormones).

In mammals, birds, the majority of reptiles, anuran amphibians, and teleost fishes, spermatogenesis takes place in seminiferous tubules; the androgens are secreted mainly by the interstitial or Leydig cells. The testes of urodele amphibians (triton, salamander) and elasmobranch fishes do not have seminiferous tubules but rather have seminiferous lobes or cysts; the interstitial tissue is generally scanty. The endocrine secretion is then mainly accomplished either by the cells associated with the cysts or their derivatives, or by cells associated with spermatogenesis.

Castrated animals differ from normal specimens of the same species; this difference has been known since ancient times. However, it was not until the end of the nineteenth century that the idea of testicular hormone secretion was first advanced. Experiments of castration and testicular grafting proved the role of the testes in maintaining male somatic features not only in mammals but also in other vertebrates. The callosites and musculature of the limbs of castrated male frogs have been observed to regress (Steinach, 1894). The classical experiments (Berthold, 1849) of castration and testicular implantation performed on birds showed the testicular influence on the whole organism.

The isolation of androgens secreted by the testes of mammals began in 1930; their chemical structure was elucidated mainly by Butenandt in Germany (Dorfman and Ungar, 1965). Natural androgens are steroids of 19 carbon atoms. Testosterone (Fig. 1), the most active of the natural androgens, is present in the testes of man, bull, boar, stallion, and rabbit; androstenedione, which has a ketone radical instead of the 17β-hydroxy group of testosterone, has been found in the same tissues. Both these components have also been isolated from peripheral blood or from the spermatic vein blood of various mammals. Numerous steroids, derivatives of testosterone, have been identified in urine, particularly androsterone, which was the first androgen isolated by Butenandt from human urine.

Since the availability of chemically pure androgens, their biological properties have been intensively studied in fishes, amphibians, reptiles, and birds (see Chapter 8). Androgens generally regulate the structure of somatic sexual characteristics as well as the physiology of reproduction of all male

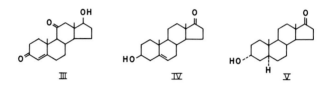

Fig. 1. Structural formulas of the principal C_{19} steroids isolated from vertebrates. I, testosterone; II, androstenedione; III, 11-ketotestosterone; IV, dehydroepiandrosterone; V, androsterone.

vertebrates. However, up to this decade, the steroid hormones had been isolated from mammals only. Some doubts still remained concerning the chemical nature of the androgens in the other classes of vertebrates. It was necessary to look elsewhere than in the mammals for the presence of the steroids and to determine their chemical structure for each species.

II. Isolation and Identification of C_{19} Steroids

A. BIOLOGICAL METHODS

Biological methods for qualitative determination of steroid hormones are generally based on the response of the somatic sexual tissues to the injections of hormones. The increase in weight of the ventral prostrate and of the seminal vesicles of a castrated or immature rat, and the variations in weight and size of a capon's comb, have permitted the qualitative and quantitative estimation of the androgenic activity of a biological extract. Hazleton and Goodrich (1937) demonstrated that the injection of testicular extracts of fishes into a castrated rooster (capon) promoted the growth of the cock's comb; in the same manner Potter and Hoar (1954) discovered androgenic activity in the testes of salmon. Valle and Valle (1943) on the basis of biological tests reported the presence of substances of androgenic character in extracts from testes of reptiles (*Crotalus terrificus terrificus, Bothrops jararaca*). Comb growth of immature chickens enabled the estimation of the endogenous male hormone secretion in this species (Breneman and Mason, 1951).

These experiments suggested, but did not prove, the presence of androgens in the testes of lower vertebrates. Indeed, biological methods reveal the presence of androgenic activity, but they do not supply any information concerning the chemical nature of the responsible substances. The first biological results only allowed the conclusion that the extracts from testes of fishes, reptiles, and birds have a biological activity which is comparable to that of the androgens obtained from the testes of mammals. The biological results must be confirmed by the chemical isolation of the steroids.

B. BIOCHEMICAL METHODS (Table I)

The first sexual steroid hormones identified with certainty from nonmammalian vertebrate tissues were estrone and estradiol-17β. Wotiz *et al.* (1960) isolated them in a crystalline form from the ovaries of *Squalus suckleyi*. Since then these estrogenic hormones have been discovered in every one of the vertebrate classes explored (see Chapter 7). Studies dedicated to the exploration of the androgenic hormones are much less numerous.

1. Fishes

a. Testes. Chieffi and Lupo (1961a) have searched for the presence of steroids in testicular extracts of *Scyliorhinus stellaris*. Analyses by paper chromatography of the neutral fraction of the extract demonstrated the presence of three spots absorbing ultraviolet light at 240 mμ and corresponding to testosterone, androstenedione, and progesterone. Testosterone and androstenedione were identified by measurement of their R_f values in various paper chromatographic systems and by the Zimmermann reaction; the spot having the same chromatographic behavior as testosterone was oxidized to androstenedione by CrO_3. The authors also reported the presence of estradiol-17β in the phenolic fraction.

Substances of chromatographic mobility similar to that of testosterone have been extracted from the testes of *Salmo irideus* and *Cyprinus carpio* (Galzigna, 1961). Chemical analysis of 1200 g of testicular tissue of the salmon *Oncorhynchus nerka* (Grajcer and Idler, 1963) revealed the presence of testosterone chiefly conjugated with glucuronic acid. The neutral fraction did not contain detectable quantities of free testosterone. However, enzymic hydrolysis by β-glucuronidase released a compound which absorbed ultraviolet light at 240 mμ, which migrated in the same manner as testosterone, and which was oxidized by CrO_3 to androstenedione; it could be acetylated

TABLE I

Isolation and Identification of C_{19} Steroids in Nonmammalian Vertebrates

Species	Steroid	Source of Steroid	Quantity	Major criteria[a]	Rating for identification	Reference
FISHES						
Torpedo marmorata	Testosterone	Plasma (before reproduction)	1.56 μg/100 ml	TLC, GLC	Su	Lupo di Prisco et al. (1967b)
Scyliorhinus stellaris	Testosterone Androst-4-ene-3,17-dione	Testes	50 μg/kg 70 μg/kg	PC, CT, Der	Su	Chieffi and Lupo (1961a)
Scyliorhinus caniculus	Testosterone	Sperm	6 μg/kg	TLC, GLC	Ex	Gottfried and Chieffi (1967)
	Testosterone	Plasma ♂				Simpson et al. (1968a)
Raja radiata	Testosterone	Plasma ♂	2.8–10.2 μg/100 ml	TLC, PC, GLC, Der, CT	Po	Idler and Truscott (1966)
	Testosterone gluc. Testosterone conjug.		4.3–6.7 μg/100 ml 0.1–0.3 μg/100 ml			
	Testosterone Testosterone gluc.	Plasma ♀	0.02–0.6 μg/100 ml 0.13 μg/100 ml			
Raja ocellata	Testosterone	Plasma ♂	2.2–20.8 μg/100 ml	TLC, PC, GLC, Der, CT	Po	Idler and Truscott (1966)
	Testosterone conjug. Testosterone	Plasma ♀	0.14–0.47 μg/100 ml 0.59 μg/ml			
Squalus acanthias	Androst-4-ene-3,17-dione Androsterone Dehydroepi-androsterone	Sperm	2 μg/100 g 5 μg/100 g 2 μg/100 g 2 μg/100 g	PC, CT, Der	Te	Simpson et al. (1963a)
Oncorhynchus nerka	Testosterone Testosterone gluc. 11-Ketotestosterone Testosterone	Plasma ♂ Plasma ♀	1.7 μg/100 ml 13.7 μg/100 ml 12. μg/100 ml 7.8 μg/100 ml	PC, CT, Der, IR	Po Po Po Po	Grajcer and Idler (1963) Idler et al. (1960b)

332

Species	Compound	Source	Amount	Method		Reference
Salmo salar	Testosterone gluc.	Plasma ♂	7.6 μg/100 ml		Po	Schmidt and Idler (1962)
	11-Ketotestosterone		0–9.6 μg/100 ml		Te	Idler *et al.* (1961b)
	Adrenosterone		2.5 μg/100 ml		Te	Grajcer and Idler (1963)
	Testosterone gluc.	Testes	30 μg/kg	PC, CT	Po	Schmidt and Idler (1962)
Mugil capito	11-Ketotestosterone	Plasma ♂	67 μg/100 ml	PC, GLC, Der, IR	Su	Eylath and Eckstein (1969)
	11-Ketotestosterone	Ovaries			Po	
	Dehydroepi-androsterone					
Gasterosteus aculeatus	Testosterone	Testes		TLC, GLC	Su	Van Mullem and Gottfried (1966)
	Androst-4-ene-3,17-dione					
	Dehydroepi-androsterone					
Serranus scriba	Testosterone	Hermaphrodite Gonads	5 μg/65 mg	AC, TLC, GLC, Der	Su	Lupo and Chieffi (1965)
	Androst-4-ene-3,17-dione		15 μg/65 mg			
	Testosterone conjug.					
Salmo irideus	Testosterone	Testes	3 μg/65 mg	PC	Ex	Galzigna (1961)
Cyprinus carpio	Testosterone	Testes		PC	Ex	Galzigna (1961)
AMPHIBIANS						
Xenopus laevis	17-Ketosteroids	Breeding water (adults)		CT	Ex	Rapola (1963)
Rana pipiens	17-Ketosteroids	Breeding water (larvae)		CT	Ex	Dale (1962)
Necturus maculosus	Testosterone	Plasma	4.2–26 μg/100 ml	PC, Der, CryC	Pr	Rivarola *et al.* (1968)
	Androst-4-ene-3,17-dione		0.05–0.35 μg/100 ml	^{3}H/^{14}C		
Pleurode waltlii	Testosterone	Plasma	4 μg/100 ml	TLC, Der, GLC	Te	Ozon and Attal (1969)
	Epitestosterone		2 μg/100 ml			
REPTILES						
Lacerta sicula	Testosterone conjug.	Testes	91 μg/kg	AC, TLC, CT, GLC	Te	Lupo di Prisco *et al.* (1967a)
	Androst-4-ene-3,17-dione		53 μg/kg			
	Androsterone		99 μg/kg			
	Dehydroepiandros-terone		454 μg/kg			

TABLE I (cont.)

Species	Steroid	Source of Steroid	Quantity	Major criteria[a]	Rating for identification	Reference
	Androst-4-ene-3,17-dione Dehydroepiandrosterone	Ovaries	6.2 µg/kg 9.4 µg/kg	PC, TLC, GLC, Der	Te	Lupo di Prisco et al. (1968)
Naja naja	Androst-4-ene-3,17-dione Dehydroepiandrosterone	Testicular incubates in vitro	1.34 µg/hr/100 mg 1.47 µg/hr/100 mg	TLC, Der GLC	Te	Gottfried et al. (1967)
BIRDS						
Steganopus tricolor Charadrius vociferus Agelaius phoeniceus	Testosterone Androst-4-ene-3,17-dione	Testes		PC, CT PC, CT	Su Su	Höhn and Cheng (1967)
Anas platyrhynchos Gallus gallus Columbia livia						
White carneau pigeon	Testosterone Androst-4-ene-3,17-dione Dehydroepiandrosterone	Plasma ♂	15–98 ng/100 ml 31–378 ng/100 ml 0–338 ng/100 ml	PC, Der, C ^{3}H/^{14}C	Te	Rivarola et al. (1968)
Gallus domesticus	Testosterone Androst-4-ene-3,17-dione	Testes	35 µg/kg 2.4 µg/kg	PC, TLC, GLC, CT, Der	Te	Delrio et al. (1967)
	Testosterone	Plasma ♀ (laying hen)	55 ng/100 ml	PC, TLC, GLC, C ^{3}H/^{14}C	Pr	O'Malley et al. (1968)
	Androst-4-ene-3,17-dione		98 ng/100 ml			
DUCK	Testosterone	Testicular Plasma	340–1580 ng/100 ml	TLC, Der, GLC	Te	Jallageas and Attal 1968 Garnier and Attal 1970

a For an explanation of abbreviations and rating system, see Chapter 3, Table I, p. VI.

and the acetate could not be separated from standard testosterone acetate. Finally, enough of the material was prepared in a pure state to permit its identification by infrared spectroscopy. Testosterone accounted for most of the biological activity of the extract. The research of Grajcer and Idler (1963) based on solid physicochemical criteria, proved the presence of testosterone in fish. It is of interest to note that the hormone was present in testes almost exclusively as the glucuronoside; the linkage is probably through the 17β position (Hadd and Rhamy, 1965).

Several steroids have been extracted from the hermaphrodite teleost fish *Serranus scriba* (Lupo and Chieffi, 1965). Testosterone, androstenedione, and androsterone (in a free state) were identified by thin-layer and gas chromatography. Again only testosterone was found in the fraction of conjugated steroids. The authors did not report the details of the techniques used for the identification. Estrone and estriol were also allegedly present in the free phenolic fraction.

The analysis of steroids in *Morone labrax* testes revealed the presence of large quantities of estrogens and traces of testosterone (Lupo and Chieffi, 1963b). More recently, Van Mullem and Gottfried (1966) using gas chromatography reported testosterone, androstenedione, and dehydroepiandrosterone in the testes of *Gasterosteus aculeatus* during the period when the interstitial tissues are well developed.

b. Sperm. C_{19} Steroids (dehydroepiandrosterone particularly) and C_{18} steroid oestrogens have been isolated from the sperm of man and bull (see Dorfman and Ungar, 1965). The sperm of the elasmobranch fish *Squalus acanthias* contains steroids in very large quantities (Simpson *et al.*, 1963a). Deoxycorticosterone was present at a concentration of 500 μg/100 g of sperm. It has been obtained in a purified crystalline form and identified by its infrared spectrum. Progesterone and pregnenolone were also present (Simpson *et al.*, 1963a). In addition to the C_{21} compounds, C_{19} steroids, androstenedione, dehydroepiandrosterone, and probably androsterone were extracted from the sperm of *Squalus acanthias*. Androstenedione was identified by several paper chromatograms, by its reduction with $NaBH_4$, by light measurements at 240mμ, and finally by color reactions. No traces of testosterone could be detected. On the other hand, dehydroepiandrosterone was demonstrated by paper chromatography and by the Zimmermann reaction, while androsterone was identified by paper chromatography only. These results, however, have to be considered as a particular case, since no steroids have been found in the sperm of four other species of elasmobranchs: *Lamna cornubica, Scyliorhinus caniculus, Galeus vulgaris*, and *Raja batis* (Simpson *et al.*, 1963b).

In a preliminary note, Gottfried and Chieffi (1967) reported the presence of testosterone and 3β, 17 α-dihydroxy-5-pregnen-20-one in the sperm of *Scyliorhinus stellaris*; these two compounds have not been conclusively identified.

   c. Blood and Plasma. Grajcer and Idler (1961) isolated testosterone from both male and female salmon (*Oncorhynchus nerka*). In both sexes testosterone existed not only in the free form, but also conjugated with glucuronic acid. The concentration of the free testosterone in a sample of plasma taken from male fish after spawning was 1.7 μg/100 ml, and hydrolysis of the plasma by β-glucuronidase released a further 13.7μg of testosterone per 100 ml. The infrared spectrum of this testosterone after acetylation corresponded exactly with the spectrum of the acetate of authentic testosterone (Grajcer and Idler, 1961, 1963). In female salmon studies at the same time, i.e., after spawning, the concentration of free testosterone was 7.8 μg/100 ml of plasma and there were 7.6 μg of glucuronic–acid–conjugated testosterone per 100 ml of plasma (Schmidt and Idler, 1962). The total plasmatic concentration was close to 15 μg/100 ml for both male and female. However, the concentration of the testosterone glucuronoside was higher in the male.

   11-Ketotestosterone has been extracted from the plasma of male salmon, *Oncorhynchus nerka* (postspawned, 12 μg/100 ml), and from female salmon during some stages of river migration as well as from the plasma of Atlantic salmon, *Salmo salar* (Idler *et al.*, 1960a; Schmidt and Idler, 1962). It was the first time that 11-Ketotestosterone, chromatographically isolated and then identified by its infrared spectrum, had been demonstrated in a vertebrate. It has not yet been reported in the plasma of any other species of salmonid. The concentration of 11-ketotestosterone and of testosterone in the blood of the sockeye salmon varied during the spawning migration and the data suggest that these steroids may play a role in triggering the river phase of the migration. Just prior to the migration to Adams River, British Columbia, the plasma of females contained less than 2.5 μg/100 ml of 11-ketotestosterone and 17.5 μg/100 ml of testosterone but after the migration had begun 11-ketotestosterone rose to 7.1 μg/100 ml and testosterone decreased to 3.2 μg/100 ml. In males the situation was reversed; testosterone levels rose and 11-ketotestosterone fell coincident with the migration. 11-Ketotestosterone was not detactable in plasma of postspawned females. In male fish, testosterone levels increased (from 4.3 to 11 μg/100 ml) and 11-ketotestosterone decreased (from 7.9 to 4.8 μg/100 ml) during the migratory phase of their life. Adrenosterone is also a plasmatic steroid of salmon (Idler *et al.*, 1961b). The plasmatic concentrations of 17α-hydroxyprogesterone and of several corticosteroids as well as testosterone and 11-ketotestosterone varied during the migration of the fish (Schmidt and Idler, 1962).

Idler and Truscott (1966) have identified testosterone in the plasma of two elasmobranch fishes: *Raja radiata* and *Raja ocellata*. The identification of testosterone was done by paper, thin-layer, and gas chromatography, the formation of derivatives (oxidation, acetylation), double-isotope analysis, and finally by aromatization of the testosterone to estradiol-17β. Although testosterone was not isolated in crystalline form, the criteria are sufficient to allow a conclusive identification. As in salmon, testosterone was present in the plasma in both free and conjugated forms; among the conjugated forms the authors identified the glucuronide of testosterone. Testosterone liberated by acid hydrolysis after the action of the β-glucuronidase was assumed to be sulfate. In *R. radiata* the concentration of plasmatic testosterone in a mature male varied from 2.8 to 10.2 μg/100 ml, while the concentration of testosterone glucuronoside was between 4.3 and 6.7 μg/100 ml. Very little testosterone (0.1 μg/100 ml) was liberated by acid hydrolysis. Plasma of a female also contained free testosterone (0.02–0.60 μg/100 ml) and 0.13 μg/100 ml of glucurono conjugate. In a subsequent study on *R. radiata* the high levels of free testosterone in the male skate were confirmed; however, female skates were also found to contain high levels of testosterone (1.6–6.2 μg/100 ml, 5 fish) (Fletcher *et al.*, 1970). This point remains to be further investigated; however, differences in skate populations and/or the season of their capture were suggested. Preliminary evidence has also been presented which indicates that a daily cycle of testosterone concentrations may be present in male and female skates (Fletcher *et al.*, 1970). These authors found that the plasma concentrations of testosterone in five males and four females were significantly lower at 5:30 P.M. than at 9:30 A.M.

Plasmatic concentrations of dehydroepiandrosterone and androsterone in *Torpedo marmorata* varied with the reproductive cycle (Buonanno *et al.*, 1964). By thin-layer and gas chromatography Lupo di Prisco *et al.*(1967b) have demonstrated the presence of testosterone (free or conjugated) in the plasma of a female *T. marmorata*. This steroid was present in immature animals (3.5 μg/100 ml), in the period preceding gestation (1.56 μg/100 ml), during gestation (0.80 μg/100 ml), and in the postgestative period (2.36 μg/100 ml). A preliminary study has indicated small quantities of testosterone and 17α-hydroxyprogesterone in the plasma of *Scyliorhinus caniculus* (Simpson *et al.*, 1968a).

d. Other Tissues. Cédard and Fontaine (1963) reported that the corpuscles of Stannius of the Atlantic salmon *Salmo salar* contained 17-ketosteroids and estrogens. From the beginning of the anadramous migration to the time of spawning the amount of androgens increased tenfold in the corpuscles of Stannius of the male.

2. Other Vertebrates

A conclusive identification of C_{19} androgens in amphibians, reptiles, and birds has not been realized as yet; preliminary experiments strongly suggest their presence in some species.

17-Ketosteroids were present in the breeding water of *Xenopus laevis*; the chemical structures of these compounds have not been established (Rapola, 1963). Dale (1962) reported the presence of 17-ketosteroids in the breeding water of *Rana pipiens* larvae after sex differentiation; a compound having the same $\overset{\circ}{R}_f$ on paper chromatograms as androsterone gave a positive Zimmerman reaction. Progesterone, estrone, estradiol-17β, and estriol have been isolated from the organ of Bidder and from testes of a toad (Chieffi and Lupo, 1961b); the authors did not report the presence of androgens.

Testosterone was identified by double-isotope dilution in the plasma of the salamander *Necturus maculosus*. The plasma concentration of testosterone ranges between 4.3 and 26 μg/100 ml. Androstenedione and dehydroepiandrosterone are also present in much lower concentrations (Rivarola *et al.*, 1968). In another urodele amphibian, *Pleurodeles waltlii*, testosterone and epitestosterone (17α-hydroxy-4-androsten-3-one) were isolated and quantified in plasma following the technique described by Attal (1970). The free steroids were purified by different chromatographies and estimated, after formation of heptafluorobutyrate derivatives, by gas chromatography with an electron capture detector; radioactive tracers were added for quantitative data. The concentration of free testosterone was in the range 4–5 μg/100 ml and that of epitestosterone was 2 μg/100 ml of plasma (Ozon and Attal, 1969).

From 35 g of testicular tissue obtained from 400 lizards (*Lacerta sicula*) Lupo di Prisco *et al.* (1967a) extracted and then analyzed by gas chromatography eight steroids, chiefly testosterone (in conjugated form) and androstenedione. Lupo di Prisco *et al.* (1968) isolated androstenedione (among eight other steroids) in the ovaries of the same lizards. Gottfried *et al.* (1967), by incubation *in vitro*, demonstrated that the testes of the cobra *Naja naja* produced from endogenous precursors androstenedione and dehydroepiandrosterone, both of which were identified by gas chromatography and the formation of derivatives (acetates). The authors reported that the adrenal tissue of cobra, in similar experimental conditions, produced testosterone and dehydroepiandrosterone. The identification of these two C_{19} steroids as well as estrone, present in the same extract, was based on insufficient criteria to allow an immediate conclusion concerning the biological role of the sex steroids of adrenal origin in the lower vertebrates.

During the period of sexual activity the female phalarope has brightly colored feathers and an aggressive attitude; the opposite of this generally occurs with birds, the male being the active sex. Höhn and Cheng (1967) examined the levels of sexual steroids in the testes and ovaries by paper chromatography and color reactions. Testosterone and androstenedione were detected in all cases. The concentration of testosterone was higher in the female than in the male and, according to the authors, this could explain the active sexual behavior of the females. Similar comparative studies have been carried out in other species of birds (Table I). The presence of testosterone and androsterone in the testes of *Gallus domesticus* was confirmed by Delrio *et al.* (1967). By gas chromatography and double-isotopic techniques, testosterone was isolated in the plasma of the laying hen (O'Malley *et al.*, 1968); androstenedione was also present. In the plasma of another bird, the white carneau pigeon, Rivarola *et al.* (1968) found testosterone, androsternedione, and dehydroepiandrosterone. Testosterone had been detected by gas chromatography in the duck and other birds (Jallageas and Attal, 1968; Garnier and Attal, 1970).

C. COMMENTS

During the last decade, steroid hormones have been isolated from non-mammalian vertebrates (for reviews see Gottfried, 1964; Ozon, 1966). Concerning the C_{19} androgens the only conclusive identification of testosterone has been done in fishes (Grajcer and Idler, 1963; Idler and Truscott, 1966). Preliminary experiments strongly suggest the presence of these hormones in amphibians, reptiles, and birds. Among the vertebrates, testosterone probably is not the only androgenic hormone. 11-Ketotestosterone, a steroid isolated from the plasma of salmon (*Oncorhynchus nerka* and *Salmo salar*), has important androgenic activity, superior or comparable to that of testosterone in the case of *Oryzias latipes*, *Oncorhynchus nerka*, and chicken (capon's comb test) (Arai, 1967; Idler *et al.*, 1961a,c.).

Pregnenolone and progesterone are the immediate precursors of androgens in the ovaries and testes of vertebrates (Fig. 2). These C_{21} steroids have been demonstrated by chromatography in the gonads of the lower vertebrates (Table II).

Estrogens, namely estradiol-17β and estrone, have been extracted from the testicular tissue of fishes (Chieffi and Lupo, 1961a; Lupo and Chieffi, 1963a, 1965), amphibians (Chieffi and Lupo, 1963), reptiles (Gottfried *et al.*, 1967), and birds (Höhn and Cheng, 1967). Further studies are necessary to confirm the secretion of C_{18} steroids by the testes of lower vertebrates.

It must be pointed out that many of these endeavors to isolate and identify steroids are based upon incomplete chemical analyses. The

TABLE II
Progesterone Isolated by Chromatography from Nonmammalian Vertebrates

Species	Origin of steroid	Concentration ($\mu g/kg$)[a]	Reference
Petromyzon marinus	Ovaries		Botticelli et al. (1963)
Squalus suckleyi	Ovaries		Wotiz et al. (1960)
Torpedo marmorata	Ovaries	15	Chieffi and Lupo (1963)
Conger conger	Ovaries	68	Lupo and Chieffi (1963a)
Protopterus annectens	Ovaries	92	Dean and Chester Jones (1959)
Serranus scriba	Hermaphrodite gonads	16	Lupo and Chieffi (1965)
Bufo vulgaris	Ovaries		Chieffi and Lupo (1963)
		Pregnenolone, 29	
Lacerta sicula	Ovaries	17α-Hydroxypregnenolone, 93	Lupo di Prisco et al. (1968)
		17α-Hydroxypregnenolone, 8.6	Höhn and Cheng (1967)
Steganopus tricolor	Ovaries		Layne et al. (1957)
Gallus domesticus	Ovaries		O'Malley et al. (1968)
	Plasma (laying hen)	126[a]	
Scyliorhinus stellaris	Testes	100	Chieffi and Lupo (1961a)
Squalus acanthias	Sperm	80	Simpson et al. (1963a)
		Pregnenolone, 140	
Morone labrax	Testes	17	Lupo and Chieffi (1963b)
Gasterosteus aculeatus	Testes		Van Mullem and Gottfried (1966)
Triturus cristatus	Testes		Della Corte and Cosenza (1965)
Bufo vulgaris	Testes + Bidder's organ		Lupo di Prisco et al. (1967a,b)
Lacerta sicula	Testes	34	
Naja naja	Testes, incubated *in vitro*	Pregnenolone, 123	Gottfried et al. (1967)
		17α-Hydroxypregnenolone, 127	
Steganopus tricolor	Testes		Höhn and Cheng (1967)
Gallus domesticus	Testes	Pregnenolone, 66.5	Delrio et al. (1967)

[a] Footnoted values in nanograms per 100 ml.

minute quantities of hormone contained in the tissues present the main difficulty in their isolation. Chromatographic methods, which have proven particularly useful for the separation of a few micrograms of purified substances, often are insufficient for an identification; for a conclusive identification a relatively large quantity (20–100 μg) of hormone should be purified. Only then can the steroid be identified by the various micromethods of physical chemistry (chemical derivatives, crystallization, melting point, infrared spectrum, mass spectrometry, and nuclear magnetic resonance spectra). Hence, great quantities of tissue have to be used and, consequently, a great number of specimens. For instance, 17 μg of testosterone were isolated from 1 kg of salmon testes (Grajcer and Idler, 1963). Extraction experiments produce only quantitative results concerning a hormone present in a certain set of animals. Physiological studies of variations of a hormone in a single animal (for instance in the blood of a frog, from which 1–2 ml samples only can be obtained) bring up complicated methodological problems which are now being tackled by gas chromatography, a method which has been found useful for quantitative studies. One must also point out that investigators have isolated only minute quantities of steroids, and their research has also been focused on the "classical" steroids already known in the mammals; for instance, estradiol-17β and testosterone generally have been isolated from lower vertebrates by methods established for mammals. It is seldom possible to detect with certainty a new steroid compound present in small quantities in a species. When an organ contains a hormone one can also question whether it secrets the hormone or is only a place for storage, finally, the hormone may be only precursor of other metabolites.

The identification of steroids in the tissues of vertebrates is not a goal in itself; it is only a static viewpoint of biochemical events. It is necessary to know the nature of the steroids which circulate in the blood, the mechanisms which control their biosynthesis, the pathway of their metabolism, as well as the means of their elimination, in the various classes of vertebrates.

III. Biosynthesis of C_{19} Steroids

In mammals several endocrine glands, including the ovaries, the testes, and the adrenal cortex, secrete steroid hormones. It is generally admitted that cholesterol is the principal precursor of the steroid hormones; the gonads and the adrenal cortex are in fact tissues rich in cholesterol and its concentration is lowered when they are stimulated by pituitary hormones.

The synthesis of cholesterol begins with the acetate radical; the principal intermediaries between acetyl-CoA and cholesterol are mevalonic acid, isopentenyl pyrophosphate, farnesyl pyrophosphate, and squalene (Dorfman and Ungar, 1965). During the next stage, cholesterol is transformed into steroids with 21 carbon atoms. Cholesterol is first hydroxylated in the 20α position and then 20α-hydroxycholesterol is transformed into 20α, 22-dihydroxycholesterol; the cleavage of the side chain gives rise to pregnenolone and isocaproic acid. The cofactor of the two hydroxylation reactions is NADPH (Ichii *et al.*, 1963). Pregnenolone can be considered as a precursor with 21 carbon atoms that is common to all hormonal steroids. Conversion

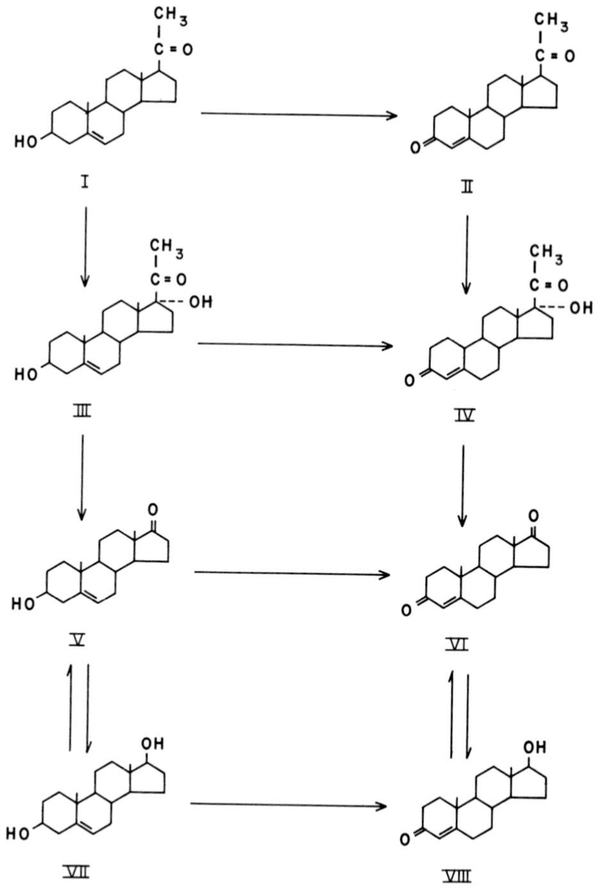

Fig. 2. Biosynthesis of C_{19} steroid hormones from C_{21} precursors in mammals. A similar sequence of reactions has been described for fishes, amphibians, reptiles and birds. I, Pregnenolone; II, progesterone; III, 17 α-hydroxypregnenolone; IV, 17α-hydroxyprogesterone; V, dehydroepiandrosterone; VI, androstenedione; VII, 5-androstene-3β, 17β-diol; VIII, testosterone.

of pregnenolone to biologically active hormones is specific to each endocrine gland.

The main pathways of biosynthesis of androgens in mammals are shown in Fig. 2; other mechanisms are also possible (Dorfman and Ungar, 1965). These have not been included because no experimental results have yet been obtained which would permit a postulation of their existence in non-mammalian vertebrates.

Since 1963, the study of the biosynthesis of androgens has been undertaken in fishes, amphibians, reptiles, and birds. These studies have in general been carried out *in vitro* using incubating techniques of testicular tissue in the presence of either neutral of radioactive precursors: acetate; cholesterol; Δ^5-3β-hydroxysteroids:pregnenolone, 17α-hydroxypregnenolone, dehydroepiandrosterone; and Δ^4-3-ketosteroids:progesterone, 17α-hydroxyprogesterone. The transformation of the Δ^5-3β-hydroxysteroids into Δ^4-3-ketosteroids, an indispensable stage in the synthesis of hormonal steroids, is catalyzed by two enzymes, 3β-hydroxysteroid oxido-reductase and $\Delta^5 \longrightarrow \Delta^4$-isomerase ($\Delta^5-3\beta$-hydroxysteroid oxido-reductase). A histochemical technique described by Wattenberg (1958) enables one to show the presence of this enzyme activity in almost all the tissues which secrete steroid hormones. Histochemistry reveals the presence of Δ^5-3β-hydroxysteroid oxido-reductase in the gonads of certain lower vertebrates (Nandi, 1967). However, one must specify that the histochemical presence (or absence) of this enzymic activity does not necessarily mean that the organ may (or may not) produce steroids. In our opinion every histological study of Δ^5-3β-hydroxysteroid oxido-reductase must be paralleled by a biochemical synthesis of the steroids. In any case it permits one to detect in the tissue the cells which actively participate in the biosynthesis of steroid hormones, thus providing valuable information indicating the site of their secretion in the gonads, a problem which cannot be perfectly solved by biological experiments alone (van Oordt, 1963).

A. THE MALE (Table III)

1. Fishes

a. In Vivo. Radioactive testosterone and 11-ketotestosterone were isolated in a free state from the plasma of a sexually mature salmon (*Oncorhynchus nerka*) $1\frac{3}{4}$ hr after *in vivo* injection of 17α-hydroxyprogesterone-4-^{14}C (Idler and Truscott, 1963). Testosterone and 11-ketotestosterone are powerful androgens in salmon and chicken (Idler *et al.*, 1961a,c). Idler and Truscott (1963) studied the precursors of this steroid. They showed that the 11-hydroxycorticosteroids (cortisol or cortisone) *in vivo* were not transformed into C_{19} steroids substituted at C-11. On the other hand, testosterone-4-^{14}C and 17α-hydroxyprogesterone-4-^{14}C were the precursors of 11-ketotestosterone. Considering the percentage of conversion, the authors, although they did not isolate the intermediates, postulated a pathway to the synthesis of 11-ketotestosterone through androstenedione, 11β-hydroxyandrostenedione, and adrenosterone in addition to a pathway via testosterone. 11β-hydroxylation appears to be more important when the substrate has a 17-ketone radical. In conclusion, a $C_{21} \longrightarrow C_{19}$ *desmolase*, 17β-hydroxysteroid oxido-reductase, 11β-hydroxylase, and 11β-hydroxysteroid oxido-reductase have all been demonstrated *in vivo* in a teleost fish, *Oncorhynchus nerka*. However, these experiments *in vivo* did not provide information about the localization of these enzymes in the tissues. In other teleosts the testicular tissue contains an active desmolase which transforms 17α-hydroxyprogesterone into androstenedione. It was of great interest to learn at which site (interrenal or testes) the 11β-hydroxylation takes place; experiments performed *in vitro* and using neutral C_{19} steroids as substrate showed that the testes of two teleost fishes contained an 11β-hydroxylase (Idler and MacNab, 1967; Arai and Tamaoki, 1967a,b).

Proof that 11-ketotestosterone and testosterone are produced *in vivo* by the testis has been provided by studies of the major androgens in testicular and peripheral plasma of the Atlantic salmon *Salmo salar* (Idler *et al.*, 1971). Blood samples were removed from male Atlantic salmon during two histologically distinct stages of their sexual development. Histological examination showed the earlier fish to be in an advanced maturing stage, as sperm cells at all stages of development were present in the testis lobules, and the later fish to be in the fully mature spawning stage. Testosterone, 11β-hydroxytestosterone, and 11-ketotestosterone were quantified in the plasma by a double-isotope derivative assay procedure. 11-Ketotestosterone was the major androgen in both testicular and peripheral plasma and the concentration greatly increased as maturation advanced. Testosterone levels in peripheral plasma remained comparatively stable, while there was a trend toward increased levels in testicular plasma. The quantities of 11-ketotestosterone and testosterone were greater in testicular than in peripheral plasma, indicating that the testis is the primary site of their production. In addition, substantial amounts of 11-ketotestosterone, testosterone, and 11β-hydroxytestosterone were present as glucuronosides. The concentration of glucuronosides was generally higher in testicular than in peripheral plasma, suggesting that these conjugates are produced in the testes. The concentration of 11-ketotestosterone and 11β-hydroxytestosterone glucuronosides was high in the more mature fish while testosterone glucuronoside changed very little in concentration. 11β-Hydroxytestosterone was isolated and identified in salmon plasma for the first time and its concentration in testicular plasma

TABLE III

Synthesis of C_{19} Steroids in Testis of Nonmammalian Vertebrates

Species	Tissue incubated *in vitro* or injection *in vivo*	Precursor steroid	Isolated steroid[a]	Reference
FISHES				
Squalus acanthias	Testes	Pregnenolone-^{14}C Progesterone-^{14}C	Progesterone 20β-Hydroxypregn-4-ene-3-one Testosterone Deoxycorticosterone 17, 21-Dihydroxypregn-4-ene-3-one	Simpson *et al.* (1964b)
	Sperm	Cholesterol-^{14}C Pregnenolone-^{14}C or progesterone-^{14}C	Progesterone Deoxycorticosterone No C_{19} steroids	Simpson *et al.* (1964a)
Scyliorhinus canaliculus	Testes and testicular cysts	Dehydroepiandrosterone	Androst-4-ene-3,17-dione	Collenot and Ozon (1964)
	Testes	Pregnenolone-^{14}C Progesterone-^{14}C	Testosterone Progesterone 20α- and 20β-Hydroxypregn-4-ene-3-one 17α-Hydroxyprogesterone Androst-4-ene-3,17-dione Testosterone	Simpson *et al.* (1969a)
Tribolodon hakonensis	Testes	Progesterone	17α-Hydroxyprogesterone Androst-4-ene-3,7-dione	Arai *et al.* (1964)
Oncorhyncus nerka	*In vivo*	17α-Hydroxyprogesterone-^{14}C	Testosterone 11-Ketotestosterone (isolated from plasma)	Idler and Truscott (1963)
Salmo salar	Testes	Testosterone-^{14}C Adrenosterone-^{3}H Androst-4-ene-3,17-dione-^{14}C	11β-Hydroxytestosterone 11-Ketotestosterone Testosterone	Idler and MacNab (1967)
	Testes	Dehydroepiandrosterone-^{3}H	11β-Hydroxytestosterone 11-Ketotestosterone 11β-Hydroxyandrost-4-ene-3,17-dione Androst-5-ene-3β,17β-diol Androst-5-ene-3β, 11β, 17β-triol	Idler *et al.* (1968)

TABLE III (cont.)

Species	Tissue incubated in vitro or injection in vivo	Precursor steroid	Isolated steroid[a]	Reference
Microstomus kitt Walbaum	Testes	Progesterone-^{14}C	17α-Hydroxyprogesterone Androst-4-ene-3,17-dione Testosterone 3-Hydroxy-5β-androstan-17-one 5β-Androstanedione	Simpson et al. (1969b)
Salmo gairdnerii	Testes	Progesterone-^{14}C	17α-Hydroxyprogesterone 17α,20β-Dihydroxypregn-4-ene-3-one Androst-4-ene-3,17-dione Testosterone	Arai and Tamaoki (1967a,b)
		Androst-4-ene-3,17-dione	Testosterone 11β-Hydroxytestosterone 11-ketotestosterone	
AMPHIBIANS *Pleurodeles waltlii*	Testes	Pregnenolone Progesterone-^{14}C or 17α-hydroxyprogesterone-^{14}C	Progesterone 17α-Hydroxyprogesterone Androst-4-ene-3,17-dione Testosterone	Ozon (1967)
Rana esculenta	Testes	Dehydroepiandrosterone	Androst-4-ene-3,17-dione Testosterone	Botte and Lupo di Prisco (1965)
Xenopus laevis	Testes	17α-Hydroxyprogesterone-^{14}C	Androst-4-ene-3,17-dione Testosterone	Rao et al. (1969)
Rana catesbeiana	In vivo	Progesterone-^{14}C	Testosterone	Dale and Dorfman (1967)
	Testes	Progesterone-^{14}C	Testosterone 20α-Hydroxypregn-4-ene-3-one Pregnane-3,20-dione	Dale and Dorfman (1967)
REPTILES Natrix sipedon	Testes	Pregnenolone-^{3}H	Progesterone Testosterone	Callard (1967)

	Tissue	Substrate	Products[a]	Reference
BIRDS				
Passer domesticus	Testes	Progesterone-^{14}C	20α- and 20β-Hydroxypregn-4-ene-3-one 17α-Hydroxyprogesterone Androst-4-ene-3,17-dione <u>Testosterone</u>	Fevold and Eik-Nes (1963)
Gallus domesticus	Testes (of 2-day-old chick)	Acetate-^{14}C	<u>Testosterone</u>	Connell *et al.* (1966)
	Testes, in culture (9-day-old embryo)	Dehydroepiandrosterone-^{14}C	Dehydroepiandrosterone Testosterone Androst-5-ene-3β,17β-diol	Cédard and Haffen (1966)
	Testes	Progesterone-^{14}C	17α-Hydroxyprogesterone Androst-4-ene-3,17-dione <u>Testosterone</u>	Subhas and Edwards (1968)
Steganopus tricolor	Testes	17α-Hydroxyprogesterone-^{14}C and Pregnenolone-^{3}H	<u>Testosterone</u> Androst-4-ene-3,17-dione	Fevold and Pfeiffer (1966)

[a]Underlined compound is the main isolated androgen.

347

increased in the late stages of maturation; this observation is consistent with the conclusion based on *in vitro* incubations that 11β-hydroxytestosterone is a precursor of 11-ketotestosterone in testes.

   b.   Testes. The testes of an elasmobranch fish, *Squalus acanthias*, possess the enzymes which catalyze the transformation of pregnenolone and progesterone into testosterone (Simpson *et al.*, 1964b). When progesterone-4-^{14}C was incubated with 12–16 g of testicular tissue, they identified by paper chromatography, after the formation of derivatives, several metabolites and indicated the percentage of conversion, e.g., 1.4% of the progesterone was transformed into testosterone. In one incubation they showed the presence of 17α,20β-dihydroxy-4-pregnen-3-one. From the absence of 17α-hydroxyprogesterone among the intermediary metabolites the authors inferred the presence of a very active C_{21} $\longrightarrow$$C_{19}$ desmolase in the testes, but this conclusion does not explain the absence of androstenedione. The great activity of a 21-hydroxylase in the sperm of this elasmobranch possibly accounts for the formation of deoxycorticosterone when pregnenolone or progesterone were incubated with testicular tissue containing ripe spermatozoa (Simpson *et al.*, 1964a). The authors did not exclude in *Squalus acanthias*, under the experimental conditions used, a route of testosterone biosynthesis bypassing 17α-hydroxyprogesterone and androstenedione. One must, however, note that the long duration of the incubations (16.5 hr) may account for the absence of known intermediates in the synthesis of testosterone.

   In another elasmobranch, *Scyliorhinus caniculus*, dehydroepiandrosterone was an active precursor of androstenedione and testosterone (Collenot and Ozon, 1964). The enzymes which bring about this transformation are present in spermatozoic cysts. On the other hand, a histochemical study showed that the Δ^5-3β-hydroxysteroid oxido-reductase is principally localized in the Sertoli cells of spermatozoic cysts and also in the spermatozoa themselves. Simpson *et al.* (1969a) have recently taken up this study, again using as precursors pregnenolone-4-^{14}C and progesterone-4-^{14}C. These two steroids were transformed into testosterone by the testes of *Scyliorhinus caniculus*. Simpson and his collaborators have isolated neither 17α-hydroxypregnenolone nor dehydroepiandrosterone after the incubation of testes in the presence of pregnenolone-4-^{14}C; however. the Δ^5-3β-hydroxysteroids are very rapidly metabolized, which may explain why they could not be isolated under these conditions. In conclusion, it is probable that the main pathway of synthesis of testosterone, beginning with pregnenolone, passes through progesterone without, however, excluding the formation of dehydroepiandrosterone as an intermediary.

   The team of Simpson (Simpson *et al.*, 1969b), has undertaken a study of the biosynthetic capabilities of the testes of the teleost *Microstomus kitt* Walbaum; as before, after incubating progesterone-4-^{14}C they have isolated 17α-hydroxyprogesterone, androstenedione, and testosterone. They have also identified in these incubations saturated compounds derived from 5β-pregnane and 5β-androstane. In a short communication Eckstein (1967) reported the conversion of ^{3}H-pregnenolone to C_{19} steroids by testes and ovaries of *Mugil cephalus*.

In 1964 Arai *et al.* showed that the testes of a cyprinid, *Tribolodon hako-nensis*, contain enzymes which *in vitro* catalyze the transformation of pro-gesterone-4-^{14}C into 17α-hydroxyprogesterone and androstenedione. However, since they did not isolate testosterone in any of their experiments, one must assume the absence or the inactivation of a 17β-hydroxysteroid oxido-reductase under the experimental conditions used. Actually, the authors incubated 5 μCi of progesterone-4-^{14}C (83 μCi/mg), which corres-ponds to about 60 μg of precursor, and this can be considered as extra-physiological. A large quantity of precursor can influence the enzymes responsible for the synthesis of androgens; particularly progesterone could possibly inhibit the activity of 17β-hydroxysteroid dehydrogenase. After incubation of progesterone-4-^{14}C the authors detected nine unidentified metabolites, one of which had a polarity similar to that of testosterone (Arai *et al.*, 1964). In the trout *Salmo gairdnerii*, Arai and Tamaoki (1967a,b), after incubation of progesterone-4-^{14}C with a testicular homogenate, obtained 17α-hydroxyprogesterone, 17α,20β-hydroxy-4-pregnen-3-one, androstene-dione, and testosterone. The metabolic pathway was similar to that of the previous study. Moreover, they showed that androstenedione-4-^{14}C was metabolized by the testes, under the same experimental conditions, to testosterone, 11β-hydroxytestosterone, and 11-ketotestosterone.

These results confirm, from a qualitative viewpoint, the *in vivo* and *in vitro* experiments of Idler and Truscott (1963) and Idler and MacNab (1967). *In vivo*, after injection of testosterone, only 11-ketotestosterone was isolated from the plasma of the salmon *Oncorhynchus nerka*. *In vitro*, testosterone-4-^{14}C and adrenosterone-1,2-^{3}H were transformed by testicular as well as interrenal tissues into 11β-hydroxytestosterone and 11-ketotestosterone (Idler and MacNab, 1967); the incubation medium contained a NADPH-generating system. Under these experimental conditions adrenosterone emerged as the best precursor of 11-ketotestosterone in both tissues. The testis, considering its size (3.3% of the total live weight), was the main source of 11-ketotestosterone synthesized from adrenosterone. Thus the presence of an active 17β-hydroxysteroid oxido-reductase was demonstrated in the testes. On the other hand, testosterone was the best precursor of 11β-hydro-xytestosterone in both the testicular and interrenal tissues. 11β-hydroxy-androstenedione was not isolated from incubations with androstenedione

(Arai and Tamaoki, 1967a,b). Figure 3 shows the proven stages in the *in vitro* formation of 11-ketotestosterone; it shows the presence in teleost testicular tissue of 11β-hydroxylase and 11β- and 17β-hydroxysteroid oxido-reductase. the results obtained by Arai and Tamaoki (1967a,b) indicate that the synthesis of 11-ketotestosterone from androstenedione by testes would pass through 11β-hydroxytestosterone. However, the experiments of Idler and MacNab (1967), although they confirmed the formation of 11β-hydroxy-testosterone, also showed that adrenosterone was the better precursor of 11-ketotestosterone.

The Halifax workers recently reported the incubation of androstene dione-[14]C (2.2 μCi) and dehydroepiandrosterone-[3]H (DHA) (10.4 μCi) with mature testes of Atlantic salmon (Idler *et al.*, 1968) in the presence of a NADPH-generating system. Radioactive testosterone, 11β-hydroxytesto-sterone, 11-ketotestosterone, 11β-hydroxyandrostenedione, 5-androstene-diol, and 5-androstenetriol were rigorously identified by establishing isopolarity and isomorphism with authentic steroids. The incubation media were analyzed at 1, 3, and 5$\frac{1}{2}$ h and the yields and [3]H:[14]C ratios were deter-mined for the above steroids and for androstenedione and DHA. No adreno-sterone was detected. In the 1 hr incubates adequate androstenedione and DHA remained and there were sufficient products to achieve constant isotope ratios. Androstenedione ([3]H:[14]C, 1:∞) was several times more efficiently converted to 11-ketotestosterone (1.3:1) than was DHA (∞:1). There was some conversion of DHA to testosterone (1:9.5); however, the data show that DHA was converted to 11β-hydroxytestosterone (1:1) via a pathway other than testosterone, i.e., via 5-androstenediol (∞:1). There was somewhat more tritium in 11-ketotestosterone (1.3:1) than in 11β-hydroxytestosterone (1:1) suggesting that 5-androstenediol was also going to 11-ketotestosterone via 5-androstenetriol. The [3]H:[14]C ratio (1:2.6) in 11β-hydroxyandrostenedione shows that androstenedione (1:∞) was not an effective precursor of this steroid under the experimental conditions. Even when 11β-hydroxyandrostenedione-^{3}H and testosterone-^{14}C were in-cubated with testes, it was not possible to isolate adrenosterone (Idler 1969). However, the [3]H:[14]C ratios in 11-hydroxytestosterone were 1:1.5 and 1:1.8 at 1.5 and 3 hr, respectively, compared with ratios of 1.1:1 and 1.2:1 in 11-ketotestosterone. The corresponding ratios in 11β-hydroxy-androstenedione were 10.3:1 and 4.9:1. From these data it seems reasonable to conclude that 11β-hydroxyandrostenedione *is* converted to 11-ketotesto-sterone via adrenosterone even though the route is not competitive with that through 11β-hydroxytestosterone under the experimental conditions. The current status of the pathways of metabolism to 11-ketotestosterone in Atlantic salmon *in vitro* is shown in Fig. 3.

When and how is adrenosterone [a plasmatic steroid in salmon (Idler *et*

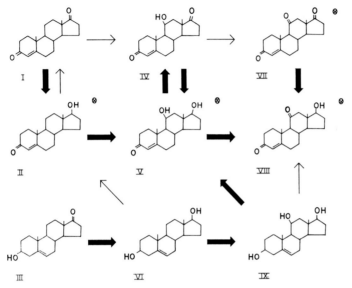

Fig. 3. Formation *in vitro* of 11-ketotestosterone in testes of *Salmo salar*. Major potential pathways, ➡; other pathways, ⟶. The pathway from androstenedione was favored over the route from DHA under the experimental conditions, which assumed equal availability of the two precursors and an efficient NADPH-generating system. I, androstenedione; II, testosterone; III, dehydroepiandrosterone; IV, 11β-hydroxyandrostenedione; V, 11β-hydroxytestosterone; VI, 5-androstene-3β, 17β-diol; VII, anrenosterone; VIII, 11-ketotestosterone; IX, 5-androstene-3β,11β,17β-triol.

al., 1961b)] synthesized? This question opens avenues for new experiments. It is known that the experimental conditions of incubations *in vitro* (temperature, duration of incubation, quantity of the precursor, cofactors, pituitary stimulation) generally modify the enzymic activities. In these previously described experiments, NADPH, a cofactor of hydroxylation of steroids, was added to the incubation medium; it probably activates 11β-hydroxylation and it can also modify the equilibrium of oxido–reduction catalyzed by hydroxysteroid oxido-reductase. Is the testicular 11β-hydroxylase specific for the C_{19} substrate? Which cells are responsible for the 11β-hydroxylation? What is the cellular location of 11β-hydroxylation, enzyme mitochondria or microsomes? The concentration of 11-ketotestosterone in the plasma varies with the sexual cycle (Schmidt and Idler, 1962); is the variation in the total amount of 11-ketotestosterone determined by the variation of the activity of 11β-hydroxylase or by the accelerated rate of inactivation of this hormone in the liver? Many questions deserve to be investigated, because it now appears likely that 11-ketotestosterone plays an important role in the sexual physiology of teleost fishes.

c. *Sperm*. Recent results have shown that sperm contains steroid hormones (Section II, B). We shall see (Section IV, D) that the sperm of several vertebrates contains enzymes which metabolize steroid hormones; hence, it is of interest to question if the spermatozoa play a role in the synthesis of androgens in the testes.

Simpson *et al*. (1964a), intrigued by the presence of steroids (mainly deoxycorticosterone) in the sperm of *Squalus acanthias*, looked for the precursors and the site of synthesis of these hormones. They were able to show that the sperm of *Squalus acanthias* contained enzymes which catalyze the synthesis of deoxycorticosterone from cholesterol (Fig. 4). The sperm contained Δ^5-3β-hydroxysteroid dehydrogenase and a very active 21-hydroxylase. There was no formation of testosterone or other steroids. The active transformation of cholesterol or pregnenolone into progesterone is proof that the sperm of this species is able to synthesize the precursors of C_{19} steroids. Where are the enzymes localized? In another elasmobranch, *Scyliorhinus caniculus*, the spermatozoa isolated by centrifugation contained Δ^5-3β-hydroxysteroid oxido-reductase (Ozon and Collenot, 1965). These results raise the question of the participation of spermatozoa, at least in the elasmobranch fishes, in the synthesis of androgenic steroids in the testes in single or multiple stages.

2. Amphibians

The presence of C_{19} steroids in testes of amphibians has not yet been demonstrated; only preliminary results suggest the presence of progesterone (Table II). The activity of Δ^5-3β-hydroxysteroid dehydrogenase has

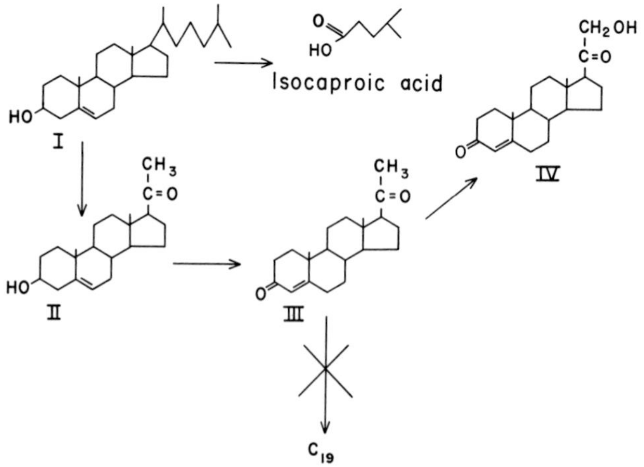

Fig. 4.   Transformation of cholesterol into C_{21}-steroids by sperm of *Squalus acanthias*.
I, cholesterol; II, pregnenolone; III, progesterone; IV, deoxycorticosterone. Details in text.

been shown by histochemical methods in testes of certain amphibians (See Nandi, 1967).

Study of the biosynthesis of C_{19} steroids from exogenous precursors in Urodela, *Pleaurodeles waltlii* Michah, showed that the testes have Δ^5-3β-hydroxysteroid oxido-reductase, 17α-hydroxylase, $C_{21} \longrightarrow C_{19}$ desmolase, and 17β-hydroxysteroid oxido-reductase (Ozon, 1967). The major transformation of pregnenolone or progesterone into testosterone took place in cells of the walls of empty cysts which constitute the glandular tissue. Desmolase and 17α-hydroxylase were localized in a microsomal fraction of the glandular tissue. More recently (Ozon, 1968) it was possible to show that progesterone-4-^{14}C and pregnenolone-7-^{3}H, when incubated simultaneously in the presence of testicular tissue of *P. waltlii*, were transformed into 17α-hydroxyprogesterone, androstenedione, and testosterone. The ratios ^{3}H:^{14}C of the formed compounds indicated the presence of two simultaneous metabolic pathways, one passing through Δ^5-3β-hydroxysteroids, the other through Δ^4-3-ketosteroids. Botte and Lupo di Prisco (1965) demonstrated the conversion *in vitro* of pregnenolone and dehydroepiandrosterone by a testicular homogenate of *Rana esculenta* into progesterone and androstenedione, respectively.

Testicular tissue of the American bullfrog *Rana catesbeiana* metabolizes progesterone-4-^{14}C to testosterone *in vitro* and *in vivo* Dale and Dorfman, 1967). These authors found, in the same incubation, a reduction of the C_{20} ketone of progesterone to the α-hydroxy configuration.

3. Reptiles

Pregnenolone-16-^{3}H was a precursor of progesterone and testosterone in the snake *Natrix sipedon pictiventris* (Callard, 1967). Histochemically, Δ^5-3β-hydroxysteroid oxido-reductase was shown to be present in the interstitial tissue.

4. Birds

The testicular tissue of the bird *Passer domesticus* was capable of synthesizing testosterone and androstenedione from progesterone-4-^{14}C (Fevold and Eik-Nes, 1962, 1963). The synthesis of the androgenic steroids, under these conditions, was similar to that in mammals. On the other hand, testes have 20α- and 20β-hydroxysteroid oxido-reductase. The formation of the reduced compounds, 20α-hydroxy-4-pregnen-3-one and its 20β isomer, could control the synthesis of testosterone; indeed, the inactivation of progesterone into 20α and 20β derivatives would lower the amount of precursor available, in this case progesterone, for the synthesis of C_{19} steroids; such inactivation could depend upon the concentration of the 17α-hydroxylase. These explanations are valid only under the condition that the pathway of testosterone synthesis proceed through progesterone, 17α-hydroxyprogesterone, androstenedione, and testosterone. The pathway through 17α-hydroxypregne-nolone, dehydroepiandrosterone, and androstenedione is not excluded, and the formation of dehydroepiandrosterone by chicken (Connell *et al.*, 1966) suggests that it also has an important role in the formation of testosterone in the testes of birds. Neither the significance of the formation of 20α-hydroxy-4-pregnen-3-one and its 20β isomer nor the formation of the 17α, 20α-dihydroxy-4-pregnen-3-one and its 20β isomer in the same incubations of the testes of *Passer domesticus* is known.

In vitro the testes of a 2-day-old chick incorporated acetate-^{14}C into testo-sterone, androstenedione, and dehydroepiandrosterone (Connell *et al.*, 1966). After 2 hr of incubation at 41°C the ratio of testosterone and andro-stenedione formed was 2.3:1.0. For the first time the authors described the influence of gonadotropins on the synthesis of C_{19} steroids in nonmammalian vertebrate testes; an injection of 100 μg intersititial-cell-stimulating hor-mone, ICSH (luteinizing hormone) into the chick 24 hr preceding the removal of testes increased the incorporation of acetate-^{14}C into the neutral C_{19} steroids and at the same time raised the ratio testosterone; androstenedione to 5.3:1.0. The identification of dehydroepiandrosterone very strongly sug-gests that testosterone can be formed by passing through the Δ^5-3β-hydroxy-steroid intermediates but the results of these authors do not indicate the importance of this pathway. The isolation of dehydroepiandrosterone by Connell *et al.* (1966) after incorporation of acetate-^{14}C warrants the assump-tion that this steroid plays a role as an intermediate in the synthesis of steroids in chicken. Cédard and Haffen (1966) showed that dehydroepian-drosterone-4-^{14}C was metabolized to testosterone by embryonic testes of chicken incubated for 16 days. The experiments were performed *in vitro* in tissue culture for 24 hr. The isolation of 5-androstene-3β,17β-diol from the culture medium suggested to the authors that the formation of testosterone occurred through the Δ^5-3β-hydroxysteroid (Fig. 5) without passing through androstenedione. In adult cockerel, progesterone-^{14}C is a precursor of an-drostenedione and testosterone. Gonadotropins influence the rate of con-version (Subhas and Edwards, 1968).

In a study similar to the experiments of Fevold and Eik-Nes (1962, 1963), Fevold and Pfeiffer (1966) showed that the testicular tissue of the phalarope bird *Steganopus tricolor* had enzymes permitting the synthesis of testosterone from progesterone.

B. The Female

Numerous experiments performed during recent years exclude any doubt that the majority, if not all, estrogens are formed by aromatization of the

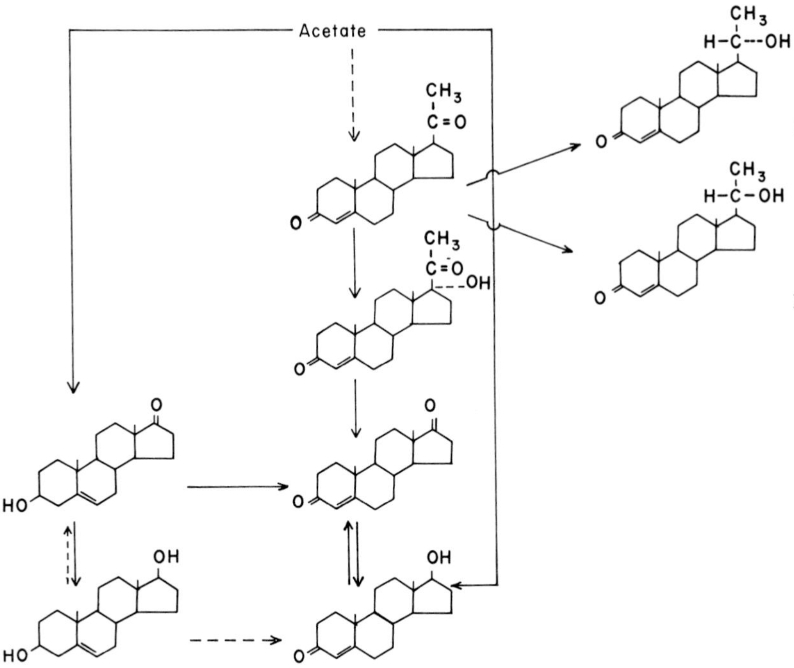

Fig. 5. Reactions occurring in the synthesis of androgens in testes of birds; the results have been obtained *in vitro* with *Passer domesticus* (adults) and *Gallus domesticus* 2-day-old chicks and 16-day-old embryos. I, 20α-hydroxypregn-4-en-3-one; II, 20β-hydroxy-4-pregnen-3-one. Details in text.

neutral C_{19} steroids. According to the results obtained to date (Breuer, 1962; Talalay, 1965) three enzymes catalyze the aromatization of the neutral C_{19} steroids into phenolic C_{18} steroids. They are 19-hydroxylase, 19-oxydase and $C_{19} \longrightarrow C_{18}$ desmolase. The latter enzyme leads to the formation of formaldehyde and estrogen in a molecular ratio close to 1 (provided the formaldehyde itself is not consequently metabolized). The existence of estrogens (see Chapter 7) in the ovarian tissues of fishes, amphibians, reptiles, and birds suggests that in the nonmammalian vertebrates aromatization very likely plays an important role and neutral C_{19} steroids are the intermediates in the synthesis of estrogens in ovaries.

The results gathered in Table IV show that testosterone is formed by the ovary of fishes, amphibians, reptiles, and birds when pregnenolone and progesterone are used as precursors. The synthesis of androgens in the ovary of the various vertebrates examined can be summarized as follows: pregne-nolone $\longrightarrow$ progesterone $\longrightarrow$ 17α-hydroxyprogesterone $\longrightarrow$ androstene-dione $\longrightarrow$ testosterone. This metabolic pathway is comparable to that which

TABLE IV

Synthesis of C_{19} Steroids in Ovaries of Nonmammalian Vertebrates

Species	Precursor steroid	Isolated steroid	Reference
FISHES			
Raja erinacea	Pregnenolone-³H	Progesterone	Callard and Leathem (1965)
	Progesterone-¹⁴C	17α-Hydroxyprogesterone	
		Testosterone	
Squalus acanthias	Pregnenolone-³H	Progesterone	Callard and Leathem (1965)
	Progesterone-¹⁴C (gestation)	Testosterone	
Torpedo marmorata	Pregnenolone	Progesterone	Lupo di Prisco *et al.* (1966)
	Dehydroepiandrosterone	Androst-4-ene-3,17-dione	
Scyliorhinus caniculus	Dehydroepiandrosterone-¹⁴C	Androst-4-ene-3,17-dione	Simpson *et al.* (1968b)
		Testosterone	
		Androst-5-ene-3β,17α-diol	
Centropistes striatus	Progesterone-¹⁴C	No C_{19} steroids	Reinboth *et al.* (1966)
Tilapia aurea	Acetate-³H	Cholesterol	Eckstein (1970)
		Pregnenolone	
		Dehydroepiandrosterone	
	Progesterone-¹⁴C +	Dehydroepiandrosterone	
	pregnenolone-³H	Androst-4-ene-3,17-dione	
		Testosterone	
	17-Hydroxyprogesterone-³H	Androst-4-ene-3,17-dione	
		Testosterone	
	Androst-4-ene-3,17-dione-³H	Testosterone	
		11-Ketotestosterone	
Mugil capito	Androst-4-ene-3,17-dione-³H	Testosterone	Eckstein and Eylath (1970)
		11-Ketotestosterone	
AMPHIBIANS			
Pleurodeles waltlii	Progesterone-¹⁴C	17α-Hydroxyprogesterone	Ozon (1967)
		Androst-4-ene-3,17-dione	
		Testosterone	

356

Species	Substrate	Products	Reference
Necturus maculosus	Progesterone-^{14}C	17α-Hydroxyprogesterone Androst-4-ene-3,17-dione Testosterone	Callard and Leathem (1966)
Xenopus laevis	17α-hydroxyprogesterone-^{14}C	Testosterone Androst-4-ene-3,17-dione	Rao *et al.* (1969)
Rana pipiens	Progesterone-^{14}C	Androst-4-ene-3,17-dione Testosterone	Callard and Leathem (1966)
Nectophrynoides occidentalis (before gestation)	Pregnenolone-^{3}H 17α-Hydroxyprogesterone-^{14}C	Progesterone Androst-4-ene-3,17-dione Testosterone	Ozon and Xavier (1968)
REPTILES			
Coluber constrictor	Pregnenolone-^{3}H	Progesterone	Callard and Leathem (1965)
Natrix pictiventris	Pregnenolone-^{3}H Progesterone-^{14}C	Progesterone 17α-Hydroxyprogesterone Androst-4-ene-3,17-dione Testosterone	Callard and Leathem (1965)
Thamnophis sirtalis	Pregnenolone-^{3}H	Progesterone 17α-Hydroxyprogesterone Testosterone	Callard and Leathem (1965)
BIRDS			
Steganopus tricolor	Pregnenolone-^{3}H 17α-Hydroxyprogesterone-^{14}C	Testosterone Androst-4-ene-3,17-dione	Fevold and Pfeiffer (1966)

is known at this time in mammals. The few results obtained do not allow the consideration of another mechanism (except the intermediary stage of the neutral C_{19} steroids) which would account for the synthesis of estrogens in the ovaries of lower vertebrates.

C. Comments

The actual secretion of a steroid by an endocrine gland cannot be proven only by the study of the biosynthesis of steroid hormones by the gland from exogenous precursors nor by the demonstration of the presence of hormones in the gland. The proof of endocrine secretion in the first place requires an analysis of the venous blood draining the gland. Because of the multiple technical difficulties, among which the size of the animals is the most obvious, such blood analyses in lower vertebrates have seldom been achieved for sex steroids. However, the incorporation of precursors of low molecular weight, acetate and mevalonate, into a steroid hormone allows the determination of the endocrine activity of a gland *in vitro* as well as the mechanisms which control it. Three studies of nonmammalian vertebrates have shown that steroid hormones can be synthesized from acetate-^{14}C:testosterone by testes of a juvenile chicken (Connell *et al.*, 1966), progesterone by the ovary of a snake, *Natrix sipedon pictiventris* (Callard, 1966), and dehydroepiandrosterone by ovary of the fish *Tilapia aurea* (Eckstein, 1970).

When the C_{21} steroids pregnenolone or progesterone are used as precursors, no basic difference from mammals is observed. In all cases testicular tissue is capable of forming neutral C_{19} steroid hormones from progesterone.

In fishes 11-ketotestosterone appears as a new, strongly androgenic, neutral C_{19} steroid. In the testes of *Salmo gairdnerii* and *Salmo salar* the presence of 11β-hydroxylase reacting with C_{19} substrate was demonstrated for the first time in fishes; in mammals under normal physiological conditions such a hydroxylation does not occur. Testicular 11β-hydroxylation should be investigated in other fishes as well as in amphibians and reptiles in order to elucidate its role in the lower vertebrates; it could be specific to a particular physiological adaptation. In another fish, *Squalus acanthias*, a 21-hydroxylase appears to be a relatively important activity (Simpson *et al.*, 1964b). However, it is not known if the testes are responsible for the 21-hydroxylation, and if such is the case which particular cells, or if the sperm only, are responsible (Simpson *et al.*, 1964a). In the testes of two fishes, *Squalus acanthias* (Simpson *et al.*, 1964b) and *Salmo gairdnerii* (Arai and Tamaoki, 1967a,b), progesterone or 17α-hydroxyprogesterone are metabolized by 20β-hydroxysteroid oxido-reductase. These results are in agreement with the isolation of $17\alpha,20\beta$-dihydroxy-4-pregnen-3-one from plasma of the salmon *Oncorhynchus nerka* (Idler *et al.*, 1960a). The testes of the bullfrog *Rana catesbeiana* metabolize progesterone to 20α-hydroxy-4-pregnen-3-one (Dale and Dorfman, 1967). Similarly, in the testis of *Passer domesticus* (Fevold and Eik-Nes, 1963) there is a 20α- and 20β-hydroxysteroid oxido-reductase. These findings were confirmed in birds by the isolation of 20α- and 20β-hydroxy-4-pregnen-3-one in the plasma of the laying hen (O'Malley *et al.*, 1968). At the present time, it is impossible to ascribe a function to these steroids.

The results suggest the formation of unusual steroids in the testes of non-mammalian vertebrates; more research is necessary, and it will likely reveal that these are not isolated cases. Not only is it likely that new steroids are acting in the lower vertebrates, but also unusual sites of secretion may exist. The cells responsible for the synthesis of C_{19} steroids vary in the testes. In elasmobranch fishes testicular cysts devoid of interstitial tissue are able to insure the synthesis of testosterone (Collenot and Ozon, 1964). In certain cases the sperm contains several enzymes intervening in their synthesis (Simpson *et al.*, 1964a,b; Ozon and Collenot, 1965). In the Urodela amphibian *Pleurodeles*, glandular tissue consisting of the walls of emptied cysts is the main site of synthesis of testosterone from progesterone (Ozon, 1967; Certain *et al.*, 1964). However, until now only the testes and ovaries have shown the ability to produce androgenic steroids from precursors. Although it has been reported that sexual androgenic steroids or estrogens were secreted by the adrenal cortex of a reptile (Gottfried *et al.*, 1967), it has never been demonstrated that this tissue is capable of synthesizing them from precursors except in the mammals. The absence of $C_{21} \longrightarrow C_{19}$ desmobase in the interrenal tissue of an amphibian can be demonstrated (Ozon and Dupuis-Certain, 1967) as well as in the adrenal capsules of a bird (Fevold and Pfeiffer, 1966).

The presence of estrogens in relatively important quantities in the testes of *Scyliorhinus stellaris* (Chieffi and Lupo, 1961a), *Bufo vulgaris* (Chieffi and Lupo, 1963), *Naja naja* (Gottfried *et al.*, 1967), *Steganopus tricolor*, and other birds (Höhn and Cheng, 1967) deserves confirmation. The routes of formation of phenolic C_{18} steroids in testes will have to be analyzed.

The role of the pituitary hormones in the control of steroidogenesis in the gonads of lower vertebrates has not yet been explored in detail. Adrenocorticotropin has a stimulating action upon the synthesis of corticosteroids by the interrenal tissues of fishes, amphibians, reptiles, and birds. It is not known if gonadotropic hormones have a comparable activity in lower vertebrates and mammals. The only experimental result known shows that ICSH increases the incorporation of acetate-^{14}C into testosterone by the testes of a juvenile chicken (Connell *et al.*, 1966). These problems are complicated and delicate because of the zoological specificity of certain gonado-tropic factors (Burzawa-Gérard and Fontaine, 1965).

Temperature affects sexual endocrinology (van Oordt, 1963). The in-corporation *in vitro* of acetate-^{14}C into testosterone by the testes of a juvenile chicken stimulated by ICSH is maximal at 41°C. In the lower vertebrates, which as a rule are poikilothermic, the influence of the temperature on the mechanism of steroid synthesis is not known.

IV. Intermediate Metabolism of C_{19} Steroids

The sexual steroids are secreted by the gonads and in some cases by the adrenal glands. The circulatory system carries them to the target organs where they exert their hormonal activity. Then, still carried by the blood, they enter the metabolic organs (mainly the liver) where they are inactivated and transformed into biologically inert compounds. The pathways of forma-tion of hormonal metabolites are specific. For instance, the metabolites of testosterone (Fig. 6) result from hydrogenation of the unsaturated carbon skeleton and the reduction of ketone radicals to hydroxyl groups. Hydro-genation of the double bond at C-4 to C-5 produces a new center of asym-metry on C-5 which leads to the formation of 5α- or 5β-steroids. There are two enzymes, a 5α-reductase, which catalyzes the formation of 5α-steroids, and a 5β-reductase for the 5β-steroids. The cellular location of these enzymes is different in the liver. In the first case it is microsomal, and in the second cytoplasmic. The reduction of ketones is also stereospecific; it is catalyzed by different enzymes according to the position of the resulting hydroxyl group on the steroid ring. The structures of the products vary according to the parent compounds.

Several metabolic reactions of C_{19} steroids, particularly the catabolism of testosterone, have been explored *in vivo* and *in vitro* in the nonmammalian vertebrates.

A. *In Vivo*

Preliminary studies (Chieffi, 1958) have shown that the larvae and adults of several amphibian species (*Rana pipiens, Rana catesbeiana, Xenopus laevis, Ambystoma maculatum, Ambystoma opacum*) transformed testo-sterone *in vivo* into 3-ketosteroid compounds which have not been identified. Breuer *et al*. (1966) showed that testosterone was oxidized *in vivo* to andro-stenedione by both male and female larvae of *X. laevis*. Female larvae oxidized testosterone more rapidly than did the male larvae. After injection

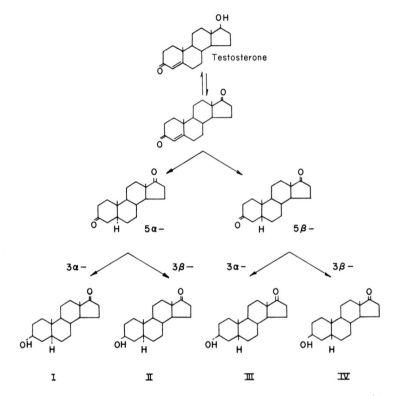

Fig. 6. Stereospecific reduction during the metabolism of C_{19} steroids. The Δ^4-3-keto structure of testosterone is reduced in two stages by two hydrogen molecules. I, Androsterone; II, epiandrosterone; III, etiocholanolone; IV, 3β-etiocholanolone.

of testosterone into the toad *Bufo bufo* (Pesonen and Rapola, 1962; Pesonen and Saure, 1963), various metabolites were isolated by thin-layer chromatography, among them epiandrosterone (3β-hydroxy-5α-androstan-17-one), 11-oxygenated 17-ketosteroids, and quite surprisingly dehydroepiandrosterone, although identification of the metabolites was less than satisfactory. From these results it is difficult to draw an outline of the catabolism of testosterone *in vivo* in the amphibians.

Stárka and Horáková (1967) investigated the metabolism *in vivo* of dehydroepiandrosterone (DHA) in *Rana esculenta*. After injection of DHA the main metabolites isolated from excreta were 5-androstene-$3\beta,17\beta$-diol, 5-androstene-$3\beta,7\alpha,17\beta$-triol, and $3\beta,7\alpha$-dihydroxy-5-androstene-17-one. The 7α-hydroxylated compounds of DHA represented the major part of the excreted compounds; in addition but in smaller quantities there were $3\beta,16\alpha$-

dihydroxy-5-androstene-17-one and 5α-androstane-3,17-dione. These results indicated that when DHA was injected *in vivo* in extraphysiological amounts, it was metabolized into Δ⁵-3β-hydroxysteroids which were rendered polar by the addition of the hydroxyl group in the 7α position and to a certain extent by conjugation with sulfuric acid. The excretion of Δ⁴-3-ketosteroids and of the derivatives of 5α-androstane was negligible. However, the dosages injected were nonphysiological and the results do not allow a strict biological interpretation.

B. LIVER

The first paper dealing with the metabolism of androgens in lower vertebrates was published by Samuels *et al.*(1950). They found that the Δ⁴-3-keto moiety of testosterone was destroyed by incubation with minced fragments of liver of fish, frog, snake, and chicken; there was no formation of 17-ketosteroids. None of the testosterone metabolites was identified. These studies were resumed by Breuer and Ozon (1965) and Lisboa and Breuer (1966), who used a method of identification including thin-layer chromatography and color reactions. The metabolism of testosterone was studied first *in vitro* by incubating liver slices of *Salmo irideus, Pleurodeles waltlii, Rana temporaria*, and chicken (*Gallus domesticus*). After incubation of testosterone with liver slices of *P. waltlii* and of *R. temporaria*, the major metabolites formed were 5α-androstanes. On the other hand, 5β-androstane compounds appeared as the major compounds in the cases of *S. irideus* and *G. domesticus*. These results clearly showed the differences in *in vitro* metabolism of testosterone in vertebrates. A more detailed study (Lisboa and Breuer, 1966) with cell fractionation made it possible to localize the enzymes responsible for this metabolism. In every species explored the 5α-reductase was localized in the microsomal fraction and the 5β-reductase in the cytoplasmic fraction. These two enzymes were active with both NAD and NADP. In the cytoplasmic or microsomal fractions, depending on the species, 3α-, 3β-, 17α-, and 17β-hydroxysteroid oxido-reductase were present. In Fig. 7 are shown the theoretically possible metabolisms of testosterone in each of the species explored.

The demonstration of an enzyme *in vitro* does not exactly reflect the *in vivo* activity of an organ; however, it clarifies the mechanisms of the metabolic reactions. For instance, it is known that the liver of a rat contains microsomal 5α-reductase and a cytoplasmic 5β-reductase and that the 5β-reductase is inhibited by the 5α-reductase (Forchielli and Dorfman, 1956). If this phenomenon is not limited to the rat alone, it could account for some difference observed in the metabolism of testosterone. In conclusion, the

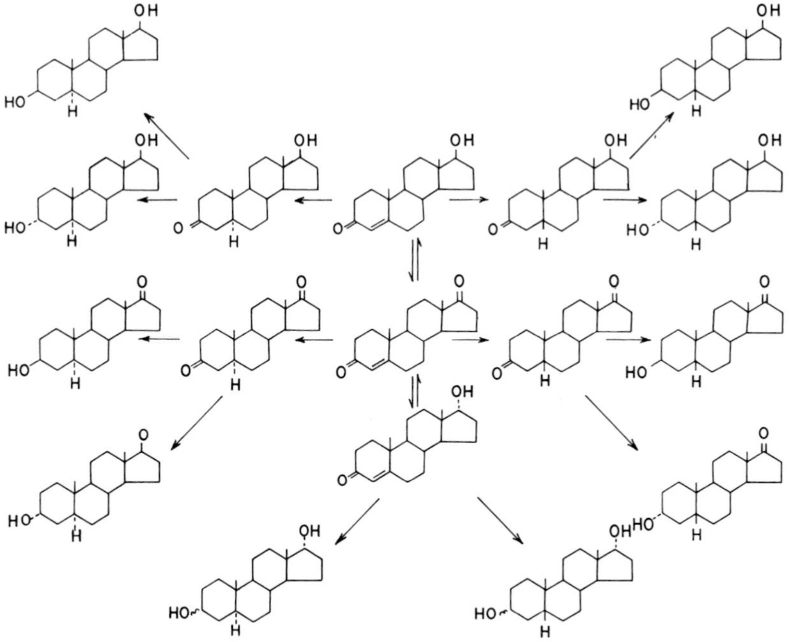

Fig. 7.   Metabolism of testosterone in liver of various vertebrates. Qualitative results obtained *in vitro* after cellular fractionation (Lisboa and Breuer, 1966).

qualitative exploration of the metabolism of C_{19} steroids (Lisboa and Breuer, 1966) has shown that the formation of the various reduced isomers depends upon the species under study and the nature of the substrate. Differences observed *in vitro* from incubation of tissue slices are primarily of a quantitative nature.

Pesonen and Saure (1963) studied *in vitro* the breakdown of testosterone by liver of the toad *Bufo bufo*. They indicated that the principal metabolites formed by the incubation of liver slices were C_{19} steroids which have a ketone or hydroxyl radical on C-11, adrenosterone being one of them. However, the identification of metabolites was not sufficiently conclusive to consider the presence of 11β-hepatic hydroxylase as certain. In addition Schneider (1965) established that the liver of *Rana catesbeiana* contained 6β-, 11α-, 15α-, 15β-, and 16α-hydroxylases with deoxycorticosterone serving as substrate. Although the hydroxylation of steroids depends on the nature of the substrate, this work would suggest that the results obtained by Pesonen and Saure (1963) be given careful consideration. The liver of *Rana esculenta* was found to contain a 7α-hydroxylase which catalyzed the hydroxylation of dehydroepiandrosterone (Stárka and Horáková, 1967).

TABLE V

Metabolism of C_{19} Steroids in Various Tissues of Nonmammalian Vertebrates

Species	Tissue or Locus of Cells	Hydroxysteroid Oxido-reductase (ol OR)	Reductase[a]	Reference
FISHES				
Raja erinacea	Ovaries	3α- or 3β-ol OR[b] 17β-ol OR	5α- or 5β-Reductase[b]	Callard and Leathem (1965)
Squalus acanthias	Ovaries	3α- or 3β-ol OR[b] 17β-ol OR	5α- or 5β-Reductase	Callard and Leathem (1965)
Scyliorhinus caniculus	Sperm	17β-ol Or		Ozon and Collenot (1965)
	Ovaries	3β-ol OR 17β-ol OR	5α-Reductase	Simpson et al. (1968)
Centropistes striatus	Ovaries	3α-ol OR	5β-Reductase	Reinboth et al. (1966)
Salmo irideus	Liver: Slices	3α-ol OR 3β-ol OR 17α-ol OR 17β-ol OR	<u>5β-Reductase and 5α-Reductase</u>	Lisboa and Breuer (1966)
	Microsomes		5α-Reductase	
	Cytoplasm		5β-Reductase	
Salmo gairdnerii	Sperm	17β-ol OR	<u>5β-Reductase[c]</u>	Hathaway (1965)
Microstomus kilt	Testes			Simpson et al. (1969b)
AMPHIBIANS				
Pleurodeles waltlii	Liver: Slices	3α-ol OR 3β-ol OR 17α-ol OR 17β-ol OR	5α-Reductase	Lisboa and Breuer (1966)

364

Species	Tissue		Enzyme	Reference
	Microsomes		5α-Reductase	
	Cytoplasm		5β-Reductase	
	Testes	17β-ol OR		Ozon (1967)
Necturus maculosus	Ovaries	3α-ol OR 17β-ol OR	5α-Reductase	Callard and Leathem (1966)
Rana pipiens	Ovaries	3α-ol OR 17β-ol OR	5β-Reductase	Callard and Leathem (1966)
Rana temporaria	Liver: Slices	3α-ol OR 3β-ol OR 17α-ol OR 17β-ol OR	5α-Reductase and 5β-Reductase	Lisboa and Breuer (1966)
	Microsomes		5α-Reductase	
	Cytoplasm		5β-Reductase	
	Testes (homogenate)	17β-ol OR	5α-Reductase	Ozon et al. (1964)
	Ovaries (homogenate)	17β-ol OR	5α-Reductase	
BIRDS Gallus domesticus	Liver: Slices	3α-ol OR 3β-ol OR 17α-ol OR 17β-ol OR	5β-Reductase and 5α-Reductase	Lisboa and Breuer (1966)
	Microsomes		5α-Reductase	
	Ctyoplasm		5β-Reductase	

[a] The main enzyme is underlined.
[b] Upon incubation of the testosterone there is formation of isoandrosterone or etiocholanolone.
[c] Upon incubation of progesterone-^{14}C.

C. Gonads

The liver is the most important metabolic organ in mammals and we have just seen that it also has metabolic activity in the nonmammalian vertebrates. However, it is not the only metabolic organ; in the nonmammalian vertebrates the gonads generally have enzymes which metabolize testosterone (Table V). Ovaries of two elasmobranch fishes (*Raja erinacea* and *Squalus acanthias*) transformed testosterone into reduced metabolites (Callard and Leathem, 1965). A very active 5β-reductase metabolized testosterone in the ovary of the teleost *Centropistes striatus* (Reinboth *et al.*, 1966).

Ovaries and testes of the frog *Rana temporaria* (Ozon *et al.*, 1964) can metabolize testosterone. Three steroids have been identified: androstenedione, 5α-androstane-3, 17-dione, and 5α-androstan-17β-ol-3-one. During incubation of testicular homogenates approximately 159 μg of testosterone per gram of tissue per hour were destroyed; while the testes very rapidly inactivated testosterone, the ovaries under the same conditions did it at a lower rate. The ovarian tissues of *Rana pipiens* transformed testosterone into 5β-steroids, and those of *Necturus maculosus* into 5α-steroids (Callard and Leathem, 1966).

D. Sperm

Are the cells responsible for testosterone metabolism in the gonads also in control of its biosynthesis? Among the vertebrates, according to the species, there are various categories of cells which intercede in the synthesis of testosterone in testes; the cells responsible for the metabolism of testosterone have not been identified. However, it is known that in certain species the sperm itself has various enzymes influencing the metabolism of C_{19} steroids. The sperm of the trout *Salmo gairdnerii* contains 17β-hydroxysteroid dehydrogenase which converts testosterone into androstenedione (Hathaway, 1965). This enzyme is also found in the sperm of *Scyliorhinus caniculus* (Ozon and Collenot, 1965). The presence of steroids (Section II, B), of enzymes that take part in the biosynthesis of steroids (Section III, A), as well as of enzymes that metabolize steroids suggests that in certain species the sperm may take part in the endocrine functions of the male.

E. Other Tissues

It is now well documented that testosterone is metabolized in target tissues from mammals. *In vivo* and *in vitro* testosterone is reduced mainly to

5α-dihydrotestosterone (17β-hydroxy-5α-androstan-3-one) and to the corresponding 3α- and 3β-diols. These reactions occur in prostate and other target tissues such as skin. Reduction to the 5α position is now considered as the first step of testosterone action in target cells (Ofner, 1968; Wilson and Gloyna, 1970). Extrahepatic metabolism of testosterone has also been studied in other vertebrates. Rongone *et al.* (1967) showed that homogenates of uropygial glands from chicken metabolized testosterone to 5α-compounds: 3α-hydroxy-5-androstan-17-one, 5α-androstane-3,17-dione, and androstanediols. Murota and Tamaoki (1967) demonstrated that tibia and femur of chicken embryos transformed testosterone to 5β-reduced compounds. Testosterone is also actively reduced by the comb of a cock (Bagget, 1962). Preliminary results in amphibians showed that testosterone as well as progesterone is actively reduced by different organs of *Pleurodeles waltlii* (skin, oviduct cloacal glands); this extrahepatic metabolism is quantitatively important. *In vitro* incubation of the seminal vesicles of the anoure amphibian *Discoglossus pictus* showed that testosterone-4-^{14}C was actively metabolized by these target organ to 5α- reduced compounds; The 5α-dihydrotestosterone was the main metabolite formed. (Ozon and Fouchet 1972).

V. Conjugation of Steroids

The androgenic hormones are transformed into metabolites in metabolic organs. In addition, it is known that in mammals these metabolites are conjugated, i.e., esterified with sulfuric acid or bound to glucuronic acid (Fig. 8). As a result of this conjugation they become water soluble and ionized, while the androgens themselves as well as their nonconjugated metabolites are fat soluble. The conjugated metabolites are eliminated from the blood

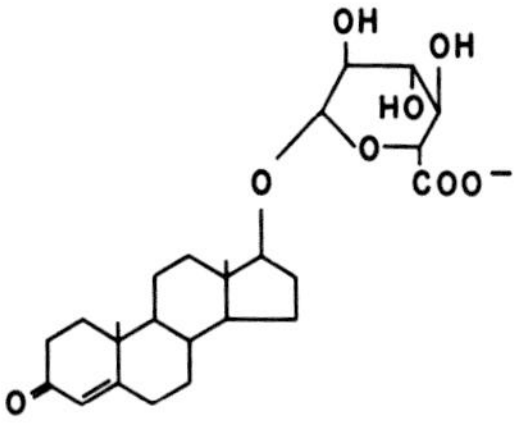

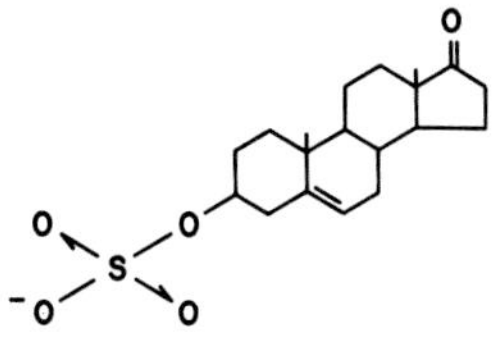

Fig. 8. Examples of conjugated C_{19} steroids. I, glucuronide of testosterone; II, sulfate of dehydroepiandrosterone.

and excreted in the urine and thus appear as hormones of elimination, devoid of biological activity.

Several excretory patterns exist in aquatic or semiaquatic vertebrates. From this viewpoint it is of interest to consider the elimination of steroids in the lower vertebrates. On the other hand conjugation does not represent exclusively a method of inactivation and elimination of steroids. Indeed, there are conjugated steroids, the sulfate of dehydroepiandrosterone for example, which have a particular function in mammals unrelated to excretion.

Conjugated steroids have been isolated in nonmammalian vertebrates. The glucuronide of testosterone was identified in the plasma of two fishes: *Raja radiata* and *Oncorhynchus nerka* (Idler and Truscott, 1966; Grajcer and Idler, 1963). Newcomer (1958) indicated that the majority of corticosteroids formed in adrenal glands of chicken were conjugated with glucuronic acid. Various authors described the liberation of steroids after acid or enzymic hydrolysis of tissue, or plasmatic extracts, but no information has been supplied concerning the nature or the site of the conjugation. Dehydroepiandrosterone injected into the frog *Rana esculenta* was partially excreted in conjugated form with sulfuric acid (Stárka and Horáková, 1967).

By injecting phenols (phenolphthalein, 8-hydroxyquinoline, α-naphthol, or *p*-nitrophenol) into a frog, *Rana pipiens*, and a toad, *Bufo marinus*, Maickel *et al*. (1958) showed that exogenous phenols are excreted by these animals conjugated with glucuronic and sulfuric acids; under the same conditions, i.e., *in vivo*, the fishes are incapable of this. Dutton (1962) performed a comparative study of the mechanism of glucuronization in the vertebrates. The formation of glucuronides is catalyzed by UDP-glucuronyltransferase. Uridine diphosphate glucuronic acid (UDPGA) is the donor of the glucuronyl group according to the reaction.

$$\text{Aglycone + UDPGA} \xrightarrow{\text{UDP-Glucuronyltransferase}} \text{aglycone glucuronide + UDP}$$

The UDPGA is formed from UDPG (uridine diphosphate glucose) in the presence of UDPG-dehydrogenase and NAD. In the mammals, UDP-glucuronyltransferase is localized in the microsomes of liver, kidneys and gut; UDPGA as well as UDP-glucuronyltransferase are present in the liver, kidney, and gut of pigeon and chicken. This enzyme (*o*-aminophenol served as the aglycone in this study) is active in the liver of the frog *Rana pipiens* (Dutton and Greig, 1957); however, it is absent in tadpoles as well as in the two entirely aquatic amphibians *Xenopus laevis* and *Necturus maculosus* (Lester and Schmid, 1961). *In vitro*, *o*-aminophenol is conjugated in small quantities with glucuronic acid by the liver of the trout *Salmo fario* (Dutton and Montgomery, 1958). The absence of UDPG-dehydrogenase might account for the inability of certain fishes to form the glucuronides (Dutton, 1962). In these experiments the steroids are not used in the same manner as the aglycone; nevertheless, it is possible that, as in mammals, the gluco conjugation of steroids having an alcohol radical proceeds by a similar enzymic mechanism. A urodele amphibian, *Pleurodeles waltlii* Michah, binds estrone and estradiol-17β with glucuronic acid *in vivo* as well as *in vitro* (Ozon and Breuer, 1966). UDP-Glucuronyltransferase is localized in a hepatic fraction of microsomes of *Pleurodele*; it uses UDPGA as donor of the glucuronic acid, but the activity of this enzyme is weak. Estrone is utilized like aglycone; Breuer and Ozon (1965) showed that UDP-glucuronyltransferase activity of hepatic microsomes is dependent upon temperature. The maximal activity of this hepatic enzyme is at 45°C in chicken, at 17°C in *Rana temporaria*, and close to 20°C in *Pleurodele*. These results confirm the thermolability of UDP-glucuronyltransferase observed in lower vertebrates (Dutton and Montgomery, 1958). In chicken (Newcomer and Heninger, 1960), cortisol, tetrahydrocortisone, and tetrahydrocortisol are conjugated to glucuronic acid in the presence of UDPGA and a fraction of adrenal gland microsomes.

It is regrettable that no study has yet been performed concerning the glucuronization of C_{19} steroids in nonmammalian vertebrates, particularly in fishes, in which group the glucuronide of testosterone has been isolated from plasma (Section II,B). In *Oncorhynchus nerka* and *Raja radiata* the plasmatic concentration of testosterone glucuronide in male is different than in female. It is of interest to compare these results with what is known about the rat (see Dutton, 1962) where a difference of activity of the UDP-glucuronyltransferase hepatic microsomes exists between the sexes. It would be of great interest to learn in which organs of fishes the glucuronization of testosterone takes place.

Conjugation of neutral C_{19} steroids was demonstrated in the gonads of two fishes. *In vitro* incubation of ovarian tissue from *Scyliorhinus caniculus* with radioactive androstenedione leads to the formation of testosterone glucuronide and traces of testosterone sulfate (Simpson *et al.*, 1968b). *In vivo* the major androgens 11-ketotestosterone, testosterone, and 11β-hydroxytestosterone were estimated in peripheral and testicular plasma of *Salmo salar*; these steroids were also present as glucuronides. The concentration of glucuronides was generally higher in testicular than peripheral plasma, suggesting that these conjugates are produced in the testes of *Salmo salar* (Idler *et al.*, 1971).

The lower vertebrates have the enzymic mechanisms which catalyze glucuronide formation but at the present time too few experimental results are available to confirm that these mechanisms account for the glucuronization of steroids in vertebrates other than mammals and in particular the neutral C_{19} steroids in fishes.

Until now only the biosynthesis and the metabolism of free steroids have been investigated in the nonmammalian vertebrates; study of the conjugated steroids opens new avenues of research. Indeed, one can ask if the conjugation of steroids in the vertebrates represents exclusively a form of inactivation and excretion.

VI. Androgen Production and Clearance *in Vivo*

With the exception of the human, very little is known about the rates at which androgens are secreted into and subsequently removed from the peripheral plasma. Clearly these parameters are of prime importance as regulators of the plasma hormone concentrations, and therefore some knowledge of them is prerequisite to our understanding of the control systems guiding androgenic action.

The metabolic clearance rate (MCR) of a steroid hormone has been defined as that volume of plasma (or blood) completely cleared of steroid in unit time (Tait and Burstein, 1964). The method of choice for measuring the MCR is to continuously infuse intravenously an isotope of the steroid in question until the plasma concentration of this isotope reaches a constant level. Once this has been attained, one assumes a steady state and therefore it follows that the rate at which the steroid is being removed from the blood must be equal to the rate at which it is being infused. The *in vivo* production rate of the hormone can then be calculated from the product of the MCR and the endogenous concentration of the hormone.

Testosterone production and metabolic clearance rates have been measured in sexually mature male and female skates, *Raja radiata* (Fletcher *et al.*, 1970). The plasma MCR's reported by these authors were 10.4 and 7.93 ml/ kg hr for females and males, respectively. These values are low when compared with the MCR of 1α-hydroxycorticosterone (92 ml/kg hr) (Idler and Truscott, 1969); the authors attributed this low rate of testosterone clearance to the fact that it is strongly bound to the plasma protein of the skate and therefore unavailable for metabolism (Section VII).

Testosterone production rates for male and female skates were very low, and the mean values obtained for the sexes did not differ significantly (males, 0.38 μg/kg body weight per hour; females, 0.33 μg/kg body weight per hour). The conclusions drawn from these data were that the high levels of plasma testosterone found in the skate were primarily the result of the low metabolic clearance rate.

VII. Protein Binding of Sex Hormones in Fishes and Amphibians*

Little has been published on the protein binding of sex hormones in fish (Idler and Freeman, 1968, 1969; Freeman and Idler, 1969; Martin and Ozon, 1971). It was originally thought that protein binding protected the animal from elevated plasma hormone levels since protein-bound steroids were thought to be biologically inactive (for a review see Sandberg *et al.*, 1966). Later, Keller *et al.* (1969) suggested that steroid-binding proteins perform an important physiological role in that they increase the specificity of the hormone system by determining the distribution of the steroid signals. Increases in the levels of binding are postulated to distribute steroid hormonal signals toward organs with protein-permeable vascular beds. Presently, protein binding of steroids is also considered as a storage and buffer system in which the steroid–protein complex serves as a biologically inert reservoir where the hormone is protected from metabolism or excretion; by dissociation the steroid may become available as a physiologically active entity (Hoffman *et al.*, 1969). Thus it appears that protein-bound steroids may play an important physiological role by assisting in the selection of receptor sites, where, by dissociation [which is determined in part by the relative affinities of the steroid for the plasma protein(s) and the protein(s) of the receptor(s)], the steroid is made available to the receptor tissue as a physiologically active agent.

Plasma testosterone levels about tenfold those found in man (Forchielli *et al.*, 1963) occur in the thorny skate *Raja radiata* (Idler and Truscott, 1966), some salmonids (Schmidt and Idler, 1962), two amphibians, *Necturus maculosus* (Rivarola *et al.*, 1968), and in *Pleurodeles waltlii* (Ozon and Attal, 1969). However, high testosterone binding by the serum proteins also occurs in at least some of these species (Table VI).

A plasma protein of high testosterone-binding activity, a "β-globulin," occurs in man (Mercier *et al.*, 1965; Mercier, 1966). This protein also binds estradiol-17β and several androgens extensively, suggesting that it may be associated with the regulation of sex hormone metabolism (Rosenbaum *et al.*, 1966; Murphy, 1968; Vermeulen and Verdonck, 1968).

A testosterone-binding protein, which in reality is a sex-hormone-binding protein (SHBP), was isolated from the serum of the mature male thorny skate (Freeman and Idler, 1969). Preliminary work has indicated a similar testosterone-binding protein in the Atlantic salmon *Salmo salar* and in the amphibian *Pleurodeles waltlii* (Ozon *et al.*, 1971; Martin *et al.*, 1971). The binding properties of the skate SHBP were found to be different from those reported for the human testosterone-binding globulin (Freeman and Idler, 1969).

*by D. R. Idler, H. C. Freeman, and R. Ozon.

TABLE VI

Binding[a] of Testosterone, 11-Ketotestosterone, and Estradiol-17β by Several Species of Fish

Species	No. of fish	Maturity and sex	Steroid	Bound (%)[b]	
				Gel filtration (4°C)	Dialysis (3°C)
Thorny skate	11	Mature female	Testosterone		95.7 ± 1.52
	7	Immature female	Testosterone		97.6 ± 0.64
	13	Mature male	Testosterone		95.9 ± 1.29
Atlantic salmon	1	Immature male	Testosterone		92.0
	5	Mature male	Testosterone	84.8 ± 3.24	99.1 ± 0.04
Bowfin	5 (pooled)	Mature male	Testosterone	85.3	98.5
Halibut	1	Immature female	Testosterone	54.9	95.1
Atlantic salmon	5	Mature male	11-Ketotestosterone	54.1 ± 3.45	94.3 ± 0.23
	5	Mature male	Estradiol-17β	60.0 ± 1.12	95.2 ± 0.07
Halibut	1	Immature female	Estradiol-17β	64.0	94.0

[a] Binding values were determined ±SE when binding was determined individually. (Compiled from data of Idler and Freeman.)
[b] Binding was determined in serum or plasma.

A. FISHES

1. Isolation of Skate SHBP

Serum from the mature male thorny skate was separated into four protein fractions (Fig. 9) by column chromatography on DEAE-cellulose (Freeman and Idler, 1969). These fractions were tested for specificity of steroid binding by equilibrium dialysis using 12 selected steroids (Table VII). Protein IV (Fig. 9) contained steroid-binding proteins which bound all the steroids tested except 11β-hydroxy-4-androstene-3,17-dione. Progesterone (95.1%), 17α-hydroxyprogesterone (93%), testosterone (89.6%), estradiol-17β (86.9%), and 11-deoxycorticosterone (82.4%) were highly bound by this fraction.

Protein IV was fractionated into one major and three minor proteins by polyacrylamide disc electrophoresis (Fig. 10) and into one major and two minor proteins by gel filtration through Sephadex G-200 at 4°C (Fig. 11). The largest protein area from Sephadex G-200 was eluted immediately after the void volume and contained principally one protein by polyacrylamide disc electrophoresis. The second and third protein areas were not completely separated and were combined. The combination was resolved into three proteins by polyacrylamide disc electrophoresis. A protein of highest

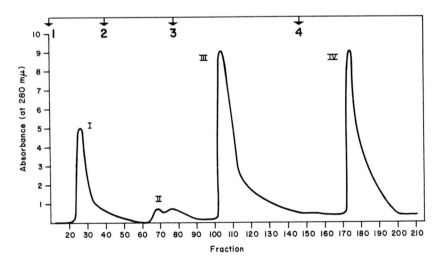

Fig. 9. DEAE-Cellulose chromatography of 5 ml of mature male thorny skate serum. A(2.5 × 25)-cm column was used at 4°C. Eluting buffers were 1,0.0175 *M* phosphate, pH 6.3 II, 0.04 *M* phosphate, pH 5.9; III, 0.10 *M* phosphate, PH 5.8; IV, 0.4 *M* phosphate, pH 5.2. Fractional elution yielded four protein fractions, I, II, III, and IV; 5-ml fractions were collected. (From Freeman and Idler, 1969.)

TABLE VII

Binding of Steroids by Thorny Skate Serum Protein Fractions from DEAE-Cellulose Chromatography[a]

Steroid	Bound (%)[b]			
	Fraction I (OD–0.246)[c]	Fraction II (OD–0.375)[c]	Fraction III (OD–1.152)[c]	Fraction IV (OD–0.392)[c]
Testosterone	0	3.8	6.5	89.6
11-Ketotestosterone	0	0	0	53.3
4-Androstene-3,17-dione	0	0	6.7	18.1
4-Androsten-11β-ol-3,17-dione	0	0	3.1	0
Estradiol-17β	2.7	8.8	39.3	86.9
Progesterone	0	0	36.4	95.1
17α-Hydroxyprogesterone	0	2.7	15.4	93.0
11-Deoxycorticosterone	0	2.6	7.8	82.4
Corticosterone	2.1	2.5	4.8	73.7
Cortisone	0	0	2.2	65.7
Cortisol	0	2.5	0	37.3
1α-Hydroxycorticosterone	0	1.7	0	9.1

[a]From Freeman and Idler (1969).
[b]One microgram of steroid and 3 ml of protein fraction were used for each binding test.
[c]The OD values were determined in a 1 cm cell at λ 280 mμ using a water reference.

testosterone-binding activity, homogenous to polyacrylamide disc electrophoresis (Fig. 12) was prepared by combining the peak fractions from several Sephadex G-200 column runs.

a. Molecular Weight of SHBP. The molecular weight of the SHBP, as determined by gel filtration and thin-layer chromatography, is 81,000–

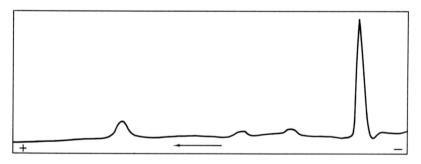

Fig. 10. Polyacrilamide electrophoresis of protein fraction IV prepared by DEAE-cellulose chromatography of skate serum. (From Freeman and Idler, 1969.)

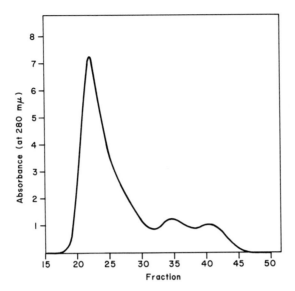

Fig. 11. Sephadex G-200 gel filtration at 4°C of DEAE-cellulose protein fraction IV. (From Freeman and Idler, 1969.)

82,000. Testosterone-binding and ultraviolet absorption (280 mμ) measurements indicated testosterone-binding proteins of molecular weights of multiples of 2, 4, and 6 times the molecular weight (80,000) of the basic protein. The testosterone-binding activities of these proteins were inversely proportional to their molecular weights. It is not known whether all the high molecular weight proteins are polymers, but association could be prevented and reversed, to some extent, by using 2-mercaptoethanol or 2-

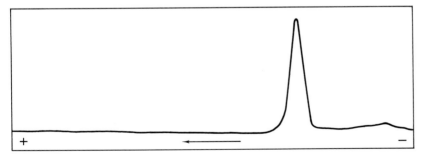

Fig. 12. Polyacrilamide electrophoresis of a homogenous protein prepared from the peak fraction of protein III from Sephadex G-200 gel filtration of DEAE-cellulose fraction IV. (From Freeman and Idler, 1969.)

dithiothreitol in the buffers during isolation; however, the testosterone-binding activity was only partially restored by the promoted disaggregation.

b. *Binding Affinity of SHBP.* The binding affinity of the SHBP was found to be high, and greater than 95% of low concentrations of testosterone were bound at 4°C. Competitive binding experiments of SHBP against high concentrations of bovine serum albumin and human serum albumin (HSA) also demonstrated a high binding affinity for testosterone.

Thorny skate serum has two testosterone-binding systems and therefore two association constants (Table VIII) (Freeman and Idler, 1970). The association constants K_1 of the high-affinity systems (SHBP) are 4.8 × 10⁷ and 8.1 × 10⁷ for three male and four female skates, respectively, and are similar to the association constants of the high-affinity binding systems in the salmon and the cod (Table VIII). Although the association constant for the skate SHBP is only about $\frac{1}{10}$ of the association constant at 25°C for testosterone-binding globulin in man (K = 4–16 × 10⁸) (Vermeulen and Verdonck, 1968) it is about 1000 times higher than that of HSA for testosterone. The SHBP has a capacity of 20–40 μg of testosterone/100 ml of serum (Freeman and Idler, 1970). The second testosterone-binding system in the skate has association constants (Table VIII) similar in magnitude to the low-affinity systems in the other fish (Table VIII) and are similar in capacity and affinity to that of HSA for testosterone. It is apparent that the skate SHBP–testosterone bond is fairly strong and therefore testosterone binding plays a prominent role in regulating testosterone metabolism in the animal (Section VI). This may explain why the skate is able to tolerate high plasma testosterone levels.

c. *Competitive Binding of Steroids by SHBP.* The competitive binding by SHBP of several selected steroids relative to testosterone is given in Table IX. 5α-Androstane-3β,17β-diol (280), 5-androstene-3β,17β-diol (138), and estradiol-17β (110) compete more effectively than testosterone for the same binding sites. The 17β-OH group in 17β-hydroxy-4-androsten-3-one (testosterone) is more competitive than is the 17α in 17α-hydroxy-4-androsten-3-one (epitestosterone). The 3β configuration in 5α-androstane-3β,17β-diol (280) caused a great increase in binding relative to the 3α configuration in 5α-androstane-3α,17β-diol (14).

d. *Specificity of SHBP.* A comparison of the noncompetitive binding of 12 selected steroids by SHBP relative to testosterone rated at 100 is given in Table X. Estradiol-17β (125), progesterone (118), and 17α-hydroxyprogesterone (108) were bound more effectively than testosterone (100). Binding is reduced by the presence of a 17α-OH group as demonstrated by

TABLE VIII

Association Constants (3°C) of Androgens Bound to Atlantic Salmon, Atlantic Cod, and Thorny Skate Plasma

Sample no.	Fish	Sex	Maturity	No. of fish	Steroid	$K_1 (\times 10^7)^a$	$K_2 (\times 10^4)^a$
1	Thorny skate	M	Immature	3	Testosterone	4.8	8.4
2	Thorny Skate	F	Immature	4	Testosterone	8.1	9.3
3	Atlantic salmon	M	Immature	31	Testosterone	9.3	9.1
4	Atlantic salmon	F	Immature	21	Testosterone	13.8	7.4
5	Atlantic salmon	M	Immature	31	11-Ketotestosterone	1.1	5.4
6	Atlantic salmon	F	Immature	21	11-Ketotestosterone	1.1	2.0
7	Atlantic cod	M	Immature	5	Testosterone	1.2	79
8	Atlantic cod	F	Immature	6	Testosterone	2.6	3.3

[a] Association constant K in liters per mole. (Freeman and Idler, 1970.)

377

TABLE IX

Competitive Binding of Steroids[a] to the Sex-Hormone-Binding Protein[b]

Steroid	Binding value
5α-Androstane-3β,17β-diol	280
5-Androstene-3β,17β-diol	138
Estradiol-17β	110
Testosterone	100
Estrone	76
4-Androsten-17α-ol-3-one	16
5α-Androstane-3α,17β-diol	14
5α-Androstan-3β-ol-17-one	12
5β-Androstan-17β-ol-3-one	5

[a] In binding tests, 100 sp. ng of steroid were used in competition with 0.1 ng of test osterone-
³H.
[b] The OD of SHBP in a 1 cm cell at λ 280 mμ using a water reference was 0.111. Table from
Freeman and Idler (1969).

TABLE X

Noncompetitive Binding of Steroids to the Sex-Hormone-Binding Protein[a] Relative
to Testosterone[b] Rated at 100[c]

Steroid	Binding value
Testosterone	100
4-Androstene-3,17-dione	2
4-Androstene-3, 17-dione	2
Estradiol-17β	125
Progesterone	118
17α-Hydroxyprogesterone	108
Corticosterone	68
11-Deoxycorticosterone	64
Cortisone	54
Cortisol	19
Tetrahydrocortisone	4
Tetrahydrocortisol	3
1α-Hydroxycorticosterone	2

[a] For each binding test 0.1 μg of steroid and 3 ml of protein were used.
[b] The OD of SHBP in a 1 cm cell at λ 280 mμ using a water reference was 0.090.
[c] From Freeman and Idler (1969).

comparing 17α-hydroxyprogesterone (108) with progesterone (118) and cortisol (19) with corticosterone (68). Cortisone (54) was bound more extensively than corticol (19) showing that the 11-ketone group conferred greater binding than the 11β-OH group. The addition of the 1α-OH group to corticosterone caused a loss in binding from 68 to 2%. In the C_{21} steroids tested, the degree of binding by skate SHBP was inversely proportional to the polarity with the exception of a minor discrepancy between 11-deoxy-corticosterone and corticosterone (Table X). Steroids, like cortisol and progesterone, which possess a lateral chain at C-17, do not compete with testosterone for human testosterone-binding globulin (Mercier and Baulieu, 1968); in this regard, it is clear that the skate SHBP is different, for it binds progesterone and 17α-hydroxyprogesterone extensively as well as corti-costerone, 11-deoxycorticosterone, and cortisone to a lesser degree. How-ever, it should be emphasized that 1α-hydroxycorticosterone, the principal interrenal corticoid of this species, is not bound to any significant extent. The virtual absence of cortisone, cortisol, and 11-deoxycorticosterone and the generally low levels of corticosterone in Elasmobranchii suggest that about the only steroids that have to be considered for protein binding in the skate are testosterone, progesterone, estradiol-17β, and 1α-hydroxycorti-costerone. The latter is bound to a very low level by skate plasma; testo-sterone, estradiol-17β, and progesterone have all been reported to occur in elasmobranchs (Wotiz *et al.*, 1960; Idler and Truscott, 1966) and this is why we have called the protein that binds these steroids a sex-hormone-binding protein (SHBP). Martin and Ozon (1971) confirmed the occurrence of a SHBP in Elasmobranchii. They isolated and partially purified a protein which binds testosterone, estradiol-17β, corticosterone and progesterone in *Scyliorhinus canicula* serum.

It is not suprising that skate SHBP is quite different from human testo-sterone-binding globulin, for Elasmobranchii have been reported to be devoid of serum albumin and some of the globulin fractions normally found in man (Irisawa and Irisawa, 1954; Sulya *et al.*, 1961). Skate SHBP is eluted from DEAE-cellulose in fraction IV, like transcortin from human plasma, whereas the human testosterone-binding globulin is eluted in fraction II, which contains the "β-globulins." Skate SHBP, although eluted in the same position as transcortin, has different binding properties and a different molecular weight. In our experiments there was a loss of SHBP binding activity during dialysis, concentration, and freeze-drying. Several investiga-tors (Pearlman *et al.*, 1967; Kato and Horton, 1968) have reported variable losses in testosterone-binding activity in human plasma caused by freezing and thawing, particularly when diluted plasma was used. Others (Forest *et al.*, 1968) have reported no loss in binding with similar treatment. Highest activity was obtained in dilute solutions of skate SHBP for, when concentrated, an association of the protein molecules occurred with a corresponding loss of binding activity. The molecular weight of skate SHBP ($\sim 80,000$) is much higher than that of human serum albumin (65,000) and transcortin (58,500). The molecular weight of the human testosterone-binding globulin has not been reported although it is eluted from a Sephadex column just before the albumin peak, which indicates that the molecular weight is greater than that of albumin.

2. Binding of Sex Hormones by Other Species

Although a sex-hormone-binding protein has been isolated from the serum of the thorny skate little has been published concerning the blood protein binding of sex hormones in other species of fish. Some binding data, on the Atlantic salmon *Salmo salar*, the halibut *Hippoglossus hippoglossus*, and the bowfin *Amia calva*, are included in Tables VI and VIII. It can be seen that total testosterone binding in these species ranges from 94 to 99%, whereas high-affinity binding is also high, ranging from 55 to 85% (Table VI). Estradiol-17β binding, both total and high-affinity binding, in the Atlantic salmon and halibut are also high. 11-Ketotestosterone binding in the mature male Atlantic salmon is 95.2% and 60% for total and high-affinity binding, respectively. It appears that these species may also possess proteins that are specific for the sex hormones.

The association constants for binding testosterone and 11-ketotestosterone in salmon plasma of both sexes are given in Table VIII. The association constants K_2 for testosterone and 11-ketotestosterone are of the same order of magnitude as $K_{25}°C$ (2.38×10^4) for HSA binding of testosterone (Vermeulen and Verdonck, 1968). The association constants K_1 (Table VIII) for the high-affinity binding system in salmon are less than the association constants (4–16×10^8, 25°C) (Vermeulen and Verdonck, 1968) for testosterone-binding globulin in man. Vermeulen and Verdonck (1968) found however that the K values for testosterone at 37°C were only about half the values reported at 25°C, which would make them at the physiological temperature nearer to the value of K_1 in the skate. It is not known whether the salmon has a specific testosterone-binding protein but preliminary information indicates that it has. The binding capacity of this high-affinity testosterone-binding protein in the salmon ranged from 25 to 55μg of testosterone/100 ml of plasma (Freeman and Idler, 1970), which is far above the normal physiological testosterone level of the peripheral plasma (0.5–1.6 μg/100 ml of plasma, 18 fish). Testosterone levels as high as 17.5 μg/100 ml were reported in the sockeye salmon *Oncorhynchus nerka* (Schmidt and Idler, 1962).

The association constants K_1 (1.1×10^7) for 11-ketotestosterone (Table VIII) for salmon of both sexes are about $\frac{1}{10}$ of the value for K_1 for testosterone in the same plasma. It is not known whether both androgens compete for the same binding sites, but if they do, the 11-keto group attached to the testosterone molecule lowers the binding affinity for the protein considerably. The binding capacity for 11-ketotestosterone ranged from 20 to 50 μg/100 ml of plasma. The 11-ketotestosterone level ranged from 0.7 to 6.7 μg/100 ml in the peripheral plasma (20 immature male fish); therefore, at normal physiological levels of 11-ketotestosterone, the binding capacity is in excess of the plasma concentration of the steroid. If both androgens, testosterone and 11-ketotestosterone, do compete for the same binding sites, the binding capacity of the system is sufficient for both at normal physiological levels.

Binding of testosterone in the male and female Atlantic cod (Table VIII) is similar to that in the salmon and the skate. Again, in both sexes there are two binding systems, one of low capacity and high affinity and one of high capacity and low affinity. The binding capacities of the high-affinity systems of the cod (both sexes) ranged from 40 to 100 μg of testosterone/100 ml of serum and, at physiological testosterone levels, the cod bound 97–98% of its serum testosterone. It is apparent that both the male and female cod have little free testosterone in their peripheral blood. It is of interest that the male cod appeared to have a higher binding capacity for the androgen than did the female.

B. AMPHIBIANS

Equilibrium dialysis experiments demonstrate that estradiol-17β, testosterone, and progesterone are bound to blood serum from male and female *Pleurodeles waltlii* (Ozon *et al.*, 1971). Binding of steroids to normal serum by dialysis at 4°C shows that 96% of estradiol-17β and 93% of testosterone are bound to serum proteins. Influence of serum dilution on the binding of estradiol-17β is represented in Fig. 13.

1. Binding Specificity

Competitive binding by serum of several steroids relative to estradiol-17β is given in Table XI; C$_{21}$ steroids do not compete with sex steroids.

2. Binding Affinity and Capacity

Association constants and binding capacity were determined by equilibrium dialysis at 4°C with diluted serum (1–80). The Scatchard plot (Fig. 14) gives constants for testosterone and estradiol-17β as indicated in Table XII. The association constants are higher than in fishes (Table VIII); the binding capacity is of the same order. The association constant of estradiol-17β with a

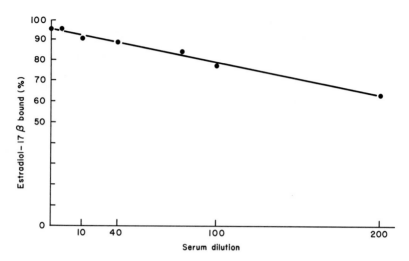

Fig. 13.   Estradiol-17β-2,4,6,7-^{3}H (1.7 $\times$ 10^{-10} M) binding to blood serum, from female *Pleurodeles waltlii*, of different dilutions.

TABLE XI

Competitive Binding of Different Steroids on Estradiol-17β-Binding Serum Protein[a]
from *Pleurodele*

Steroids	Bound (%)	B/U[b]
	91	10.1
Estradiol-17β	70	2.3
Testosterone	78	3.5
5α-Androstan-17β-ol-3-one	79	3.7
5α-Androstane-3β,17β-diol	83	4.9
Estradiol-17α	88	7.3
Dehydroepiandrosterone (DHA)	88.5	7.7
Androst-4-en-17α-ol-3-one	89	8.1
Progesterone	89	8.1
Estriol	89	8.1
Cortisol	89	8.1
17-Hydroxyprogesterone	90	9
Androst-4-ene-3,17-dione	90	9
5β-Androstane-3α,17β-diol	90	9
Corticosterone	90	9
11-Deoxycorticosterone	90	9
Cortisone	90	9
Estrone	91	10.1

[a]Equilibrium dialysis of 1 ml of diluted serum ($\frac{1}{10}$) against 10^{-10} M estradiol-17β-^{3}H and 10^{-7} M unlabeled steroids.
[b]Estradiol-17β-^{3}H bound, B; estradiol-17β-^{3}H unbound, U.

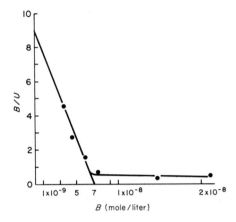

Fig. 14. Influence of estradiol-17β concentration on specific binding of diluted serum (1/80). Scatchard type of plot (B/U) versus B (B, estradiol-17β bound to protein; U, estradiol-17β not bound; binding capacity $= 7 \times 10^{-9} \times 80 = 5.6 \times 10^{-7}$ mole/liter; $K = 1.3 \times 10^9$ liters/mole).

purified protein fraction after Sephadex G-200 chromatography has also been determined by equilibrium dialysis and Scatchard plot (Fig. 15).

3. Purification of an Amphibian SHBP

Chromatography on CM-cellulose of an undiluted serum sample equilibrated with tritiated estradiol-17β is represented in Fig. 16a; when radioactive fractions eluted from this first column were rechromatographed on DEAE-32-cellulose the diagram given in Fig. 16b was obtained. It shows, first, a good separation of transferrin and amphibian SHBP, and, second, a microheterogeneity of this protein system. A nearly identical elution pattern is obtained when tritiated testosterone is used instead of estradiol-17β. Further purification is now being undertaken. Experiments with tritiated progesterone demonstrated that this C_{21} steroid is not eluted in the same fractions after DEAE-cellulose chromatography, as are sex steroids.

TABLE XII

Association Constants of Testosterone and Estradiol-17β Determined by Equilibrium Dialysis, Bound to Serum from Female *Pleurodeles waltlii*

Steroid	Association constant $K_{4\,°C}$ (liters/mole)	Binding capacity (moles/liter)
Estradiol-17β	1.3×10^9	5.6×10^{-7}
Testosterone	5.4×10^8	1.7×10^{-6}

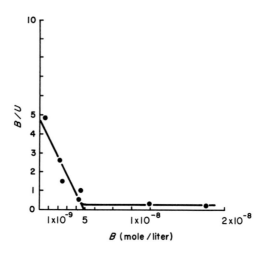

Fig. 15. Influence of estradiol-17β concentration on specific binding of purified serum fractions after Sephadex G-200 chromatography ($K = 1.0 \times 10^9$ liters/mole).

VIII. Conclusions

An androgenic steroid hormone formed from precursors in the gonads (mainly testes) enters the blood stream where it attaches itself to the plasmatic proteins. Carried by the blood it reaches the target organ where it exerts its effect. From there the blood carries it further to the metabolic organs. There, by chemical modifications, it is transformed into metabolites which usually are rendered water soluble by conjugation in order to aid in

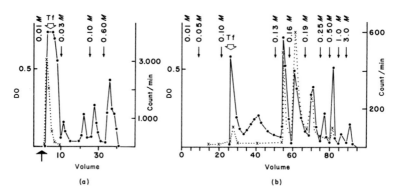

Fig. 16. Ion-exchange chromatography of *Pleurodeles waltlii* serum. (a) CM-Cellulose chromatography of 1.5 ml of serum equilibrated with 1.7×10^{-9} M estradiol-17 β-³H, pH 7.4; (b) DEAE-cellulose chromatography of fraction 3 and 4 eluted at 0.01 M in the first chromatography, pH 8 (Tf, transferrin).

its urinary excretion. That is the scheme known in mammals for the metabolism of steroid hormones and androgens in particular. The analysis of each category of steroid hormones requires a multidisciplined approach. For androgens of nonmammalian vertebrates, the major aspects thus far emphasized have been isolation and identification, biosynthesis, and intermediary metabolism.

Examination of studies mentioned in this survey does not reveal fundamental differences across the vertebrate phylum. Testosterone is the most common C_{19} steroid. The majority of enzymic mechanisms controlling the synthesis and the transformations of the hormones in mammals are also present in fishes, amphibians, reptiles, and birds. However, the discovery of unusual enzymes, e.g., 11β-hydroxylase in the testes of teleost fishes, suggests the existence of certain qualitative differences. However, too few species have been explored to permit the formation of an idea of the singularity and role of such differences.

In conclusion, the biosynthesis and the transformations of sexual steroid hormones, which are molecules of low molecular weight derived from cholesterol, are comparable from one species to another; this is of no surprise since they represent the chemical foundation of the sex. On the other hand, the control of their metabolism by macromolecules, the enzymic proteins, varies. Other aspects of androgen C_{19} steroid studies which must be considered in order to evaluate fully the role of steroids in the vertebrates are (a) their functions and their biological properties (it is not excluded that the functions of the same androgenic steroid may vary from one species to another) and (b) their mechanism of action in the target organs.

REFERENCES

Arai, R. (1967). *Annot. Zool. Jap.* **40**, 1.
Arai, R., and Tamaoki, B. I. (1967a). *Gen. Comp. Endocrinol.* **8**, 305.
Arai, R., and Tamaoki, B. I. (1967b). *Can. J. Biochem.* **45**, 1191.
Arai, R., Shikita, M., and Tamaoki, B. (1964). *Gen. Comp. Endocrinol.* **4**, 68.
Attal, J. (1970). "Mesure des Oestrogénes et des androgénes Testiculaires et Plasmatiques dans l'Espece Ovine par des Micromethodes de Chromatographie en Phase Gazeuse. Influence de l'Age de la Saison et du Cycle Diurne." Thesis, Paris.
Bagget, B. (1962). *Fed. Proc. Fed. Amer. Soc. Exp. Biol. 46th Annu. Meet. Abstr.*, 211.
Berthold, A. A. (1849). *Arch. Anat. Physiol. Physiol. Abt.* **16**, 42.
Botte, V., and Lupo di Prisco, C. (1965). *Gen. Comp. Endocrinol.* **5**, 665.
Botticelli, C. R., Hisaw, F. L., Jr., and Roth, W. D. (1963). *Proc. Soc. Exp. Biol. Med.* **114**, 225.
Breneman, W. R., and Mason, R. C. (1951). *Endocrinology* **48**, 752.
Breuer, H. (1962). *The Metabolism of the Natural Estrogens. Vitamins, and Hormones.* **20**, 285.
Breuer, H., and Ozon, R. (1965). *Arch. Anat. Microsc. Morphol. Exp.* **54**, 17.
Breuer, H., Dahm, K., Mikamo, B., and Witschi, E. (1966). *Excerpta Med. Found. Int. Congr. Ser.* **111**, 215.

Buonanno, C., Chieffi, G., and Imparato, E. (1964). *Pubbl. Sta. Zool. Napoli* **34**, 66.

Burzawa-Gérard, E., and Fontaine, Y. A. (1965). *Gen. Comp. Endocrinol.* **5**, 87.

Callard, I. P. (1966). *Amer. Zool.* **6**, 587.

Callard, I. P. (1967). *J. Endocrinol.* **37**, 105.

Callard, I. P., and Leathem, J. H. (1965). *Arch. Anat. Microsc. Morphol. Exp.* **54**, 35.

Callard, I. P., and Leathem, J. H. (1966). *Gen. Comp. Endocrinol.* **7**, 80.

Cédard, L., and Fontaine, M. (1963). *C.R. Acad. Sci.* **257**, 3095.

Cédard, L., and Haffen, K. (1966). *C.R. Acad. Sci.* **263**, 430.

Certain, P., Collenot, G., Collenot, A., and Ozon, R. (1964). *C.R. Soc. Biol.* **158**, 1040.

Chieffi, G. (1958). *Proc. Int. Congr. Zool., 15th,* 600.

Chieffi, G., and Lupo, C. (1961a). *Nature (London)* **190**, 169.

Chieffi, G., and Lupo, C. (1961b). *Atti Accad. Naz. Lincei Cl. Sci. Fis. Mat. Natur. Rend.* **30**, 399.

Chieffi, G., and Lupo, C. (1963). *Gen. Comp. Endocrinol.* **3**, 149.

Collenot, G., and Ozon, R. (1964). *Bull. Soc. Zool. Fr.* **89**, 577.

Connell, G. M., Connell, C. J., and Eik-Nes, K. B. (1966). *Gen. Comp. Endocrinol.* **7**, 158.

Dale, E. (1962). *Gen. Comp. Endocrinol.* **2**, 171.

Dale, E., and Dorfman, R. I. (1967). *Gen. Comp. Endocrinol.* **9**, 313.

Dean, S. D., and Chester Jones, I. (1959). *J. Endocrinol.* **18**, 366.

Della Corte, F., and Cosenza, L. (1965). *Gen. Comp. Endocrinol.* **5**, 679.

Delrio, G., Lupo di Prisco, C., and Chieffi, G. (1967). *Experientia* **23**, 594.

Dorfman, R. I., and Ungar, F. (1965). "Metabolism of Steroid Hormones." Academic Press, New York.

Dutton, G. J. (1962). *Proc. Int. Pharmacol. Meet., 1st, 1961* **6**, 39.

Dutton, G. J., and Greig, C. G. (1957). *Biochem. J.* **66**, 52P.

Dutton, G. J., and Montgomery, J. P. (1958). *Biochem. J.* **70**, 17P.

Eckstein, B. (1967). *Gen. Comp. Endocrinol.* **9**, 447.

Eckstein, B. (1970). *Gen. Comp. Endocrinol.* **14**, 303.

Eckstein, B., and Eylath, U. (1970). *Gen. Comp. Endocrinol.* **14**, 396.

Eylath, U., and Eckstein, B. (1969). *Gen. Comp. Endocrinol.* **12**, 58.

Fevold, H. R., and Eik-Nes, K. B. (1962). *Gen. Comp. Endocrinol.* **2**, 500.

Fevold, H. R., and Eik-Nes, K. B. (1963). *Gen. Comp. Endocrinol.* **3**, 335.

Fevold, H. R., and Pfeiffer, E. W. (1966). *Excerpta Med. Found. Int. Congr. Ser.* **111**, 369.

Fletcher, G. L., Hardy, D. C., and Idler, D. R. (1970). *Endocrinology* **85**, 552.

Forchielli, E., and Dorfman, R. I. (1956). *J. Biol. Chem.* **223**, 443.

Forchielli, E., Sorcini, G., Nightingale, M. S., Brust, N., Dorfman, R. I., Perloff, W. H., and Jacobson, G. (1963). *Anal. Biochem.* **5**, 416.

Forest, M. G., Rivarola, M. A., and Migeon, C. J. (1968). *Steroids* **12**, 323.

Freeman, H. C., and Idler, D. R. (1969). *Gen. Comp. Endocrinol.* **13**, 83.

Freeman, H. C., and Idler, D. R. (1970). *Steroids* **17**, 233.

Galzigna, L. (1961). *Atti Accad. Naz. Lincei Cl. Sci. Fis. Mat. Natur. Rend.* **31**, 92.

Garnier, D. H., and Attal, J. (1970). *C. R. Acad. Sci.* **270**, 2472.

Gottfried, H. (1964). *Steroids* **3**, 219.

Gottfried, H., and Chieffi, G. (1967). *J. Endocrinol.* **37**, 99.

Gottfried, H., Huang, D. P., Lofts, B., Phillips, J. G., and Tam. W. H. (1967). *Gen. Comp. Endocrinol.* **8**, 18.

Grajcer, D., and Idler, D. R. (1961). *Can. J. Biochem. Physiol.* **39**, 1585.

Grajcer, D., and Idler, D. R. (1963). *Can. J. Biochem. Physiol.* **41**, 23.

Hadd, H. E., and Rhamy, R. K. (1965). *J. Clin. Endocrinol. Metab.* **25**, 876.

Hathaway, R. R. (1965). *Amer. Zool.* **5**, 211.

Hazleton, L. W., and Goodrich, F. J. (1937). *J. Amer. Pharmacol.* **26**, 420.
Hoffman, W., Forbes, T. R., and Westphal, U. (1969). *Endocrinology* **85**, 778.
Höhn, E. O., and Cheng, S. C. (1967). *Gen. Comp. Endocrinol.* **8**, 1.
Ichii, S., Forchielli, E., and Dorfman, R. I. (1963). *Steroids* **2**, 631.
Idler, D. R., (1969). Unpublished data.
Idler, D. R. and Freeman, H. C. (1968). *Gen. Comp. Endocrinol.* **11**, 366.
Idler, D. R., and Freeman, H. C. (1969). *Gen. Comp. Endocrinol.* **13**, 75.
Idler, D. R., and MacNab, H. C. (1967). *Can. J. Biochem.* **45**, 581.
Idler, D. R., and Truscott, B., with the collaboration of Freeman, H. C., Chang, V., Schmidt, P. J., and Ronald, A. P. (1963). *Can. J. Biochem. Physiol.* **41**, 875.
Idler, D. R., and Truscott, B. (1966). *Gen. Comp. Endocrinol.* **7**, 375.
Idler, D. R., and Truscott, B. (1969). *Gen. Comp. Endocrinol. Suppl.* **2**, 325.
Idler, D. R., Fagerlund, U. H. M., and Ronald, A. P. (1960a). *Biochem. Biophys. Res. Commun.* **2**, 133.
Idler, D. R., Schmidt, P. J., and Ronald, A. P. (1960b). *Can. J. Biochem. Physiol.* **38**, 1053.
Idler, D. R., Schmidt, P. J., and Biely, J. (1961a). *Can. J. Biochem. Physiol.* **39**, 317.
Idler, D. R., Schmidt, P. J., and Bitner, I. (1961b). *Can. J. Biochem. Physiol.* **39**, 1653.
Idler, D. R., Bitners, I. I., and Schmidt, P. J. (1961c). *Can. J. Biochem. Physiol.* **39**, 1737.
Idler, D. R., Truscott. B., and Stewart, H. C. (1968). *Excerpta Med. Found. Int. Congr. Ser.* **184**, 724.
Idler, D. R., Horne, D. A., and Sangalang, G. B. (1971). *Gen. Comp. Endocrinol.* In press.
Irisawa, H., and Irisawa, A. G. (1954). *Science* **120**, 849.
Jallageas, M., and Attal, J. (1968). *C. R. Acad. Sci.* **267**, 341.
Kato, T., and Horton, R. (1968). *J. Clin. Endocrinol. Metab.* **28**, 1160.
Keller, N., Richardson, U. I., and Yates, F. E. (1969). *Endocrinology* **84**, 49.
Layne, D. S., Common, R. H., Maw, W. A., and Fraps, R. M. (1957). *Proc. Soc. Exp. Biol. Med.* **94**, 528.
Lester, R., and Schmid, R. (1961) *Nature (London)* **190**, 452.
Lisboa, B. P., and Breuer, H. (1966). *Gen. Comp. Endocrinol.* **6**, 114.
Lupo, C., and Chieffi, G. (1963a). *Nature (London)* **197**, 596.
Lupo, C., and Chieffi, G. (1963b). *Atti Accad. Naz. Lincei Cl. Sci. Fis. Mat. Natur. Rend.* **34**, 443.
Lupo, C., and Chieffi, G. (1965). *Gen. Comp. Endocrinol.* **5**, 698.
Lupo di Prisco, C., Botte, V., and Chieffi, G. (1966). *Excerpta Med. Found. Int. Congr. Ser.* **111**, 368.
Lupo di Prisco, C., Chieffi, G., and Delrio, G. (1967a). *Experientia* **23**, 73.
Lupo di Prisco, C., Vellano, C., and Chieffi, G. (1967b). *Gen. Comp. Endocrinol.* **8**, 325.
Lupo di Prisco, C., Delrio, G., and Chieffi, G. (1968). *Gen. Comp. Endocrinol.* **10**, 292.
Maickel, R. P., Jondorf, W. R., and Brodie, B. B. (1958). *Fed. Proc. Fed. Amer. Soc. Exp. Biol.* **17**, 390.
Martin, B., and Ozon, R. (1971). *C. R. Acad. Sci.* **273**, 390.
Martin, B., Ozon, R., and Boffa G. A., (1971). *C.R. Acad Sci.* **272**, 1413.
Mercier, C., (1966). *Excerpta Med. Found. Int. Congr. Ser.* **111**, 269.
Mercier, C., and Baulieu, E. E. (1968). *Ann. Endocrinol.* **29**, 159.
Mercier, C., Alfsten, A., and Baulieu, E. E. (1965). *Excerpta Med. Found. Int. Congr. Ser.* **101**, 212.
Murota, S. I., and Tamaoki, B. (1967). *Biochim. Biophys. Acta* **137**, 347.
Murphy, B. E. P. (1968). *Can. J. Biochem.* **46**, 299.
Nandi, J. (1967). *Amer. Zool.* **7**, 115.

Newcomer, W. S. (1958). *Amer. J. Physiol.* **196**, 276.

Newcomer, W. S., and Heninger, R. W. (1960). *Proc. Soc. Exp. Biol. Med.* **105**, 32.

Ofner, P. (1968). *Vitam. Horm.* (*New York*) **26**, 237.

O'Malley, B. W., Krischner, M. A., and Wayne Bardin, C. (1968). *Proc. Soc. Exp. Biol. Med.* **127**, 521.

Ozon, R. (1966). *Ann. Biol. Anim. Biochim. Biophys.* **6**, 537.

Ozon, R. (1967). *Gen. Comp. Endocrinol.* **8**, 214.

Ozon, R. (1968). Unpublished results.

Ozon, R., and Attal, J. (1969). Unpublished data.

Ozon, R., and Breuer, H. (1966). *Gen. Comp. Endocrinol.* **6**, 295.

Ozon, R., and Collenot, G. (1965). *C.R. Acad. Sci.* **261**, 3204.

Ozon, R., and Dupuis-Certain, P. (1967). *Gen. Comp. Endocrinol.* **9**, Abstr. 130.

Ozon, R., and Fouchet, C. (1972). *Gen. Comp. Endocrinol.* in press.

Ozon, R., and Xavier, F. (1968). *C.R. Acad. Sci.* **266**, 1173.

Ozon, R., Breuer, H., and Lisboa, B. P. (1964). *Gen. Comp. Endocrinol.* **4**, 577.

Ozon, R., Martin, B., and Boffa, G. A. (1971). *Gen. Comp. Endocrinol.* **17**, 566.

Pearlman, W. H., Crepy, I., and Murphy, M. (1967). *J. Clin. Endocrinol. Metab.* **27**, 1012.

Pesonen, S., and Rapola, J. (1962). *Gen. Comp. Endocrinol.* **2**, 425.

Pesonen, S., and Saure, A. (1963). *Arch. Soc. Zool. Bot. Fenn. Vanamo* **18**, 1.

Potter, G. D., and Hoar, W. S. (1954). *J. Fish. Res. Bd. Can.* **11**, 63.

Rao, G. S., Breuer, H., and Witschi, E. (1969). *Gen. Comp. Endocrinol.* **12**, 119.

Rapola, J. (1963). *Gen. Comp. Endocrinol.* **3**, 412.

Reinboth, R., Callard, I. P., and Leathem, J. H. (1966). *Gen. Comp. Endocrinol.* **7**, 326.

Rivarola, M. A., Snipes, C. A., and Migeon, C. J. (1968). *Endocrinology* **82**, 115.

Rongone, E. L., Hill, M., and Burns, R. (1967). *Steroids* **10**, 425.

Rosenbaum, W., Christy, N. P., and Kelly, W. G. (1966). *J. Clin. Endocrinol. Metab.* **26**, 1399.

Samuels, L. T., Sweat, M. L., Levedahl, B. M., Pottner, M. M., and Helmreich, M. L. (1950). *J. Biol. Chem.* **183**, 231.

Sandberg, A. A., Rosenthal, U. I., Schneider, S. L., and Slaunwhite, W. R. (1966). *In* "Steroid Dynamics" (G. Pincus, T. Nakao, and J. F. Tait, eds.) pp. 1–61. Academic Press, New York.

Schmidt, P. J., and Idler, D. R. (1962). *Gen. Comp. Endocrinol.* **2**, 204.

Schneider, J. J. (1965). *Biochemistry* **4**, 689.

Simpson, T. H., Wright, R. S., and Gottfried, H. (1963a). *J. Endocrinol.* **26**, 489.

Simpson, T. H., Wright, R. S., and Hunt, S. V. (1963b). *J. Endocrinol.* **27**, 131.

Simpson, T. H., Wright, R. S., and Renfrew, J. (1964a). *J. Endocrinol.* **31**, 11.

Simpson, T. H., Wright, R. S., and Hunt, S. V. (1964b). *J. Endocrinol.* **31**, 29.

Simpson, T. H., Wright, R. S., and Hunt, S. V. (1968a). Personal communication.

Simpson, T. H., Wright, R. S., and Hunt, S. V. (1968b). *J. Endocrinol.* **42**, 519.

Simpson, T. H., Wright, R. S., and Hunt, S. V. (1969a). Personal communication.

Simpson, T. H., Wright, R. S., and Wardle, O. (1969b). Personal communication.

Stárka, L., and Horáková, E. (1967). *Endocrinol. Exp.* **I**, 209.

Steinach, E. (1894). *Pfluegers Arch. Gesamte Physiol. Menschen Tiere* **56**, 304.

Subhas, S., and Edwards, H. M. (1968). *Fed. Proc. Fed. Amer. Soc. Exp. Biol.* **27**, 623.

Sulya, L. L., Box, B. E., and Gordon, G. (1961). *Amer. J. Physiol.* **200**, 152.

Tait, J. F., and Burstein, S. (1964). *In* "The Hormones" (G. Pincus, K. V. Thimann, and E. B. Astwood, eds.), Vol. 5, p. 518. Academic Press, New York.

Talalay, P. (1965). *Annu. Rev. Biochem.* **34**, 347.

Valle, J. R., and Valle, L. A. R. (1943). *Science* **97**, 400.

Van Mullem, P. J., and Gottfried, H. (1966). *Excerpta Med. Found. Int. Congr. Ser.* **111**. 368.

van Oordt, G. J. (1963). *In* "Comparative Endocrinology" (U. S. Euler and H. Heller, eds.), pp. 154–207. Academic Press, New York.

Vermeulen, A., and Verdonck, L. (1968). *Steroids* **11**, 609.

Wattenberg, L. W. (1958). *J. Histochem. Cytochem.* **6**, 225.

Wilson, J. D., and Gloyna, R. E. (1970). *Recent Progr. Horm. Res.* **29**, 309.

Wotiz, H. H., Botticelli, C. R., Hisaw, F. L., Jr., and Olsen, A. G. (1960). *Proc. Nat. Acad. Sci. U.S.* **46**, 580.

Chapter 7

ESTROGENS IN FISHES, AMPHIBIANS, REPTILES, AND BIRDS

R. OZON

I. Introduction

It was known about 40 years ago that the ovary of vertebrates contains a factor which produces estrus in immature or castrated mice. Since 1939 three compounds with estrogenic activity have been isolated in crystalline form from mammals: estradiol-17β, estrone, and estriol (Dorfman and Ungar, 1965). For two further decades these were the only known estrogenic steroids. More recently other estrogens occurring mainly during the gestation period have been isolated from mammals; studies of their biosynthesis and metabolism have resulted in a number of publications (Breuer, 1962; Dorfman and Ungar, 1965; Breuer and Knuppen, 1969).

The estrogens are derived from cholesterol, contain 18 carbon atoms, and have a phenolic group at position 3 (Fig. 1). It should be noted that estrogenic activity is not a characteristic of all phenolic steroids, particularly of the recently isolated compounds. In the same manner there are certain analogs which have estrogenic activity without having the chemical structure of the C_{18} estrogens (e.g., coumestrol, genisteine and derivatives of stilbene).

In mammals, estrogens constitute a group of hormones which are responsible for the development and maintenance of the genital tract and the somatic sexual characteristics of the female. Their production varies with the sexual cycle characteristic of each species and they play a quantitatively important role during pregnancy. The main source of estrogens is the ovary. In some cases the C_{18} steroids are produced by the adrenal cortex. In certain species, and particularly in humans during pregnancy, the placenta becomes the predominant source of phenolic steroids.

Is the presence of phenolic steroids limited exclusively to mammals? Certainly not. Indeed, parallel to the research performed on mammals it has been demonstrated that (a) the ovaries of fishes, amphibians, reptiles, and birds contain some factors which have estrogenic activity when they are tested in mammals (Forbes, 1961; van Tienhoven, 1961); (b) the crystalline phenolic steroids have biological properties in nonmammalian vertebrates. They act upon the female genital tract and they modify the somatic sex characteristics of the female. These results suggest a positive answer to

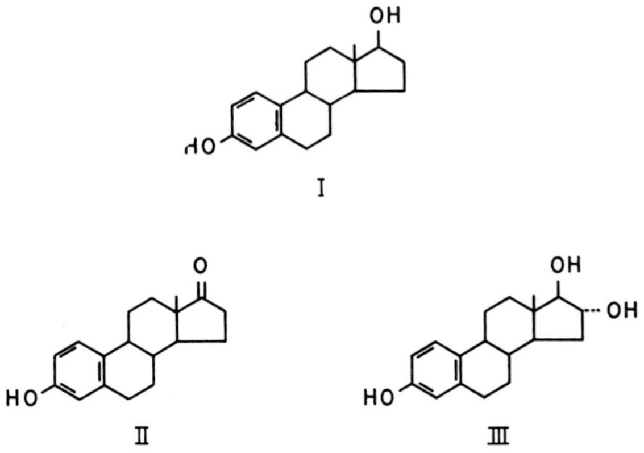

Fig. 1.   Plane formulas of the three classical estrogens. I, Estradiol-17β; II, estrone; III, estriol.

our question without, however, providing a single clue concerning the chemical nature of these compounds.

Conclusive proof of the presence of phenolic steroids in nonmammalian vertebrates was provided 10 years ago. Wotiz *et al.*, (1960) isolated estradiol-17β from the ovary of an elasmobranch, *Squalus suckleyi*, and MacRae *et al.*, (1959) isolated estradiol-17β from the excreta of a laying hen. In both cases the steroids were isolated and identified by infrared spectrometry. These initial results opened the way to much comparative research concerned with the occurrence, synthesis, and metabolism of phenolic steroids in nonmammalian vertebrates.

It is not our intention to offer in this chapter a complete review of the literature dealing with estrogens and nonmammalian vertebrates, but rather to show, in the light of recently acquired data, the state of our knowledge and to assess the opportunities opened by comparative endocrinology for the study of biochemistry and physiology of estrogenic sex steroids.

II. Isolation, Identification, and Quantification

A. OVARY

It was noted above that biological tests suggested the presence of C_{18} steroids in the ovary of nonmammalian vertebrates. Table I summarizes the current literature. We will not discuss the various results in detail since several reviews have been published recently on this subject (Gottfried, 1964; Chieffi, 1966; Ozon, 1966; Barr, 1968). The criteria of identification are those described in Chapter 2 (Tables I–III) and used in the preceding chapters. Difference in techniques employed probably accounts for the considerable variation in the quantitative results. The majority of these publications must be considered as preliminary reports and not as conclusive proof for the presence of a particular steroid in a given species. All the estimations have been performed on large quantities of tissue taken from a great number of animals. They indicate the presence of phenolic steroids in a particular species without providing precise physiological information concerning their possible functions (see Chapter 6, Section II,C).

According to some authors (Table I) estriol appears to be the most important C_{18} steroid isolated from ovarian tissue; however, we must note that not a single positive identification of estriol, not even by chromatography, has been reported (Lisboa and Diczfalusy, 1962; Knuppen, 1963). The problem of the isolation of estriol from ovarian tissue of lower vertebrates remains unsolved. On the other hand it is advisable to speak of polar phenolic

TABLE I

Isolation and Identification of Estrogens in Fish, Amphibians, Reptiles, and Birds

Species	Source of steroid	Steroid	Quantity ($\mu g/kg$)	Identity rating[a]	Reference
FISH					
Petromyzon marinus	Ovary (568 g)	Estradiol-17β	16	Su	Botticelli et al. (1963)
		Estrone			
Squalus suckleyi	Oocyte plus follicle	Estradiol-17β	100	Ex	Wotiz et al. (1958)
	Ovary (7.9 kg)	Estradiol-17β	120	Po (IR)	Wotiz et al. (1960)
		Estrone			
Squalus acanthias	Ovary	Estradiol-17β	32		Simpson et al. (1964)
		Estrone	3–4		
Scyliorhinus caniculus	Ovary (415 g)	Estradiol-17β	19	Te	Simpson et al. (1963)
		Estrone	19		
Torpedo marmorata	Ovary (600 g)	Estradiol-17β	38	Su	Chieffi and Lupo (1963)
		Estriol	55	Ex	
Salmo irideus	Ovary	Estradiol-17β		Ex	Galzigna (1961)
Cyprinus carpio	Ovary	Estradiol-17β		Ex	Galzigna (1961)
		Estriol ?			
		16-Epiestriol ?			
Anguilla anguilla	Ovary	Estradiol-17β		Ex	Penso and Galzigna (1963)
Gadus callarias	Ova (10 kg)	Estradiol-17β	4.8	Te	Gottfried et al. (1962)
		Estrone	1		
Conger conger	Ovary	Estradiol-17β	80	Su	Lupo and Chieffi (1963)
		Estrone	50	Ex	
		Estriol		Ex	
Oncorhynchus nerka	Ovary	Estradiol-17β	36	Su	Botticelli and Hisaw (1964)
		Estrone			
Ictalurus punctatus	Ovary (684 g)	Estradiol-17β		Su	Eleftheriou et al. (1966)
		Estradiol-17α		Ex	
		Estrone		Su	

TABLE I (cont.)

Species	Source of steroid	Steroid	Quantity (μg/kg)	Identity rating[a]	Reference
Serranus scriba	Gonad Hermaphrodite (65 g)	Estriol ?		Ex	Lupo and Chieffi (1965)
		16-Epiestriol ?		Ex	
		16-Ketoestradiol-17β		Ex	
		Estradiol-17β	122	Ex	
		Estrone	426	Ex	
Protopterus annectens	Ovary	Estriol?			Dean and Chester Jones (1959)
		Estradiol-17β	70	Ex	
		Estriol?	700	Ex	
AMPHIBIANS					
Xenopus laevis	Ovary	Estradiol-17β	9	Ex	Gallien and Chalumeau-Le-Foulgoc (1960)
		Estrone	11		
Rana pipiens	Immature larvae	Estradiol-17β	60	Ex	Dale (1962)
Bufo vulgaris	Bidder's organ	Estradiol-17β	60	Ex	Chieffi and Lupo (1961)
		Estrone	150	Ex	
		Estriol?		Ex	
	Ovary (250 g)	Estradiol-17β	40	Su	Chieffi and Lupo (1963)
		Estrone	41	Su	
		Estriol?	60	Ex	
REPTILES					
Lacerta sicula	Ovary (128 g)	Estradiol-17β	21	Su	Lupo di Prisco et al. (1968)
		Estrone	81		
BIRDS					
Gallus domesticus	Ovary	Estradiol-17β		Ex	Layne et al. (1958)
		Estrone			
	Feces	Estradiol-17β		Po (IR)	MacRae et al. (1959)
	Urine	Estrone		Po	Ainsworth and Common (1962)

Species	Tissue	Compound	Rating	Reference
		Estradiol-17β	Po	Hertelendy et al. (1965)
		16-Epiestriol	Po	Hertelendy and Common (1964)
		Estriol	Te	Mathur and Common (1967)
		16,17-Epiestriol	Te	Mathur and Common (1967)
Steganopus tricolor and other birds	Ovary	Estradiol-17β	Su	Höhn and Cheng (1967)
		Estrone		

[a]For an explanation of abbreviations and rating system, see Chapter 2, Tables I–IV.

395

TABLE II

Isolation and Identification of Estrogens in the Plasma of Fish, Amphibians, and Birds

Species	Method		Estradiol-17β (μg/100 ml)	Estrone (μg/100 ml)	Other estrogens (μg/100 ml)	Reference
	Hydrolysis	Estimation [a]				
FISH						
Scyliorhinus caniculus	No	PC, CT	0.3–0.4	0.05–0.1		Simpson et al. (1963)
Torpedo marmorata	Yes, β-gluctro-nidase	TLC, GLC		0.8–2.96	Estriol, 91–217	Lupo di Prisco et al. (1967)
Anguilla anguilla	Yes, HCl	AC, AcFl	1.5–1.7	2.5–3.6		Cédard and Nomura (1961)
Conger conger	Yes, HCl	AC, AcfL	1.1–2.2	0.7–3.2		Cédard and Nomura (1961)
Murena helena	Yes, HCl	AC, AcFl	7.2	11.7		Cédard and Nomura (1961)
Cyprinus carpio	Yes, HCl	AC, AcFl	0.5–2.5	1.5–4.5		Cédard and Nomura (1961)
Salmo salar	Yes, HCl	AC, AcFl	0.2–2.2	0–0.45	Estriol, 0.9–2.9	Cédard et al. (1961)
Ictalurus punctatus	No	TLC, AcFl	2–14	1.5–5.7	Estiol, 4–14; 16-Epiestriol, 2–7; 16-Ketoestradiol-17β, 6–20; Estradiol-17α, 1.5–6	Eleftheriou et al. (1966)
AMPHIBIANS						
Pleurodeles waltlii	No	TLC, GLC, Der	0.06	0.06		Ozon and Attal (1969)
Xenopus laevis	Yes, HCl	AC, AcFl	Total estrogens, 4			Gallien and Chalumeau-Le-Foulgoc (1960)

Rana temporaria	Yes, HCl	AC, AcFl	0.3–0.5	0.1	Polar estrogens, 0.3–0.7	Cédard and Ozon (1962)
Rana esculenta	No	TLC, GLC	11–23		Estriol, 11–36	Polzonetti-Magni *et al.* (1970)
BIRDS						
Gallus domesticus	Yes	PC	Present	Present		Layne *et al.* (1958)
	Yes, HCl	AC, TLC, AcFl	0.2	2	16-Epiestriol, present	Ozon (1965)
	Yes, HCl	DIDA	Present	Present		O'Grady and Heald (1965)

[a]For an explanation of abbreviations, see Chapter 2, Table IV.

TABLE III

Biosynthesis *in Vitro* or C_{18} Steroids from Precursors in the Ovary

Species	Precursor	C_{18} Steroid isolated	References
Scyliorhinus caniculus	Androst-4-ene-3,17-dione-4-^{14}C	Testosterone Estradiol-17β Estrone	Simpson *et al.* (1968)
Pleurodeles waltlii	Testosterone-4-^{14}C	Androst-4-ene-3,17-dione Estradiol-17β Estrone	Ozon (1967)
Xenopus Laevis	Androst-4-ene-3,17-dione-4-^{14}C	Testosterone 5α-Androstane-3-one-17β-ol Estrone Estradiol-17β	Redshaw and Nicholls (1971)
Rana temporaria	Testosterone	Androst-4-ene-3,17-dione Estradiol-17β Estrone	Ozon and Breuer (1964) Breuer and Ozon (1965)
Nectophrynoides occidentalis	Testosterone-7α-^{3}H	Androst-4-ene-3,17-dione Estradiol-17β	Xavier and Ozon (1971)

Gallus domesticus
  Organotypic cultures
  of embryonic gonads
	Acetate-1-^{14}C	Estradiol-17β	Cédard *et al.* (1968)

Adult	Acetate-1-^{14}C	Progesterone Androst-4-ene-3,17-dione Testosterone Estradiol-17β	Bouceck and Savard (1970)

steroids since estrogen steroids are now known with substitutions on carbon 2, 6α, 6β, 11β, 15α, 15β, 16β, and 18 which exhibit only slight differences in their chromatographic behavior (Breuer and Knuppen, 1969). These facts invite caution before the identification of a phenolic estrogen is claimed. A more physiological approach to the role of steroids in nonmammalian vertebrates (after isolation and identification) is the estimation of their concentration in blood.

B. PERIPHERAL BLOOD

Research on plasma estrogens has been undertaken in some species of nonmammalian vertebrates (Table II); the quantitative results vary greatly from one species to another. Differences in methodology account to a certain extent for these variations. It is important to note that (a) in some cases only the fraction of free phenolic steroids was analyzed whereas in other instances the estimation was made after enzymic or acid hydrolysis of the plasma and (b) purification of the steroids before their quantitative estimation was inadequate in nearly all instances.

Much research has been devoted to the determination of plasma estrogens in humans. Until recently the determinations were performed using fluorescence or color reactions. The presence of nonspecific fluorescent material in plasma is conducive to overestimates when fluorometric methods are employed; nevertheless this method was a sensitive one. Since 1967 new and more sensitive methods have been developed: gas–liquid chromatography (GLC) with electron capture detectors (Attal and Eik-Nes, 1968; Attal, 1970), double-isotope derivative assay (Baird and Guevara, 1969), protein binding assay (Korenman *et al.*, 1969), and radioimmunological assay (Ábrahám, 1969). Taking the determination of estradiol-17β in human plasma as an example, we see that its measurements in a female during her cycle gave, by fluorometric methods, values varying from 0.7 to 9 μg/liter. By contrast methods involving double-isotope derivatives, protein binding, and radioimmunology gave values ranging from 0.03 to 0.5 μg/liter depending on the period of the cycle. This example shows clearly that an improvement of methods results in an increased sensitivity and specificity of determinations which in turn lead to a better assessment of the true values. The very low levels of estrogens in human plasma invite us to consider with caution the results obtained in other vertebrate classes.

Table II illustrates results obtained by either fluorescence or GLC; due to the presence of nonspecific material in plasma the results obtained by fluorescence can only be too high. Considering all factors it appears reasonable not to overestimate their biological significance but rather to consider them as a preliminary identification of plasma estrogens.

Lupo di Prisco *et al.* (1967) as well as Polzonetti-Magni *et al* (1970) determined various plasma steroids by gas chromatography using a strontium-90 argon detector. One may be surprised by the very high values for estriol reported by the authors. The specificity and scope of the method used remain under discussion (Eik-Nes and Horning, 1968). This method is no longer used for the determination of C_{19} and C_{18} plasma steroids. A more specific method for the determination of estradiol-17β and estrone involves the formation of pentafluorophenylhydrazone and measurement by GLC with an electron capture detector after addition of a radioactive internal standard (Attal and Eik-Nes, 1968). The sensitivity is approximately 1 ng per sample; the amount of blood necessary for a determination lies between 10 and 20 ml. The values obtained in the pleurodele (0.06 μg/100 ml) are at the limit of sensitivity of the method. In conclusion, the results shown in Table II provide a biochemical confirmation (rather inadequate) of the presence of C_{18} steroids in nonmammalian vertebrates; it is premature to attribute a physiological significance to these results.

C. OTHER TISSUES

Cédard and Fontaine (1963) reported that corpuscles of Stannius of the Atlantic salmon *Salmo salar* contained estrogens as well as 17-ketosteroids (see Chapter 6). The concentration of estriol was scarcely doubled in the corpuscles of Stannius of the female from the beginning of the anadromous migration to the time of spawning, while the amount of androgens increased tenfold in the corpuscles of Stannius of the male.

III. Biosynthesis

The androgens are formed from precursor Δ^5- and Δ^4-C_{21} steroids; similarly it is well established that the Δ^4-C_{19} compounds androstenedione and testosterone are the immediate precursors of estrogens (Chapter 6, Section III,B). Figure 2 summarizes the route of this transformation (Breuer, 1962; Dorfman and Ungar, 1965; Talalay, 1965). 19-Hydroxytestosterone and 19-nortestosterone are intermediates in aromatization in the ovary of mammals (Axelrod and Goldzieher, 1969).

A. CONVERSION OF C_{21} STEROIDS TO C_{19} STEROIDS

The experimental results are shown in Table IV of Chapter 6, Section III,B. Although the metabolic pathways are comparable to those described

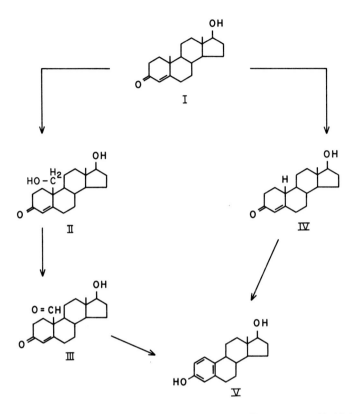

Fig. 2. Aromatization of C_{19} steroids to C_{18} steroids. I, Testosterone; II, 19-hydroxytestosterone; III, 19-oxotestosterone; IV, 19-nortestosterone; V, estradiol-17β. (According to Dorfman and Ungar, 1965; Breuer and Knuppen, 1969; Axelrod and Goldzieher, 1969.)

for mammals, some remarks are pertinent. First we shall discuss the research of Eckstein (1970) on the teleost *Tilapia aurea*. The ovary of this species is capable of synthesizing cholesterol, pregnenolone, and dehydroepiandrosterone from acetate-^{3}H. This is an important finding which again confirms the existence of common mechanisms of steroid synthesis in all vertebrates. In the same publication Eckstein discussed the *in vitro* transformation of C_{21} Steroids into C_{19} steroids by the ovary (Chapter 6, Table IV). From experiments in which double isotopes were used (progesterone-4-^{14}C, specific activity 35 mCi/mmole, and pregnenolone-7α-^{3}H, specific activity 1 Ci/mmole) he concluded that 17α-hydroxylation is not a necessary intermediate stage between progesterone and testosterone; the acetate of testosterone, a possible intermediate, was not isolated. However, this conclusion must be reviewed with some reservations. First, the whole homogenates were incubated without prior centrifugation and this could give rise to inactivation by proteolytic enzymes. Furthermore it is important to take into account the amount of precursors used in a double-isotope experiment. Calculation reveals that about 80 μg of progesterone-^{14}C but only 1 μg of pregnenolone-7α-^{3}H was incubated; this situation detracts considerably from any comparison of ratios of ^{3}H/^{14}C in the metabolites formed. Also, 80 μg of progesterone is probably a nonphysiological dose, which may lead to inhibition of one or more reactions involved in the synthesis of steroids. The identification of 11-ketotestosterone in the ovary of *Mugil capito* (Eckstein and Eylath, 1970) could be foreseen from the results of Schmidt and Idler (1962), who isolated 11-ketotestosterone from plasma of female Salmon (*Oncorhynchus nerka*). Of particular interest is the demonstration of 11β-hydroxylase in the ovary of two teleosts: *Tilapia aurea* (Eckstein, 1970) and *Mugil capito* (Eckstein and Eylath, 1970). The authors showed that the endogenous concentrations of 11-ketotestosterone as well as the activity of the 11β-hydroxylase depend on the medium in which this euryhaline fish lives. Indeed the mullet does not reproduce in fresh water; in this medium the *in vitro* activity of 11β-hydroxylase is much higher than in seawater mullets at the stage of reproduction. 11-Ketotestosterone is an extremely potent androgen for some fish and it might inhibit the mechanism of ovulation. These results show that different ecological conditions can influence the metabolism of steroids in the ovary and can cause physiological modifications in reproduction (Eckstein and Eylath, 1970).

The toad *Nectophrynoides occidentalis* is the only viviparous anuran known; its gestation period is 9 months. The intrauterine development of embryos corresponds with the presence of postovulatory ovarian corpuscles, i.e., corpora lutea. The metabolism of pregnenolone and 17α-hydroxyprogesterone have been studied *in vitro* (Ozon and Xavier, 1968; Xavier and Ozon, 1971). During gestation pregnenolone is transformed into progesterone; the corpora lutea are mainly responsible for this conversion. The amount of progesterone produced *in vitro* is at its maximum at the beginning of gestation, then decreases considerably towards parturition. Incubations of ovary performed during the first part of gestation showed that neither progesterone nore 17α-hydroxyprogesterone were metabolized. This indicates inhibition or absence of 17α-hydroxylase and desmolase in the ovary when functional yellow bodies are present. On the other hand after parturition C_{21} steroids are actively transformed into C_{19} steroids. The results establish that at different physiological periods there are qualitative and quantitative differences in metabolic activity. The research of Eckstein and Eylath (1970) and of Xavier and Ozon (1971) emphasized the fundamental importance of physiological and ecological conditions in influencing the mechanisms of biosynthesis of ovarian steroids in lower vertebrates.

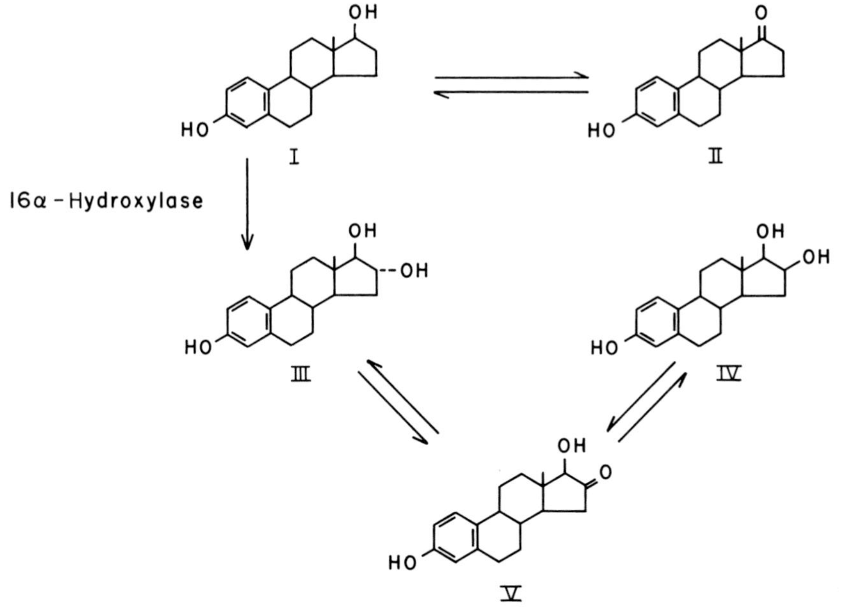

Fig. 3.   Reactions of intermediate metabolism of estrogens in lower vertebrates. I, Estradiol-17β; II, estrone; III, estriol; IV, 16-epiestriol; V, 16-ketoestradiol-17β. (According to Breuer *et al.*, 1963; Ozon and Breuer, 1963.)

B. Conversion of C_{19} Steroids to C_{18} Steroids

The main results are shown in Table III. The aromatization of C_{19} to C_{18} steroids is a mechanism common to the ovary of all vertebrates. The intermediary stages have not been thoroughly investigated, but 19-hydroxytestosterone could be an intermediate in *Pleurodeles waltlii* (Ozon, 1967). The yield from aromatization is low; Callard and Leathem (1965, 1966) did not find any transformation of C_{21} steroids to estrogens using ovaries of several elasmobranchs, reptiles, and amphibians. Eckstein (1970) did not isolate estrogen after incubation of the ovary of *Tilapia aurea* in the presence of 17α-hydroxyprogesterone. The negative results are possibly due to the low conversion of C_{19} steroids to C_{18} steroids. Eckstein (1970) did not look for phenolic steroids after the incubation of ovaries in the presence of androstenedione-7-^{3}H; consequently these results do not necessarily indicate that estrogens are not formed in the ovary. Indeed Simpson *et al.* (1968), Ozon (1967), Ozon and Breuer (1964), Xavier and Ozon (1971) and Redshaw and Nicholls (1971) have shown that estrogens are synthesized in the ovary of one elasmobranch and four amphibians. The low yield of aro-

TABLE IV

Summary of Known Enzyme Reactions in the Intermediate Metabolism of Estrogens in Nonmammalian Vertebrates

Enzyme	In vivo occurrence	In vitro occurrence (liver)	Enzyme system		Species	Reference
			Cellular localization	Cofactor requirement		
Oxidoreductases						
6α-		+	Soluble fraction	$NADH_2$	*Pleurodeles waltlii*	Breuer *et al.* (1963)
		+	Soluble fraction	$NADPH_2$	*Rana temporaria*	Breuer *et al.* (1963)
		+			*Gallus domesticus*	Ozon and Breuer (1965)
6β-		+			*G. domesticus*	Ozon and Breuer (1965)
16α-		+	Soluble fraction	$NADH_2$, $NADPH_2$	*Salmo irideus*, *P. waltlii*, *R. temporaria*	Breuer *et al.* (1963)
	+	+	Soluble fraction		*G. domesticus*	Ozon and Breuer (1965)
					G. domesticus	MacRae *et al.* (1960)
16β-		+	Soluble fraction	$NADH_3$ $NADPH_2$	*S. irideus*	Breuer *et al.* (1963)
		+	Soluble fraction	$NADH_2$ $NADPH_2$	*P. waltlii*, *R. temporaria*	Breuer *et al.* (1963)
	+				*G. domesticus*	Ozon and Breuer (1965)
					G. domesticus	MacRae *et al.* (1960)
17α-	+	+	Soluble fraction	$NADH_2$, $NADPH_2$	*P. waltlii*	Ozon and Breuer (1966)
17β-	+	+	Soluble fraction	$NADH_2$, $NADPH_2$	*P. waltlii*	Ozon and Breuer (1966)
			Soluble fraction		*G. domesticus*	Ozon and Breuer (1965), Renwick and Engel (1967)
	+				*G. domesticus*	Mulay and Common (1968)
	+				*Torpedo marmorata* *Crenilaberus ocellatus*	Breuer and Breuer (1968) Itrich (1962)
		+	Soluble fraction	$NADH_2$, $NADPH_2$	*S. irideus*,	Breuer *et al.* (1963)

404

Hydroxylases			Preparation	Cofactor	Species	Reference [a]
6α-	+	+	Microsomes	NADPH₂	P. waltlii, R. temporaria, G. domesticus	Ozon and Breuer (1965)
	+				P. waltlii	Ozon (1963)
					Xenopus laevis	Breuer et al. (1966)
	+				G. domesticus	MacRae et al. (1959)
	+	+	Microsomes	NADPH₂	P. waltlii, R. temporaria	Ozon and Breuer (1963)
15α-	+	+	Microsomes	NADPH₂	X. laevis	Rao et al. (1968)
16α-	+	+	Microsomes	NADPH₂	X. laevis	Rao et al. (1968)
	+	+			Anguilla anguilla	Ozon (1964)
	+	+			P. waltlii, R. temporaria	Ozon and Breuer (1963)
					G. domesticus	Ozon and Breuer (1965), Mitchell and Hobkirk (1959)
16β-	+	+	Microsomes	NADPH₂	X. laevis	Rao et al. (1968)
	+				G. domesticus	Ozon and Breuer (1965)
					G. domesticus	MacRae et al. (1960)

[a] Key to references:

405

matization *in vitro* and the physiological stage at which the incubations were performed probably account for the first negative results.

IV. Intermediate Metabolism of C$_{18}$ Steroids

Like the androgens, the estrogens are metabolized by nonmammalian vertebrates (Fig. 3). Several enzymes which metabolize estrogens have been discovered (Table IV). *In vivo* estradiol-17β is metabolized by fishes and amphibians after injection or addition to the breeding water (Ittrich, 1962; Ozon, 1963; Breuer *et al.*, 1966). The main metabolites are estrone, estriol, and polar compounds which are seldom identified. During the past decade the *in vivo* metabolism of estrogens was studied in the laying hen by Common's group (Mulay and Common, 1968; Mathur and Common, 1968a,b); the results obtained are of fundamental importance to comparative physiology. In the hen estradiol-17α and 16-epiestriol are urinary metabolites (Tables I and IV).

The interconversion of estrone and estradiol-17β *in vitro* is catalyzed by a 17β-hydroxysteroid oxidoreductase; this activity has been discovered in the ovary of every species investigated (Table III). Quantitatively liver is the most important site of metabolism. Various hepatic metabolic reactions have been studied in a fish, *Salmo irideus*, and in two amphibians, *Pleurodeles waltlii* and *Rana temporaria* (Breuer *et al.*, 1963). The activities of a 16α-, 16β-, and 17β-hydroxysteroid oxidoreductase have been compared. The enzymes are localized in the supernatant fraction of the cytoplasm after centrifuging at 100,000 *g* (Fig. 4). Precipitation by ammonium sulfate allows the purification and partial fractionation of enzymes bound to NAD from those bound to NADP. These results establish that estrogen-metabolizing enzymes in nonmammalian vertebrates are comparable to those in mammals; differences are probably quantitative. Phenolic steroids not only can be metabolized by enzymes of oxidoreduction but they also can be hydroxylated (Ozon and Breuer, 1963). In the species investigated, estriol appeared to be the main product of hepatic hydroxylation of estradiol-17β. In *Anguilla anguilla*, *P. waltlii*, and *R. temporaria* 16α-hydroxylase is localized in microsomes and requires oxygen and NADPH$_2$. Various metabolic reactions of estrogens have been studied in the chick (Fig. 5). The most interesting results are the discovery of a 16β-hydroxylase localized in the hepatic microsome fraction (Ozon and Breuer, 1965) and a 17α-hydroxysteroid oxidoreductase and a 17β-hydroxysteroid oxidoreductase in liver cytosol (Ozon and Breuer, 1965; Renwick and Engel, 1967). The two oxidoreductases are localized in the soluble fraction after centrifugation at 100,000 *g*; a partial fractionation has been achieved by ammonium sulfate precipitation and chromatography on Sephadex G-200.

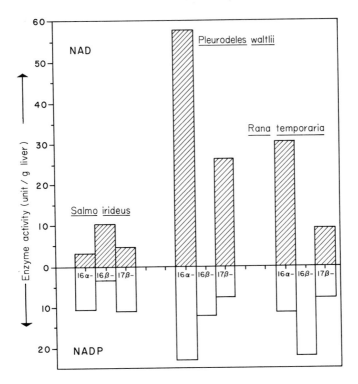

Fig. 4. Activity of 16α-, 16β-, and 17β-hydroxysteroid oxidoreductases in the liver of *Salmo irideus, Pleurodeles waltlii,* and *Rana temporaria*; unit of enzymic activity is micrograms of steroid formed $\times$ 10 per 60 mn. Hatched columns: coenzymes $NAD/NADH_2$; white columns: coenzymes $NADP/NADPH_2$. (According to Breuer *et al.*, 1963.)

The presence of conjugated estrogens has been demonstrated in non-mammalian vertebrates. The enzymic systems responsible for the glucuronization of estradiol and estrone have been discovered in the liver of *Pleurodeles waltlii* (Ozon and Breuer, 1966). The mechanisms of conjugation are discussed in Chapter 6. Recent studies of Mathur *et al.* (1969) show that estrogens are conjugated *in vivo* with sulfuric acid in the hen; the di- and monosulfates have been isolated from urine.

V. Concluding Remarks

Phenolic estrogens are present in fishes and other vertebrates and probably range from cyclostomes to humans. The ovary is the main source of C_{18}

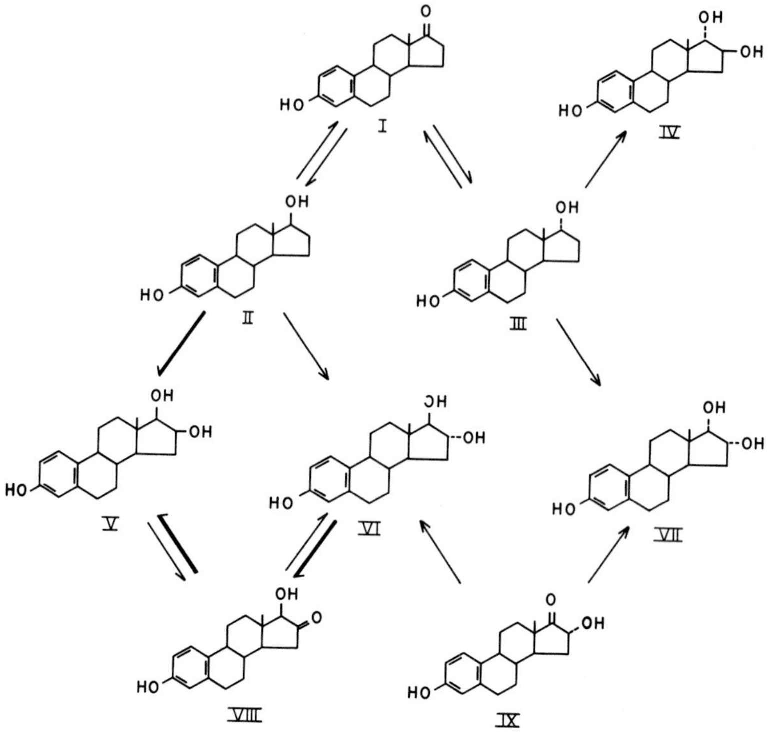

Fig. 5. Intermediate metabolism of estrogen steroids in hen according to experiments performed *in vivo* and *in vitro* (see text). I, Estrone; II, estradiol-17β; III, estradiol-17α; IV, 16, 17-epiestriol; V, 16-espiestriol; VI, estriol; VII, 17-epiestriol; VIII 16-ketoestradiol-17β; IX, 16α-hydroxyestrone.

steroids; however, the production of estrogens by adrenal tissues or testes should not be excluded in the case of certain vertebrates (Gottfried *et al.*, 1967; Chieffi, 1966). The pathways of biogenesis and intermediate metabolism of C_{18} as well as of C_{19} steroids are similar in all vertebrates; most of the enzymic mechanisms described for mammals have been found in non-mammalian species investigated to date. Species are characterized by qualitative and quantitative differences, by the presence or absence of certain activity (e.g., the absence or the presence of 17α-hydroxysteroid oxidoreductase in the liver), or by enzymic activities of different biochemical characteristics (Fig. 4). These differences account for the urinary metabolites varying from one species to another as well as for the different C_{18} plasma steroids; the case of the hen clearly shows that the excretion of 16-epiestriol corresponds to high activities of 16β-hydroxylase and 16β-hydroxysteroid oxidoreductase in the liver.

Comparative study of steroid metabolism has shown that in some cases it is possible to link a particular metabolic activity to a certain physiological state. In the case of the female teleost *Mugil capito* (Eylath and Eckstein, 1969) 11-ketotestosterone is synthesized and accumulated when the animals are in fresh water, i.e., in a medium in which they do not reproduce. In the viviparous amphibian *Nectophrynoides occidentalis* the enzymic activity of the ovary *in vitro* differs during the period of ovogenesis from that during gestation (Xavier and Ozon, 1971). Too few species have been investigated to allow the formulation of a complete picture of the variations in steroid metabolism, particularly of the estrogens, with respect to species and ecological factors. There is no doubt that these studies, when more numerous, will allow us to reconsider, from a different angle, the evolution of the biochemical mechanisms which control the physiology of reproduction. A particularly interesting aspect of comparative studies is that they suggest favorable models for research on enzymic reactions related to steroid metabolism.

The concentration of phenolic steroids in mammalian plasma is very low. The level of estradiol-17β is 5–40 ng/100 ml of plasma. Too few investigations have been performed to allow us to form a precise idea of the true situation in the nonmammalian vertebrates.

The binding of steroids by plasma proteins is a new domain for research in comparative endocrinology. Seal and Doe (1965) studied the distribution of transcortin in vertebrates. Their results show a considerable variation among the species (see, however, Chapter 4). Idler and Freeman (1969) and Freeman and Idler (1969) have demonstrated the existence of protein (sex-hormone-binding protein) which binds C_{18} and C_{19} steroids in the skate *Raja radiata*. A similar protein occurs in several teleost species (Chapter 6, Section VII, A). A protein which binds estradiol-17β and testosterone in the amphibian *Pleurodeles waltlii* has been demonstrated by Ozon *et al.*, (1971). The physicochemical characteristics of these proteins differ in fish, amphibians, and mammals. However, it is important to point out that in fishes and amphibians the association constants $K_{4°C}$ are comparable (or less than) those for mammals, while the binding capacity in fishes and amphibians reaches 20–50 μg/100 ml of plasma compared to only 1.5 μg/100 ml in mammals.

At the present time the mechanism of action of estrogenic hormones is being studied intensely. The presence of a specific protein which plays a role of receptor has been discovered in the uterus of mammals. This protein, which is present in very low concentration, has a very strong affinity for estradiol-17β. It is possible that this protein plays a fundamental role in the initial stages of the mechanism of action of estradiol-17β in the target cells. Experiments similar to those of Jensen and Jacobson (1962) have been per-

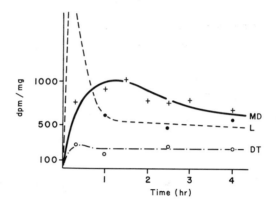

Fig. 6. Distribution of radioactivity in the tissues of a *Pleurodeles waltlii* female (cast-rated 4 months previously) after injection *in vivo* of 8 μCi(0.2 μg) of estradiol-17β- 6, 7-^{3}H (MD, Mullerian duct; L, liver; DT, digestive tube).

formed with the amphibian *Pleurodeles waltlii* (Fig. 6). The binding of estra-diol-17β is specific in the oviduct (Martin and Ozon, 1969). Preliminary results have oriented us to perform experiments *in vivo* and *in vitro*. They showed that estradiol-17β is bound to a protein located in the cytosol of Muller's duct; this protein has a sedimentation coefficient of 4 S in sucrose gradient (Martin *et al.*, 1970). These results show that the interaction of the hormone and receiving protein in target cells is a common mechanism in vertebrates. In a similar way O'Malley investigated the action of proges-terone in the õviduct of a hen (O'Malley *et al.*, 1969). Recently he has shown that progesterone is bound by a proteinaceous receptor within the oviduct of the hen (O'Malley, 1970).

REFERENCES

Ábrahám, G. E. (1969). *J. Clin. Endocrinol. Metab.* **29**, 866.
Ainsworth, L., and Common, R. H. (1962). *Nature (London)* **195**, 77.
Attal, J. (1970). Mesure des oestrogènes et des androgènes testiculaires et plasmatiques dans l'espece ovine par des minomethodes de chromatographie en phase gazeuse: influence de l'âge, de la saison et du cycle diurne. Thesis, Faculté des Sciences, Paris.
Attal, J., and Eik-Nes, K. B. (1968). *Anal. Biochem.* **26**, 398.
Axelrod, L. R., and Goldzieher, J. W. (1969). *Biochim. Biophys. Acta* **187**, 450.
Baird, D. T., and Guevara, A. (1969). *J. Clin. Endocrinol. Metab.* **29**, 149.
Barr, W. A. (1968). *In* "Perspectives in Endocrinology: Hormones in the Lives of Lower Vertebrates" (E. J. W. Barrington and C. B. Jørgensen, eds.), pp. 164–237. Academic Press, New York.
Botticelli, C. R., and Hisaw, F. L., Jr. (1964). *Amer. Zool.* **4**, 297.

Botticelli, C. R., Hisaw, F. L., Jr., and Roth, W. D. (1963). *Proc. Soc. Exp. Biol. Med.* **114**, 255.

Bouceck, R. J., and Savard, K. (1970). *Gen. Comp. Endocrinol.* **15**, 6.

Breuer, H. (1962). *Vitam. Horm.* (*New York*) **20**, 285.

Breuer, J., and Breuer, H. (1968). *Naturwissenschaften* **8**, 391.

Breuer, H., and Knuppen, R. (1969). *In* "Methods in Enzymology. Steroids and Terpenoids" (R. B. Clayton, ed.), Vol. 15, pp. 691–735. Academic Press, New York.

Breuer, H., and Ozon, R. (1965). *Arch. Anat. Microsc. Morphol. Exp.* **54**, 17.

Breuer, H., Ozon, R., and Mittermayer, C. M. (1963). *Z. Physiol. Chem.* **333**, 272.

Breuer, H., Dahm, K., Mikamo, B., and Witschi, E. (1966). *Excerpta Med. Found. Int. Congr. Ser.* **111**, 215.

Callard, I. P., and Leathem, J. H. (1965). *Arch. Anat. Microsc. Morphol. Exp.* **54**, 35.

Callard, I. P., and Leathem, J. H. (1966). *Gen. Comp. Endocrinol.* **7**, 80.

Cédard, L., and Fontaine, M. (1963). *C.R. Acad. Sci.* **257**, 3095.

Cédard, L., and Nomura, T. (1961). *Bull. Inst. Oceanogr.* **1196**, 1.

Cédard, L., and Ozon, R. (1962). *C.R. Soc. Biol.* **156**, 1805.

Cédard, L., Fontaine, M., and Nomura, T. (1961). *C.R. Acad. Sci.* **252**, 2656.

Cédard, L., Haffen, K., and Guichard, A. (1968). *C.R. Acad. Sci.* **267**, 118.

Chieffi, G. (1966). *Excerpta Med. Found. Int. Congr. Ser.* **132**, 1047.

Chieffi, G., and Lupo, C. (1961). *Atti Accad. Naz. Lincei Cl. Sci. Fis. Mat. Natur. Rend.* **30**, 399.

Chieffi, G., and Lupo, C. (1963). *Gen. Comp. Endocrinol.* **3**, 149.

Dale, E. (1962). *Gen. Comp. Endocrinol.* **2**, 171.

Dean, S. D., and Chester Jones, I. (1959). *J. Endocrinol.* **18**, 366.

Dorfman, R. I., and Ungar, F. (1965). "Metabolism of Steroid Hormones." Academic Press, New York.

Eckstein, B. (1970). *Gen. Comp. Endocrinol.* **14**, 303.

Eckstein, B., and Eylath, U. (1970). *Gen. Comp. Endocrinol.* **14**, 396.

Eik-Nes, K. B., and Horning, E. C. (1968). "Gas Phase Chromatography of Steroids." Springer-Verlag, Berlin and New York.

Eleftheriou, B. E., Boehlke, K. W., and Tiemeier, O. W. (1966). *Proc. Soc. Exp. Biol. Med.* **121**, 85.

Eylath, U., and Eckstein, B. (1969). *Gen. Comp. Endocrinol.* **12**, 58.

Forbes, T. R. (1961). *In* "Sex and Internal Secretions" (W. C. Young, ed.), Vol. 2, pp. 1035–1087. Baillière, London.

Freeman, H. C., and Idler, D. R. (1969). *Gen. Comp. Endocrinol.* **13**, 83.

Gallien, L., and Chalumeau-Le-Foulgoc, M. T. (1960). *C.R. Acad. Sci.* **251**, 460.

Galzigna, L. (1961). *Atti Accad. Naz. Lincei Cl. Sci. Fis. Mat. Natur. Rend.* **31**, 92.

Gottfried, H. (1964). *Steroids* **3**, 219.

Gottfried, H., Hunt, V. H., Simpson, T. H., and Wright, R. S. (1962). *J. Endocrinol.* **24**, 425.

Gottfried, H., Huang, D. P., Lofts, B., Phillips, J. G., and Tam, W. H. (1967). *Gen. Comp. Endocrinol.* **8**, 18.

Hertelendy, F., and Common, R. H. (1964). *Can. J. Biochem.* **42**, 1177.

Hertelendy, F., Taylor, T. G., Mathur, R. S., and Common, R. H. (1965). *Can. J. Biochem.* **43**, 1379.

Höhn, E. O., and Cheng, S. C. (1967). *Gen. Comp. Endocrinol.* **8**, 1.

Idler, D. R., and Freeman, H. C. (1969). *Gen. Comp. Endocrinol.* **13**, 75.

Ittrich, G. (1962). Personal communication cited in Breuer (1962).

Jensen, E. V., and Jacobson, H. I. (1962). *Recent Progr. Horm. Res.* **18**, 387.

Knuppen, R. (1963). *Z. Vitam. Hormon Fermentforsch.* **5**, 355.

Korenman, S. G., Perrin, L. E., and McCallum, T. P. (1969). *J. Clin. Endocrinol. Metab.* **29**, 879.

Layne, D. S., Common, R. H., Mann, W. A., and Fraps, R. M. (1958). *Nature (London)* **181**, 351.

Lisboa, B. P., and Diczfalusy, E. (1962). *Acta Endocrinol. (Copenhagen)* **40**, 60.

Lupo, C., and Chieffi, G. (1963). *Nature (London)* **197**, 596.

Lupo, C., and Chieffi, G. (1965). *Gen. Comp. Endocrinol.* **5**, 698.

Lupo di Prisco, C., Vellano, C., and Chieffi, G. (1967). *Gen. Comp. Endocrinol.* **8**, 325.

Lupo di Prisco, C., Delrio, G., and Chieffi, G. (1968). *Gen. Comp. Endocrinol.* **10**, 292.

MacRae, H. F., Zaharia, W., and Common, R. H. (1959). *Poultry Sci.* **38**, 318.

MacRae, H. F., Dale, D. G., and Common, R. H. (1960). *Can. J. Biochem.* **38**, 523.

Martin, B., and Ozon, R. (1969), *C.R. Acad. Sci. Ser. D* **268**, 132.

Martin, B., Rochefort, H., and Ozon, R. (1970). Unpublished data.

Mathur, R. S., and Common, R. H. (1967). *Can. J. Biochem.* **45**, 531.

Mathur, R. S., and Common, R. H. (1968a). *Steroids* **12**, 475.

Mathur, R. S., and Common, R. H. (1968b). *Steroids* **12**, 725.

Mathur, R. S., Common, R. H., Collins, D. C., and Layne, D. S. (1969). *Biochim. Biophys. Acta* **176**, 394.

Mitchell, J. E., and Hobkirk, R. (1959). *Biochem. Biophys. Res. Commun.* **1**, 72.

Mulay, S., and Common, R. H. (1968). *Can. J. Biochem.* **46**, 965.

O'Grady, J. E., and Heald, P. J. (1965). *Nature (London)* **205**, 390.

O'Malley, B. W. (1970). *Excerpta Med. Found. Int. Congr. Ser.* **210**, 29.

O'Malley, B. W., McGuire, W. L., Kohler, P. O., and Korenman, S. G. (1969). *Recent Progr. Horm. Res.* **25**, 105.

Ozon, R. (1963). *C.R. Acad. Sci.* **257**, 2332.

Ozon, R. (1964). Unpublished results.

Ozon, R. (1965). *C.R. Acad. Sci.* **261**, 5664.

Ozon, R. (1966). *Ann. Biol. Anim. Biochim. Biophys.* **6**, 537.

Ozon, R. (1967). *Gen. Comp. Endocrinol.* **8**, 214.

Ozon, R., and Attal, J. (1969). Unpublished data.

Ozon, R., and Breuer, H. (1963). *Z. Physiol. Chem.* **333**, 282.

Ozon, R., and Breuer, H. (1964). *Z. Physiol. Chem.* **337**, 61.

Ozon, R., and Breuer, H. (1965). *Z. Physiol. Chem.* **341**, 239.

Ozon, R., and Breuer, H. (1966). *Gen. Comp. Endocrinol.* **6**, 295.

Ozon, R., and Xavier, F. (1968), *C.R. Acad. Sci. Ser. D* **266**, 1173.

Ozon, R., Martin, B., and Boffa, G. A. (1971). *Gen. Comp. Endocrinol.* **17**, 566.

Penso, G., and Galzigna, L. (1963). *Atti Accad. Naz. Lincei Cl. Sci. Fis. Mat. Natur. Rend.* **35**, 365.

Polzonetti-Magni, A., Lupo di Prisco, C., Rastogi, R. K., Bellini-Cardellini, L., and Chieffi, G. (1970). *Gen. Comp. Endocrinol.* **14**, 212.

Rao, G. S., Breuer, H., and Witschi, E. (1968). *Experientia* **24**, 1258.

Redshaw, M. R., and Nicholls, T. J. (1971). *Gen. Comp. Endocrinol.* **16**, 85.

Renwick, A. G. G., and Engel, L. L. (1967). *Biochim. Biophys. Acta* **146**, 336.

Schmidt, P. J., and Idler, D. R. (1962). *Gen. Comp. Endocrinol.* **2**, 204.

Seal, U. S., and Doe, R. P. (1965). *Steroids* **5**, 827.

Simpson, T. H., Wright, R. S., and Hunt, S. V. (1963). *J. Endocrinol.* **26**, 499.

Simpson, T. H., Wright, R. S., and Hunt, S. V. (1964). Cited in Gottfried (1964).

Simpson, T. H., Wright, R. S., and Hunt, S. V. (1968). *J. Endocrinol.* **42**, 519.

Talalay, P. (1965). *Annu. Rev. Biochem.* **34**, 347.

van Tienhoven, A. (1961). *In* "Sex and Internal Secretions" (W. C. Young, ed.), Vol. 2, pp. 1088–1169. Baillière, London.

Wotiz, H. H., Botticelli, C. R., Hisaw, F. L., Jr., and Ringler, I. (1958). *J. Biol. Chem.* **231**, 589.

Wotiz, H. H., Botticelli, C. R., Hisaw, F. L., Jr., and Olsen, A. G. (1960). *Proc. Nat. Acad. Sci. U.S.* **46**, 580.

Xavier, F., and Ozon, R. (1971). *Gen. Comp. Endocrinol.* **16**, 30.

Chapter 8

BIOLOGICAL ACTIONS OF STEROID HORMONES IN NONMAMMALIAN VERTEBRATES

I. CHESTER JONES, D. BELLAMY,
D. K. O. CHAN, B. K. FOLLETT,
I. W. HENDERSON, J. G. PHILLIPS, and
R. S. SNART

I. Actions of Adrenocorticosteroids

The adrenocortical hormones are known to affect many mammalian processes. In nonmammalian vertebrates many of the same hormones are secreted, but in most instances their precise physiological role remains to be examined. The almost classical subdivision of adrenal steroids into those affecting glycogen, protein, and intermediary metabolism (the so-called "glucocorticoids") and those affecting water and electrolyte metabolism (the so-called "mineralocorticoids") is being eroded, as it is now apparent that there is considerable overlap of their actions in many species. Much research in recent years has been concentrated on steroidal effects on electrolyte homeostasis and in many ways has taken preference over the other diverse actions of the hormones. Structures such as the skin and bladder of amphibians, the gills of teleosts and cyclostomes, the rectal gland of elasmobranchs, the nasal gland of birds and reptiles, and the renal tubule have all been examined from the viewpoint of adrenal steroidal control of sodium transport and water movement. In contrast, comparative aspects concerning growth, protein metabolism, and other actions have received regrettably scant attention.

A. Metabolism

The metabolic role of corticosteroids may be investigated in three ways:

1. Remove the adrenocortical tissue and observe deficiency symptoms and the effects of steroid replacement.
2. Inject pure steroids or adrenocorticotropin (ACTH) into normal animals or add them to tissue preparations.
3. Observe changes in the concentration of plasma corticosteroids and relate these to coincident physiological and biochemical events in intact animals.

Although a wide range of lower vertebrates has not been examined, the available evidence from experiments of type 1 and 2 fits the pattern established for mammals. That is to say, the results obtained for animals from fish to man are consistent with the view that corticosteroids of the cortisol type promote gluconeogenesis and that this process underlies their major role in intermediary metabolism (Hartman and Brownell, 1949; Pickford and Atz, 1957; Segal and Kim, 1963; Robertson *et al.*, 1963; Hazelwood, 1965; Bentley and Follett, 1965; Falkmer and Matty, 1966).

With regard to experiments of type 3 there have been few investigations even in the common laboratory animals. Difficulties here are linked with technical problems in measuring steroid hormones in small amounts of blood and of establishing a normal unstressed state in the experimental animal. The fullest investigations of this type have been carried out on the salmonid fish in which a high level of circulating corticosteroids is often associated with the nonfeeding spawning migration. The concentration of cortisol is increased in salmon when they are very active (Fagerlund, 1967) and it appears that the state of hyperadrenocorticism is associated with an internal rearrangement of tissue leading to a fall in muscle mass and an increase in the size of the gonads (Robertson *et al.*, 1961a, 1963).

A system for ensuring an efficient utilization of tissue protein when dietary protein is at a premium would appear to be a fundamental requirement for the maintenance of organisms. Further, it would be anticipated that the necessary endocrine system would have been established early in the evolution of the vertebrates. Indeed, a requirement for adrenocortical hormones may be general throughout the vertebrates when food is in short supply and there is a natural suppression of feeding activity.

The evolution of adrenocortical function has been examined in detail elsewhere (Bellamy and Chester Jones, 1965). At this point we may ask if there is a unifying pattern for the action of corticosteroids throughout the vertebrates. Cortisol-like hormones have been implicated either directly, or by association, with the breakdown of selected tissues when the animal has to maintain itself independently of its environment and quantitatively the major catabolic action appears to be on skeletal muscle. The resultant amino acids may be used for the synthesis of new tissue elsewhere in the body, as in migratory teleost fish (Robertson *et al.*, 1961a,b) and the metamorphosing tadpole (Dale, 1962; Rapola, 1963), for tissue maintenance and energy production as in, for example, starved fish and mammals (White and Dougherty, 1947; Bondy, 1949; Kline, 1949; Mathies *et al.*, 1951; Hunter and Johnson, 1960; Robertson *et al.*, 1963; Bellamy *et al.*, 1968), and perhaps for protein secretion or lactation (Nandi and Bern, 1961; Gala and Westphal, 1965). Taking this into consideration, as a working hypothesis it may be assumed that there is a common mode of action of cortisol-like steroids throughout the vertebrates.

When vertebrate muscle is utilized normally or under the influence of small doses of exogenous corticosterone, the biochemical changes indicate that the tissue is being degraded without a change in gross composition. That is to say, not only is the protein being lost, but all cell constituents associated with it are lost in their normal proportions. It seems that cellular units are being destroyed, possibly at the level of the fibril. Two kinds of experiment concerned with the action of cortisol on skeletal muscle in rat and goldfish illustrate this point.

The normal young growing rat injected with small amounts of cortisol at first shows a falling off in growth. When the dose is increased the animal loses weight, which is reflected by the decrease in the mass of skeletal muscle. Palmer (1966) showed, in this type of experiment, that there was a 40% decrease in the mass of the vastus lateralis muscle. However, this was not associated with marked alteration in the composition of the remaining muscle, although the glycogen content rose. Starvation brings about a similar fall in muscle mass which is associated with the combined action of the adrenal cortical and thyroid hormones (Bellamy *et al.*, 1968). Again there was no change in the proportion of the major constituents, protein and water.

The reaction of mammalian tissues to corticosteroids is well documented but there is little for comparison from submammalian vertebrates. In the goldfish, after 8 days starvation, there is a 15% decrease in body weight due almost entirely to the loss of parietal muscle (Table I). Again there appears to be no change in the composition of the remaining muscle. Cortisol treatment for 4 days, which produced the same weight loss as starvation, also had no effect on muscle composition. It is interesting that when the amount of tissue water lost by the fish (obtained from the weight loss) is related to the extra potassium excreted in each condition, the ratio of potassium to water is the same in both starved and cortisol-treated animals and similar to that

TABLE I

Effect of Cortisol on Body Weight, Muscle Water Content, and Liver Glycogen Content of Fed and Starved Goldfish[a,b]

	Fed		Starved	
	Control	Cortisol	Control	Cortisol
Body weight (% increase or decrease)				
4 days	+5.91	−4.21	−5.78	−9.58
	(15)	(11)	(13)	(11)
8 days	+13.8	+1.98	—	—
	(15)	(11)		
Muscle water (%)				
8 days	77.8 ±0.22	77.8 ±0.18	79.2 ±0.63	79.1 ±0.49
	(6)	(6)	(7)	(11)
Liver glycogen (mg/100 mg liver wet weight)				
4 days	11.0 ±1.29	10.7 ±0.94	9.41 ±0.96	5.83 ±0.97
	(8)	(10)	(7)	(12)

[a]Storer (1967).
[b]Number of animals is given in parentheses.

expected for the ratio of potassium to water in the intracellular fluid compartment (Stimpson, 1965; Storer, 1967).

The effect of cortisol on muscle depends on the dose, large amounts producing considerable alterations in the composition of skeletal muscle. For example, in the young chick it is possible to increase the percentage of water, alter the ratio of sodium and potassium, and lower the percentage of protein (Bellamy and Leonard, 1965). These gross changes in muscle composition are not observed in normal animals.

Lymphoid tissue is another site of action of corticosteroids and here the overall effect is similar to that in skeletal muscle. There is a fall in tissue mass and a decrease in the number of cells. The kinetics of the process and the changes in chemical composition and tissue ultrastructure suggest that cells disintegrate at random without a deterioration in all cells at the same time (Bellamy *et al.*, 1966).

Detailed work on the interaction of corticosteroids with lymphoid tissue has been carried out with birds and mammals. Little is known of this response in other vertebrates (see Pickford and Atz, 1957) but the catabolic effects of corticosteroids on both lymphoid tissue and muscle suggests that there is a fundamental reaction of associated cells in tissues. Such evidence as exists indicates a common mode of action; it also suggests that the overall response takes place in a stepwise manner and is more complicated than can be explained by a change in a single enzyme. Further, the action of cortisol in promoting the utilization of tissues clearly poses problems of cell–cell interactions and suggests the presence of factors which delay the onset of the endocrine response in individual cells (Bellamy *et al.*, 1966).

Apart from skeletal muscle and lymphoid tissue the other important target for the long-term action of cortisol-like hormones is liver. This is particularly true in mammals, birds, and amphibians in which the liver responds to cortisol treatment by increase in mass (Goodland and Munro, 1959; Bellamy and Leonard, 1965; Janssens, 1967). The change in weight is due, initially, to an increase in cell size but in the long term there is also a rise in cell number. The biological significance of this change is difficult to assess. The absolute quantity of hepatic enzymes concerned with transamination does not appear to limit amino acid catabolism, and a direct connection with the production of urea or uric acid has not been established (Bellamy and Leonard, 1965; Adams, 1968). Also, the rise in liver weight is not always a characteristic of natural conditions when there is an enhanced level of plasma cortisol or corticosterone, although in mammals, at least, the adrenal gland is necessary for the maintenance of the maximal liver–body weight ratio.

There is a large gap in our knowledge of corticosteroid–liver interactions at the level of the teleosts. So far, fish liver has not been observed to increase in size after treatment with corticosteroids, and may decrease in *Poecilia* (Chester Jones *et al.*, 1969). Another difference between the response of the liver of fish and higher vertebrates lies in the pattern of enzyme induction. The inconsistency first appears at the level of the reptiles (Chan and Cohen, 1964a,b).

The significance of these variations in the response of liver to cortisol is not known. Recent work indicates that the liver of teleosts plays a role similar to that in the mammal except that there appears to be less emphasis on amino acid deamination (Kenyon, 1967). Perhaps a change in the role of the liver underlies the evolution of its response to cortisol. In this connection there is the possibility that liver weight increase in higher vertebrates is connected with the metabolism of the excessive amounts of adrenal hormones that are necessary to bring about the response.

B. WATER AND ELECTROLYTES

Animals have morphological and physiological adaptations to the various environmental niches of the earth. Yet, despite such variations, vertebrates maintain a dynamic equilibrium of the body fluids. Thus, with the exception of the Elasmobranchii and Myxinoidea, blood osmolarity is about 300 mosmol/kg water. Marine vertebrates, in seas containing about 1 osmol/kg water, face passive forces along concentration gradients, thereby tending toward water depletion and solute concentration. In contrast, freshwater animals are concerned with water influx and salt depletion across permeable surfaces. On land, vertebrates are subject to water loss, its evaporation tending toward concentration of the body fluids. However the vertebrate body maintains homeostasis and the kidney is the major organ in the regulation of fluid balance. In addition there are various accessory structures, such as fish gills, the amphibian skin and bladder, and the nasal gland of reptiles and birds, which aid in the control of the composition of the body fluids.

1. Fishes

Fishes may be stenohaline (restricted to one environment) or euryhaline (able to survive in fresh, brackish, or seawater). Some euryhaline fish migrate. Thus the anadromous salmon and lamprey move from the sea to river to spawn, while catadromous species after various periods in fresh water spawn in the sea. Some of the osmoregulatory processes have been known for some time and have recently been reviewed (Parry, 1966; Motais, 1967; Maetz, 1964, 1970; Potts, 1968; Conte, 1969; Hickman and Trump, 1969). Certain organs, both endocrine and *incertae sedis*, have been implicated, namely the adrenal cortex (discussed below), the neurophypophysis, adenohypophysis, urophysis, and the corpuscles of Stannius, and their possible roles have been reviewed (Ball and Ensor, 1968; Chester Jones *et al.*, 1969; Perks, 1969; Chan *et al.*, 1969; Maetz, 1970).

a. Cyclostomata. The living members of the superclass Agnatha comprise the class Cyclostomata, which consists of two orders, Petromyzontia and Myxinoidea. The latter group, the hagfishes, are very different from the former, the lampreys.

The Myxinoidea maintain the electrolyte composition of plasma at levels similar to those of the environmental seawater but with lower concentrations of divalent ions (Robertson, 1954; McFarland and Munz, 1958, 1965; Bellamy and Chester Jones, 1961; Morris, 1965; Rall and Burger, 1967). Renal tubular structures are not extensive and there may well be neither net absorption of water, with the inulin urine/plasma ratio at one, nor net reabsorption of sodium (Munz and McFarland, 1964; Rall and Burger, 1967), although Morris (1965) found urinary sodium concentration less than that of plasma. It may be that extrarenal structures are of prime importance for ionic regulation—the skin by copious mucus secretion, the liver, especially in regard to organic acid and magnesium, and the gills (Fänge, 1963; Morris, 1965; Rall and Burger, 1967). Adrenocorticosteroids occur in Myxinoidea (see Chapter 5) but their function is not known. Adrenocortical cells have been tentatively described and injections of aldosterone and deoxycorticosterone acetate (DOCA) alter electrolyte composition in *Myzine* (Chester Jones *et al.*, 1962). Further investigation of this order is required.

The Myxinoidea may represent the early condition of vertebrates rather than comprising a secondary modification. If this is true, then ionic regulation rather than osmoregulation was the primary condition. It can be argued, in view of the apparent absence of renal tubular function in respect to water and electrolyte control, that the liver is of prime importance as a regulatory structure. In evolution, then, the adrenocorticosteroids impinged, in the first place, on hepatic regulation and only later, with the occurrence of more complex kidneys, on renal function.

In contrast to the Myxinoidea, the lampreys, Petromyzontia, fall into the general vertebrate patterns (Chester Jones, 1957). In fresh water, the lampreys excrete significant amounts of dilute urine (Morris, 1960; Bentley and Follett, 1963). Aldosterone administration reduces the overall loss of sodium, that is from both renal and extrarenal sources, with the latter predominating (Bentley and Follett, 1962). The renal tubules reabsorb much of the filtered load of solutes and water but it is not known whether this is mediated by the adrenocortical or neurohypophysial hormones (Hickman and Trump, 1969). In the sea, the lamprey may not have detectable corticosteroids (Weisbart and Idler, 1970) but in the freshwater *Lampetra fluviatilis* adrenocortical cells are apparently discernible and corticosteroids occur (Sandor *et al.*, 1970). It is anticipated that further research will demonstrate a role of the adrenocortical secretions similar, in principle, to those described for other fish such as the Teleostei.

b. *Elasmobranchii.* Elasmobranchs are predominantly marine but they do occur in fresh water (Smith, 1953). The total osmolarity of the plasma is generally greater than that of seawater, achieved principally by high circulating levels of urea and trimethylamine oxide (Smith, 1929). Uremia is the normal physiological condition of the seawater elasmobranch, although urea retention occurs in other vertebrates in response to various environmental changes (Pickford and Blake Grant, 1967; Janssens and Cohen, 1968; Forster and Goldstein, 1969). Involvement of the endocrine system in this process, or in the movements of water and electrolytes, is not known or even conjectured. Here, the plasma concentrations of sodium, potassium, chloride, magnesium and calcium are almost always higher than those found in other gnathostomes but lower than those of seawater. Sodium flux in marine elasmobranchs is low compared with that of marine teleosts (Maetz and Lahlou, 1966; Burger and Tosteson, 1966; Horowitz and Burger, 1968). Excess sodium may be excreted by the rectal gland, which can be influenced by corticosteroids (Chan *et al.*, 1967a), although it is perhaps not the major pathway (Burger, 1965).

Elasmobranchs do not keep well in laboratory conditions so that the sequelae of operations are often difficult to interpret. Thus adrenalectomy does not appear to have any effects which can be separated from those occurring in sham-operated controls (Hartman *et al.*, 1944; Idler and Szeplaki, 1968). In brief, therefore, the action of corticosteroids in cartilaginous fishes has yet to be delineated. Uremia might be controlled at intermediary sites of synthesis, by changes in renal clearance, or by alteration of gill permeability, all possible sites of corticosteroid action (cf. Idler and Szeplaki, 1968).

c. *Teleostei.* The physiological mechanisms of adaptation by teleosts to environments with different osmotic properties require, *inter alia*, both humoral and hemodynamic controls (Chester Jones *et al.*, 1967, 1969; Potts, 1968; Maetz, 1968; Maetz and Rankin, 1969; Henderson *et al.*, 1970). Earlier work using exogenous corticosteroids was not helpful in the elucidation of physiological processes (for a review see Holmes *et al.*, 1963; Maetz, 1968; Chester Jones *et al.*, 1969; Holmes and Donaldson, 1969). However the adrenalectomized eel has provided much useful data. The consequences of adrenalectomy on the electrolyte composition of eels adapted to fresh water and seawater are given in Table II. In the freshwater eel, concentra-

TABLE II

Effects of Adrenalectomy on Serum Electrolyte Composition of Silver Eels[a]

Group	No. of eels	Serum concentration (mM)				
		Na	K	Ca	Mg	PO$_4$
Freshwater adapted						
Sham operated	25	150	1.75	2.29	2.13	1.50
		±1	±0.15	±0.05	±0.22	±0.14
Adrenalectomized	8	121[b]	1.89	1.89[b]	1.88	1.94[b]
		±4	±0.16	±0.17	±0.22	±0.15
Seawater adapted						
Sham operated	16	183	3.22	2.37	3.74	1.45
		±3	±0.20	±0.08	±0.30	±0.15
Adrenalectomized	11	222[b]	3.24	4.23[b]	10.3[b]	1.93
		±13	±0.39	±0.57	±1.9	±0.32

[a]Mean ± SE; from Chan *et al.* (1969).
[b]Significant change ($p < 0.05$).

tions of serum sodium, calcium, and phosphate fall, with inconsistent changes in magnesium. In neither the fresh- nor seawater eel does serum potassium concentration change significantly after adrenalectomy, reflecting extracellular–intracellular water changes and perhaps the absence of a positive kaliuretic agent since aldosterone has not been identified in this species. Adrenalectomy is followed by a progressive increase in body weight in the freshwater eel, principally by intracellular water accumulation, and by a decrease in the seawater eel (Fig. 1) (Chan *et al.*, 1967b, 1969). In the latter, there is an increase in the concentrations of serum sodium, calcium, and magnesium and the amount of intracellular muscle water declines with concomitant accumulation of intracellular sodium and potassium.

Adrenalectomy of the freshwater eel results in altered renal and branchial functions. Thus, there is a decline in urine flow to about 70% of normal values 5–6 days postoperatively. Urinary sodium, calcium, and magnesium concentrations rise but that of potassium does not change (Fig. 2). There is impaired uptake of sodium by the gills (Henderson and Chester Jones, 1967; Mayer and Maetz, 1967; Chan *et al.*, 1969). Both extrarenal and renal function in the adrenalectomized freshwater eel can be restored to normal by injection of cortisol at 20 μg/100 g body weight although high doses (5–10 mg/100 g body weight) induce sodium loss. 11-Deoxycortisol, 11-deoxycorticosterone, and aldosterone were almost ineffective in restoring renal function although the latter acts extrarenally (Henderson and Chester Jones, 1967; Chan *et al.*, 1969). Aldosterone, however, has not been identified in the eel and its position as a hormone in teleosts has yet to be clarified.

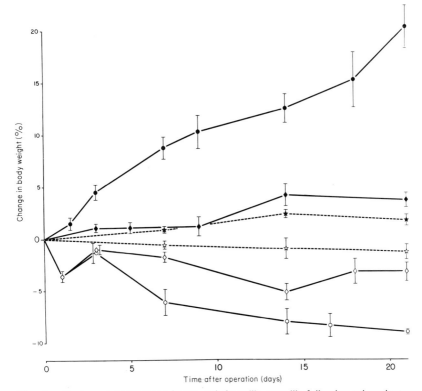

Fig. 1.   Body weight changes in the eel *Anguilla anguilla* following adrenalectomy, removal of the corpuscles of Stannius, or sham operation. Vertical bars represent standard errors. Freshwater eels: ●, adrenalectomized; ♦, stanniectomized; ★, sham operated. Seawater eels: ○, adrenalectomized; ◇, Stanniectomized; ☆, sham operated. (From Chester Jones *et al.*, 1969.)

Adrenalectomy of the seawater eel results in a lowered rate of sodium efflux across the gills which can be restored by cortisol (Mayer *et al.*, 1967). In contrast to the effects of corticosteroids on gill fluxes of sodium (outflux in seawater eels, influx in freshwater eels) the passive components of sodium movement appear to be independent of adrenal secretions. Thus seawater eels transferred to fresh water show an immediate reduction in sodium efflux whether the animal is adrenalectomized or injected with cortisol (Fig. 3). The possible mechanisms have been fully discussed by Motais *et al.* (1966), Maetz *et al.* (1967a,b). and Maetz (1970).

Reference must be made briefly to the corpuscles of Stannius, as these glandular structures occurring in the kidney have been considered as part of the adrenocortical system (see Chester Jones *et al.*, 1969). The pertinence of the corpuscles of Stannius to this chapter lies in the similarity of the

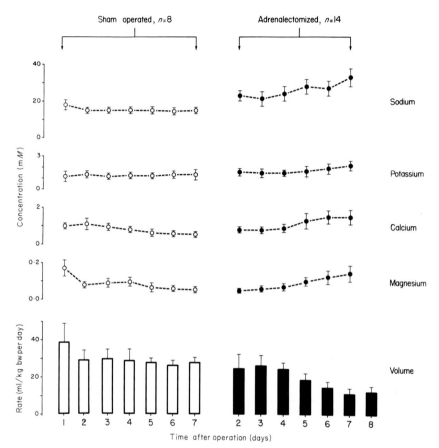

Fig. 2. Renal response of the freshwater silver eel to adrenalectomy; *n*, number of animals; bw, body weight; vertical line represents standard error (Chan *et al.*, 1969).

consequences of their removal to those following adrenalectomy (Fontaine, 1964; Chester Jones *et al.*, 1965). Indeed, only careful analysis has revealed a dichotomy of the effects of the two operations. Thus removal of the corpuscles of Stannius from freshwater eels is not followed by a significant change in body weight (Fig. 1). The serum potassium and calcium concentrations increase in contrast to their changes following adrenalectomy. Other changes in serum composition are similar to those following adrenalectomy (Table III). Adrenalectomy together with removal of the corpuscles of Stannius appears to override some of the effects of corpuscular removal (Chan *et al.*, 1967b). Furthermore the observed changes after removal of the corpuscles of Stannius seem to depend to a large extent on the length of time after surgery. Thus the rise in serum potassium and calcium concentrations

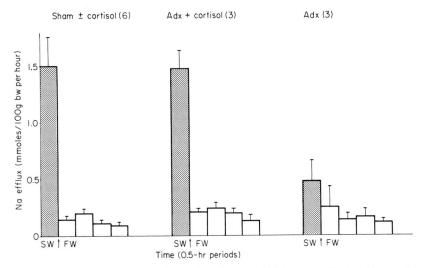

Fig. 3. Effect of sham operation, adrenalectomy (Adx), and cortisol replacement on sodium efflux during transfer of seawater (SW), silver eels to fresh water (FW). Number in parentheses indicates number of animals; bw, body weight; vertical line represents standard error (Mayer *et al.*, 1967).

TABLE III

Effect of Stanniectomy, With or Without Adrenalectomy, on Serum Electrolyte Composition of Eels[a]

Group	No. of eels	Serum concentration (mM)				
		Na	K	Ca	Mg	PO$_4$
Freshwater adapted						
Control	9	143	2.26	2.31	3.04	1.56
		±3	±0.25	±0.18	±0.43	±0.12
Stanniectomized	9	110[b]	3.34[b]	3.54[b]	2.10	1.80
(3 weeks)		±5	±0.14	±0.33	±0.24	±0.13
Adrenalectomized and						
Stanniectomized	4	112[b]	3.10	3.47	1.78	
(1 week)		±2	±0.53	±0.72	±0.21	
Seawater adapted						
Control	16	183	3.22	2.37	3.74	1.45
		±3	±0.20	±0.08	±0.30	±0.15
Stanniectomized	18	184	4.33[b]	4.05[b]	9.63[b]	1.40
(3 weeks)		±6	±0.18	±0.25	±2.8	±0.10
Adrenalectomized						
and Stanniectomized	9	205[b]	4.08	4.65[b]	10.8[b]	
(2 weeks)		±7	±0.54	±0.46	± 1.2	

[a]Mean ±SE; from Chan *et al.* (1967b).
[b]Value statistically different from controls at $p < 0.05$.

reaches a peak after 3 weeks and thereafter returns toward normal (Fontaine, 1967; Chan and Chester Jones, 1968; Chan, 1968; Tentatively it seems that an interaction between adrenocortical function with that of the corpuscles of Stannius exists. Recent work has shown that removal of the corpuscles of Stannius affects adrenocortical secretion *in vitro* (Leloup-Hatey, 1970a,b). This may suggest either a direct "tropic" action or it may be a reflection of the change in plasma calcium concentration.

In this section we have confined discussion to biological actions of corticosteroids very strictly. It is obvious however that no endocrine secretion can work in isolation. The adrenocorticosteroids may interact or indeed be controlled by the secretion(s) of the corpuscles of Stannius; the tropic influence of the pituitary (ACTH) has been established (see Chester Jones *et al.*, 1969, for a review). Apart from ACTH, the pituitary prolactin also interacts with cortisol in the maintenance of body fluid homeostasis in the eel (Chan *et al.*, 1968).

The precise picture of the biological actions of adrenocorticosteroids upon osmoregulation in teleost fishes remains incomplete. It is unwise at the present time to draw too firm conclusions concerning normal physiology from studies that, it must be admitted, are largely pharmacological. However some of the data demonstrate corticosteroid effects in both marine and freshwater eels. Among the target organs are the gill transporting systems (both influx and outflux, depending on the environmental salinity), the kidney of the freshwater preparation, and probably the cell membranes throughout the body. It is also apparent that the adrenocortical secretions form part of a highly integrated endocrine system whose secretions have a delicate interplay with one another.

It is not possible at the moment to elect one adrenal steroid as a primary regulator of electrolyte metabolism. Cortisol at least can strongly influence the sodium, and possibly water, movements both between the body fluids and environment and within the various fluid compartments of the body. The sporadic occurrence of aldosterone and our lack of information concerning adrenocortical secretion rates under different water and salt regimens make it difficult to assess whether there is an aldosteronelike steroid in bony fish generally. By analogy with mammalian physiology, it might be that sodium-regulating surfaces of teleost fishes require more than one corticosteroid to achieve "ideal" regulation. It might, for example, be profitable to examine in greater detail the degrees to which cortisol alters overall permeability of the branchial epithelium and directly alters sodium transport. It is within the realm of possibility that another steroid is capable of stimulating sodium uptake in fresh water, only when the water permeability has been decreased by the presence of cortisol, such as has been observed in the mammalian distal tubule. If it is postulated that membrane permeability is itself a local regulator of sodium movement, then clearly a whole range of peptides might severely alter a given teleost's response to exogenous corticosteroids or adrenalectomy.

2. Amphibia

Little is known about the action of corticosteroids in the intact animal (see Maetz, 1968) although there is a considerable literature on *in vitro* effects. The plasma levels and secretion rates of corticosteroids are influenced by environmental salinity (Crabbé, 1963a; Ulick and Feinholtz, 1968) and by factors similar to those having tropic influences on the mammalian adrenal cortex, including ACTH and the renin–angiotensin system (Cartensen *et al.*, 1961; Johnston *et al.*, 1967; Crabbé, 1966; Piper and Deroos, 1967). Ulick and Feinholtz, 1968. Surgical adrenalectomy is followed by hyponatremia and hyperkalemia. The responses show seasonal variation, with "winter" frogs surviving the operation well and "summer" frogs dying rapidly (Chester Jones, 1957), probably dependent on temperature and changed metabolic rates. It is anticipated, but still to be definitely shown, that, *in vivo*, corticosteroids act on renal function, the skin, and urinary bladder to maintain homeostasis of electrolytes (Maetz, 1968). Some evidence is provided by the use of inhibitors of corticosteroidogenesis, such as metyrapone and aminoglutethimide, which gives altered water and electrolyte balances (Edwards, 1969). Exogenous administration of corticosteroids increases skin permeability and sodium uptake, resulting in a net gain of sodium by the animal (Crabbé, 1963b; 1964; Alvarado and Kirschner, 1964; Socino and Ferreri, 1965). Aldosterone increased urinary osmolarity in *Bufo marinus* kept in saline but not when in distilled-water (Crabbé, 1961a). This suggests that the distilled-water animals were already retaining sodium maximally; those in saline might have had lower levels of circulating aldosterone rendering them more sensitive to exogenous administration. On the other hand Middler *et al.* (1969), using the same species, did not obtain clear effects of aldosterone on renal function or on sodium generally.

It is clear from this brief review of the literature concerning actions of corticosteroids in amphibian salt and water homeostasis that much more information is required. The sites of action, secretion rates with environmental changes, and the control over the secretion rates have all to be examined in a wider range of species. The lack of direct *in vivo* evidence for an action of aldosterone as a sodium-retaining steroid is a curious anomaly. The total response to aldosterone is not known; for example, if aldosterone acts to promote sodium uptake through the skin and bladder, there will be a net sodium retention and a renal natriuresis might then occur. In addition, potassium does not appear to be altered

TABLE IV

Effect of Adrenalectomy (adx) and Adrenocortical Steroids on Excretion of Electrolytes by Nasal gland of duck *Anas platyrhynchos* in Response to Single Load of Hypertonic Sodium Chloride[a]

Group	Time of onset of secretion (min)	Initial rate (output/hr) Vol (ml)	Na (meq)	K (meq)	Total output Vol (ml)	Na (meq)	K (meq)	Na:K	Concentration Na (meq/l)	K (meq/l)
Intact control	52.8 ±11.3	2.1 ±0.8	1.2 ±0.4	0.03 ±0.01	28.9 ±3.5	17.1 ±1.6	0.44 ±0.06	36.8 ±2.8	602.6 ±13.9	17.3 ±0.5
Unilateral adx	116.6 ±9.4	5.8[b] ±1.3	3.3[b] ±0.7	0.84[b] ±0.02	15.5[b] ±3.9	8.6[c] ±2.2	0.21[b] ±0.05	32.3 ±7.4	571.3 ±25.0	14.4[b] ±1.2
Total adx	270	. . . . .	. . . . .	. . . . .	. . . . .	Trace	. . . . .	. . . . .	. . . . .	. . . . .
Total adx plus cortisol	30.2 ±14.8	5.4[b] ±0.7	2.6 ±0.6	0.07[b] ±0.01	48.1 ±11.4	19.5 ±7.1	0.63 ±0.17	38.5 ±3.9	486.9[c] ±24.1	13.1[c] ±1.0
Cortisol (5 mg)	16.0 ±6.5	7.1[c] ±1.1	3.6[b] ±0.4	0.09[c] ±0.02	59.0[c] ±5.1	31.3[c] ±2.4	0.89[c] ±0.06	35.6 ±0.8	534.0[b] ±14.8	15.2[c] ±0.4
11-Deoxycorticosterone (5 mg)	24.0 ±6.5	6.5[c] ±0.8	3.1[c] ±0.4	0.09[c] ±0.004	54.6[c] ±4.6	27.9[c] ±2.8	0.92[c] ±0.09	31.2 ±2.8	511.2[c] ±11.9	16.8 ±1.1
Aldosterone (250 µg)	14.0 ±3.3	6.7[b] ±2.7	3.7 ±1.4	0.08 ±0.03	82.1[c] ±3.8	45.9[c] ±2.2	1.08[c] ±0.04	42.8 ±0.8	560.4[b] ±13.8	13.2[c] ±0.6
ACTH, 6 daily 20-IU doses	11.4 ±1.9	8.2[c] ±1.9	3.7[c] ±0.6	0.11[c] ±0.02	40.3[b] ±4.2	21.5 ±1.7	0.66 ±0.10	35.7 ±1.6	541.9[b] ±19.8	15.3[b] ±0.8

[a]Mean ±SE; from Holmes *et al.* (1963).
[b]Value statistically different from the corresponding controls at $p < 0.05$.
[c]Value statistically different from the corresponding controls at $p < 0.01$.

428

in the *in vitro* isolated amphibian membranes, but it is not known how far the well-established kaliuresis seen in mammalian renal function applies to amphibians. Finally, it is worth emphasizing that aldosterone is produced in relatively large quantities in amphibians and this group could, as in the past, provide many answers to problems involved in understanding the physiology of other vertebrates.

3. Reptiles and Birds: The Nasal Gland

Certain aquatic birds are able to secrete a fluid, originating in the supra-orbital nasal glands, through the external nares. It chiefly comprises a sodium chloride solution hypertonic to plasma and it is considered to donate a survival value to those species which normally ingest food containing sodium chloride hypertonic to the body fluids (Holmes *et al.*, 1961).

Adrenocorticosteroids appear to be essential for the normal functioning of the nasal glands (Table IV). Thus the nasal glands of adrenalectomized ducks which were loaded with sodium chloride solution, did not secrete and the normal response was restored by cortisol (Phillips *et al.*, 1961). After unilateral adrenalectomy, birds gave less than normal secretory levels. On the other hand, administration of exogenous corticoid or ACTH to normal birds, simulating hyperadrenocorticism, gave an enhanced nasal secretory response (Holmes *et al.*, 1961). The principal steroid involved is corti-costerone (Phillips and Bellamy, 1962). An anticipated correlation between the peripheral levels of circulating corticosteroids and the response of the nasal gland was not shown (Macchi *et al.*, 1967) despite possible increased steroidogenesis with high salt intake (Holmes, 1965). In the duck after salt loading, the nasal gland takes up, intracellularly, significantly greater amounts of corticosterone than do such tissues as muscle, liver, and Harder-ian gland (Bellamy and Phillips, 1966). Under these conditions, with increas-ed rate of removal of corticosterone from the circulation by the nasal gland and increased plasma volume, the tendency would be for a fall in the peri-pheral concentrations of corticosterone. This would lead to activation of the hypothalamico-hypophysial-adrenocortical axis to reestablish corticos-terone at near normal levels. The parasympathetic nervous system activates the nasal gland via acetylcholine (Fänge *et al.*, 1958; Schmidt-Nielsen, 1960). The mode of action might be by vasodilation of the vascular bed of the gland, leading to a greater blood flow per unit time with consequent in-creased presentation of corticosterone (Fänge *et al.*, 1963; Phillips and Bellamy, 1966).

It is very possible but not definitively shown that adrenocorticosteroids, that is the presence of functional adrenal glands, are necessary for the active elimination of excess sodium by the nasal glands (Phillips *et al.*, 1961;

Holmes *et al.*, 1969). Certainly the endocrine status of the animal is important (Holmes *et al.*, 1969) and associated with changes in glandular cells (Ernst and Ellis, 1969).

The sodium of the hypertonic nasal fluid is secreted against a bioelectric potential (Thesleff and Schmidt-Nielsen, 1962). Sodium ions which are moved against both an electrical and chemical gradient, involve active transport (Ussing, 1960). The nasal gland, as other organs such as the toad bladder and kidney, is rich in Na–K-activated ATPase (Hokin, 1963; Bonting and Canady, 1964; Bonting *et al.*, 1964), which is involved in the active transport of cations across biological membranes (Katz and Epstein, 1967). There is supporting evidence that this enzyme is involved in the active transport of sodium by the nasal gland. In the gull, injection of ouabain into the nasal gland duct abolished the positive potential which normally develops, and sodium secretion ceased (Thesleff and Schmidt-Nielsen, 1962). Bonting *et al.* (1964) assayed the ATPase activity in the nasal glands of gulls which had been kept on fresh water for 7 weeks. This group showed a decline in nasal gland size and a diminution of the Na–K ATPase activity per unit weight of the gland. The nasal gland of the domestic duck was found to possess only 6% of the Na–K ATPase activity found in the wild gull. These findings contrast with those of Hokin (1963), who showed that there was no difference between the nasal gland activity with regard to ATPase activity in Great Lakes' gulls adapted to fresh water and that of gulls given a 1.5% salt solution. It must be recognized, however, that the latter diet is only half seawater. If, however, the ATPase system is responsible for the active transport of Na$^+$ by the nasal gland then it would be expected that the activity of the enzyme system would correlate with the secretory capacity of the gland. Studies on ducks maintained for periods of up to 30 days on a diet containing saline drinking water (284 mM Na$^+$, 6 mM K$^+$) followed by a return to fresh water (2.0 mM Na$^+$, 0.07 mM K$^+$) and subsequently exposed for a second time to saline drinking water have shown that the Na$^+$-transporting capacity of the nasal gland is correlated both in quantitative and temporal terms with the activity of the ATPase system (Fletcher *et al.*, 1967). Moreover, the Na$^+$-transporting capacity of the glands from birds fully adapted to the hypertonic regimen was significantly and positively correlated with the tissue ATPase activity.

Similar studies have shown (Holmes and Stewart, 1968) that the protein: DNA and RNA:DNA ratios show increases following exposure to hypertonic saline and revert to normal values following return to fresh water. Concomitant with these changes at the cellular level in the nasal gland is an accumulation within the cell of corticosteroids (Phillips and Bellamy, 1967) and an increased corticosterone secretory rate (Donaldson and Holmes, 1965). These changes suggest a DNA- and RNA-dependent protein synthesis induced in the nasal gland which may be responsible for the increasing capacity of the epithelium to transport Na⁺ and that the adrenocortical hormones may be involved. Holmes *et al.* (1969) have pointed out that the observed changes in the nasal gland are reminiscent of the changes which occur in the toad bladder before the onset of active Na⁺ transport under the influence of aldosterone. In this tissue, a 60–90 min delay precedes the onset of active Na⁺ transport stimulated by aldosterone (Crabbé, 1961b) and it is possible that, during this delay period, protein synthesis is taking place under the influence of aldosterone (Edelman *et al.*, 1963). It is attractive to speculate that the increased ATPase activity is associated with the synthesis of new protein induced hormonally, but no firm evidence exists. In the toad bladder, aldosterone did not affect the Na–K-dependent ATPase activity (Bonting and Canady, 1964) although there may be regulation of the levels of this enzyme in the mammalian kidney by glucocorticoids (Chignell *et al.*, 1965; Chignell and Titus, 1966; Landon *et al.*, 1966) (see Section II).

Adrenocorticosteroids cannot be the sole influence on nasal gland function. Thus administration of glucose together with the intravenous salt load in the duck gives an increased nasal secretion. The gland may therefore be sensitive to changes in the amounts of available substrate, in part brought about by ACTH and the corticosteroids (Holmes *et al.*, 1969).

Reptiles have nasal glands (Schmidt-Nielsen, 1960; Templeton, 1964, 1966; Norris and Dawson, 1964; Dunson and Taub, 1967). Little is known of their control by hormones although adrenocorticosteroids seem to be involved (Holmes, 1965).

With regard to adrenocorticosteroids and kidney function, not enough is known to make discussion profitable but work is starting on this aspect (see Elizondo and LeBrie, 1969; LeBrie and Elizondo, 1969).

II. Physicochemical Aspects

A. BINDING IN PLASMA AND TARGET TISSUES

A specific plasma protein that binds corticosteroids, corticosteroid-binding globulin (CBG), has been demonstrated and its binding capacity shown for some nonmammalian vertebrates (Seal and Doe, 1963, 1966). The various methods for quantitative measurement of CBG (Sandberg, *et al.*, 1966) are generally based on the techniques of gel filtration, which has limitations (Quincey and Gray, 1963), or equilibrium dialysis (Daughaday *et al.*, 1962). Snart (1969) has proposed a more simple method for the determination of binding capacity. While the level of free rather than total steroids in plasma may reflect the biological activity of corticosteroids (Mills, 1961; Matsui and Plager, 1966), the dynamics of the relationship between free and bound is important (Yates and Urquhart, 1962). The binding characteristics and thermal stability of CBG in the nonmammalian vertebrates so far studied were found to be similar to those of mammals by Seal and Doe (1966), to whom reference should be made for a discussion of the general vertebrate spectrum (see also Chapters 4 and 6 of this volume).

Circulating steroids in the plasma act upon target tissues in which they interact with cellular macromolecular structures. One approach is to study the binding characteristics in order to determine the nature of the active binding sites, and here most progress has been made for aldosterone in relationship to the toad bladder (Edelman *et al.*, 1963; Sharp *et al.*, 1966; Snart, 1967). It has been shown that toad bladder takes up aldosterone maximally within 0.5 hr and that 95% is released by 1 hour after bathing in Ringer's solution (Edelman *et al.* 1963; Sharp *et al.*, 1966). The biological response to aldosterone, however, takes considerably longer than the time taken for such washing-out procedures and may still occur after a lag period, even after washing-out 5 min after treatment (Edelman *et al.*, 1963; Sharpe and Leaf, 1963). It has been shown that more than 8 hr preincubation of toad bladder is required for maximal sensitivity to aldosterone (Edelman *et al.*, 1963; Porter and Edelman, 1964). It would thus seem that a small fraction of bladder tissue has a tight binding capacity for aldosterone and constitutes a physiological receptor. The product of the interaction of steroid and receptor is then responsible for the observed increase in the rate of sodium transport.

The nature of the receptor for aldosterone has been investigated (Sharp *et al.*, 1966). Snart (1967) used a displacement binding technique for toad bladder where there are a good number of sites of low affinity to provide a constant distribution of steroid over a reasonably large concentration range. It is then possible to displace bound labeled with unlabeled steroid from the limited number of tight binding sites without displacing steroid from the larger set of sites with low affinity for aldosterone. Separate Scatchard plots can then be obtained for the high-affinity sites. Using this method, values were obtained for bound/free aldosterone-^{3}H for each set of sites to give a graph shown in Fig. 4. Analysis shows that the binding sites may be characterized by three association constants, $K_A = 5.4 \times 10^{10}$ liters/mole, $K_B = 2.1 \times 10^8$, liters/mole, and $K_C = 1.0 \times 10^4$ liters/mole, which correspond to free energies of association for the sites $\Delta G_A = 14.4$ kcal/mole, $\Delta G_B = 11.2$ kcal/mole, $\Delta G_C = -5.4$ kcal/mole. Nonspecific adsorption of steroid to protein has been shown (Snart, 1964) to have an association constant of the same order as K_C, which is too weak to carry bound steroid through a gel or column. It was therefore supposed that activity in the electrophoretic and chromatographic systems is moving with a high molecular weight protein possibly corresponding to the second set of binding sites, $K_B = 2.1 \times 10^8$ liters/mole (Fig. 4). The association constant for the interaction of aldosterone with this set of sites may be compared with that reported for transcortin with cortisol (Mills, 1962; Paterson and Hills, 1967).

The localization of the active binding sites in the tissue has been investigated using a technique of high-resolution radioautography (Edelman *et al.*, 1963). At low magnification it was found that tritium-labeled aldosterone gave heavy labeling of the mucosal cells but it was less intense in the submucosal and serosal layers. At high magnification, heavy labeling was seen in the nuclei but only occasionally in the cytoplasm. In contrast, the use of labeled progesterone gave rise to widely scattered intensity over the whole tissue (Porter *et al.*, 1964). The nature of the tight binding sites can be further

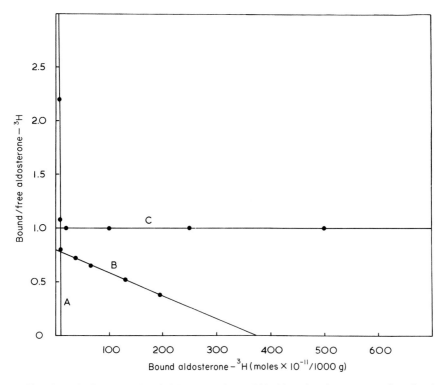

Fig. 4. Binding capacity of aldosterone in toad bladder, showing separate Scatchard plots for the three sets of binding sites revealed by a displacement binding technique. Association constants (in liters per mole): $K_A = 5.4 \times 10^{10}$, $K_B = 2.1 \times 10^8$, $K_C = 1.0 \times 10^4$. Binding capacity (in moles per 1000 g): $n_A = 9 \times 10^{-11}$, $n_B = 4 \times 10^{-9}$, $n_C = 1 \times 10^{-4}$ (Snart, 1967).

elucidated by work on rat liver in which, using corticosterone, it has been found that they are similar to those for aldosterone in toad bladder (Snart *et al.*, 1969). These sites occur in the buffer soluble fraction and correspond to protein units having molecular weights of the order of 200,000, 100,000, and 50,000. The latter two may be subunits of the larger protein and may be identified with the two binding sites revealed by the studies on tissue binding. Other work, for example, on cytosol and nuclear binding of estradiol in rat uterus, shows a similar pattern in that the cytoplasmic receptor, which may be readily dissociated into two subunits, further changes on entering the nucleus to form a receptor unit of intermediate size (Jensen *et al.*, 1969; Rochefort and Baulieu, 1969). Further, the nuclear uptake of this hormone is linked to cellular metabolism (Shyamala and Gorski, 1969). There has been some confusion as to whether the binding sites for aldosterone occur in the cytoplasm (Snart, 1967; Sharp and Dempsey, 1969) or in the nucleus (Edelman *et al.*, 1963). Such variable reports about the nuclear localization of receptors (Ausiello and Sharp, 1968; Sanyal and Snart, 1968) may be due to different procedures leading to variation in nuclear uptake (see Alberti and Sharp, 1969).

B. ALDOSTERONE

The well-documented induction of protein synthesis by steroids (Kenney and Kull, 1963) is regarded as the initial action of aldosterone. Supporting evidence comes from such observations as the lag period of 90 min before the response to aldosterone is shown by the toad bladder (Sharp and Leaf, 1964), during which time there is enhanced synthesis of protein (Fanestil and Edelman, 1966). The site of action of aldosterone may be the nucleus, influencing the genetic control of the cell (Edelman *et al.*, 1963). Such compounds as actinomycin D, believed to inhibit specifically the synthesis of RNA, inhibit the stimulation of sodium transport by aldosterone, whereas it has no effect on that produced by glucose or vasopressin (Fanestil and Edelman, 1966). Further, tritiated uridine is incorporated to an increased extent in the nuclei of toad bladder stimulated by aldosterone (Porter *et al.*, 1964).

Given, then, that aldosterone affects protein synthesis, there are at least three possibilities to occasion the stimulation of sodium transport: (a) an increase in the permeability of the mucosal or serosal surface of the epithelial cell membrane to sodium, (b) increased capacity of $Na^+ - K^+$-activated ATPase, (c) increased rate of production of high-energy intermediates. Crabbé (1963a,b) and Sharp and Leaf (1964) suggested that aldosterone increases sodium transport by affecting the permeability of the serosal surface.

Dalton and Snart (1967), using the effects of hormones on the temperature coefficients of active transport, support the theory that the protein induced by aldosterone affects permeability in a way similar to that given by amphoterocin B and vasopressin. It is supposed that pore size in the mucosal membrane is altered and this would facilitate the movement of sodium into epithelial cells (Leaf and Dempsey, 1960; Frazier and Hammer, 1963; Snart and Sanyal, 1968). However, the maximal increase in short-circuit current obtained with aldosterone is greater than that with vasopressin. This may be taken to indicate that proteins induced by aldosterone also have an effect on the sodium pump, and Fanestil *et al.* (1967) concluded that aldosterone increases the output of the sodium pump independently of effects on permeability. On the other hand, some experiments suggest that the principal mechanism of action of aldosterone is to stimulate the production of high-energy intermediates. Thus, addition of substrate to depleted toad bladders was followed by an increase in sodium transport by about 50% (Edelman *et al.*, 1963), although this was not confirmed by Sharp *et al.* (1965). Aldosterone does not affect the $Na^+-K^+-Mg^{2+}$-activated ATPase in toad bladder (Bonting and Canady, 1964; Dalton and Snart, 1969) but its induced protein may influence tricarboxylic acid production (Fimognari *et al.*, 1967). It is clear that the problem of separating the effects of aldosterone on the production of high-energy intermediates from a possible action on the sodium pump remains unresolved.

Dalton and Snart (1969) investigated the relationship between aldosterone and respiration by the toad bladder. The dose-response characteristics indicated that stimulation of both K_A and K_B sites led to respiration changes in the tissue. This meant that respiration changes occurred at doses of aldosterone that were unable to stimulate sodium transport to a comparable extent. The stimulation associated with lower doses of the hormone was identified with increased succinate dehydrogenase activity of the mitochondrial fractions. This agrees with the increase in several mitochondrial enzyme activities produced by the addition of aldosterone to toad bladder preparations (Kirsten *et al.*, 1968). From this kind of evidence, Dalton and Snart (1969) suggested that the mechanism of action of aldosterone involves the induction of two proteins, both affecting permeability to sodium, one acting on the mucosal surface of the epithelial cells of the toad bladder, the other acting on the surface of the mitochondrial membranes. Further work is required to examine the validity of this suggestion.

III. Actions of Sex Steroids

It is impracticable to consider comprehensively the vast number of articles which have been devoted to the actions of sex steroids in the submammalian vertebrates. Nor perhaps is it necessary since a number of authoritative reviews are available which summarize most of the relevant studies (e.g., Bretschneider and Duyvène de Wit, 1947; Adams, 1950; Gallien, 1954a, 1962; Dodd, 1955, 1960a, b; Fraps, 1955; Pickford and Atz, 1957; Ball, 1960; Turner, 1960; Parkes and Marshall, 1960; Forbes, 1961; Burns, 1961; Chester Jones and Ball, 1962; Hoar, 1962, 1965; Atz, 1964; Foote, 1964; Baggerman, 1966, 1968; Barr, 1968; Lofts, 1968). These extensive surveys emphasize one of the central problems in the field, namely that much of the literature is confusing and sometimes contradictory. It is extremely difficult to make a definitive and consistent statement about the biological action of a particular steroid. The inconsistencies would seem to arise from a combination of factors. First, there is a clear species specificity toward any one drug (Witschi and Crown, 1937; Puckett, 1939, 1940; Egami, 1960a; Dodd *et al.*, 1960; Amanuma, 1963a; Egami and Arai, 1964). In addition, the state of sexual maturity of the experimental animal, the precise protocol followed, as well as various environmental characteristics (e.g., temperature, salinity, lighting, season of the year) almost certainly influence the end point of the experiment (Adams, 1946; Penhos, 1953 Egami, 1954a, 1955a; Asayama and Miyamori, 1957; Dodd, 1960b; Urist and Schjeide, 1961; Egami and Nambu, 1961; Hanaoka, 1963; Kambara, 1964; Fleming *et al.*, 1964; Fontaine *et al.*, 1964; Segura and D'Agostino, 1965; Egami *et al.*, 1965; Yamamoto *et al.*, 1966; Oguri and Takada, 1967). The routes of drug administration have been another variable parameter. Often the preparations have been dissolved in the experimental water, making it difficult to compare dosages in such experiments with those employing parenteral routes. There have been a number of studies demonstrating the minimal external concentration required for a particular effect, although again how these compare with ip or im doses is unknown (Duyvène de Wit, 1940; Turner, 1942a; Cummings, 1943; Mintz *et al.*, 1945; Grobstein, 1948; Sangster, 1948; Ashby, 1959; Yamamoto, 1959a; Fachini, 1964; Hishida, 1965; Mintz and Witschi, 1966). The lack of effect of some steroids dissolved in the water could well be due to lack of penetration into the animal.

Finally, and perhaps most importantly, the problems of interpretation are compounded by a general lack of knowledge not only of the exact chemical nature of the steroids secreted by the gonads of lower vertebrates but also of the normal circulating levels of these hormones and of their half-lives in the vascular system. While certain of the more "classical" steroidal hormones occur at all levels, such as testosterone and estradiol-17β, it is also clear that nonmammalian vertebrates possess hormonal steroids which have yet to be described in mammals (e.g. Idler *et al.*, 1961a,b). The recent intro-duction of gas–liquid chromatography and "protein binding" methods to measure circulating levels of hormone promises much in this regard but already the results show much specific variation. For example, Idler and Truscott (1966) reported a mean circulating level of androgens in the skate *Raja radiata* of 74 ng/ml whereas in the quail the level rarely exceeds 1 ng/ml in sexually mature males. Such levels suggest that much of the pub-lished work has been carried out with excessive quantities of administered steroid and may ultimately explain many of the apparent discrepancies among results.

It is tempting to seek a common pattern of action for the sex steroids throughout the vertebrates and much of the research in the past has tended to concentrate on target organs and effects which are known to be influenced by gonadal steroids in mammals. This approach has been reasonably suc-cessful, particularly in the male where the reproductive processes have undergone relatively minor changes and the testes of all vertebrates have as their primary function the production of large quantities of spermatozoa. However, reproduction in the female has evolved much more extensively as a result of tendencies to produce fewer mature oocytes and to provide a better food supply and protection for the embryo. It is to be expected *a priori* that additional and different target organs for the female sex steroids have evolved in association with the refinements of both oviparity and viviparity. This is well illustrated by the fact that a primary target organ in oviparous female vertebrates is the liver where estrogens induce the synthesis of the future yolk proteins. The female gonoduct appears to be a target organ for estrogens and progestogens in most vertebrates and yet the role of these hormones in oviparous forms where they cause the production of the pro-tective coats surrounding the fully formed oocyte is very different from their roles in the mammalian uterus. In these instances, however, the ultimate effect of the sex steroid appears to be as an anabolic hormone increasing the level of RNA formation and hence of new protein material.

It should be emphasized that the terms "estrogenic," "androgenic," and "progestational" are related to the activities of the steroidal hormones in standard mammalian bioassays and do not necessarily refer to their activi-ties in the particular experimental animal. For example, ethynyltestosterone (pregneninolone) has characteristic progestational activity in mammals, while in lower vertebrates it has activities more akin to those of androgenic steroids (Regnier, 1941; Eversole, 1941; Hopper, 1949; Thiebold, 1955; Mohsen, 1958). In the sections which follow, most of the major actions of the sex steroids are considered with the exception of their roles in sexual dif-ferentiation of the gonads and gonoducts. This topic is thoroughly covered in reviews by Dodd (1960a,b), Burns (1961), and Atz (1964). Some of the experimental results in this field are summarized in Tables V–IX for fish and amphibians and Table X for reptiles.

A. The Gonads (Tables V–VIII)

The conclusion that androgens have a direct and beneficial effect on spermatogenesis has been arrived at only after many reversals of opinion. The problem may be illustrated by three experiments which have been carried out on a number of occasions in the rat. A low dose of testosterone causes testicular atrophy in the intact animal while a large dose maintains spermatogenesis (Albert, 1961). Testosterone in large amounts maintains spermatogenesis in hypophysectomized rats (Albert, 1961) and restores gametogenesis in testes which have been allowed to regress fully following hypophysectomy (Boccabella, 1963). It is now clear that these anomalous effects arise from whether just enough steroid is administered to suppress pituitary gonadotropin secretion, in which case the testes atrophy, or whether the dose is so large that the lack of gonadotropins is masked by a stimulatory action of testosterone on the germinal epithelium. In lower vertebrates the problems are the same and in only a few instances are unequivocal data available. The topic has been well reviewed by Dodd and Wiebe (1968) and by Lofts (1968).

Among the fishes only two species, a killifish *Fundulus heteroclitus* and a catfish *Heteropneustes fossilis*, have been studied adequately. In both, androgens stimulate the regressed testes of hypophysectomized animals and within a few weeks of treatment there are increases in testicular size and degree of spermatogenesis (Burger, 1942; Pickford and Atz, 1957; Lofts, *et al.*, 1966; Sundararaj and Nayyar, 1967). Maturation can be completed with androgens and after 8 weeks of treatment with methyltestosterone spermatozoa may be seen in the efferent testicular ducts of the hypophysectomized killifish (Lofts *et al.*, 1966). Some evidence suggests that the effect of androgens may be exerted in postspermatogonial development (see Dodd, 1960a; Dodd and Wiebe, 1968). Whether the effects seen after exogenous hormone treatment reflect a role for endogenous androgens during the breeding cycle remains unknown.

Experiments with amphibians have been more confusing. A stimulation of spermatogenetic activity with androgens has been reported in *Bufo fowleri* (Blair, 1946), *B. arenarum* (Penhos, 1953, 1956), and *Triturus pyrrhogaster* (Iwasawa, 1957) while inhibitory effects seemed to dominate in experiments with *Leptodactylus chaquensis* (Cei *et al.*, 1955), *Rana temporaria* (van Oordt and Basu, 1960), *R. esculenta* (van Oordt and Schouten, 1961), *R. tigrina* (Basu, 1962a), *B. melanostictus* (Basu, 1962b), and *Triturus cristatus cristatus* (Walton, 1963). Most of these inhibitory responses probably result from suppression of gonadotropin secretion since exogenous mammalian gonadotropins can often prevent the testicular atrophy induced by androgens (Cei and Acosta, 1953; Cei *et al.*, 1955; Walton, 1963). However, Basu and

TABLE V

Effects of Androgens on the Male Reproductive System of Fish and Amphibia

Species	Hormone	Effect	Reference
CYCLOSTOMATA			
Lampetra fluviatilis	Testosterone	Slight stimulation of spermatogenesis	Knowles (1939)
	Testosterone	No deleterious effects on spermatogenesis	Evennett (1963)
Lampetra planeri	Testosterone propionate[a]	No effect on testis	Hardisty and Taylor (1965)
ELASMOBRANCHII			
Scyliorhinus caniculus	Testosterone propionate (into yolk sac)	Feminization of testis; inhibition of gonadal medulla of genetic males	Chieffi (1959)
	Testosterone propionate, ethynyltestosterone (into yolk sac)	Feminization of testis in genetic males; tendency toward intersexuality	Thiebold (1952, 1955)
TELEOSTEI			
Anguilla anguilla L.	Testosterone propionate	Slight regression of testis	D'Ancona (1957)
Fundulus heteroclitus	Testosterone propionate	In hypophysectomized fish, slight testicular stimulation, little effect in intact fish	Burger (1942)
Heteropneustes fossilis	Methyltestosterone	In hypophysectomized fish, increased spermatogenesis	Lofts et al. (1966)
	Testosterone propionate	Stimulated seminal vesicle and testis, restored spermatogenesis in hypophysectomized fish	Sundararaj and Goswami (1965a,b) Sundararaj and Nayyar (1967)
Hippocampus hippocampus	Ethynyltestosterone[a]	Disturbed incubation of young in male fish	Boisseau (1965)
Lebistes reticulatus	Testosterone propionate, Ethynyltestosterone[a]	Stimulated testis, causing eventual exhaustion and degeneration	Eversole (1941)
	Ethynyltestosterone[a]	Stimulated testis; precocious maturation	Regnier (1942)
	Testosterone propionate	Stimulated testis	Svärdson (1943)
Oncorhynchus nerka	11-Ketotestosterone	Increased spermatogenesis	Idler et al. (1961a,b)
Oryzias latipes	Methyltestosterone	Sex reversal in genetic males	Yamamoto (1958)
Phoxinus laevis	Testosterone propionate	Induction of spermatogenesis	Bullough (1942)

TABLE V (cont.)

Species	Hormone	Effect	Reference
Salmo trutta	Testosterone propionate[a]	Inhibition of testis; accelerated development of vas deferens	Ashby (1959)
Tilapia aurea	Methyltestosterone[a] or testosterone[a]	No effect on testis	Eckstein and Spira (1965)
Xiphophorus maculatus	Methyltestosterone	Stimulated testis	Laskowski (1953)
	Ethynyltestosterone[a]	Stimulated testis; precocious maturation	Tavolga (1949)
	Ethynyltestosterone[a]	Stimulated testis	Cohen (1946)
Xiphophorus variatus	Methyltestosterone	Stimulated testis	Laskowski (1953)
AMPHIBIA			
Acris gryllus	Testosterone propionate (implants)	No change in gonadal structure; enlarged seminal vesicle	Greenberg (1942)
Alytes obstetricans	Ethynyltestosterone	No effect on gonadal differentiation	Witschi and Allison (1950)
Ambystoma punctatum	Testosterone propionate	Slight inhibition of testis; hypertrophy of mesonephric duct; vas deferens not affected	Burns (1939)
Ambystoma opacum	Methyltestosterone[a]	Suppression and feminization of testis	Bruner and Witschi (1954)
Bufo americanus	Methyltestosterone	Slight testicular regression	Chang (1955)
	Methyltestosterone[a]	Reduction in size only of testis	Chang (1955)
	Testosterone propionate	No effect on testis	Puckett (1939, 1940)
Bufo arenarum	Testosterone propionate	Increase in testis weight	Penhos (1953)
Bufo fowleri	Testosterone propionate or androsterone	Stimulated spermatogenesis, but damaged tubules resulting in reduction of testis size; hypertrophy of Müllerian duct	Blair (1946)
Bufo melanostictus	Testosterone	Inhibited mitosis at the secondary spermatogonia stage	Basu (1962a,b)
Hynobius nebulosus	Methyltestosterone	Suppression of gonadal medulla	Amanuma (1963a)
Leptodactylus chaquensis	Testosterone propionate	Inhibited mitosis at the second spermatogonia stage; degeneration of primary spermatocytes	Cei *et al.* (1955)

Species	Hormone	Effect	Reference
Pleurodeles waltlii	Testosterone propionate	Inhibition of testis	Cei and Acosta (1953)
	Testosterone propionate[a]	Suppression of mesonephric blastema and gonadal medulla; feminization of testis	Mintz and Gallien (1954), Gallien (1954b)
Rana esculenta	Testosterone (implants)	Inhibited mitosis at secondary spermatogonial stage	van Oordt and Schouten (1961)
Rana japonica	Methyltestosterone	Slight retardation of formation of seminiferous tubules	Amanuma (1963a)
Rana pipiens	Testosterone (implants)	Inhibition of mitosis of late secondary spermatogonia but speed-up of spermiogenesis	Basu (1965)
Rana temporaria	Testosterone (implants)	Inhibition of mitosis of late secondary spermatogonia but no effect on development of spermatocytes and spermatids	van Oordt and Basu (1959, 1960)
Rana tigrina	Testosterone (implant)	Inhibition of mitosis of late secondary spermatogonia but no effect on development of spermatocytes and spermatids	Basu (1962a,b)
Rhacophorus schlegelii	Methyltestosterone[a]	Depression of formation of seminiferous tubules; feminization of gonad	Amanuma (1963b)
Triturus pyrrhogaster	Methyltestosterone[a]	Suppression of mesonephric blastema; sex reversal	Asayama and Matsuzaki (1958)

[a]Hormone dissolved in environmental water or in diet; otherwise hormones implanted in pellet form or injected.

TABLE VI

Effect of Androgens on the Female Reproductive System of Fish and Amphibia

Species	Hormone	Effect	Reference
CYCLOSTOMES			
Lampetra planeri	Testosterone propionate[a]	No effect on ovary	Hardisty and Taylor (1965)
TELEOSTEI			
Chaenogobius annularis	Testosterone[a]	Stimulated unpaired fins in both ♂ and ♀	Egami (1960b)
Gambusia affinis	Testosterone	Sex reversal	Okada and Yamashita (1944)
Halichoerus poecilopterus	Testosterone propionate	Sex reversal	Hamon (1945a,b)
	Testosterone propionate	Sex reversal	Okada (1964)
Lebistes reticulatus	Testosterone propionate, Ethynyltestosterone[a]	Inhibited ovary; partial sex reversal	Eversole (1939, 1941)
	Ethynyltestosterone	Partial sex reversal	Mohsen (1958)
Oryzias latipes	Methyltestosterone[a]	Stimulated ♂ characters in females; inhibited by X irradiation	Egami et al. (1956)
Phoxinus laevis	Testosterone propionate	Degeneration of ovary; thickening of oviduct	Bullough (1940)
Salmo trutta	Testosterone[a]	Inhibition of ovarian germinal epithelium; hypertrophy of oviducal epithelium	Ashby (1965)
Xiphophorus helleri	Testosterone propionate	Sex reversal; spermatogenesis	Regnier (1937)
	Testosterone propionate[a]	Resorption of large eggs and abortion in pregnant female fish	Witschi and Crown (1937)
	Testosterone propionate	Sex reversal; induction of spermatogenesis	Baldwin and Goldin (1939)
	Testosterone	Induced spermatogenesis in young female; no effect on mature female	Vallowe (1957)
Xiphophorus maculatus	Ethynyltestosterone	Degeneration of ovary; inhibited yolk formation	Cohen (1946)
	Ethynyltestosterone[a]	Degeneration of ovary; ♂ gonopodia developed	Tavolga (1949)
Various species	Testosterone (+ PMS[b])	Sterile hybrids rendered fertile	Oztan (1960)

AMPHIBIA

Acris gryllus	Testosterone propionate (implants)	Enlargement of oviduct; no effect on gonad	Greenberg (1942)
Alytes obstetricans	Ethynyltestosterone	No effect on gonad	Witschi and Allison (1950)
Ambystoma sp.	Testosterone propionate (into ova)	Inhibition of ovary; intersex	Burns (1939)
Hyla arborea japonica	Methyltestosterone[a]	Cortical regression; diminution of number of germ cells	Takahashi (1958)
Hyla nebulosus	Methyltestosterone[a]	Inhibited oogenesis and gonadal medulla	Amanuma (1963a)
Rana catesbeiana and *Xenopus laevis*	Testosterone injected or in culture	Sex reversal in *R. catesbeiana in vitro* and *in vivo*; no effect in *Xenopus*	Foote and Foote (1959)
Rana climitans	Testosterone propionate[a]	Complete sex reversal due to cortical atrophy	Mintz *et al.* (1945)
Rana japonica	Methyltestosterone[a]	Sex reversal	Kawamura and Yokota (1959)
		Complete sex reversal	Amanuma (1963a)
Rana pipiens	Testosterone propionate[a]	Complete sex reversal	Witschi and Crown (1937), Foote (1938)
Rana sylvatica	Testosterone propionate[a]	Complex sex reversal	Mintz and Witschi (1966)
	Ethynyltestosterone	Complete sex reversal	Witschi and Allison (1950)
Rhacophorus schlegelii arborea	Methyltestosterone[a]	Inhibited ovarian differentiation and oogenesis; complete masculinization not observed	Amanuma (1963a,b)
Triturus pyrrhogaster	Testosterone	Partial sex reversal	Iwasawa (1958)
	Testosterone	Increase in alkaline phosphatase in oviduct epithelium	Kambara (1964)
	Testosterone propionate (intraovary ± testicular extract)	Increased number of germ cells but not differentiation of columnar epithelium of germinal patch; with testicular extract, columnar epithelium differentiated into seminiferous tubules	Hanaoka (1965)
Triturus viridescens	Testosterone propionate	Stimulation of ovary	Adams *et al.* (1964)
Xenopus laevis	Ethynyltestosterone	No effect on ovary	Witschi and Allison (1950), Chang and Witschi (1955, 1956)

[a]Hormone dissolved in environmental water or in diet; otherwise hormones implanted in pellet form or injected.
[b]Pregnant mare serum.

443

TABLE VII

Effect of Estrogenic Agents on the Male Reproductive System of Fish and Amphibia

Species	Hormone	Effect	Reference
ELASMOBRANCHII			
Scyliorhinus caniculus	Estradiol	Feminization of ♂ embryos	Thiebold (1954)
TELEOSTEI			
Anguilla anguilla	Estradiol dipropionate	Partial sex reversal	D'Ancona (1957)
Gambusia holbrooki	Estradiol benzoate	Feminization of males of all ages	Hamon (1945c, 1946)
Gambusia sp.	Estradiol benzoate	Sex reversal	Chambolle (1965)
Halichoerus poecilopterus	Estradiol benzoate	Reduction of testis	Okada (1964)
Heteropneustes fossilis	Estradiol benzoate	No effect on spermatogenesis or seminal vesicle	Sundararaj and Goswami (1966a)
Lebistes reticulatus	Estradiol benzoate	Inhibition of spermatogenesis but no oocytes	Regnier (1938)
		Incomplete sex reversal; ovotestis	Berkowits (1941)
Misgurnus anguillicaudatus	Ethynylestradiol[a]	Sex reversal	Miyamori (1962, 1964)
		Sex reversal	Kobayaski (1951), Egami (1954d)
Oryzias latipes	Estrone[a]	Sex reversal	Okada and Yamashita (1944)
	Estrone[a]	Sex reversal	Yamamoto (1953, 1955, 1959a,b 1969)
	Stilbestrol[a]	Sex reversal	Yamamoto and Matsuda (1963)
	Estrone (into egg), Stilbestrol (into egg)	Sex reversal in genetic males	Hishida (1964)
Phoxinus laevis	"Estrin"	Partial sex reversal	Egami (1955b)
		Degeneration of testis; on stopping injection testis recovered	Bullough (1940)
Salmo trutta	Estradiol[a]	Inhibition of germinal tissue; accelerated vas deferens development	Ashby (1957, 1959, 1965)

444

Species	Hormone	Effect	Reference
Tilapia aurea	Stilbestrol	Reduction of testis	Eckstein and Spira (1965)
Xiphophorus helleri	"Estrogen"	Decreased spermatogenesis	Baldwin and Li (1945)
	Estradiol benzoate	Partial sex reversal: ovotestis; suppression of germ cells and atrophy of testis	
	Estrogen	Inhibition of spermatogenesis, but no oocytes	Regnier (1938)
	Estradiol benzoate	Induced oogenesis in young male, no effect on testis of mature male	Vallowe (1957)
Xiphophorus maculatus	Estradiol benzoate	Inhibition of spermatogenesis; ovotestis in young males	Cohen (1946)
	Estradiol benzoate[a]	Inhibited testis	Tavolga (1949)
	Estradiol[a]	Stimulated testis in large (over 19 mm) males	Taylor (1948)
Xiphophorus–Platypoecelius hybrids	Estradiol	Inhibited testis without altering external characteristics	
AMPHIBIA			
Alytes obstetricans	Estradiol	Feminized testis	Witschi and Allison (1950)
Bufo americanus	Estradiol[a]	Feminized testis	Chang (1955)
Hyla arborea japonica	Estradiol[a]	Partial feminization of testis	Takahashi (1959)
Hynobius nebulosus	Estradiol[a]	No effect on testis	Asayama and Miyamori (1957)
Pleurodeles waltlii	Estradiol benzoate[a]	Sex reversal	Gallien (1954b)
	Estradiol benzoate[a]	Inhibited Δ^5-3β-hydroxysteroid dehydrogenase in testis	Collenot (1964)
Rana clamitans	Estradiol dipropionate	Distention of proximal part of rete apparatus; no effect on gonad	Mintz et al. (1945)
Rana esculenta	Estradiol	Stimulated 3β-hydroxysteroid dehydrogenase in testis	Botte and Delrio (1967)
	Estrone[a]	Partial sex reversal	Foote (1938)
Rana pipiens	Estradiol benzoate	No effect on testis of newly metamorphosed frog	Schreiber and Rugh (1945)
Triturus pyrrhogaster	Estradiol benzoate[a]	Sex reversal	Hanaoka (1963)
Triturus viridescens	Stilbestrol	Atrophy of testis; hypertrophy of Müllerian duct; also affected certain male characteristics of kidney	Adams (1945)
Xenopus laevis	Estradiol[a]	Feminized testis, complete sex reversal in genetic males	Witschi and Allison (1950), Chang and Witschi (1955, 1956)
	Estradiol benzoate	Complete sex reversal	Gallien (1955)

[a]Hormone dissolved in environmental water or in diet; otherwise hormones implanted in pellet form or injected.

TABLE VIII

Effect of Estrogenic Agents on the Female Reproductive System of Fish and Amphibia

Species	Hormone	Effect	Reference
CYCLOSTOMES			
Lampetra planeri	Estradiol benzoate [a]	Degeneration of growing oocytes	Hardisty and Taylor (1965)
ELASMOBRANCHII			
Scyliorhinus caniculus	Estradiol benzoate (into vitelline sac)	Intersexuality; stimulation of Wolffian duct	Thiebold (1953a,b)
	Estradiol benzoate (implants)	No effect on immature ; mature oviducts and cloaca stimulated	Dodd and Goddard (1961)
TELEOSTEI			
Anguilla anguilla	Estradiol, hexestrol + HCG[b]	Stimulated ovarian growth	Boetius *et al.* (1962)
Ctenopharyngodon idellus	Estradiol benzoate	Stimulated ovarian development	Kawamoto (1950)
Halichoerus poecilopterus	Estradiol benzoate	Inhibition of ovary	Okada (1964)
Heptatus heptatus	Estradiol	Small dose feminized gonad; large dose masculinized gonad	Padoa (1939)
Lebistes reticulatus	Estradiol benzoate [a]	Inhibition of yolk deposition	Berkowitz (1941)
	Ethynylestradiol[a]	Accelerated ovarian development	Miyamori (1962)
	Estradiol benzoate	Maintained oviducal epithelium in ovariectomized animals	Chambolle (1965)
Misgurnus anguillicaudatus	Estrone benzoate	Inhibition of ovarian growth	Kobayashi (1951), Egami (1954c)
Oncorhynchus nerka	Estradiol	Increased ovarian mass	Idler *et al.* (1961a)
Oryzias latipes	Estradiol	Stimulated ovarian growth and oviposition	Egami (1954e, 1955c)
	Estrone [a]	Inhibited yolk deposition	Okada and Yamashita (1944)
	Estrone (± dessicated frog pituitaries)	Estrone + frog pituitary reduced oocyte production, while pituitary after estrone stimulated oocyte production	Egami (1954b)

446

Phoxinus laevis	Estrone	Stimulated mitosis and formation of small oogonia; inhibited development of primary oocytes	Bullough (1942)
Salmo trutta	Estradiol benzoate [a]	Inhibited ovarian development; hypertrophy of oviducal epithelium and cilia	Ashby (1965)
Salmo uridens	Estrone	No effect on ovary	Padoa (1939)
Tilapia aurea	Stilbestrol	Inhibition of ovary	Eckstein and Spira (1965)
Xiphophorus maculatus	Estradiol benzoate [a] or estradiol	Inhibited yolk deposition and caused ovarian degeneration	Tavolga (1949)
AMPHIBIA			
Bufo arenarum	Estradiol benzoate	Maintained oviduct after castration	Galli-Mainini (1950)
Bufo bufo gregarizans	Estradiol benzoate	No effect on oviduct secretion	Wang (1963)
Bufo fowleri	Estradiol benzoate	Hypertrophy of Mullerian duct	Blair (1946)
Rana clamitans	Estradiol dipropionate	Some oocyte degeneration	Mintz *et al.* (1945)
Rana esculenta	Estradiol	Increased alkaline phosphatase but decreased acid phosphatase and acid proteinase of oviduct	Chieffi *et al.* (1966)
			Botte and Delrio (1967)
Rana pipiens	Estradiol	Stimulated Mullerian duct weight	Basu *et al.* (1967)
	Estradiol benzoate	Stimulated gonoduct but slightly inhibited ovarian growth	Schreiber and Rugh (1945)
Triturus pyrrhogaster	Pregneninolone [a]	Stimulated oviduct and Wolffian ducts	Eversole and D'Angelo (1943)
	Estriol, estrone, or diethylstilbestrol	Stimulated oviduct epithelium alkaline phosphatase but inhibited the enzyme-activating effect of progesterone in ovariectomized animals	Kambara (1964)
Triturus viridescens	Diethylstilbestrol	Stimulated ovarian growth (atretic follicles), then decreased; oviduct increased in weight	Adams (1950)

[a] Hormone dissolved in environmental water or in diet; otherwise hormones implanted in pellet form or injected.
[b] Human chorionic gonadotropin.

Nandi (1965) feel that androgens may also have a direct suppressive action on the amphibian testis since gonadotropins could not counteract the collapse of the germinal epithelium caused by testosterone in *Rana pipiens*. Further, it appeared that spermatogenetic inhibition was even greater in hypophysectomized frogs treated with testosterone; in all cases the formation of new secondary spermatogonia was impaired. Little is known of the effects of androgens on the reptilian testis although Eyeson (cited in Dodd and Wiebe, 1968) found that testosterone treatment of the hypophysectomized lizard *Agama agama* had no effect on spermatogenesis. On the other hand, testosterone appears to stimulate the testis in intact *Sceloporus* (Forbes, 1941) and in intact immature *Crocodylus palustris* and *Varanus monitor* (Ramaswami and Jacob, 1963, 1964). These authors also reported an inhibitory effect of testosterone propionate (5 mg/day) on mature but sexually quiescent *Uromastix hardwickii* (see also Table X).

The effects obtained with androgens in birds seem to depend on both the dose and when the steroid was administered during the gonadal cycle. Thus, androgens maintain starlings, sparrows (Pfeiffer, 1947), and weaver-finches, *Quelea quelea* (Lofts, 1962), in breeding condition and prevent the seasonal testicular regression which occurs when the birds become refractory. In fully mature male *Coturnix*, injections of testosterone propionate of 10 and 100 μg/day do not induce testicular regression while a dose of 1 mg/day results in testicular atrophy. However, a dose of testosterone of 100 μg/day given at the start of the testicular growth cycle inhibits further development. Lofts (1962) reported similar results in *Quelea*. If the injections of androgen are delayed until the seminiferous tubules are producing primary spermatocytes the same dose of androgen will actually enhance testicular development (Lofts, 1962). The conclusions that might be drawn from these types of experiment are that if androgens do play a role in avian spermatogenesis it is one which occurs in the later stages of development. There is no doubt that androgens can stimulate testicular growth since they promote gametogenesis in the testes of hypophysectomized pigeons (Chu, 1940; Chu and You, 1946) and in intact weaver finches and house sparrows (Lofts, 1968) when in the middle of their refractory period.

Although it is possible to speculate on the possible sites where estrogens could modify oogenesis directly there is little evidence to support such a role. In most cases the administration of estrogens results in ovarian collapse, presumably because they block gonadotropin secretion (Barr, 1968).

B. Secondary Sexual Characters (Tables IX and X)

It is well established that the sex steroids play a primary role in eliciting the growth and development of the secondary sexual characters. Many target organs have evolved, and androgens induce changes as diverse as the degree of nuptial coloration in fishes and amphibians, comb growth and feather pigmentation in birds, external genital structures such as the gonopodia of certain fishes, and the gonoducts themselves. Secondary sexual characters are often less well developed in females but estrogens have an essential function in stimulating the growth of the oviduct. The reader is referred to the many reviews of this topic for more detail (Pickford and Atz, 1957; Dodd, 1960a; Parkes and Marshall, 1960; Forbes, 1961; van Tienhoven, 1961; Barr, 1968) (See also Tables V–X). One of the few target organs which have been studied at more than a superficial level is the avian oviduct. Estrogen treatment leads to a large increase in size and weight which is accompanied by gross changes in the levels of DNA, RNA, and protein (Noble and Wurm, 1940; Adams and Herrick, 1955; Brant and Nalbandov, 1956; Breneman, 1956; Steele and Hinde, 1963; Vyas and Ramaswami, 1967). At a cytological level the first event to occur following estrogen administration is an edema of the stromal tissues lying beneath the mucosal epithelium and an increase in the size of the stromal capillaries. After 24 hrs the number of mitoses in the epithelial cells is seen to increase and this is followed sequentially by enlargement of the nucleus and nucleolus and a progressive development of an elaborate rough endoplasmic reticulum in the newly formed tubular gland cells (Kohler *et al.*, 1969). Biochemically these changes are paralleled by an increase in the activity of DNA dependent RNA polymerase (McGuire and O'Malley, 1968) and, between 2 and 5 days, by the emergence of new species of nuclear RNA (O'Malley *et al.*, 1967a; O'Malley and McGuire, 1968a; Hahn *et al.*, 1968). Ovalbumin synthesis increases over the same period (O'Malley *et al.*, 1967b and by immunofluorescent studies can be seen to occur only within the tubular gland cells (Kohler *et al.*, 1968). In many respects the underlying changes in nucleic acid and protein metabolism are similar to those which take place in the mammalian uterus following estrogen stimulation (Hamilton, 1968). Also like the uterus the chicken oviduct is able to take up selectively estrogens both *in vivo* and *in vitro* (Jonsson and Terenius, 1965; Terenius, 1969). This suggests that an underlying action of estrogens throughout the vertebrates is to act anabolically on the oviduct to stimulate protein synthesis and secretion, the many changes in the nature of the oviducal secretions perhaps reflecting the stimulation of different parts of the genome. A comparative study of this problem should prove both fascinating and illuminating.

TABLE IX

Effect of Androgens and Estrogens on Secondary Sexual Characters and Reproductive Behavior in Male and Female Fish and Amphibia

Species	Hormone	Effect	Reference
CYCLOSTOMES			
Lampetra fluviatilis	Testosterone	Cloacal swelling	Knowles (1939)
ELASMOBRANCHII			
Raja radiata	Testosterone propionate	Stimulation of claspers in immature ♂; slight stimulation in body growth	Dodd (1955)
Scyliorhinus caniculus	Testosterone propionate	Hyperplasia of mesonephric tubules in anterior kidney (male character) in both ♂ and ♀ embryos	Thiebold (1963)
TELEOSTEI			
Acheilognathus intermedium	Extract of testis[a]	Precocious nuptial coloration in ♂	Owen (1937)
Acheilognathus lanceolata	Methyltestosterone,[a] testosterone,[a] methyl-androstenediol,[a]	Development of pearl organs(?), ovipositor (male organ) in male and female	Arai (1964)
Anguilla anguilla	Estradiol or hexestrol + HCG[b]	Ovarian growth associated with secondary sexual changes in skin, jaws, and eyes	Boetius et al. (1962)
	Testosterone propionate[a]	Stimulation of seminal vesicle secretions in hypophysectomized ♂	Slicher (1961)
Fundulus heteroclitus	Testosterone propionate	Induced nuptial color in intact and hypophysectomized fish	Burger (1942)
	Methyltestosterone	Induced nuptial coloration in hypophysectomized fish	Lofts et al. (1966)
Gambusia affinis	Ethynyltestosterone,[a] methyltestosterone[a]	Induced ♂ type of gonopodium in young ♀ and in castrated young	Turner (1960)
	Methyltestosterone,[a] ethynyltestosterone[a]	Induced anal gonopod in female	Turner (1941, 1942a,b,c,)
Gambusia holbrooki	Testosterone propionate	Precocious development of secondary sexual character	Hamon (1954a)
Gambusia sp.	Estrone[a]	Stimulated and maintained gravid spot of female	Ishii (1963)

450

Species	Hormone	Effect	Reference
Gasterosteus aculeatus	Methyltestosterone[a] (or intraperitoneally)	In both intact and castrated males and females; full male coloration, prespawning aggressive, and territorial behavior; in males, also nest-building behavior	Hoar (1962) Wai and Hoar (1963)
	Methyltestosterone[a]	Induced nuptial color in half the castrated fish; induced "sand-digging" behavior in castrate	Smith and Hoar (1967)
Halichoerus poecilopterus	Testosterone propionate	No change in skin color in females despite androgen-induced sex reversal (change in skin color occurred in natural sex reversal)	Okada (1964)
Heteropneustes fossilis	Testosterone propionate	Stimulated seminal vesicle in intact and hypophysectomized male fish	Sundararaj and Goswami (1965a,b, 1966a,b); Sundararaj and Nayyar (1966, 1967)
	Estradiol benzoate	No effect on seminal vesicle secretion or spermatogenesis in males	Sundararaj and Nayyar (1966)
Hippocampus hippocampus	Estradiol benzoate	Disturbed incubation of young in males	Boisseau (1965)
	Testosterone propionate[a]	Disturbed incubation of young in males	Boisseau (1965)
Lebistes reticulatus	Testosterone propionate	Induced gonopodia in female fish	Eversole (1939), Mohsen (1958)
	Ethynyltestosterone[a] Testosterone propionate[a]	Stimulated color and gonopod in male fish	Regnier (1941), Hopper (1951)
	Methyltestosterone[a]		
	Methyltestosterone[a]	In female induced male secondary sexual character	Hindemann (1954)
	Estradiol benzoate[a]	Elongation of anal fin	Cohen (1962)
	Methyltestosterone	Mosaic male and female secondary characters	Berkowitz (1941)
Misgurnus anguillicaudatus		Induced secondary sexual characters in castrates	Kobayashi (1951)
Molliensia latipinna	Testosterone propionate	Induction of incomplete gonopod in female	Cummings (1943)
Oncorhynchus nerka	11-Ketotestosterone	Increased skin thickness; decreased flesh color (male characters) in both males and females	Idler et al. (1961a)
Oryzias latipes	Methyldihydrotestosterone, testosterone propionate[a]	Stimulated male secondary characteristics in female fish	Egami (1954a, 1955a)

451

TABLE IX (cont.)

Species	Hormone	Effect	Reference
	Testosterone or testosterone propionate[a]	Increase in leucophores in castrated males or intact females	Arai and Egami (1961)
	Methyltestosterone,[a] methyltestosterone,[a] methylandrostenediol[a]	Induced papillary processes in anal fin rays	Arai (1964)
	Methyltestosterone	Stimulated male nuptial coloration in castrate	Niwa (1965a)
	Methyltestosterone	Stimulated papillary process in anal fin rays and leucophores	Egami et al. (1965)
	Estradiol,[a] methyltestosterone[a]	Methyltestosterone induced nuptial coloration in spayed ♀; inhibited by estradiol	Niwa (1965a)
	Methyltestosterone[a]	Induction of nuptial coloration in castrated ♂, ♀, and intact ♀	Niwa (1965b)
	Estradiol	Inhibited methyltestosterone-induced nuptial coloration	Niwa (1965b)
Phoxinus laevis	Testosterone propionate	Induction of male nuptial coloration in female	Bullough (1940)
	"Estrin"	Produced female light coloration in males	Bullough (1940)
Rhodeus amarus	Testosterone[a]	Ovipositor reaction	Duyvène de Wit (1940)
Xiphophorus helleri	Testosterone propionate	Enhanced body color, gonopod, and sword	Baldwin and Goldin (1939)
	Testosterone propionate[a]	Stimulated male color; gonopod and sword in male and female	Witschi and Crown (1937)
	Testosterone	Stimulation of ♂ coloration and tail sword	Regnier (1937)
	Testosterone[a]	Ovipositor reaction	Duyvène de Wit (1940)
Xiphophorus maculatus	Estradiol benzoate	Prevented gonopod development in males; lost aggressiveness and pursued by normal males	Cohen (1946)
	Estradiol benzoate[a]	No effect on female secondary characters	
	Estradiol[a]	Stimulated partial to complete gonopod development in male and female	Tavolga (1949)

Species	Hormone	Effect	Reference
	Testosterone propionate	Development of ♂ characters in ♀	Rubin and Gordon (1953)
	Ethynyltestosterone	Induced gonopod in male and female, tiny sword in female, and male courtship behavior in female	Cohen (1946)
Xiphophorus sp.	Ethynyltestosterone [a]	Stimulated gonopod in male and female	Tavolga (1949)
	Methyltestosterone	Induction of gonopod and tail sword	Dzwillo (1963)
AMPHIBIA			
Acris gryllus	Testosterone propionate (implants)	Induced nuptial color in both sexes; stimulated vocal sac in male	Greenberg (1942)
Ambystoma punctatum	Testosterone propionate	Hypertrophy of mesonephric duct; modified "collecting duct" of sexual kidney	Burns (1939)
Bufo arenarum	Estradiol benzoate	Decreased Bidder's organ and potentiated testosterone propionate effect on digital callosity and thumb pad	Penhos (1957)
	Testosterone propionate	Development of digital callosity	Penhos (1953)
Bufo fowleri	Testosterone propionate	Precocious development of thumb pad, dark throat, chirp, and vibration in both male and female	Blair (1946)
Pleurodeles waltlii	Testosterone propionate [a]	Slight stimulation of male secondary sexual characters despite testicular feminization	Mintz and Gallien (1954)
Rana pipiens	Testosterone	Stimulated Müllerian duct weight	Basu et al. (1967)
Triturus viridescens	Testosterone propionate	Stimulated oviductal growth	Adams et al. (1941)
Xenopus laevis	Ethynyltestosterone	Induced precocious development of male secondary sexual characters in male and female	Witschi and Allison (1950)

[a] Hormone dissolved in environmental water or in diet; otherwise hormones implanted in pellet form or injected.
[b] Human chorionic gonadotropin.

TABLE X

Effect of Sex Steroids on the Reproductive System of Reptiles

Species	Hormone	Effect	Reference
Agama agama	Estradiol hexahydro-benzoate (1.25–4.25 mg)	Inhibits spermatogenesis; direct inhibition of interstitial cells of testes	Charnier (1965)
Alligator sp.			
Immature ♀	Testosterone propionate (10 mg/11 weeks)	Oviducts increased in length and diameter; clitorides enlarged	Forbes (1938a)
Immature ♂	Testosterone propionate (10 mg/11 weeks)	Penes hypertrophy; gonadal changes minimal	Forbes (1938a)
Immature ♀	Estrone (46,000 IU/80 days)	Hypertrophy of oviducts	Forbes (1938b)
Immature ♂	Estrone (46,000 IU/80 days)	Development of prominent Mullerian ducts; clitoris and penis unaffected	Forbes (1938b)
Anguis fragilis ♀	Testosterone propionate	Stimulates urinogenital connections and mesonephric duct; little effect in male	Pieau and Raynaud (1966)
Anolis carolinensis ♀	Testosterone propionate	Hypertrophy of ovaries (but no change in ovulation sequence); hypertrophy of oviduct	Noble and Greenberg (1941b)
	Spaying	Also causes hypertrophy of oviduct	Noble and Greenberg (1941b)
Immature and mature ♀	Testosterone propionate (pellet)	Hypertrophy of oviduct, enlargement of ovary; increases ova production.	Noble and Greenberg (1940)
Castrated male	Testosterone propionate (pellet)	Maintains epididymis and ductus deferens	Noble and Greenberg (1940)
Calotes versicolor	Castration	Lack of activity in sexual segment of kidney; reduction of hemipenes	Thapliyal and Singh (1959)
Crocodylus palustris (immature)	Testosterone propionate (5.0 mg/day for 5 days)	Increase in size of testes and induction	Ramaswami and Jacob (1964)
Emys leprosa ♀	Folliculin	Promotes development of oviduct	Kehl (1930)

454

Species	Hormone	Effect	Reference
Hemidactylus flaviviridis	Testosterone propionate	Stimulation of sexual segment of kidney	Prasad and Sanyal (1963)
Malacemmys centrata (immature)	Testosterone propionate	Masculinization	Sanyal *et al.* (1966)
	Estradiol benzoate	Increase in oviduct development	Risley (1941)
Sceloporus occidentalis ♂	Theelin, testosterone	Reduced size of epididymes; increased size of Wolffian duct	Gorbman (1939)
	Theelin, testosterone	Increased diameter of oviduct and thickness of oviduct wall	Gorbman (1934)
Uromastix hardwickii (mature but sexually quiescent)	Testosterone propionate	Decrease in size of testes and in diameter of seminiferous tubules	Ramaswami and Jacob (1963)
Uromastix occidentalis ♀ (adult in repose after spring breeding cycle)	Progesterone	Twofold increase in size of oviducal mucosa; thickening of epithelium	Kehl (1940)
	Androsterone benzoate (2 mg)	Stimulates sexual segment of the kidney	Kehl (1938)
Varanus monitor (immature)	Testosterone propionate	Increase in size of testes and stimulation of spermatogenesis	Kehl (1938)

The behavioral patterns during the breeding season are greatly influenced by steroid secretions from the gonad and probably also directly by pituitary hormones. Recent reviews are available which cover this topic in the fishes (Baggerman, 1968) and birds (Lehrman, 1961; Hinde and Steel, 1966). In the latter group much research has been carried out on pigeons and doves and perhaps the most complete analyses are available for these animals (see Lehrman, 1958, 1961; Vowles and Harwood, 1966; Ericksen *et al.*, 1967; Murton *et al.*, 1969; see also Table XI).

C. Hypothalamic–Pituitary Axis

A prime function of sex steroids in mammals is to regulate the output of gonadotropins by acting on the hypothalamic–pituitary axis. In a relatively straightforward situation as in the male mammal, negative-feedback effects predominate and a rising androgen titer reduces gonadotropin secretion. In females negative feedback occurs during much of the ovarian cycle but at one point the sex steroids are thought to have a positive effect and stimulate a surge release of luteinizing hormone (LH), which induces ovulation. Present views consider both the pituitary and hypothalamus to be target sites for feedback effects although the latter appears more important for fine regulation of the system.

To what extent feedback of steroids occurs generally through the vertebrates remains unknown although there is much indirect evidence for its existence. Castration stimulates the output of gonadotropins and is often used by cytologists to identify the gonadotropin-secreting cells of the pituitary (see van Oordt, 1968). It can also result in changes in hypothalamic metabolism indicative of increased secretory activity (Uemura, 1964; Kobayashi and Farner, 1966). Large systemic doses of sex steroids often induce testicular or ovarian regression although, as mentioned previously, the effects of androgens are complicated by a likely duality of action whereby they can both stimulate spermatogenesis directly and inhibit gonadal function indirectly by suppressing gonadotropin secretion. The final result is influenced not merely by the dose of steroid used but also by the reproductive status of the animal at the time of the experiment. Much of the conflicting information in the literature may be explicable if these factors are taken into account. More direct evidence has recently become available for steroid feedback from experiments in which the steroids have been implanted in the basal hypothalamus and median eminence. Lisk (1967) found that implants of testosterone or estradiol in the median eminence inhibited the seasonal maturation of gonads in the desert iguana *Dipsosaurus dorsalis*

TABLE XI

Effect of Sex Hormones on Behavior of Reptiles and Birds

Species	Hormone	Effect	Reference
REPTILES			
Anolis carolinensis			
Female	Testosterone propionate (pellet 5.0 mg)	Appearance of male courtship behavior including attempted copulation	Noble and Greenberg (1941b)
Immature male	Testosterone propionate (pellet 5.0 mg)	Induced both male and female behavior	Noble and Greenberg (1940, 1941a)
Female	Spayed	Affects reaction time to strange female placed in cage	Evans (1937)
Female	Spayed	Increase in fighting behavior, suggesting that ovarian hormones inhibit fighting behavior	Evans (1936)
BIRDS			
Anas platyrhynchos			
Male	Castration	Disappearance of sexual and display activities and warning cries; general passive behavior	Etienne and Fischer (1964)
Female	Castration	More active than male; tends to increase aggressiveness; loss of mating behavior	Etienne and Fischer (1964)
Male	Testosterone propionate	Aggressiveness reappeared first, followed by sexual and display activities	Etienne and Fischer (1964)
Female	Testosterone propionate	Increased aggressiveness; reinforced female behavior but also male fighting and sexual behavior	Etienne and Fischer (1964)
Male and female	*In vivo* production of testosterone	During the breeding season, males produce more gonadal testosterone than females, reflecting former's dominance	Höhn and Cheng (1967)
Columbia livia (males)	Testosterone propionate	Enhanced aggressive components in courtship behavior; tended to inhibit nest demonstration behavior; inhibited twig collection and nest building	Murton *et al.* (1969)
	Progesterone	Depressed bowing but allowed attacking and driving to be expressed; inhibited nest demonstration, twig collection, and nest building	Murton *et al.* (1969)

457

TABLE XI (cont.)

Species	Hormone	Effect	Reference
Gallus domesticus			
Chick	Estradiol benzoate	Suppressed aggression; elevated nest demonstration behavior, inhibited twig collection and nest building	Murton *et al.* (1969)
	Testosterone propionate (250 mg/20 g)	Induction of crowing	Andrew (1963)
	Preoptic implants of androgen	Induction of mating	Gardner and Fischer (1968)
Capons	Testosterone propionate (pellet)	Induction of copulatory behavior	Barfield (1964)
Male	Progesterone (40 mg/week)	Inhibited mating behavior	Herrick and Adams (1956)
Male and female	Progesterone and diethylstilbestrol	Induced female behavior	Herrick and Adams (1956)
Larus argentatus (immature male intacts and castrates)	Androgens	Promote aggressive behavior, territorial defense, and nest building; also appearance of male vocalization	Boss (1943)
Meleagris gallopavo			
Immature	Diethylstilbestrol	Development of strutting behavior	Simpson *et al.* (1965)
Male	Castration	No vocalization	Smith and Smythe (1963)
Nycticorax nycticorax (immature or gonadectomized female)	Testosterone propionate	Induced male sexual behavior	Noble and Wurm (1940)
Steganopus tricolor	*In vivo* production of testosterone	During the breeding season females produce more gonadal testosterone than males; this can be correlated with the aggressive dominance of the female in this species	Höhn and Cheng (1967)

458

Species	Treatment	Effect	Reference
Streptopelia risoria	Progesterone (0.1 mg) or diethylstilbestrol (0.4 mg)	Immediate initiation of incubatory behavior	Lehrman (1958)
	Progesterone or progesterone + estrogen	Increase in defensive behavior toward other birds; increased defensive behavior toward a predator	Vowles and Harwood (1966)
	Progesterone	Increased aggressive behavior	Vowles and Harwood (1966)
	Estrogen	Stimulates "nest-cooing" behavior	Vowles and Harwood (1966)
	Castration	Disappearance of mating calls	Vowles and Harwood (1966)
	Testosterone propionate (0.1 mg/day)	Reappearance of mating calls (inhibited by progesterone)	Vowles and Harwood (1966)
	Progesterone (100 µg/day)	Suppressed male courtship behavior	Komisaruk (1967)
	Progesterone (100 µg/day); placed in preoptic nucleus, or lateral forebrain system)	Induced incubation and suppressed male courtship behavior (suggested these regions of the brain directly sensitive to progesterone)	Komisaruk (1967)
	Hypothalamic implants of testosterone	Initiates courtship in castrates	Hutchinson (1967)
Turdus merula	*In vivo* production of testosterone	During the breeding season, males produce more gonadal testosterone than females; this may be correlated with the aggressive dominance of the male	Höhn and Cheng (1967)

dorsalis. Implants in the adenohypophysis or basal hypothalamus were less effective in blocking gonadal development although such animals showed some degree of inhibition compared with those bearing testosterone or estrogen implants in the optic chiasma or cholesterol implants in the median eminence. A more specific effect has been reported by Callard and Mc-Connell (1969), who found that while intrahypothalamic implants of estradiol suppressed ovulation and oviduct weight in *Sceloporus cyanogenys* follicular development did not appear to be arrested, perhaps indicating that LH secretion can be selectively inhibited. In birds, implants of testosterone in the basal hypothalamus can block photoperiodically induced gonadal development or induce testicular regression (Gogan, 1968). While these experiments adduce strong evidence for hypothalamic steroid receptors they are not yet conclusive and further studies are required to see whether there are hypothalamic structures akin to those in mammals which selectively take up testosterone from the circulation. Hawkins *et al.* (1969a, b) were unable to show an accumulation of radioactive estradiol within the hypothalamus or median eminence of the domestic fowl; uptake tended to be greatest in the adenohypophysis. Finally, mention must be made of the results of Ralph and Fraps (1960), who found that progesterone implants in the anterior hypothalamus of the laying hen induced premature ovulation.

In mammals, sex steroids have an important role in the fetus or neonate of differentiating the hypothalamus into either the "male" or "female" type (for a review, see Harris and Campbell, 1966). Whether this function operates in lower vertebrates is unclear.

D. Estrogens and Vitellogenesis

It has been known for some time that estrogenic hormones are intimately involved in stimulating the formation of yolk in oviparous vertebrates. The process of yolk deposition or vitellogenesis occurs at a relatively late stage in oocyte maturation and in many species, particularly birds, is confined to the period just prior to ovulation. The amount of yolk within a mature oocyte varies widely from the relatively small quantity found in most fishes and amphibians to the extremely large quantity found in reptile and bird eggs. At its most extreme the scale of the changes involved in vitellogenesis may be judged from the fact that an ovum of the domestic fowl undergoes a thousandfold increase in weight in the course of but a few days before ovulation. During the course of a week a laying hen may be expected to produce about 100 g of yolk, equivalent to a dry lipid and protein weight of about 50 g. The changes are less pronounced in lower vertebrates but are still marked. In the ribbon snake *Thamnophis sauritus* vitellogenesis begins when the oocytes weigh about 40 mg while ovulation occurs with the mature ova weighing about 1 g (Dessauer and Fox, 1959). During the phase of yolk deposition in the toad *Xenopus laevis* the gross weight of the ovary increases in an average specimen by about 12 g, virtually all of this increase being yolky material (Gitlin, 1939).

Much controversy has centered on the site of origin of the yolk proteins but it now seems that the vast bulk is made in the liver and transported to the oocyte where it is absorbed and deposited as yolk. This does not of course exclude the oocyte as a site for protein synthesis (see Smith *et al.*, 1966); indeed, the chemical conversion of plasma proteins into yolk may well require enzymes made within the oocyte. Much of the evidence for an extraovarian source of yolk proteins came from studies on the chemical composition of the blood during vitellogenesis when large increases were found in the levels of plasma proteins, notably "serum vitellin," protein-bound phosphorus and calcium, and lipids. Much of the early work is summarized in Riddle (1942); more recent studies, particularly on the laying hen, include those of Urist *et al.* (1958), Dessauer and Fox (1959), Roos and Meyer, (1961), Chung-Wai Ho and Vanstone (1961), Heald and Badman (1963), Heald and Mc-Lachlan (1963a), Heald *et al.* (1964), and Clark (1967). Physical, chemical, and serological techniques have established the very close relationships between these compounds and the lipid and protein components of the yolk itself (e.g., Roepke and Bushnell, 1936; Flickinger and Rounds, 1956; Mok *et al.*, 1961; Schjeide *et al.*, 1963; Wallace and Dumont, 1968; Follett *et al.*, 1968).

The pattern of changes that occur during natural vitellogenesis can be readily induced by treatment with estrogens and although the number of species studied remains small it includes representatives of all the major classes of oviparous vertebrates. Estrogens do not induce such changes in mammals or apparently in the ovoviviparous shark *Triakis semifasciatus* (Urist and Schjeide, 1961).

Five species of teleost fishes have been treated with estrogens and the plasma changes recorded. Urist and Schjeide (1961) injected male bass (*Paralabrax clathratus*) with a very large dose of estrone (10 mg) and found within 5 days a hypertrophy of the liver together with much increased plasma levels of calcium, protein, phosphorus, phospholipid, and lipids. Most of these components were associated with a new protein complex in the blood of treated fish which was not present in the controls. In the ultracentrifuge this complex gave a single peak with a sedimentation constant 17 S. Bailey (1957) obtained rather similar results with goldfish (*Carassius auratus*) and noted the directly proportional increases between calcium and phosphorus. Using very much smaller doses of estradiol benzoate (10 μg/100 g body weight per day) Chuang-Wai Ho and Vanstone (1961) found increases in many plasma lipid and protein components in both male and female sockeye salmon (*Oncorynchus nerka*). Chan and Chester Jones (1968) reported a rise in bound calcium in the blood of eels (*Anguilla anguilla*) treated with pre-marin, a synthetic conjugated estrogen. The only other species studied is the cod *Gadus morrhua* in which Plack and Pritchard (1968) found that estra-diol increased plasma phospholipids and Woodhead (1969) reported a 29% increase in plasma calcium within 5 days of giving a dose of 1 mg/kg. The latter author was also able to induce a slight hypercalcemia in oviparous dog-fishes (*Scyliorhinus caniculus*) with estradiol. The liver of vitellogenic teleosts is often characteristic in appearance and this may be induced in males by treatment with estrogens (Kobayashi, 1953; Clavert and Zahnd, 1956, 1960).

In their comparative study Urist and Schjeide (1961) used male *Rana catesbeiana* as representatives of the Amphibia. Estrone treatment (10 mg) resulted in rather more drastic changes than in bass, with plasma calcium being elevated fourteenfold and protein sixfold within 5 days. There were concomitant elevations in various lipid fractions and in protein-bound phos-phorus. Recently a more complete study has been made of the vitellogenic response in the South African clawed toad *Xenopus laevis* (for a review, see Wallace and Dumont, 1968; Follett *et al.*, 1968; Wallace and Jared, 1969; Follett and Redshaw, 1970). Estradiol treatment of female toads results in a number of changes associated with the appearance in the plasma of a large molecular weight, calcium-binding lipophosphoprotein (SLPP). There is also a transient increase in unesterified fatty acids possibly related to lipid mobilization, and in other lipid components such as triglyceride and choles-terol esters which are not bound to the SLPP (Follett and Redshaw, 1968; Munday *et al.*, 1968).

The response can also be induced indirectly by stimulating endogenous estrogen production with mammalian gonadotropins (Wallace and Jared, 1968a, 1969). Interestingly this treatment results in only a relatively minor rise in SLPP concentration while the level continues to increase steadily if animals are maintained under constant estradiol treatment. The difference between responses arises because gonadotropins have a further role in vitel-logenesis; that is, apart from stimulating estrogen formation (Redshaw and Nicholls, 1970), they stimulate the incorporation of SLPP into the oocyte. Both human chorionic gonadotropin (HCG) and mammalian follicle-stimu-lating hormone (FSH) cause the uptake of radioactively labeled SLPP into the yolk platelet proteins where it may be identified chromatographically and by amino acid analysis as phosvitin and lipovitellin (Follett *et al.*, 1968; Wallace and Dumont, 1968). The response to injected estrogens is dose dependent and of the three commonly occurring hormones estradiol-17β is the most potent, being 3.9 times more active than estrone and 13.7 times more active than estriol (Redshaw *et al.*, 1969). The minimally effective dose of estradiol which causes measurable chemical changes in the plasma is about 1 μg/day although Wallace and Jared (1968b) believe that any quantity will cause the synthesis of at least some SLPP. The effects are readily inducible in males and in hypophysectomized females (Wallace and Jared, 1968b; Follett and Redshaw, 1968).

The site of SLPP synthesis and the target organ for estrogens is considered to be the liver. Only this tissue taken from estrogen-treated males was capable of synthesizing and secreting phosvitin *in vitro* (Rudack and Wallace, 1968). This test system has been developed further and liver slices from vitellogenic females have been shown to incorporate tritiated amino acids or sodium phosphate-^{32}P into a protein identifiable as SLPP (Wallace and Jared, 1969). The rate of release of SLPP from the liver tissue was much greater for vitellogenic females and estrogen-treated males than for normal females. Normal males showed no lipophosphoprotein synthesis. Estradiol administered *in vitro* could not stimulate SLPP synthesis by the liver slices. These biochemical results are supported by the cytological studies of Nicholls *et al.* (1968). Within 24 hrs of estradiol administration the hepatic ultrastructure of both male and female *Xenopus* undergoes profound modifications. In all liver cells there is a considerable proliferation of granular endoplasmic reticulum together with hypertrophy of the nucleus and an increase in electron density of the nucleolus. These changes could be correlated with the emergence in the plasma of SLPP, as measured by immunological methods. Nonestrogenic hormones such as testosterone, progesterone, or cortisone acetate did not elicit either SLPP synthesis or the hepatic structural changes (Nicholls *et al.*, 1968; Redshaw *et al.*, 1969). Finally, an odd aspect of the response in *Xenopus* is that the SLPP is a green chromoprotein which contains biliverdin (Redshaw *et al.*, 1970). Presumably the biliverdin is derived from heme metabolism but whether estrogens affect this indirectly or directly is unknown. However, its presence can be demonstrated in the mature oocytes of normal females so that its binding to SLPP appears to be of some physiological significance.

In the reptiles there is a slight qualitative change in the pattern of responses to estradiol, reflecting perhaps the rather more yolky eggs which this group produces. Estrogens again cause hypertrophy of the liver and a rise in calcium, phosphorus, and protein components. This has been demonstrated in turtles (Urist and Schjeide, 1961; Clark, 1967), snakes (Dessauer and Fox, 1959), lizards (Hahn, 1967; Suzuki and Prosser, 1968), and crocodiles (Prosser and Suzuki, 1968). The major preyolk protein in the plasma appears to be generally similar to that in fishes and amphibians and normally exists as a single component with a sedimentation constant of about 17 S (Urist and Schjeide, 1961). The liver is the site of synthesis of this complex, and Hahn *et al.* (1969a) have shown that estradiol treatment of the lizard *Uta stansburiana* stimulates the synthesis of RNA prior to vitellogenesis. Most forms of RNA seem stimulated but a particular part of the population of molecules has been shown to be different from that found in normal untreated lizards.

Lipid mobilization as judged by the appearance in the plasma of a β-lipoprotein (Urist and Schjeide, 1961) appears to be more pronounced in reptiles than in amphibians following estrogen treatment. However, great care must be taken in drawing comparisons since all workers have employed different doses of estrogens for varying periods of time. The source of the lipids may well include the fat body. Hahn (1967) was able to demonstrate that the release of fatty acids *in vitro* from the fat bodies of estrogen-treated *Uta stansburiana* was markedly faster than from nontreated females. *In vivo*, estradiol caused a rapid decrease in weight of the fat body, an effect which normally occurs during natural vitellogenesis (Hahn and Tinkle, 1966).

The vitellogenic responses to estrogens in birds are generally similar to those in lower vertebrates except that the lipid components are relatively more important. Not surprisingly perhaps, in view of their economic importance and readiness to ovulate in captivity, most work has been carried out on domestic fowls and the following remarks are mainly restricted to this species (for reviews, see Riddle, 1942; Schjeide *et al.*, 1963; Simkiss, 1967).

Following estrogen treatment there are rises in plasma calcium, protein, and phosphorus (e.g., Riddle, 1942; Clegg *et al.*, 1951; McKinley *et al.*, 1954; Schjeide and Urist, 1956; Urist *et al.*, 1958; Urist and Schjeide, 1961) associated with the synthesis and secretion into the blood of two new proteins, phosvitin and lipovitellin (Schjeide and Urist, 1956, 1960; Common and Mok, 1959; Heald and McLachlan, 1963b, 1964). In contrast with lower vertebrates these proteins exist as separate entities in the plasma and may be separated on the ultra-centrifuge or by chromatography (Schjeide *et al.*, 1963). This is not possible with the plasma preyolk protein complex of *Xenopus* (SLPP) although it is clear that both components are present since SLPP on incorporation into the oocyte cleaves to yield chemically identifiable phosvitin and lipovitellin in the yolk platelet proteins (Follett *et al.*, 1968; Wallace and Dumont, 1968). Why the two proteins occur separately in avian plasma remains obscure. There is adequate evidence that the liver is the site of yolk protein synthesis. Hepatectomy of the domestic fowl prevents the typical plasma changes which follow estrogen treatment (Ranney and Chaikoff, 1951; Vanstone *et al.*, 1957), while liver slices from laying hens will synthesize phosvitin *in vitro* (Heald and McLachlan, 1965). At least part of the estrogen action on the liver cells appears to occur at a transcription level and estrogens induce the synthesis of new RNA prior to the emergence into the blood of phosvitin after about 24 hr treatment (Schjeide and Wilkins, 1964; Greengard and Acs, 1964). The synthesis of new templates for phosphoprotein production occurs within the first few hours following treatment, since actinomycin D blocks phosvitin synthesis if given simultaneously with estrogens, but is much less effective if the injection is delayed by 4–6 hrs (Greengard *et al.*, 1964). Only after this initial period of RNA synthesis is puromycin, a specific inhibitor of protein synthesis, effective in suppressing phosvitin formation (Greengard and Acs, 1964; Greengard *et al.*, 1964). By the use of DNA–RNA hybridization techniques Hahn *et al.* (1969b) have shown that within 105 min of administering estrone to immature pullets the liver contains most if not all the RNA species present in the liver of the laying hen. The identity of the new species being formed is unknown but probably includes ribosomal RNA since estrogens cause proliferation of the granular endoplasmic reticulum (Schjeide *et al.*, 1963; Hosoda and Abe, 1965). There is also a change in the distribution of transfer RNA in the liver with pronounced increases in those specific for serine and phosphoserine (Carlsen *et al.*, 1964; Schjeide, 1967). These might be expected to increase more markedly since about one-half of all the amino-acid residues in phosvitin are serine or its phosphorylated derivative.

Rises in the levels of plasma lipids following estrogen treatment of chickens are even more pronounced than those of the protein components. Heald and Rookledge (1964) reported a twenty- to fortyfold increase in total plasma lipids after injections for 2 weeks of estradiol propionate into immature pullets. Unesterified fatty acids are also greatly increased, suggesting that as in mammals these materials are precursors of the plasma triglycerides (Heald and Rookledge, 1964). In the pheasant *Phasianus colchicus*, egg laying is accompanied by rises in the levels of both plasma "clearing factor" and total lipids. Roos and Meyer (1961) suggested that this lipase might be responsible for the mobilization of depot lipids. While some of the plasma lipids in estrogenized birds are attached to lipovitellin the great majority, primarily triglycerides, appear to be carried in association with a light β-lipoprotein. This protein is normally present in the plasma of nonlaying hens (cf. phosvitin and lipovitellin) but its concentration is greatly increased in laying hens or after estrogen treatment (Urist and Schjeide, 1961; Schjeide *et al.*, 1963). The specific lipid effects can be induced separately from those involving the synthesis of yolk proteins (Schjeide *et al.*, 1963) and it is perhaps justifiable to consider them as involving separate mechanisms. Estrogens greatly stimulate triglyceride synthesis by the liver (Hawkins and Heald, 1966; de Vellis and Schjeide, 1967) and this action, as that on yolk protein synthesis, can be prevented with actinomycin D. Malic enzyme may be the key enzyme responsible for the increased lipogenesis since its activity rises following estrogen treatment but the rise does not occur in the presence of actinomycin D (de Vellis and Schjeide, 1967).

A further role for estrogens and possibly androgens is in the laying down and resorption of calcium from the skeleton of laying birds. Controversy still surrounds these suggested actions and the experiments are equivocal. The problem is discussed thoroughly in Simkiss (1967).

E. PROGESTOGENIC STEROIDS

Reactions to the administration of progestational steroids have been varied and include their ability to feminize gonads (e.g., Gallien, 1950; Witschi and Allison, 1950), to cause growth of the ovipositor in bitterlings (see Pickford and Atz, 1957), to induce "broodiness" in cichild fishes (Noble *et al.*, 1938), and when given in very large doses to induce ovulation in some amphibians (see Barr, 1968). In addition some viviparous forms seem to need progestins for the maintenance of gestation (Ishii, 1961; Boisseau, 1965). It is unclear whether these effects are a direct or an indirect response to the hormone.

Rather more convincing evidence implicates progesterone in a number of reproductive processes in the female bird. Results in this group with exogenously administered progesterone are supported by reasonable biological (Fraps *et al.*, 1948; Layne *et al.*, 1957) and chemical (O'Malley *et al.*, 1968; Furr, 1969) evidence for the existence of progesterone in the plasma of the domestic fowl. The most interesting and controversial function ascribed to progesterone is a role in controlling ovulation in birds, an effect akin to that which has been described recently in mammals. In low doses progesterone induces premature ovulation in the domestic fowl (Rothchild and Fraps, 1949). This action seems to operate via the central nervous system since adrenergic and cholinergic blocking agents inhibit progesterone-induced ovulation (Zarrow and Bastian, 1953; van Tienhoven, 1955) while the implantation of progesterone in the preoptic area of the hypothalamus results in premature ovulation (Ralph and Fraps, 1960). On the basis of these results Fraps (1955) described a possible role for preovulatory progestins, produced by the maturing oocytes, in inducing LH release from the adenohypophysis. The presence of high concentrations of progesterone in preovulatory follicles and of cycles in the plasma levels in laying hens (Furr, 1969) supports Frap's general hypothesis, but conclusive evidence is still lacking.

A series of recent experiments by O'Malley and his colleagues shows that progesterone specifically induces the formation and secretion of avidin by the chicken oviduct. The early growth of the oviduct is estrogen dependent and following hormone treatment three types of cells are differentiated: tubular gonad cells, ciliated cells, and goblet cells. Progesterone acts on the developed goblet cells to cause the synthesis of avidin (Kohler *et al.*, 1968). The actual mechanism whereby progesterone induces avidin synthesis is not yet proven (O'Malley and McGuire, 1968b) although there is much evidence that an effect of transcription of nuclear DNA is dominant. Actinomycin D largely inhibits progesterone-induced avidin synthesis (O'Malley, 1967; Korenman and O'Malley, 1968) while a number of biochemical parameters associated with *de novo* RNA synthesis such as the specific activity of nuclear RNA and the level of DNA-dependent RNA polymerase (McGuire and O'Malley, 1968) are increased by progesterone treatment. Techniques involving DNA–RNA hybridization indicate that following administration of progesterone but prior to avidin synthesis there is formation of new species of RNA (O'Malley and McGuire, 1968c, 1969; Hahn *et al.*, 1968). The oviduct is an ideal experimental system in which to study the cellular action of steroidal hormones not only because progesterone induces the synthesis of a particular protein but also because it will induce avidin synthesis in both short- and long-term cultures of estrogen-pretreated oviduct cells (O'Malley, 1967; O'Malley and Kohler, 1967).

The oviduct of at least some amphibians appears also to be a target organ for progestins, and injected progesterone causes the release of jelly from the oviducal gonads into the ducts of *Bufo* (Galli-Mainini, 1950, 1962; Lodge and Smith, 1960; Thornton and Evennett, 1969). The effect is not absolutely specific to progesterone since deoxycorticosterone acetate will also cause jelly release *in vivo* (Thornton and Evennett, 1969). However, in the physiology of the normal organism it is probable that a progestin derived from the ovary is responsible for the effect. Thornton (1970) has recently detected a progestin (probably progesterone) in the plasma of toads prior to ovulation. An interesting point which remains to be determined is whether the progestins cause both the synthesis and release of the jelly or only the latter. Present information (Thornton, 1970) suggests that estrogens are responsible for the development of the oviducal glands and that the cells are filled with jelly prior to the action of progesterone. This control of jelly release may not be a general phenomenon in amphibians. Thornton and Evennett (1969) have found that secretion of oviducal jelly in the urodele *Triturus cristatus* (which lays only a small number of eggs over a long period) is a response to the passage of the oocytes down the oviduct rather than to an ovarian secretion.

Progestins not only act on the oviduct of amphibians but also provoke the maturation division of the oocyte (Masui, 1967; Schuetz, 1967; Thornton and Evennett, 1969). This effect may be induced both *in vivo* and *in vitro* and again is not completely specific to progesterone although this steroid is more effective than deoxycorticosterone acetate and 17-hydroxyprogesterone. A careful analysis of the time relationships involved in gonadotropin-induced ovulation in *Bufo* indicates that progestin secretion from the ovary occurs about 12–15 hrs before ovulation. In that period jelly secretion from the oviducal glands rises to a maximum and the maturation divisions of the oocyte are completed (Thornton and Evennett, 1969).

A number of observations suggest that progestins may influence behavioral patterns. For example, progesterone induces ring doves to commence incubation (see Lehrman, 1961) although the degree and rate of the response is dependent upon the individual's experience of incubation behavior. Implants of progesterone in the preoptic nucleus or lateral forebrain bundle of ring doves also induce incubation (Komisaruk, 1967). More general changes in aggressive and defensive behaviour following progesterone treatment have been reported (Vowles and Harwood, 1966; Komisaruk, 1967). Finally, progesterone may play some part in brood patch development although most of the changes are more readily induced by estrogens acting in combination with other hormones such as prolactin (Hinde and Steel, 1966; Selander and Yang, 1966). Testosterone can also cause growth of the brood patch when given with prolactin (Johns and Pfeiffer, 1963).

REFERENCES

Adams, B. M. (1968). *J. Endocrinol.* **20**, 145.
Adams, E. A. (1945). *Anat. Rec.* **91**, 263.
Adams, E. A. (1946). *J. Exp. Zool.* **101**, 1.
Adams, E. A. (1950). *J. Exp. Zool.* **113**, 463.
Adams, E. A., Gay, H. and Terzian, A. (1941). *Anat. Rec.* **79**, 67.
Adams, J. L., and Herrick, R. B. (1955). *Poultry Sci.* **34**, 117.
Albert, A. (1961). *In* "Sex and Internal Secretions" (W. C. Young, ed.), pp. 305–365. Williams & Wilkins, Baltimore, Maryland.
Alberti, K. G. M. M., and Sharp, G. W. G. (1969). *Biochim. Biophys. Acta* **192**, 335.
Alvarado, R. H., and Kirschner, L. B. (1964). *Nature (London)* **202**, 922.
Amanuma, A. (1963a). *J. Biol. Osaka City Univ.* **14**, 25.
Amanuma, A. (1963b). *J. Biol. Osaka City Univ.* **14**, 15.
Andrew, R. J. (1963). *J. Comp. Physiol. Psychol.* **56**, 933.
Arai, R. (1964). *Bull. Nat. Sci. Mus. Tokyo* **1**, 91.
Arai, R., and Egami, N. (1961). *Annot. Zool. Jap.* **34**, 185.
Asayama, S., and Matsuzaki, H. (1958). *Zool. Mag.* **67**, 133.
Asayama, S., and Miyamori, H. (1957). *J. Inst. Polytech. Osaka City Univ. Ser. D* **8**, 129.
Ashby, K. R. (1957). *J. Embryol. Exp. Morphol.* **5**, 225.
Ashby, K. R. (1959). *Riv. Biol.* **51**, 453.
Ashby, K. R. (1965). *Riv. Biol.* **58**, 139.
Atz, J. W. (1964). *In* "Intersexuality in Vertebrates Including Man" (C. N. Armstrong and A. J. Marshall, eds.), pp. 145–232. Academic Press, New York.
Ausiello, A., and Sharp, G. W. G. (1968). *Endocrinology* **82**, 1163.
Baggerman, B. (1966). *Symp. Soc. Exp. Biol.* **20**, 427.
Baggerman, B. (1968). *In* "Perspectives in Endocrinology: Hormones in the Lives of Lower

Vertebrates" (E. J. W. Barrington and C. B. Jørgensen, eds.), pp. 351–404. Academic Press, New York.

Bailey, R. E. (1957). *J. Exp. Zool.* **136**, 455.

Baldwin, F. M., and Goldin, H. S. (1939). *Proc. Soc. Exp. Biol. Med.* **42**, 813.

Baldwin, F. M., and Li, M. H. (1945). *Amer. Natur.* **79**, 281.

Ball, J. N. (1960). *Symp. Zool. Soc. (London)* **1**, 105.

Ball, J. N., and Ensor, D. M. (1968). *Colloq. Int. Cent. Nat. Rech. Sci.* **177**, 216.

Barfield, R. J. (1964). *Amer. Zool.* **4**, 301.

Barr, W. A. (1968). *In* "Perspectives in Endocrinology: Hormones in the Lives of Lower Vertebrates" (E. J. W. Barrington and C. B. Jørgensen, eds.), pp. 164–238. Academic Press, New York.

Basu, S. L. (1962a). *Naturwissenschaften* **49**, 188.

Basu, S. L. (1962b). *Folia Biol. (Warsaw)* **12**, 203.

Basu, S. L. (1965). *Naturwissenschaften* **52**, 143.

Basu, S. L., and Nandi, J. (1965). *J. Exp. Zool.* **159**, 93.

Basu, S. L., Bern, H. A., and Chan, H. (1967). *Anat. Rec.* **151**, 441.

Bellamy, D., and Chester Jones, I. (1961). *Comp. Biochem. Physiol.* **3**, 175.

Bellamy, D., and Chester Jones, I. (1965). *Excerpta Med. Found. Int. Congr. Ser.* **83**, 153.

Bellamy, D., and Leonard, R. A. (1965). *Gen. Comp. Endocrinol.* **5**, 402.

Bellamy, D., and Phillips, J. G. (1966). *J. Endocrinol.* **36**, 97.

Bellamy, D., Janssens, P. A., and Leonard, R. A. (1966). *J. Endocrinol.* **35**, 19.

Bellamy, D., Leonard, R. A., Dulieu, K., and Stevenson, A. (1968). *Gen. Comp. Endocrinol.* **10**, 119.

Bentley, P. J., and Follett, B. K. (1962). *Gen. Comp. Endocrinol.* **2**, 329.

Bentley, P. J., and Follett, B. K. (1963). *J. Physiol. (London)* **169**, 902.

Bentley, P. J., and Follett, B. K. (1965). *J. Endocrinol.* **31**, 127.

Berkowitz, P. (1941). *J. Exp. Zool.* **87**, 233.

Blair, A. P. (1946). *J. Exp. Zool.* **103**, 365.

Boccabella, A. V. (1963). *Endocrinology* **72**, 787.

Boetius, J., Boetius, L., Hemmingeen, A. M., Brunn, A. F., and Møller-Christensen, E. (1962). *Medd. Dan. Fisk. Havunders* **3**, 183.

Boisseau, J. P. (1965). *C.R. Acad. Sci.* **260**, 313.

Bondy, P. K. (1949). *Endocrinology* **45**, 605.

Bonting, S. L., and Canady, D. M. (1964). *Amer. J. Physiol.* **207**, 1005.

Bonting, S. L., Caravaggio, L. L., Canady, M. R., and Hawkins, N. M. (1964). *Arch. Biochem. Biophys.* **106**, 49.

Boss, W. R. (1943). *J. Exp. Zool.* **94**, 181.

Botte, V., and Delrio, G. (1967). *Gen. Comp. Endocrinol.* **9**, 110.

Brant, J. W. A., and Nalbandov, A. V. (1956) *Poultry Sci.* **35**, 692.

Breneman, W. R. (1956). *Endocrinology* **58**, 262.

Bretschneider, L. H., and Duyvène de Wit, J. J. (1947). "Sexual Endocrinology of Non-mammalian Vertebrates," 146 pp. *Monographs on Progress of Research in Holland.* Elsevier, Amsterdam.

Bruner, J. A., and Witschi, E. (1954). *Anat. Rec.* **120**, 99.

Bullough, W. S. (1940). *J. Exp. Zool.* **85**, 475.

Bullough, W. S. (1942). *J. Endocrinol.* **3**, 211.

Burger, J. W. (1942). *Biol. Bull.* **82**, 233.

Burger, J. W. (1965). *Physiol. Zool.* **38**, 191.

Burger, J. W., and Tosteson, D. (1966). *Comp. Biochem. Physiol.* **19**, 649.

Burns, R. K. (1939). *Anat. Rec.* **73**, 73.

Burns, R. K. (1961). *In* "Sex and Internal Secretions" (W. C. Young, ed.), pp. 75–158. Williams & Wilkins, Baltimore, Maryland.

Callard, I. P., and McConnell, W. F. (1969). *Gen. Comp. Endocrinol.* **13**, 496.

Carlsen, E. N., Trelle, G. J., and Schjeide, O. A. (1964). *Nature (London)* **202**, 984.

Carstensen, H., Burgess, A. C. J., and Li, C. H. (1961). *Gen. Comp. Endocrinol.* **1**, 37.

Cei, G., and Acosta, D. I. (1953). *C.R. Soc. Biol.* **147**, 250.

Cei, J. M., Androezzi, M. L., and Acosta, D. I. (1955). *Arch. Farm. Bioquim. Tucuman* **7**, 119.

Chambolle, P. (1965). *C.R. Acad. Sci,* **261**, 2761.

Chan, D. K. O. (1968). *Excerpta Med. Found. Int. Congr. Ser.* **184**, 709.

Chan, D. K. O., and Chester Jones, I. (1968). *J. Endocrinol.* **42**, 109.

Chan, D. K. O., Phillips, J. G., and Chester Jones, I. (1967a). *Comp. Biochem. Physiol.* **23**, 185.

Chan, D. K. O., Chester Jones, I., Henderson, I. W., and Rankin, J. C. (1967b). *J. Endocrinol.* **37**, 297.

Chan, D. K. O., Chester Jones, I., and Mosley, W. (1968). *J. Endocrinol.* **42**, 91.

Chan, D. K. O., Rankin, J. C., and Chester Jones, I. (1969). *Gen. Comp. Endocrinol. Suppl.* **2**, 342.

Chan, S. K., and Cohen, P. P. (1964a). *Arch. Biochem. Biophys.* **104**, 335.

Chan, S. K., and Cohen, P. P. (1964b). *Arch. Biochem. Biophys.* **104**, 331.

Chang, C. Y. (1955). *Anat. Rec.* **123**, 467.

Chang, C. Y., and Witschi, E. (1955). *Proc. Soc. Exp. Biol. Med.* **89**, 150.

Chang, C. Y., and Witschi, E. (1956). *Proc. Soc. Exp. Biol. Med.* **93**, 140.

Charnier, M. (1965). *C.R. Soc. Biol.* **159**, 1822.

Chester Jones, I. (1957). "The Adrenal Cortex." Cambridge Univ. Press, London and New York.

Chester Jones, I., and Ball, J. N. (1962). *In* "The Ovary" (S. Zuckerman, ed.), Vol. 1, pp. 331–360. Academic Press, New York.

Chester Jones, I., Phillips, J. G., and Bellamy, D. (1962). *Gen. Comp. Endocrinol. Suppl.* **1**, 36.

Chester Jones, I., Henderson, I. W., and Butler, D. G. (1965). *Arch. Anat. Microsc. Morphol. Exp.* **54**, 453.

Chester Jones, I., Henderson, I. W., Chan, D. K. O., and Rankin, J. C. (1967). *Excerpta Med. Found. Int. Congr. Ser.* **132**, 136.

Chester Jones, I., Chan, D. K. O., Henderson, I. W., and Ball, J. N. (1969). *In* "Fish Physiology" (W. S. Hoar and D. J. Randall, eds.), Vol. II, pp. 322–376. Academic Press, New York.

Chieffi, G. (1959). *Arch. Anat. Microsc. Morphol. Exp.* **48**, 21.

Chieffi, G., Bellini-Cardellini, L., and Polzonetti-Magni, A. (1966). *Ric. Sci.* **36**, 283.

Chignell, C. F., and Titus, E. O. (1966). *J. Biol. Chem.* **241**, 5083.

Chignell, C. F., Roddy, P. M., and Titus, E. O. (1965). *Life Sci.* **4**, 599.

Chu, J. P. (1940). *J. Endocrinol.* **2**, 21.

Chu, J. P., and You, S. S. (1946). *J. Endocrinol.* **4**, 431.

Chung-Wai Ho, F., and Vanstone, W. E. (1961). *J. Fish. Res. Bd. Can.* **18**, 859.

Clark, N. B. (1967). *Comp. Biochem. Physiol.* **20**, 823.

Clavert, J., and Zahnd, J. D. (1956). *C.R. Soc. Biol.* **150**, 1261.

Clavert, J., and Zahnd, J. D. (1960). *C.R. Ass. Anat.* **46**, 171.

Clegg, R. E., Sanford, P. E., Hein, R. E., Andrews, A. C., Hughes, J. S., and Mueller, C. D. (1951). *Science* **114**, 437.

Cohen, H. (1946). *Zoologica (New York)* **31**, 121.

Cohen, R. R. (1962). *Nature (London)* **194**, 601.

Collenot, A. (1964). *C.R. Acad. Sci.* **259**, 2535.

Common, R. H., and Mok, C. C. (1959). *Nature (London)* **183**, 1811.
Conte, F. P. (1969). *In* "Fish Physiology" (W. S. Hoar and D. J. Randall, eds.), Vol. 1, pp. 241–292. Academic Press, New York.
Crabbé, J. (1961a). *Endocrinology* **69**, 673.
Crabbé, J. (1961b). *J. Clin. Invest.* **40**, 2102.
Crabbé, J. (1963a). "The Sodium-Retaining Action of Aldosterone," 119 pp. Editions Arscia, Brussels.
Crabbé, J. (1963b). *Nature (London)* **200**, 787.
Crabbé, J. (1964). *Endocrinology* **75**, 809.
Crabbé, J. (1966). *Ann. Endocrinol.* **27**, 501.
Cummings, J. B. (1943). *J. Exp. Zool.* **94**, 351.
Dale, E. (1962). *Gen. Comp. Endocrinol.* **2**, 171.
Dalton, T., and Snart, R. S. (1967). *Biochim. Biophys. Acta* **135**, 1059.
Dalton, T., and Snart, R. S. (1969). *J. Endocrinol.* **47**, 159.
D'Ancona, U. (1957). *Pubbl. Sta. Zool. Napoli* **29**, 307.
Daughaday, W. H., Adler, R. E., Mariz, I. K., and Rasinski, D. C. (1962). *J. Clin. Endocrinol, Metab.* **22**, 704.
Dessauer, H. C., and Fox, W. (1959). *Amer. J. Physiol.* **197**, 360.
de Vellis, J., and Schjeide, O. A. (1967). *Progr. Biochem. Pharmacol.* **2**, 276.
Dodd, J. M. (1955). *Mem. Soc. Endocrinol.* **4**, 166.
Dodd, J. M. (1960a). *In* "Marshall's Physiology of Reproduction" (A. S. Parkes, ed.), Vol. 1, Part ii, pp. 417–582. Longmans, Green, London.
Dodd, J. M. (1960b). *Mem. Soc. Endocrinol.* **7**, 17.
Dodd, J. M., and Goddard, C. K. (1961). *Proc. Zool. Soc. London* **137**, 325.
Dodd, J. M., and Wiebe, J. P. (1968). *Arch. Anat. Histol. Embryol.* **51**, 157.
Dodd, J. M., Evennett, P. J., and Goddard, C. K. (1960). *Symp. Zool. Soc. (London)* **1**, 77.
Donaldson, E. M., and Holmes, W. N. (1965). *J. Endocrinol.* **32**, 329.
Dunson, W. A., and Taub, A. M. (1967). *Amer. J. Physiol.* **213**, 975.
Duyvène de Wit, J. J. (1940). *J. Endocrinol.* **2**, 141.
Dzwillo, M. (1963). *Zool. Anz. Suppl.* **26**, 152.
Eckstein, B., and Spira, M. (1965). *Biol. Bull.* **129**, 328.
Edelman, I. S., Bogoroch, R., and Porter, G. A. (1963). *Proc. Nat. Acad. Sci. U.S.* **50**, 1169.
Edwards, B. R. (1969). "Some Hormonal Influences on Water and Electrolyte Changes in *Xenopus laevis* Daudin." Ph.D. thesis, University of Sheffield, England.
Egami, N. (1954a). *J. Fac. Sci. Univ. Tokyo* **7**, 281.
Egami, N. (1954b). *Annot. Zool. Jap.* **27**, 13.
Egami, N. (1954c). *J. Fac. Sci. Univ. Tokyo* **7**, 113.
Egami, N. (1954d). *J. Fac. Sci. Univ. Tokyo* **7**, 121.
Egami, N. (1954e). *Endocrinol. Jap.* **1**, 75.
Egami, N. (1955a). *Annot. Zool. Jap.* **27**, 122.
Egami, N. (1955b). *Jap. J. Zool.* **11**, 21.
Egami, N. (1955c). *Endocrinol. Jap.* **2**, 89.
Egami, N. (1960a). *J. Fac. Sci. Univ. Tokyo* **9**, 67.
Egami, N. (1960b). *Annot. Zool. Jap.* **33**, 104.
Egami, N., and Arai, R. (1964). *Excerpta Med. Found. Int. Congr. Ser.* **83**, 146.
Egami, N., and Nambu, M. (1961). *J. Fac. Sci. Univ. Tokyo* **9**, 263.
Egami, N., Ohshima, T., and Nakanishi, Y. H. (1965). *Jap. J. Zool.* **14**, 31.
Elizondo, R. S., and LeBrie, S. J. (1969). *Amer. J. Physiol.* **217**, 419.
Ericksen, C. J., Bruder, R. H., Kamisaruk, B. R., and Lehrman, D. S. (1967). *Endocrinology* **81**, 39.

Ernst, S. A., and Ellis, R. A. (1969). *J. Cell Biol.* **40**, 305.
Etienne, A., von, and Fischer, H. (1964). *Z. Tierphysiol. Tierernaehr. Futtermittelk.* **21**, 348.
Evans, L. T. (1936) *J. Genet. Psychol.* **48**, 217.
Evans, L. T. (1937). *Physiol. Zool.* **10**, 456.
Evennett, P. J. (1963). *Nature (London)* **197**, 715.
Eversole, W. J. (1939). *Endocrinology* **25**, 328.
Eversole, W. J. (1941). *Endocrinology* **28**, 603.
Eversole, W. J., and D'Angelo, S. A. (1943). *J. Exp. Zool.* **92**, 215.
Fachini, G. (1964). *Rev. Idrobiol.* **3**, 3.
Fagerlund, U. H. N. (1967). *Gen. Comp. Endocrinol.* **8**, 197.
Falkmer, S., and Matty, A. J. (1966). *Gen. Comp. Endocrinol.* **6**, 334.
Fanestil, D. D., and Edelman, I. S. (1966) *Fed. Proc. Fed. Amer. Soc. Exp. Biol.* **25**, 912.
Fanestil, D. D., Porter, G. A., and Edelman, I. S. (1967). *Biochim. Biophys. Acta* **135**, 74.
Fänge, R. (1963). *In* "Biology of Myxine" (A. Brodal and R. Fänge, eds.), pp. 516–529. Oslo Univ. Press, Oslo.
Fänge, R., Schmidt-Nielsen, K., and Robinson, M. (1958). *Amer. J. Physiol.* **195**, 321.
Fänge, R., Krog, J., and Reite, O. (1963). *Acta Physiol. Scand.* **58**, 40.
Fimognari, G., Porter, G. A., and Edelman, I. S. (1967). *Biochim. Biophys. Acta* **135**, 89.
Fleming, W. R., Stanley, J. G., and Meier, A. H. (1964). *Gen. Comp. Endocrinol.* **4**, 61.
Fletcher, G. L., Stainer, I. M., and Holmes, W. N. (1967). *J. Exp. Biol.* **47**, 375.
Flickinger, R. A., and Rounds, D. E. (1956). *Biochim. Biophys. Acta* **22**, 38.
Follett, B. K., and Redshaw, M. R. (1968). *J. Endocrinol.* **40**, 439.
Follett, B. K., and Redshaw, M. R. (1970). *In* "Physiology of the Amphibia" (B. Lofts, ed.). In press, Academic Press, New York.
Follett, B. K., Nicholls, T. J., and Redshaw, M. R. (1968). *J. Cell. Physiol.* **72**, Suppl., p. 91.
Fontaine, M. (1964). *C.R. Acad. Sci.* **259**, 875.
Fontaine, M. (1967). *C.R. Acad. Sci.* **264**, 736.
Fontaine, M., Bertrand, E., Lopez, E., and Callamand, O. (1964). *C.R. Acad. Sci.* **259**, 2907.
Foote, C. L. (1938) *Anat. Rec.* **72**, 120.
Foote, C. L. (1964). *In* "Intersexuality in Vertebrates Including Man" (C. N. Armstrong and A. J. Marshall, eds.), pp. 233–272. Academic Press, New York.
Foote, C. L., and Foote, F. M. (1959) *Arch. Anat. Microsc. Morphol. Exp.* **48**, 71.
Forbes, T. R. (1938a). *Anat. Rec.* **75**, 51.
Forbes, T. R. (1938b). *J. Exp. Zool.* **28**, 335.
Forbes, T. R. (1941). *J. Morphol.* **68**, 31.
Forbes, T. R. (1961). *In* "Sex and Internal Secretions" (W. C. Young and G. W. Corner, eds.), Vol. 1, pp. 1035–1087. Williams & Wilkins, Baltimore, Maryland.
Forster, R. P., and Goldstein, L. (1969). *In* "Fish Physiology" (W. S. Hoar and D. J. Randall, eds.), Vol. 1, pp. 313–350. Academic Press, New York.
Fraps, R. M. (1955). *Mem. Soc. Endocrinol.* **4**, 205.
Fraps, R. M., Hooker, C. W., and Forbes, T. R. (1948). *Science* **108**, 86.
Frazier, H. S., and Hammer, E. I. (1963). *Amer. J. Physiol.* **205**, 718.
Furr, B. J. A. (1969). "A Study of Gonadotrophins and Progestins in the Domestic Fowl." Ph.D. thesis, University of Reading, England.
Gala, R. R., and Westphal, U. (1965). *Endocrinology* **76**, 1079.
Gallien, L. (1950). *Arch. Anat. Microsc. Morphol. Exp.* **39**, 337.
Gallien, L. (1954a). *Rev. Suisse Zool.* **61**, 349.
Gallien, L. (1954b). *Bull. Biol. Fr. Belg.* **88**, 1.
Gallien, L. (1955). *C.R. Acad. Sci.* **240**, 913.
Gallien, L. (1962). *Gen. Comp. Endocrinol. Suppl.* **1**, 346.

Galli-Mainini, C. (1950). *C.R. Soc. Biol.* **145**, 133.

Galli-Mainini, C. (1962). *Sem. Med.* **120**, 1575.

Gardner, J. E., and Fischer, A. E. (1968). *Physiol. Behav.* **3**, 709.

Gitlin, G. (1939). *S. Afr. J. Med. Sci.* **4**, Suppl., p. 41.

Gogan, F. (1968). *Gen. Comp. Endocrinol.* **11**, 316.

Goodland, G. A. J., and Munro, H. N. (1959). *Biochem. J.* **73**, 343.

Gorbman, A. (1939). *Proc. Soc. Exp. Biol. Med.* **42**, 811.

Greenberg, B. (1942). *J. Exp. Zool.* **91**, 435.

Greengard, O., and Acs, G. (1964). *Proc. Int. Congr. Biochem., 6th., 1964*, 57.

Greengard, O., Gordon, M., Smith, M. A., and Acs, G. (1964). *J. Biol. Chem.* **239**, 2079.

Grobstein, C. (1948). *J. Exp. Zool.* **109**, 215.

Hahn, W. E. (1967). *Comp. Biochem. Physiol.* **23**, 83.

Hahn, W. E., and Tinkle, D. W. (1966). *J. Exp. Zool.* **158**, 79.

Hahn, W. E., Church, R. B., Gorbman, A., and Wilmot, L. (1968). *Gen. Comp. Endocrinol.* **10**, 438.

Hahn, W. E., Church, R. B., and Gorbman, A. (1969a). *Endocrinology* **84**, 738.

Hahn, W. E., Schjeide, O. A., and Gorbman, A. (1969b). *Proc. Nat. Acad. Sci. U.S.* **62**, 112.

Hamilton, T. H. (1968). *Science* **161**, 649.

Hamon, M. (1945a). *C.R. Soc. Biol.* **139**, 108.

Hamon, M. (1945b). *C.R. Soc. Biol.* **139**, 110.

Hamon, M. (1945c). *C.R. Soc. Biol,* **139**, 761.

Hamon, M. (1946). *Bull. Soc. Hist. Natur. Afr. Nord* **37**, 122.

Hanaoka, K. I. (1963). *Embryologia* **7**, 306.

Hanaoka, K. I. (1965). *Embryologia* **9**, 49.

Hardisty, M. W., and Taylor, J. R. (1965). *Life Sci.* **4**, 743.

Harris, G. W., and Campbell, H. J. (1966). *In* "The Pituitary Gland" (G. W. Harris and B. T. Donovan, eds.), Vol. 2, pp. 99–165. Butterworth, London.

Hartman, F. A., and Brownell, K. A. (1949). "The Adrenal Gland" Kimpton, London.

Hartman, F. A., Lewis, L. A., Brownell, K. A., Angerer, C. A., and Sheldon, F. F. (1944). *Physiol. Zool.* **17**, 228.

Hawkins, R. A., and Heald, P. J. (1966). *Biochim. Biophys. Acta* **116**, 51.

Hawkins, R. A., Heald, P. J., and Taylor, P. (1969a). *Acta Endocrinol. (Copenhagen)* **60**, 199.

Hawkins, R. A., Heald, P. J., and Taylor, P. (1969b). *Acta Endocrinol. (Copenhagen)* **60**, 210.

Hazelwood, R. L. (1965). *In* "Avian Physiology" (P. D. Sturkie, ed.), 2nd ed. pp. 313–371. Baillière, London.

Heald, P. J., and Badman, H. G. (1963). *Biochim. Biophys. Acta* **70**, 381.

Heald, P. J., and McLachlan, P. M. (1963a). *Biochem. J.* **87**, 571.

Heald, P. J., and McLachlan, P. M. (1963b). *Nature (London)* **199**, 487.

Heald, P. J., and McLachlan, P. M. (1964). *Biochem. J.* **92**, 51.

Heald, P. J., and McLachlan, P. M. (1965). *Biochem. J.* **94**, 32.

Heald, P. J., and Rookledge, K. A. (1964). *J Endocrinol.* **30**, 115.

Heald, P. J., Badman, H. G., Wharton, J., Wulwick, C. M., and Hooper, P. I. (1964). *Biochim. Biophys. Acta* **84**, 1.

Henderson, I. W., and Chester Jones, I. (1967). *J. Endocrinol.* **37**, 319.

Henderson, I. W., Chan, D. K. O., Sandor, T., and Chester Jones, I. (1970). *Mem. Soc. Endocrinol.* **23**, 31.

Herrick, R. B., and Adams, J. L. (1956). *Poultry Sci.* **35**, 1269.

Hickman, C. P., and Trump, B. F. (1969). *In* "Fish Physiology" (W. S. Hoar and D. J. Randall, eds.), Vol. 1, pp. 91–239. Academic Press, New York.

Hildemann, W. H. (1954). *J. Exp. Zool.* **126**, 1.

Hinde, R. A., and Steel, E. (1966). *Symp. Soc. Exp. Biol.* **20**, 401.
Hishida, T. (1964). *Embryologia* **8**, 234.
Hishida, T. (1965). *Gen. Comp. Endocrinol.* **5**, 137.
Hoar, W. S. (1962). *Anim. Behav.* **10**, 247.
Hoar, W. S. (1965). *Annu. Rev. Physiol.* **27**, 51.
Höhn, E. O., and Cheng, S. C. (1967). *Gen. Comp. Endocrinol.* **8**, 1.
Hokin, M. R. (1963). *Biochim. Biophys. Acta* **77**, 108.
Holmes, W. N. (1965). *Arch. Anat. Microsc. Morphol. Exp*, **54**, 491.
Holmes, W. N., and Donaldson, E. M. (1969). *In* "Fish Physiology". (W. S. Hoar and D. J. Randall, eds.), Vol. 1, pp. 1–89. Academic Press, New York.
Holmes, W. N., and Stewart, D. J. (1968). *J. Exp. Biol.* **48**, 509.
Holmes, W. N., Phillips, J. G., and Butler, D. G. (1961). *Endocrinology* **69**, 483.
Holmes, W. N., Phillips, J. G., and Chester Jones, I. (1963). *Recent Progr. Horm. Res.* **19**, 619.
Holmes, W. N., Phillips, J. G., and Wright, A. (1969). *Gen. Comp. Endocrinol. Suppl.* **2**, 358.
Hopper, A. F. (1949). *J. Exp. Zool.* **111**, 393.
Hopper, A. F. (1951). *Pap. Mich. Acad. Sci. Arts Lett.* **35**, 109.
Horowicz, P., and Burger, J. W. (1968). *Amer. J. Physiol.* **214**, 635.
Hosoda, T., and Abe, T. (1965). *Jap. Poultry Sci.* **2**, 11.
Hunter, N. W., and Johnson, C. E. (1960). *J. Cell. Comp. Physiol.* **55**, 275.
Hutchinson, J. B. (1967). *Nature (London)* **216**, 591.
Idler, D. R., and Szeplaki, B. J. (1968). *J. Fish. Res. Bd. Can.* **25**, 2549.
Idler, D. R., and Truscott, B. (1966). *Gen. Comp. Endocrinol.* **7**, 375.
Idler, D. R., Bitners, I. I., and Schmidt, P. J., (1961a). *Can. J. Biochem. Physiol.* **39**, 1737.
Idler, D. R., Schmidt, P. J., and Piely, H. (1961b). *Can J. Biochem. Physiol.* **39**, 317.
Ishii, S. (1961). *J. Fac. Sci. Univ. Tokyo* **9**, 279.
Ishii, S. (1963). *Zool. Mag.* **72**, 235.
Iwasawa, H. (1957). *Zool. Mag.* **66**, 416.
Iwasawa, S. (1958), *J. Fac. Sci. Niigata Univ. Ser.* 11, **2**, 180.
Janssens, P. A. (1967). *Gen. Comp. Endocrinol.* **8**, 94.
Janssens, P. A., and Cohen, P. P. (1968). *Comp. Biochem. Physiol.* **24**, 887.
Jensen, E. V., Suzuki, T., Namata, M., Smith, S., and DeSombre, E. R. (1969). *Steroids* **13**, 417.
Johns, J. E., and Pfeiffer, E. W. (1963). *Science* **140**, 1225.
Johnston, C. I., Davis, J. O., Wright, F. S., and Howards, S. S. (1967). *Amer. J. Physiol.* **213**, 393.
Jonsson, C. E., and Terenius, L. (1965). *Acta Endocrinol. (Copenhagen)* **50**, 289.
Kambara, S. (1964). *Proc. Jap. Acad.* **40**, 536.
Katz, A. I., and Epstein, F. H. (1967). *Isr. J. Med. Sci.* **3**, 155.
Kawamoto, N. Y. (1950). *Jap. J. Ichthyol.* **1**, 8.
Kawamura, T., and Yokota, R. (1959). *J. Sci. Hiroshima Univ. Ser. B* **18**, 31.
Kehl, R. (1930). *C. R. Soc. Biol.* **105**, 512.
Kehl, R. (1938). *C. R. Soc. Biol.* **127**, 142.
Kehl, R. (1940). *C. R. Soc. Biol.* **135**, 1475.
Kenney, F. T., and Kull, F. J. (1963). *Proc. Nat. Acad. Sci. U.S.* **50**, 493.
Kenyon, A. J. (1967). *Comp. Biochem. Physiol.* **22**, 169.
Kirsten, E., Kirsten, R., Leaf, A., and Sharp, G. W. G. (1968). *Pfluegers Arch.* **300**, 213.
Kline, D. L. (1949). *Endocrinology* **45**, 596.
Knowles, F. G. W. (1939). *J. Exp. Biol.* **16**, 535.
Kobayashi, H. (1951). *Annot. Zool. Jap.* **24**, 212.
Kobayashi, H. (1953). *Annot. Zool. Jap.* **26**, 213.

Kobayashi, H., and Farner, D. S. (1966). *Gen. Comp. Endocrinol.* **6**, 443.
Kohler, P. O., Grimley, P. M., and O'Malley, B. W. (1968). *Science* **160**, 86.
Kohler, P. O., Grimley, P. M., and O'Malley, B. W. (1969). *J. Cell Biol.* **40**, 8.
Komisaruk, B. R. (1967). *J. Comp. Physiol. Psychol.* **64**, 219.
Korenman, S. G., and O'Malley, B. W. (1968). *Endocrinology* **83**, 11.
Landon, J. E., Jayabon, N., and Forte, L. (1966). *Amer. J. Physiol.* **211**, 1050.
Laskowski, W. (1953). *Arch. Entwicklungsmech. Organismen* **146**, 137.
Layne, D. S., Common, R. H., Maw, W. A., and Fraps, R. M. (1957). *Proc. Soc. Exp. Biol. Med.* **94**, 528.
Leaf, A., and Dempsey, E. (1960). *J. Biol. Chem.* **235**, 2160.
LeBrie, S. J., and Elizondo, R. S. (1969). *Amer. J. Physiol.* **217**, 426.
Lehrman, D. S. (1958). *J. Comp. Physiol. Psychol.* **51**, 142.
Lehrman, D. S. (1961). *In* "Sex and Internal Secretions" (W. C. Young, ed.), pp. 1268–1382. Williams & Wilkins, Baltimore, Maryland.
Leloup-Hatey, J. (1970a). *Gen. Comp. Endocrinol.* **15**, 388.
Leloup-Hatey, J. (1970b). *Comp. Biochem. Physiol.* **32**, 353.
Lisk, R. D. (1967). *Gen. Comp. Endocrinol.* **8**, 258.
Lodge, P. D. B., and Smith, C. L. (1960). *Nature (London)* **185**, 774.
Lofts, B. (1962). *Gen. Comp. Endocrinol.* **2**, 394.
Lofts, B. (1968). *In* "Perspectives in Endocrinology: Hormones in the Lives of Lower Vertebrates" (E. J. W. Barrington and C. B. Jørgensen, eds.), pp. 239–304. Academic Press, New York.
Lofts, B., Pickford, G. E., and Atz, J. W. (1966). *Gen. Comp. Endocrinol.* **6**, 74.
Macchi, I. A., Phillips, J. G., and Brown, P. (1967). *J. Endocrinol.* **38**, 319.
McFarland, W. N., and Munz, F. W. (1958). *Biol. Bull.* **114**, 348.
McFarland, W. N., and Munz, F. W. (1965). *Comp. Biochem. Physiol.* **14**, 383.
McGuire, W. L., and O'Malley, B. W. (1968). *Biochim. Biophys. Acta* **157**, 187.
McKinley, W. P., Maw, W. A., Oliver, W. F., and Common, R. H. (1954), *Can. J. Biochem. Physiol.* **32**, 189.
Maetz, J. (1964). *Extract du Bulletin d'Information Scientifique et Technique du Commisariat à l'Energie Atomique* **86**, 11–70.
Maetz, J. (1968). *In* "Perspectives in Endocrinology: Hormones in the Lives of Lower Vertebrates" (E. J. W. Barrington and C. B. Jørgensen, eds.), pp. 47–162. Academic Press, New York.
Maetz, J. (1970). *Mem. Soc. Endocrinol.* **23**, 3.
Maetz, J, and Lahlou, B. (1966). *J. Physiol. (Paris)* **58**, 249.
Maetz, J., and Rankin, J. C. (1969). *Colloq. Int. Cent. Nat. Rech. Sci.* No. 177, 45.
Maetz, J., Mayer, N., and Chartier-Baraduc, M. M. (1967a). *Gen. Comp. Endocrinol.* **8**, 177.
Maetz, J., Sawyer, W. H., Pickford, G. E., and Mayer, N. (1967b). *Gen. Comp. Endocrinol.* **8**, 163.
Masui, Y. (1967). *J. Exp. Zool.* **166**, 365.
Mathies, J. C., Palm, L., and Gaebler, O. H. (1951) *Endocrinology* **49**, 571.
Matsui, N., and Plager, J. E. (1966). *Endocrinology* **78**, 1159.
Mayer, N., and Maetz, J. (1967). *C. R. Acad. Sci.* **264**, 1632.
Mayer, N., Maetz, J., Chan, D. K. O., Forster, M., and Chester Jones, I. (1967). *Nature (London)* **214**, 1118.
Middler, S. A., Kleeman, C. R., Edwards, E., and Brody, D. (1969). *Gen. Comp. Endocrinol.* **12**, 290.
Mills, I. H. (1961). *Mem. Soc. Endocrinol.* **11**, 81.
Mills, I. H. (1962). *Brit. Med. Bull.* **18**, 127.

Mintz, B., and Gallien, L. (1954). *Anat. Rec.* **119**, 493.
Mintz, B., and Witschi, E. (1966). *Anat. Rec.* **96**, 526.
Mintz, B., Foote, C. L., and Witschi, E. (1945). *Endocrinology* **37**, 286.
Miyamori, H. (1962). *Zool Mag.* **71**, 191.
Miyamori, H. (1964). *J. Biol. Osaka City Univ.* **15**, 1.
Mohsen, T. (1958). *Nature (London)* **181**, 1074.
Mok, C. C. Martin, W. G., and Common, R. H. (1961) *Can. J. Biochem. Physiol.* **39**, 109.
Morris, R. (1960). *Symp. Zool. Soc. (London)* **1**, 1.
Morris, R. (1965). *J. Exp. Biol.* **42**, 359.
Motais, R. (1967). *Ann. Inst. Océanogr. (Monaco)* **45**, 1.
Motais, R., Garcia Romeu, F., and Maetz, J. (1966). *J. Gen. Physiol.* **50**, 391.
Munday, K. A., Ansari, A. Q., Oldroyd, D., and Akhtar, M. (1968). *Biochim. Biophys. Acta* **166**, 748.
Munz, F. W., and McFarland, W. N. (1964). *Comp. Biochem. Physiol.* **13**, 381.
Murton, R. K., Thearle, R. J. P., and Lofts, B. (1969). *J. Anim. Behav.* **17**, 286.
Nandi, S., and Bern, H. A. (1961). *Gen. Comp. Endocrinol.* **1**, 195.
Nicholls, T. J., Follett, B. K., and Evennett, P. J. (1968). *Z. Zellforsch. Mikrosk. Anat. Abt. Histochem.* **80**, 19.
Niwa, H. S. (1965a). *Jap. J. Ichthyol.* **4**, 193.
Niwa, H. S. (1965b). *Embryologia* **8**, 299.
Noble, G. K., and Greenberg, B. (1940). *Proc. Soc. Exp. Biol. Med.* **44**, 460.
Noble, G. K., and Greenberg, B. (1941a). *Proc. Soc. Exp. Biol. Med.* **47**, 32.
Noble, G. K., and Greenberg, B. (1941b). *J. Exp. Zool.* **88**, 451.
Noble, G. K., and Wurm, N. (1940). *Endocrinology* **26**, 837.
Noble, G. K., Kumpf, K. F., and Billings, V. N. (1938). *Endocrinology* **23**, 353.
Norris, K. S., and Dawson, W. R. (1964). *Copeia* **1964**, 638.
Oguri, M., and Takada, N. (1967). *Bull. Jap. Soc. Sci. Fish.* **33**, 161.
Okada, Y. K. (1964). *Proc. Jap. Acad.* **40**, 541.
Okada, Y. K., and Yamashita, H. (1944). *J. Fac. Sci. Univ. Tokyo, Sect. 4* **6**, 589.
O'Malley, B. W. (1967). *Biochemistry* **6**, 2546.
O'Malley, B. W., and Kohler, P. O. (1967). *Proc. Nat. Acad. Sci. U.S.* **58**, 2359.
O'Malley, B. W., and McGuire, W. L. (1968a). *Proc. Nat. Acad. Sci. U.S.* **60**, 1527.
O'Malley, B. W., and McGuire, W. L. (1968b). *J. Clin. Invest.* **47**, 654.
O'Malley, B. W., and McGuire, W. L. (1968c). *Biochem. Biophys. Res. Commun.* **32**, 595.
O'Malley, B. W., and McGuire, W. L. (1969). *Endocrinology* **84**, 63.
O'Malley, B. W., McGuire, W. L., and Korenman, S. G. (1967a). *Biochem. Biophys. Acta* **145**, 204.
O'Malley, B. W., McGuire, W. L., and Middleton, P. A. (1967b) *Endocrinology* **81**, 677.
O'Malley, B. W., Kirschner, M. A., and Bardin, C. W. (1968). *Proc. Soc. Exp. Biol. Med.* **127**, 521.
Owen, S. E. (1937). *Endocrinology* **21**, 689.
Oztan, N. (1960). *Istanbul Univ. Fen Fak. Mecm. Seri B* **25**, 27.
Padoa, E. (1939). *Monit Zool. Ital.* **50**, 129.
Palmer, B. G. (1966). *J. Endocrinol.* **36**, 73.
Parkes, A. S., and Marshall, A. J. (1960). *In* "Marshall's Physiology of Reproduction" (A. S. Parkes, ed.), Vol. I, Part ii, pp. 583–706. Longmans, Green, London.
Parry, G. (1966). *Biol. Rev. Cambridge Phil. Soc.* **41**, 392.
Paterson, J. Y. F. and Hills, F. J. (1967). *J. Endocrinol.* **37**, 261.
Penhos, J. C. (1953). *Rev. Soc. Argent. Biol.* **29**, 200.
Penhos, J. C. (1956). *Acta Physiol. Lat. Amer.* **6**, 95.

Penhos, J. C. (1957). *Rev. Soc. Argent. Biol.* **33**, 121.
Perks, A. M. (1969). *In* "Fish Physiology" (W. S. Hoar and D. J. Randall, eds.), Vol. II, pp. 112–206. Academic Press, New York.
Pfeiffer, C. A. (1947). *Endocrinology* **41**, 92.
Phillips, J. G., and Bellamy, D. (1962). *J. Endocrinol.* **24**, vi.
Phillips, J. G., and Bellamy, D. (1966). *J. Endocrinol.* **36**, 97.
Phillips, J. G., and Bellamy, D. (1967). *Excerpta Med. Found. Int. Congr. Ser.* **132**, 1065.
Phillips, J. G., Holmes, W. N., and Butler, D. G. (1961). *Endocrinology* **69**, 958.
Pickford, G. E., and Atz, J. W. (1957) "The Physiology of the Pituitary Glands of Fishes" New York Zoological Society, New York.
Pickford, G. E., and Blake Grant, F. (1967). *Science* **155**, 568.
Pieau, C., and Raynaud, A. (1966). *Arch. Anat. Microsc. Morphol. Exp.* **55**, 331.
Piper, G. D. and de Roos, R. (1967). *Gen. Comp. Endocrinol.* **8**, 135.
Plack, P. A., and Pritchard, D. J. (1968). *Biochem. J.* **106**, 257.
Porter, G. A., and Edelman, I. S. (1964). *J. Clin. Invest.* **43**, 611.
Porter, G. A., Bogoroch, R., and Edelman, I. S. (1964). *Proc. Nat. Acad. Sci. U.S.* **52**, 1326.
Potts, W. T. W. (1968). *Annu. Rev. Physiol.* **30**, 73.
Prasad, M. R. N., and Sanyal, M. K. (1963). *Naturwissenschaften* **50**, 311.
Prosser, R. L., and Suzuki, H. K. (1968). *Comp. Biochem. Physiol.* **25**, 529.
Puckett, W. O. (1939). *Anat. Rec.* **75**, 127.
Puckett, W. O. (1940). *J. Exp. Zool.* **84**, 39.
Quincey, R. V., and Gray, C. H. (1963). *J. Endocrinol.* **26**, 500.
Rall, D. P., and Burger, J. W. (1967). *Amer. J. Physiol.* **212**, 354.
Ralph, C. L. and Fraps, R. M. (1960). *Endocrinology* **66**, 269.
Ramaswami, L. S., and Jacob, D. (1963). *Naturwissenschaften* **50**, 453.
Ramaswami, L. S., and Jacob, D. (1964). *Experientia* **21**, 206.
Ranney, R. E., and Chaikoff, I. L. (1951). *Amer. J. Physiol.* **165**, 600.
Rapola, J. (1963). *Gen. Comp. Endocrinol.* **3**, 412.
Redshaw, M. R., and Nicholls, T. J. (1971). *Gen. Comp. Endocrinol.* **16**, 85.
Redshaw, M. R., Follett, B. K., and Nicholls, T. J. (1969). *J. Endocrinol.* **43**, 47.
Redshaw, M. R., Follett, B. K., and Lawes, G. J. (1971). *Int. J. Biochem.* **2**(7), 80.
Regnier, M. T. (1937). *C. R. Acad. Sci.* **205**, 1451.
Regnier, M. T. (1938). *Bull. Biol. Fr. Belg.* **72**, 385.
Regnier, M. T. (1941). *C. R. Acad. Sci.* **213**, 537.
Regnier, M. T. (1942). *C. R. Soc. Biol.* **136**, 202.
Riddle, O. (1942). *Endocrinology* **31**, 498.
Risley, P. L. (1941). *J. Exp. Zool.* **87**, 477.
Robertson, J. D. (1954). *J. Exp. Biol.* **31**, 424.
Robertson, O. H., Krupp, M. A., Thomas, S. F., Favour, C. B., Hane, S., and Wexler, B. C. (1961a). *Gen. Comp. Endocrinol.* **1**, 472.
Roberston, O. H., Krupp, M. A., Favour, C. B., Hane, S., and Thomas, S. F. (1961b). *Endocrinology* **68**, 735.
Robertson, O. H., Hane, S., Wexler, B. C., and Rinfret, A. P. (1963) *Gen. Comp. Endocrinol.* **3**, 422.
Rochefort, H., and Baulieu, E. E. (1969). *Endocrinology* **84**, 108.
Roepke, R. R., and Bushnell, L. D. (1936). *J. Immunol.* **30**, 109.
Roos, T. B., and Meyer, R. K. (1961). *Gen. Comp. Endocrinol.* **1**, 392.
Rothchild, I., and Fraps, R. M. (1949). *Endocrinology* **44**, 141.
Rubin, A. A., and Gordon, M. (1953). *Proc. Soc. Exp. Biol. Med.* **83**, 646.
Rudack, D., and Wallace, R. A. (1968). *Biochim. Biophys. Acta.* **155**, 299.

Sandberg, A. A., Rosenthal, H., Schneider, S. L., and Slaunwhite, W. R. (1966). *In* "Steroid Dynamics" (G. Pincus, T. Nakao, and J. F. Tait, eds.), pp. 1–62. Academic Press, New York.

Sandor, T., Henderson, I. W., and Chester Jones, I. (1970). Unpublished observations.

Sangster, W. (1948). *Physiol Zool.* **21**, 134.

Sanyal, N. N., and Snart, R. S. (1968). *J. Endocrinol.* **40**, xvi.

Sanyal, M.K., Prasad, M. R. N., and Misra, U. K. (1966). *Steroids* **7**, 391.

Schjeide, O. A. (1967), *Progr. Biochem. Pharmacol.* **2**, 265.

Schjeide, O. A., and Urist, M. R. (1956). *Science* **124**, 1242.

Schjeide, O. A., and Urist, M. R. (1960). *Nature (London)* **188**, 291.

Schjeide, O. A., and Wilkins, M. (1964). *Nature (London)* **201**, 42.

Schjeide, O. A., Wilkins, M., McCandless, R., Munn, R. Peterson, M., and Carben, G. (1963). *Amer. Zool.* **3**, 167.

Schmidt-Nielsen, K. (1960). *Circulation* **21**, 955.

Schreiber, S. S., and Rugh, R. (1945). *J. Exp. Zool.* **99**, 93.

Schuetz, A. W. (1967). *J. Exp. Zool.* **166**, 347.

Seal, U. S., and Doe, R. P. (1963). *Endocrinology* **73**, 371.

Seal, U.S., and Doe, R. P. (1966). *In* "Steroid Dynamics" (G. Pincus, T. Nakao, and J. F. Tait, eds.), pp. 63–88. Academic Press, New York.

Segal, H. L., and Kim, Y. S. (1963). *Proc. Nat. Acad. Sci. U.S.* **50**, 912.

Segura, E. T., and D'Agostino, S. A. (1965). *Gen. Comp. Endocrinol.* **5**, 278.

Selander, R. K., and Yang, S. Y. (1966). *Gen. Comp. Endocrinol.* **6**, 325.

Sharp, G. W. G., and Dempsey, E. (1969). Personal communication.

Sharp, G. W. G., and Leaf, A. (1963). *J. Clin. Invest.* **42**, 978.

Sharp, G. W. G., and Leaf, A. (1964). *Nature (London)* **202**, 1185.

Sharp, G. W. G., Lichtenstein, N. S., and Leaf, A. (1965). *Biochim. Biophys. Acta* **111**, 329.

Sharp, G. W. G., Komack, C. L., and Leaf, A. (1966). *J. Clin. Invest.* **45**, 450.

Shyamala, G., and Gorski, J. (1969). *J. Biol. Chem.* **244**, 1097.

Simkiss, K. (1967). "Calcium in Reproductive Physiology." Chapman & Hall, London.

Simpson, C. F., Harms, R. G., and Wilson, H. R. (1965). *Proc. Soc. Exp. Biol. Med.* **119**, 435.

Slicher, A. M. (1961). *Bull. Bingham Oceanogr. Collect. Yale Univ.* **17**, 3.

Smith, H. W. (1929). *J. Biol. Chem.* **81**, 407.

Smith, H. W. (1953). "From Fish to Philosopher." Little, Brown, Boston.

Smith, L. D., Ecker, R. E., and Subtelny, S. (1966). *Proc. Nat. Acad. Sci. U.S.* **56**, 1724.

Smith, R. J. F., and Hoar, W. S. (1967). *Anim. Behav.* **15**, 342.

Smith, R. T., and Smythe, J. R., Jr. (1963). *Poultry Sci.* **42**, 418.

Snart, R. S. (1964). *Excerpta Med. Found. Int. Congr. Ser.* **83**, 1313.

Snart, R. S. (1967). *Biochim. Biophys. Acta* **135**, 1056.

Snart, R. S. (1969). *Biochem. J.* **111**, 254.

Snart, R. S., and Sanyal, N. N. (1968). *Biochem. J.* **108**, 369.

Snart. R. S., Sanyal, N. N., and Agarwal, N. K. (1969). *J. Endocrinol.* **47**, 149.

Socino, M., and Ferreri, E. (1965). *Biochem. Biol. Sper.* **4**, 161.

Steel, E. A., and Hinde, R. A. (1963). *J. Endocrinol.* **26**, 11.

Stimpson, J. H. (1965). *Comp. Biochem. Physiol.* **15**, 187.

Storer, J. H. (1967). *Comp. Biochem. Physiol.* **20**, 939.

Sundararaj, B. I., and Goswami, S. V. (1965a). *Naturwissenschaften* **52**, 114.

Sundararaj, B. I., and Goswami, S. V. (1965b). *Gen. Comp. Endocrinol.* **5**, 464.

Sundararaj, B. I., and Goswami, S. V. (1966a). *J. Exp. Zool.* **161**, 287.

Sundararaj, B. I., and Goswami, S. V. (1966b). *J. Exp. Zool.* **163**, 49.

Sundararaj, B. I., and Nayyar, S. K. (1966). *Anat. Rec.* **154**, 491.

Sundararaj, B. I., and Nayyar, S. K. (1967). *Gen. Comp. Endocrinol.* **8**, 403.
Suzuki, H. K., and Prosser, R. L. (1968). *Proc. Soc. Exp. Biol. Med.* **127**, 4.
Svärdson, G. (1943). *Medd. Undersoknanst. Sotvatten Fisk. Stockholm* **21**, 48.
Takahashi, H. (1958). *J. Fac. Sci. Hokkaido Univ. Ser. 4* **14**, 92.
Takahashi, H. (1959). *J. Fac. Sci. Hokkaido Univ. Ser. 4* **14**, 210.
Tavolga, M. C. (1949). *Zoologica* **34**, 215.
Taylor, A. B. (1948). *Trans. Amer. Microsc. Soc.* **67**, 155.
Templeton, J. R. (1964). *Comp. Biochem. Physiol.* **11**, 223.
Templeton, J. R. (1966). *Comp. Biochem. Physiol.* **18**, 563.
Terenius, L. (1969). *Acta Endocrinol.* **60**, 79.
Thapliyal, J. P., and Singh, G. S. (1959). *J. Zool Soc. (India)* **14**, 21.
Thesleff, S., and Schmidt-Nielsen, K. (1962) *Amer. J. Physiol.* **202**, 597.
Thiebold, J. J. (1952). *C. R. Acad. Sci.* **235**, 1551.
Thiebold, J. J. (1953a). *C. R. Soc. Biol.* **147**, 480.
Thiebold, J. J. (1953b). *C. R. Acad. Sci.* **236**, 2174.
Thiebold, J. J. (1954). *Bull. Biol. Fr. Belg.* **88**, 130.
Thiebold, J. J. (1955). *C. R. Soc. Biol.* **149**, 1036.
Thiebold, J. J. (1963). *Cah. Biol. Mar.* **4**, 183.
Thornton, P. J. (1970). "Endocrine Control of Oocyte Meiosis and Oviduct Function in the Toad *Bufo bufo* (L)." Ph. D. thesis, University of Leeds, England.
Thornton, V. F., and Evennett, P. J. (1969). *Gen. Comp. Endocrinol.* **13**, 268.
Turner, C. L. (1941). *Biol. Bull.* **80**, 371.
Turner, C. L. (1942a). *Physiol. Zool.* **15**, 263.
Turner, C. L. (1942b). *Biol. Bull.* **83**, 389.
Turner, C. L. (1942c). *J. Exp. Zool.* **91**, 167.
Turner, C. L. (1960). *Trans. Amer. Microsc. Soc.* **79**, 320.
Uemura, H. (1964). *Endocrinol. Jap.* **11**, 185.
Ulick, S., and Feinholtz, E. (1968). *J. Clin. Invest.* **47**, 2523.
Urist, M. R., and Schjeide, A. O. (1961). *J. Gen. Physiol.* **44**, 743.
Urist, M. R., Schjeide, O. A., and McLean, F. C. (1958). *Endocrinology* **63**, 570.
Ussing, H. H. (1960). *In* "Handbuch der Experimentellen Pharmakologie" Vol. 13. Springer-Verlag, Berlin and New York.
Vallowe, M. H. (1957). *Biol. Bull.* **112**, 422.
van Oordt, P. G. W. J. (1968). *In* "Perspectives in Endocrinology: Hormones in the Lives of Lower Vertebrates" (E. J. W. Barrington and C. B. Jørgensen, eds.), pp. 405–468. Academic Press, New York.
van Oordt, P. G. W. J., and Basu, S. L. (1959). *Acta Physiol. Pharmacol.* **8**, 281.
van Oordt, P. G. W. J., and Basu, S. L. (1960). *Acta Endocrinol.* **33**, 103.
van Oordt, P. G. W. J., and Schouten, S. C. M. (1961). *J. Reprod. Fert.* **2**, 61.
Vanstone, W. E., Dale, D. G., Oliver, W. F., and Common, R. H. (1957). *Can. J. Biochem. Physiol.* **35**, 659.
van Tienhoven, A. (1955). *Endocrinology* **56**, 667.
van Tienhoven, A. (1961). *In* "Sex and Internal Secretions" (W. C. Young and G. W. Corner, eds.), Vol. I, pp. 1088–1172. Williams & Wilkins, Baltimore, Maryland.
Vowles, D. M., and Harwood, D. (1966). *J. Endocrinol.* **36**, 33.
Vyas, D. K., and Ramaswami, L. S. (1967). *J. Endocrinol.* **37**, 101.
Wai, E. H., and Hoar, W. S. (1963). *Can. J. Zool.* **41**, 611.
Wallace, R. A., and Dumont, J. N. (1968). *J. Cell. Physiol.* **72**. Suppl. p. 73.
Wallace, R. A., and Jared, D. W. (1968a). *Can. J. Biochem.* **46**, 953.
Wallace, R. A., and Jared, D. W. (1968b). *Science* **160**, 91.

Wallace, R. A., and Jared, D. W. (1969). *Develop. Biol.* **19**, 498.

Walton, K. (1963). "Endocrine Control of Spermatogenesis in the Newt, *Triturus cristatus*." Ph.D. thesis, University of Leeds, England.

Wang, Y. T. (1963). *Acta Biol. Exp. Sinica* **8**, 518.

Weisbart, M., and Idler, D. R. (1970). *J. Endocrinol.* **46**, 29.

White, A., and Dougherty, T. F. (1947). *Endocrinology* **41**, 230.

Witschi, E., and Allison, J. (1950). *Anat. Rec.* **108**, 589.

Witschi, E., and Crown, E. N. (1937). *Anat. Rec. Suppl.* **1**, 70.

Woodhead, P. M. J. (1969). *J. Mar. Biol. Ass. U.K.* **49**, 939.

Yamamoto, K., Nagahama, Y., and Yamazaki, F. (1966). *Bull. Jap. Soc. Sci. Fish.* **32**, 977.

Yamamoto, T. (1953). *J. Exp. Zool.* **123**, 571.

Yamamoto, T. (1955). *Genetics* **40**, 406.

Yamamoto, T. (1958). *J. Exp. Zool.* **137**, 227.

Yamamoto, T. (1959a). *J. Exp. Zool.* **141**, 133.

Yamamoto, T. (1959b). *Genetics* **44**, 739.

Yamamoto, T. (1968). *Gen. Comp. Endocrinol.* **10**, 8.

Yamamoto, T. (1969). *In* "Fish Physiology" (W. S. Hoar and D. J. Randall, eds.), Vol. III, pp. 117–175. Academic Press, New York.

Yamamoto, T., and Matsuda, N. (1963). *Gen. Comp. Endocrinol.* **3**, 101.

Yates, F. E., and Urquhart, J. (1962). *Physiol. Rev.* **42**, 359.

Zarrow, M. X., and Bastian, J. W. (1953). *Proc. Soc. Exp. Biol. Med.* **84**, 457.

AUTHOR INDEX

Numbers in italics refer to the pages on which the complete references are listed.

SUBJECT INDEX

ACTH, *see* Adrenocorticotropin
Adrenalectomy, biological effects on
 corticosteroids in fish, 236
 electrolytes in amphibia, 427
 nasal gland of reptiles, birds, 428, 429
 water and electrolytes in *Anguilla*, 422–426
Adrenocortical tissue
 anatomy and histology of, 94–105
  amphibians, 102–104
  birds, 105
  fish, 94–102
  reptiles, 104–105
 cytology and cytochemistry of, 105–112
 functional control of, 116
 histophysiology of, 105–116
 organization of, 93–94
 seasonal changes in, 113–116
 zonation of, 112–113, 304
Adrenocorticotropin
 activity in pituitary, 175, 235, 247, 280,
  290, 294
 effect on corticosteroidogenesis
  in amphibia, 257, 259, 262, 264,
   265, 267, 270
  in birds, 286, 288–291, 293–297, 300, 301
  in fish, 131, 176–184, 212, 213, 228, 230,
   234–236, 240–243
  in reptiles, 277–282
 mechanism of action, 255, 256
Adrenosterone, 333, 336, 351
Agnatha, *see* cyclostomes
Aldosterone, 315
 adrenal mitochondria, synthesis by,
  316–322

biosynthesis of
 in amphibia, 257–274
 in birds, 286–288, 293–303
 in fish, 134, 150, 216, 218, 229, 230
 in reptiles, 275–285
 effect on electrolytes, 420, 427
 18-hydroxycorticosterone as precursor,
  321
 mechanism of action, 434, 435
 occurrence
  in amphibia, 257–260, 262, 263
  in birds, 287–292
  in fish, 154, 161, 236, 238, 250
 production rate in amphibia, 259
 protein binding of, 432–434
Amphibians
 adrenocortical tissue, 102
 corticosteroids, 256–263
  biosynthesis of, 256–260, 264–274, 317,
   318
 ovary, morphology of, 76–83
 sex steroids, 333, 338, 340, 394, 396, 397,
  398
  biosynthesis of, 346, 353, 356, 357,
   360–367, 402, 406
  effect on reproductive systems, 438, 440,
   441, 443, 445, 447, 453
 testis, morphology of, 49–57
 water and electrolyte metabolism, 427
Anesthetics, 129, 165, 170–172
Androgenic agents
 effect on reproductive system of,
  amphibia 440, 441, 443
  fish, 439, 440, 442